MEDICINE

PERSPECTIVES IN HISTORY AND ART

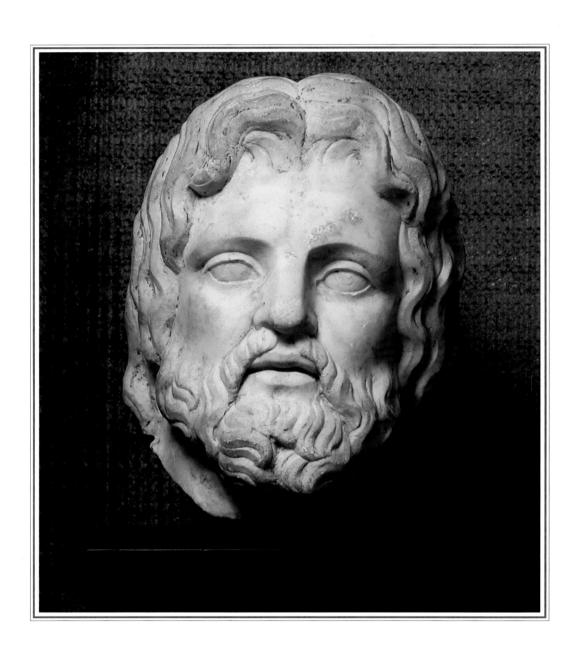

MEDICINE

PERSPECTIVES IN HISTORY AND ART

ROBERT E. GREENSPAN, MD

PONTEVERDE PRESS ~ Alexandria, Virginia

I wrote, edited, and published this book. I also took all the pictures not identified in the illustrations credit page. When I began writing, I knew nothing about how to do any of this, and I hope that fact does not occur to you as you read the following pages. I tried as much as possible to avoid interfering with those contributing most to this effort—the men and women who were both the providers and recipients of medical care in ages gone by.

—ROBERT E. GREENSPAN, MD

Design: McKnight Design, LLC
Line Editor: Robert A. Poarch
Typesetting: Blue Heron Typesetting
Printed and bound in Singapore by CS Graphics Pte. Ltd.

Greenspan, Robert E.
Medicine: perspectives in history and art / Robert
E. Greenspan.—1st ed.
Includes bibliographical references and index.
LCCN 2004094525
ISBN 0972448608

1. Medicine—History. 2. Medicine and art. I. Title.
R133.G695 2004   610'.9
QBI04 200335

First edition, first issue

Frontispiece. Aesculapius (second century), near life-size marble sculpture

p. vi. Praying skeleton (1830?), ink and watercolor by William Cheselden

p. vii. Hemisected skull in *Traité complet d'anatomie de l'homme,* 2nd ed. (1866–1871), by J.M. Bourgery, Claude Bernard, and N.H. Jacob

PONTEVERDE PRESS

7922 Washington Avenue
Alexandria, VA 22308
1-888-Hx of Med (496-3633)
www.MedicalHistoryandArt.com

"Where there is love for man, there is also love for the art."

Hippocrates (460–377 B.C.)
On Precepts

This book is dedicated to Richard B. Greenspan (1913–2001) and Hyman Rubin (1916–1994), whose guidance in my life has been immeasurable; they are very much missed.

This book is dedicated to Bonnie, Emily, Sarah, Rachel, and Matthew, without whom this book could not have been written (though it would have been finished a lot sooner).

And finally, this book is dedicated to Theodore E. Woodward, MD, MACP (1914–2005), former Chief of Medicine at the University of Maryland School of Medicine (1954–1981). Dr. Woodward practiced medicine with a grace and dignity that inspired generations of physicians fortunate enough to learn the art of medicine under his guidance. All physicians trained by Dr. Woodward can recite his simple advice regarding the formulation of a differential diagnosis: "When you hear hoof beats, don't expect to see a zebra." As a young medical student, I had just written one of my first orders only to be surprised to find Dr. Woodward behind me, observing over his half-glasses. I had begun my order with the word "please," and my courtesy was commended by the Chief of Medicine. I have never forgotten that, and I still feel Dr. Woodward looking over my shoulder as I write my orders today. These were Dr. Woodward's concluding remarks to aspiring medical students at the Franklin & Marshall College on September 23, 1995:

> Finally, in closing, let us all continue to nurture our aspirations and values so that they can serve as well whether the road is rough, or smooth, or even too quick for our own good. On the conduct of our lives, rely on the principles of love and affection for family, the enjoyment and warm fellowship of friends, devoted service for the welfare of others, and a touch of sentiment. Fulfillment of these ideals will return one of life's most precious rewards, the respect of our fellow man.

"By any standard, his intellect, his circle of friends, his concept of values, ideals, and willingness to share with others, (were) enormous." — Philip A. Mackowiac, MD

Many helped in the preparation of this book, though I wanted to especially thank the following:

Beverly Bacon, MBA
Camille Bacon, PhD
Melanie Bacon, RN, MPH
Dave Burgevin
Regina Butler, RN
Stanley B. Burns, MD
Judy M. Chelnick
James Connor, PhD
Charles Crenshaw
Rainer M. Engel, MD
Bonnie B. Greenspan, RN, MBA
Emily Greenspan
Rachel Greenspan
Sarah Greenspan
John M. Hyson Jr., DDS, MS, MA
Olgierd Lindan, MD, PhD
Samuel Littlepage
Bob McCoy
Linda McKnight
Elizabeth Mullen
Franco Musio, MD, FACP
Jeremy Norman
Lawrence E. and Linda G. Rubin
Debra Scarborough
Michael Simons, MA
Scott Swank, DDS
Ben Z. Swanson Jr., DDS
Benedek Varga, PhD
and
Matthew Greenspan, who is very glad that this "stupid book" is finally finished.

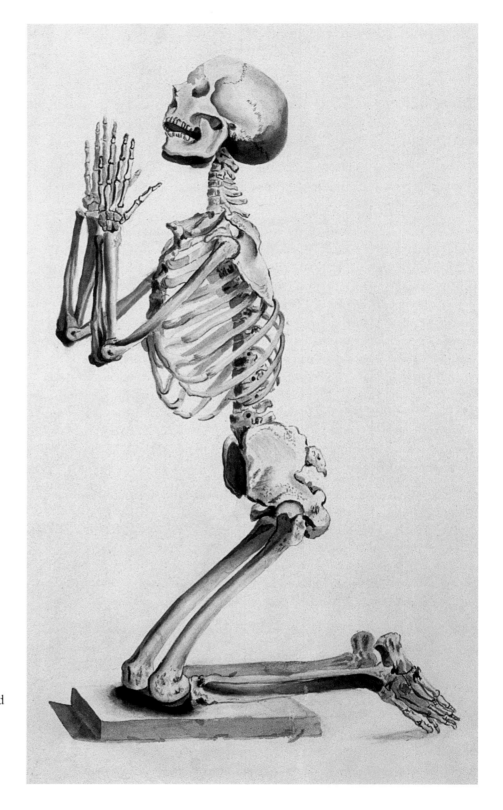

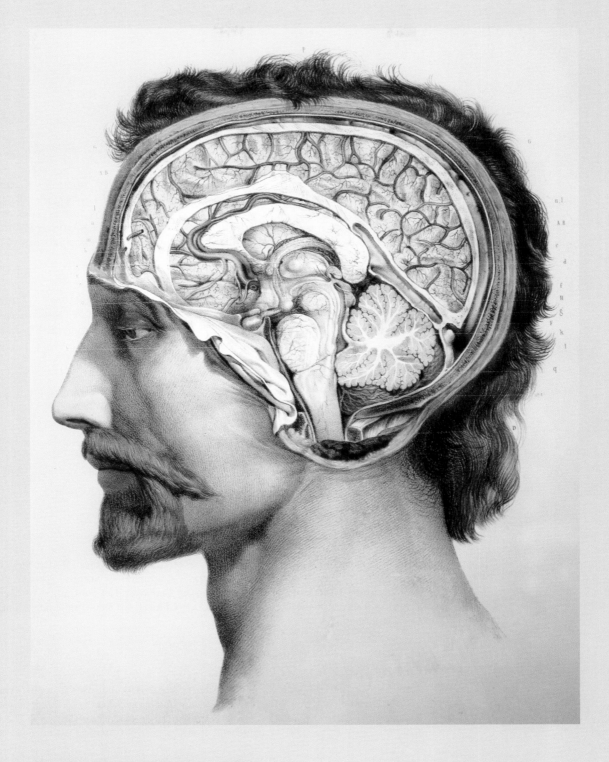

For the mind and for the heart . . .

"Life is too important to be taken seriously."
OSCAR WILDE (1854–1900)

"The steps aren't enough—feel the music."
JOHNNY CASTLE in *Dirty Dancing* (1987)

CONTENTS

X INTRODUCTION

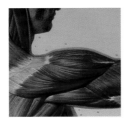

2 ANATOMY
Hippocrates of Cos • Anatomy According to Galen • Medical Illustration • Renaissance Art • The First Modern Medical Classic • A Missed Opportunity • Looking for a Subject and a Purpose • Medicine Becomes a Science • Art and Physiology • A Seventeenth Century Controversy • Structure and Function • Wonderful Medical Art • Anatomic Models • At the Dissecting Table • Postmortem Instruments • Microscopic Anatomy • Embalming

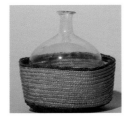

56 PHYSICAL DIAGNOSTICS
Inspection • The Pulse • Recording the Temperature • Auscultation • Percussion • Uroscopy • Observation: When the end is near . . . • Communicating the Diagnosis

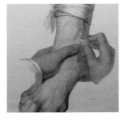

80 BLEEDING
The Four Humors • Bloodletting – It's Good for You • Leeches • Nursing Responsibilities • A Risky Procedure • Instrumentation • The Bleeding of George Washington • Transfusion • Other Uses for Blood • Counterirritation and Cupping • The Seton • The Life Awakener

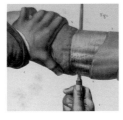

122 GENERAL SURGERY
Surgery in Ancient Egypt • Rome • Middle Eastern Surgery • From Barber-Surgeons to Patron Saints • Surgery Becomes a Profession • Amputation • Surgical Sets and Manufacturers • The Control of Bleeding • The Cautery • The Tourniquet • Surgical Asepsis • Anesthesia • Laughing Gas • Ether • Chloroform • An Immediate Controversy • Local Anesthesia

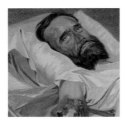

198 TRAUMA SURGERY
Neurosurgery • Orthopedic Surgery • Alternatives to Amputation • Gunshot Wounds; Bell and the Bullet • Civil War Medicine • A Life Saving Amputation • *The Medical and Surgical History of the War of the Rebellion* • Sepsis among the Troops • Pain Control • The Battle of Cold Harbor • Letters: "If we could only live in peace..." • Medical Advances from the War

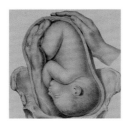

238 OBSTETRICS AND GYNECOLOGY
Obstetrics • The Role of the Midwife • A (Secret) Landmark Discovery • The Dangers of Delivery • Medical Abortion • Instruments of Destruction • After the Blessed Event • Instruments Designed for Women

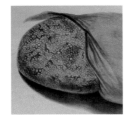

270 UROLOGY
Early Medical Therapy • Kidney Stones – The Cause • The Medical Treatment of Stones • The Surgical Treatment of Stones • Of Bladder Stones and Nursery Rhymes • Early Urologic Surgery • The Moveable Kidney • Bright's Disease

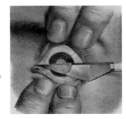

294 OPHTHALMOLOGY AND OTOLARYNGOLOGY
OPHTHALMOLOGY • Cataract Surgery • Always a Place for Bleeding • An Explosion of Instrumentation • OTOLARYNGOLOGY • The Ear • The Nose • The Throat

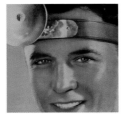

326 MEDICINE
Ancient Chinese Medical Care • Ancient Indian Medical Care • Religion and the Roots of Western Medicine • Early Hospitals • INFECTIOUS DISEASE • The Plague • Malaria • Leprosy • The French Pox • Consumption • Typhoid Mary • Ignaz Semmelweis: Medicine's Unsung Hero • Immunization: Smallpox, Rabies, and Tetanus • Growth of the Germ Theory • PULMONARY MEDICINE • Tobacco • GASTROENTEROLOGY • Purging the System • The Therapeutic Clyster • Early Forms of Intervention • A CLASSIC DESCRIPTION

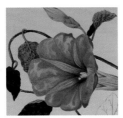

404 PHARMACY
Strange Ingredients • Medical Botany • Theories of Therapy • Self-Experimentation • Homeopathy • The Drug Trade • The Apothecary Shoppe • Put on the Brakes

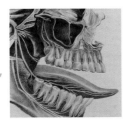

454 DENTISTRY
The Tooth Worm • A Patron Saint • Early Therapy of Dental Disease • Pull a Tooth, Cure a Patient • Dentistry Becomes a Profession • The Amalgam Wars (1840-1850) • Prosthetics • Dental Equipment and Furniture • Personal Dental Hygiene • The End of an Era

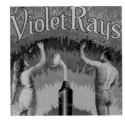

488 QUACK MEDICINE
Quacks Become Legit – Perkins Tractors • Phrenology • Healing and the Elements • Water Therapy • Vibration and Massage Therapy • Dr. Mesmer and His Magnets • Electricity • King of the Quacks • Ruth Drown: A Queen Ascends the Throne • Radioactivity • The Sanitarium • Victorian Prohibitions • John Brinkley: The Goat Gland Doctor • Miscellaneous Therapies • The Future?

573 GLOSSARY

579 ILLUSTRATION CREDITS

581 BIBLIOGRAPHY

585 INDEX

"There is nothing men will not do, there is nothing they have not done, to recover their health, and save their lives. They have submitted to be half drowned in water, and half choked with gases, to be buried up to their chins in earth, to be seared with hot irons like galley slaves, to be crimped with knives like codfish, to have needles thrust into their flesh, and bonfires kindled on their skin, to swallow all sorts of abominations, and to pay for all of this as if to be singed and scalded were a costly privilege, as if blisters were a blessing and leeches a luxury. What more can be asked to prove their honesty and sincerity?"

This statement was made in the nineteenth century by the great Harvard professor Oliver Wendell Holmes, MD, and accurately describes the value given to medical care from the beginning of recorded history. It is not surprising, then, that physicians have gone to great lengths in order to address the needs of the suffering and the debilitated. The variety of therapy offered to patients throughout the centuries, however, has been enormous since there was never a scientific basis on which to judge success. Even after the discovery of a new and effective treatment, communication was often poor, and sometimes the dissemination of information was inhibited by proprietary concerns. Bizarre procedures (by modern standards) remained popular for centuries frequently because some conditions improved spontaneously regardless of what was done. In addition, many patients improved by placebo effect. Some therapy was actually helpful, leaving members of the medical community free to provide whatever care they fancied. Physicians often remained adrift in a sea of human suffering with only superstition, anecdotal evidence, placebo "cures," and religious doctrine to guide their way.

Throughout history, various forms of therapy have come into and out of vogue with the resultant confusion presenting an opportunity to both the well-meaning and the dishonest, leaving patients the difficult task of choosing between the two. One example of a courageous physician might be Ignes Simmelweiss, a Hungarian obstetrician who first applied the germ theory and reduced the staggering incidence of post-partum mortality in his hospital from eighteen percent to one percent. In appreciation for his demonstration of the importance of simple hand washing, Simmelweiss' chief not only ridiculed him, but forced him out of his hospital. After several stops in different parts of the world, Simmelweiss was subsequently confined to a mental institution, and, by some accounts, ironically died of infection. For the finest in nobility and honor, one must look to Sir William Osler, who wrote the first "modern" textbook of medicine and revolutionized medical instruction by bringing it to the bedside. His interest in patient care went well beyond the study of pathophysiology: "The practice of medicine is an art, not a trade, a calling, not a business, a calling in which your heart will be exercised equally with your head."

One hopes that medical choices are in the interest of the suffering, though there have always been physicians eager to profit at the expense not only of their patients, but of medical progress as well. Those whose greed exceeded their judgment have included William Morton, DDS, a pioneer of one of the greatest breakthroughs in the history of medicine—anesthesia. He named his finding "Letheon" and then tried to patent the use of this wondrous gas by charging fees to anyone who used it. There were the unscrupulous, exemplified by Dr. Albert Abrams, the "King of the Quacks," who produced a large number of electrotherapy devices that remained popular until the early twentieth century and the enactment of federal oversight. Abrams represents many physicians who recognized a good business opportunity in health care and then took advantage, often to the detriment of the very ill and dependent. His box of nonfunctional tubes and wires was leased to physicians only with the written agreement that it would never be opened for inspection. And then there were physicians guilty of conceit, with the famous Dr. Robert Liston a good example. Before the availability of anesthesia, Liston, after whom many of his own surgical instruments were named, prided himself on his ability to amputate a limb in less than two minutes, sometimes attempting to break his own speed record in a manner detrimental to his patients' care.

The craftsmanship of artisans has always been more advanced than the medical care available at the time. Highly ornamented instruments often led to infection, while chemicals and potions sometimes themselves caused suffering and death. Though much of the therapy was often primitive by modern standards, one can only marvel at the skill exhibited by those who came before us—the artistry of da Vinci, Rembrandt, Kalkar, Gautier D'Agoty, and Bourgery, the prose of William Shakespeare, Mark Twain, and Oliver Wendell Holmes, and the craftsmanship of instrument manufacturers like Charrière, Aubry, Tiemann, Weiss, and Maw. As the practice of medicine became more advanced, so did the artifacts. The history of medicine can be reviewed from the perspective of the wonderful art and craftsmanship that was applied to the healing sciences. Unfortunately, the skill exhibited by these magnificent ivory, ebony, porcelain, and blued-steel instruments is frequently overshadowed by their misuse and the unintended harm they caused as a result of the infection they introduced.

This is not an academic text of the history of medicine, nor is it a review of medical art and craft, since history is not meaningful when related through the collection and display of ivory, canvas, and parchment. It is only by meeting those who found themselves on both sides of carefully sharpened scalpels and magically mixed potions that the past can be properly appreciated. In order to understand the heights and depths of their emotions, one must read the words of the men and women who either suffered the effects of untreatable diseases or were thrilled by the discovery of a treatment that could save the lives of millions. Some patients were cured while others were publicly ridiculed, enduring frequently horrifying therapy with only the dimmest hope of lasting relief. It was not until the twentieth century and the discovery of the scientific method that new discoveries could be found to cure illnesses that had plagued mankind from the beginning of recorded history. Ancient voices here relate the pain suffered from devastating diseases we don't see today through quotes and letters, sometimes to the amusement, sometimes to the horror, but always to the wonder of later generations.

I am not presumptuous enough to call myself a historian, and I have tried to stay out of the way as much as possible. I have relied heavily on original illustrations and quotes so that those in the past may "speak" to the reader and add texture to a history that can be at times so elusive. The case histories of desperate patients are touching and their treatment seems bizarre, though when viewed in the context of contemporary medical care, many forms of therapy were, in fact, quite sensible. This is an opportunity to understand the reasoning we now find so unusual and at the same time give great physicians from the past a chance to influence the way in which medicine is practiced today. Certainly the quote by holistic physician and philosopher Maimonides (1135–1204) will always remain relevant to the proper provision of medical care: *"quoniam medicus non curabat speciem aegritudinis sed individuum ipsius"* ("the physician should treat the patient and not the disease"). I have, in fact, attempted to adopt this profound advice as an author in writing the following pages.

After spending five years in preparing this book, I have come to the conclusion that it is impossible to write such a work and cover the territory in a truly comprehensive way. Some of the most historically significant events are not included, nor is there a complete list of medical instrumentation and art. It would have taken several lifetimes to research the necessary original documents, so I have had to depend on others. Where there have been differences of opinion regarding the facts, I have tried to include what is generally accepted, though I do apologize to the reader when I have failed. Problems arise as one attempts to sort out the accounts of those who are secondary or tertiary sources, and whose interpretations of the past vary. In order to provide a truly accurate account of the history of medicine, one has to have been there to see the events take place and to have spoken directly to the participants. I am reminded of the childhood game of passing a simple piece of information from one to another in a line of several people. The story told by the last rarely resembles the story told by the first.

This being my first effort at writing, I have learned a great deal. Most importantly, I have learned to take nothing at face value since it is only through relentless questioning that one can approach the truth. I have found that history is really not as boring as when I went to school, and that everyone is usually motivated by the same interests, sometimes to great discovery, while at other times to great embarrassment. My purpose in taking on the formidable task of writing this book was not to achieve the former, though hopefully the latter will not be my fate.

I will end by giving you the two pieces of advice that I have given each of my children as I have sent them off to college:

1. No one is as smart as you think they are.
2. Take at least one course in philosophy.

—ROBERT E. GREENSPAN, MD

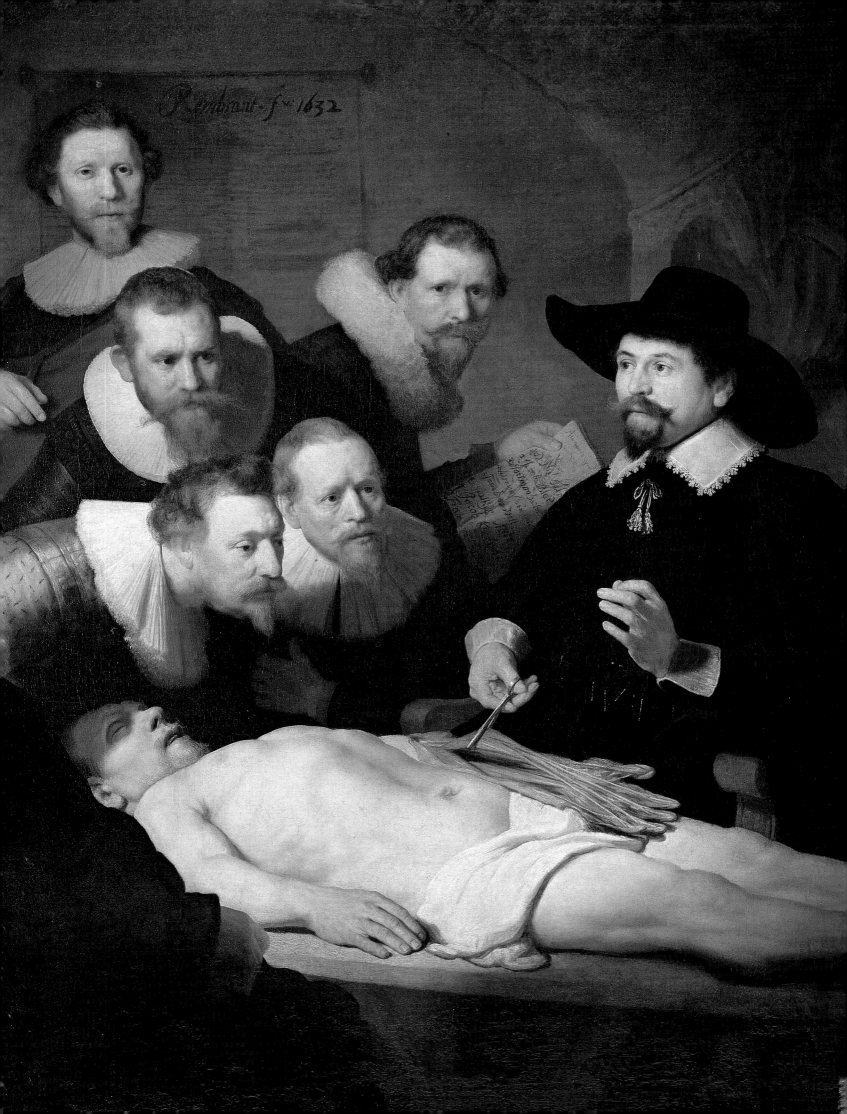

Reinbrant f. 1632

ANATOMY

Whenever you shall be so unhappy as to fail, in your Endeavours to relieve; let it be your constant Aim to convert particular Misfortunes into general Blessings, by carefully inspecting the Bodies of the Dead, inquiring into the Causes of their Diseases, and thence improving your own Knowledge, and making further and useful Discoveries in the healing Art.

A Discourse upon the Duties of a Physician
presented by Samuel Bard, MD
at the King's College commencement,
16th of May, 1769

Detail, *The Anatomy Lesson of Dr. Nicholaes Tulp* (1632), oil on canvas by Rembrandt van Rijn

Most medical careers begin at the dissecting table, so it is appropriate to open any discussion of medical history, art, and instrumentation with the study of anatomy. The earliest referral to this discipline is found in the Georg Ebers papyrus, which was written in Egypt in the early sixteenth century B.C. Religious restrictions prohibited any detailed study of organ systems, though the brain, heart, lungs, spleen, and anus were clearly identified. Egyptians described the circulatory system in a rudimentary way, and they believed that vessels carried not only blood but tears, mucus, urine, semen, and air (the word *artery* meaning "air tube" in Greek): "46 vessels go from the heart to every limb. There are 4 vessels to his nostrils, 2 give mucus and 2 give blood; there are 4 vessels in the forehead; there are 6 vessels that lead to the arms; there are 6 vessels that lead to the feet; there are 2 vessels to the testicles (and) it is they which give semen; there are 2 vessels to the buttocks."

HIPPOCRATES OF COS

Hippocrates of Cos (460–377 B.C.) is considered the "Father of Medicine" (figure 1). He elevated the practice of medical care from the realm of mystery, magic, and religion to become the first physician to employ common sense and logic in the treatment of his patients. He believed that one could understand the causes of various illnesses (and thereby discover their cure), only after the careful observation and study of the human body. From the beginning of recorded medical history, physicians and religious leaders had given the heart a unique role as the source of "thought, memory, and consciousness." It was not until Hippocrates in the fourth century B.C. that the brain was considered the center of mental function.

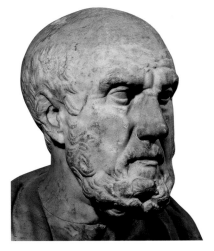

1. Marble bust of Hippocrates (ca. sixth century B.C.)

A great medical reformer, Hippocrates rejected previous superstitions suggesting that disease was the result of displeasure by the gods and the anger of evil spirits. His beliefs were recorded in the *Corpus Hippocraticum,* or Hippocratic Collection, brought together in the fourth century B.C. by Ptolemy, one of Alexander's generals. According to Hippocrates, "To know is one thing; merely to believe one knows is another. To know is science, but merely to believe one knows is ignorance." He carefully observed the progress of his patients and emphasized the importance of bedside diagnosis with a treatment plan based on the holistic approach of cleanliness, fresh air, and a simple diet. Hippocrates recognized the value of the relationship between science and art in medicine, and he established that association as the distinguishing characteristic of all great clinicians that followed.

Hippocrates founded his famous school of medicine on the Greek island of Cos, where he created a code of ethics, the Hippocratic Oath, which is still recited at many medical school graduation ceremonies (figure 2). The first half of the oath relates to the duties of a pupil toward his teacher, while the second remains quite controversial because it mentions abortion and suicide, topics that continue to be debated today. Discussions regarding the ethics of these issues is not new since both practices were not uncommon at the time the document was written centuries ago, probably accounting for the fact that there were many subsequent interpretations of the oath. Extensive instruction regarding the techniques of abortion and the "use of the knife" found in the *Corpus Hippocraticum* is inconsistent with the oath of Hippocrates, making multiple authorship of the latter a probability. This has led most scholars to believe that the oath, initially recorded in the first century A.D., was later modified according to contemporary religious thinking. This is one of the more popular translations of the Hippocratic Oath, written by Ludwig Edelstein in 1943:

2. Oath of Hippocrates from a tenth-century Urbinas text

I swear by Apollo the Physician and Aesculapius and Hygeia and Panaceia and all the gods and goddesses, making them my witnesses, that I will fulfill according to my ability and judgment this oath and this covenant:

To hold him who has taught me this art as equal to my parents and to live my life in partnership with him, and if he is in need of money to give him a share of mine, and to regard his offspring as equal to my brothers in male lineage and to teach them this art—if they desire to learn it—without fee and covenant; to give a share of precepts and oral instruction and all the other learning to my sons and to the sons of him who has instructed me and to pupils who have signed the covenant and have taken an oath according to the medical law, but no one else.

I will apply dietetic measures for the benefit of the sick according to my ability and judgment; I will keep them from harm and injustice.

I will neither give a deadly drug to anybody who asked for it, nor will I make a suggestion to this effect. Similarly I will not give to a woman an abortive remedy. In purity and holiness I will guard my life and my art.

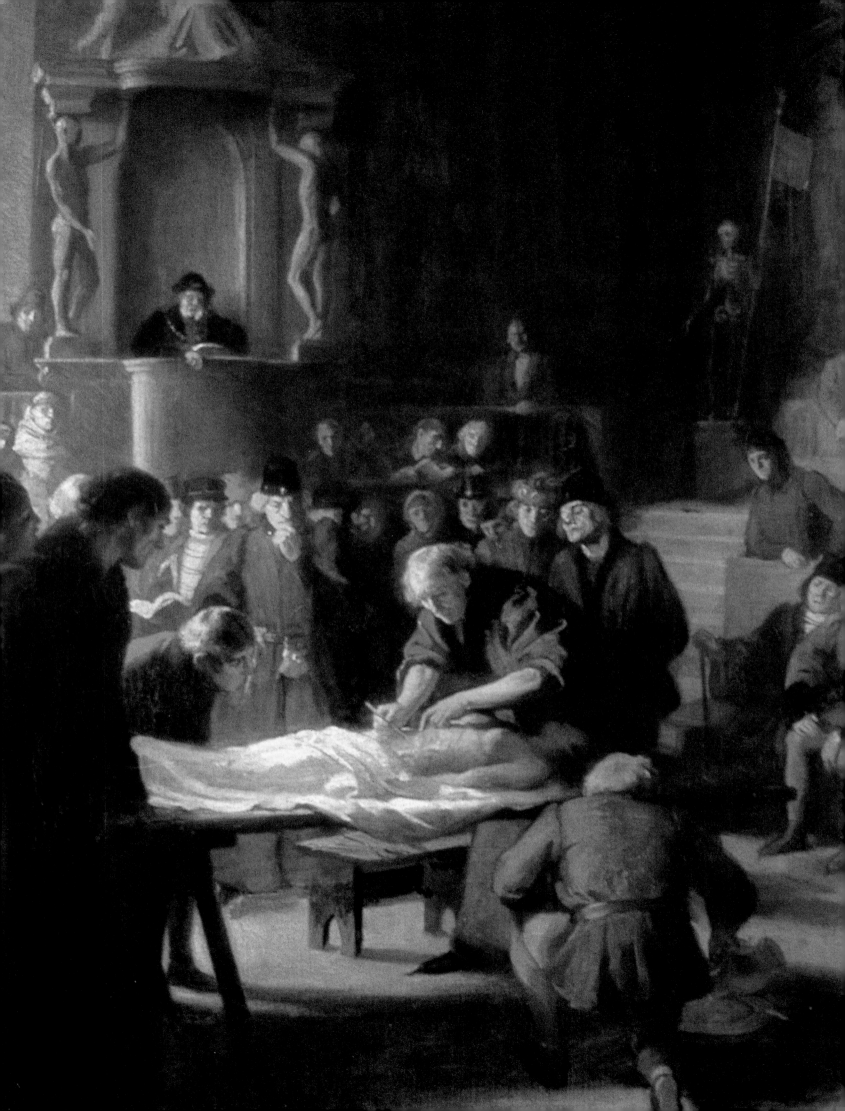

I will not use the knife, not even on sufferers from the stone, but will withdraw in favor of such men as are engaged in this work.

Whatever houses I may visit, I will come for the benefit of the sick, remaining free of all intentional injustice, of all mischief and in particular of sexual relations with both female and male persons, be they free or slaves.

What I may see or hear in the course of the treatment or even outside of the treatment in regard to the life of men, which on no account one must spread abroad, I will keep to myself, holding such things shameful to be spoken aloud.

If I fulfill this oath and do not violate it, may it be granted to me to enjoy life and art, being honored with fame among all men for all time to come; if I transgress it and swear falsely, may the opposite of all this be my lot.

The understanding of anatomy was not extensive when the oath of Hippocrates was written, though surgeons practicing in Alexandria, Egypt, soon after the time of Hippocrates did show an early interest in the structure of the body. Their dissection of criminals was recorded in the important text *De Medicina*, written by Aulus Cornelius Celcus (25 B.C.–A.D. 50) :"They hold that Herophilos and Erasistratos did this in the best way by far, when they laid open men whilst alive—criminals received out of prison from the kings—and whilst these were still breathing, observed parts which beforehand nature had concealed, their position, color, shape, size, arrangement, hardness, softness, smoothness, relation, processes and depression of each, and whether any part is inserted into or is received into another. For when pain occurs internally, neither is it possible for one to learn what hurts the patient, unless he has acquainted himself with the position of each organ or intestine. . . ."

ANATOMY ACCORDING TO GALEN

Claudius Galen of Pergamum (A.D. 120–200) was a prominent Greek physician whose contributions to health care made him one of the most important figures in the history of medicine. He was initially a physician to the gladiators and subsequently attended emperors Marcus Aurelius and Lucius Verus. Galen was the most skilled physician of his time, and in fact he established the experimental method in medicine, a discovery that languished until practiced by William Harvey in the seventeenth century. Galen systematized medical knowledge in over four hundred treatises, and his ideas remained influential for over 1,500 years, despite the fact that religious doctrine and superstition continued to play a significant role in

3. Dissection performed by Mondino de Cuzzi in Bologna in 1318, late nineteenth century oil on canvas by Ernest Board

anatomic study and medical care. In addition to the major contributions he made to medicine, Galen's success was a direct result of the hubris he exhibited as a medical authority: "Never as yet have I gone astray, whether in treatment or in prognosis, as have so many other physicians of great reputation. If anyone wishes to gain fame . . . all that he needs is to accept what I have been able to establish."

Some of the first recorded anatomic descriptions have been attributed to Galen, and while correct in most cases, there were a number of inaccuracies resulting from the fact that most of his dissections were based on animal rather than human specimens. According to Galen, the circulation was thought to be in two closed systems, the "natural" and the "vital." The natural system began in the liver, which was felt to be the seat of the soul and the source of blood that ebbed and flowed to the rest of the body for nourishment. The vital system contained the spirits originating in the heart with that organ's purpose to distribute heat and life to all parts of the body. Blood that was formed in the liver was strengthened by the natural spirit (*pneuma physicon*) for nutrition and metabolism, and then moved on to the lungs for the vital spirit (*pneuma zoticon*), where it was also cooled. The blood was mixed and heated in the heart, the animal spirit (*pneuma psychian*) was added in the brain for perception, and then those animal spirits moved out through the nerves to empty in the veins. Some of Galen's human material for dissection had come from criminals suffering a violent death whose arterial system was (normally) empty and whose veins were filled with clotted blood, thus supporting his theory that blood was produced in the liver, and then consumed in the body. In order to make the whole theory work, Galen postulated a connection between the two systems by way of small pores separating the right and left sides of the heart. Unfortunately, many of the errors formulated by Galen were perpetuated without question into the sixteenth century.

MEDICAL ILLUSTRATION

It was well into the twelfth century before anatomy became a legitimate part of the study of medicine. Many countries had political and religious laws restricting the use of human specimens for study, while cadavers for dissection were difficult to come by and preservation was inadequate. Most define the Dark Ages as the period from 500 to 1050, and with the end of the Roman Empire, medical literature moved east to Arabian countries where it was translated into Hebrew and held for centuries. It was in the medical community of Salerno in southern Italy that the study of medicine reawakened following the beginning of trade with Constantinople. The school at Salerno, the *Civitas Hippocratica*, attracted currents of medical thought from all over Europe and the Middle East, and it was there that animal dissections were first introduced into medical courses late in

4. Opposite. *Fasciculus Medicinae* (1493) by Johannes de Ketham

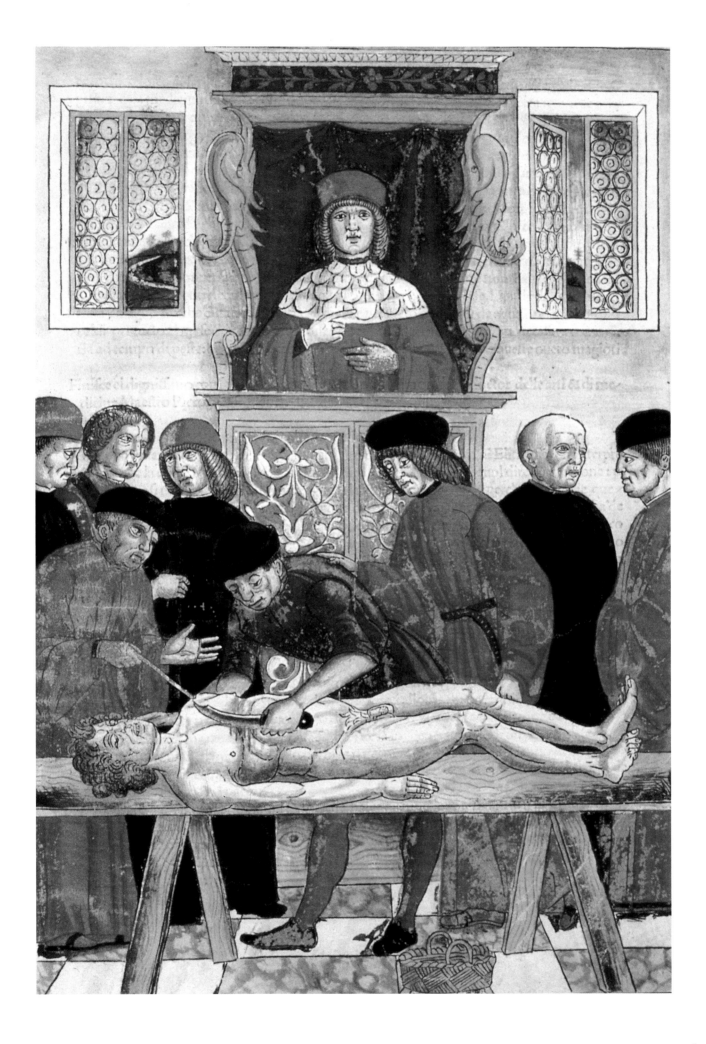

the twelfth century. The first to demonstrate Galen's teachings was Mondino de Cuzzi (1275–1326) of Bolognia when he dissected a human cadaver in about 1315, this famous lesson now a landmark in the history of medicine (figure 3). Johannes de Ketham illustrated the event in *Fasciculus Medicinae* (1493), and thereby became the author of the first anatomic illustration ever to appear in print. (figure 4) The gentleman sitting in the chair at the center of the woodcut orchestrated the procedure while he read from one of Galen's anatomic texts. This illustration is believed to be the origin of the term "chairman of the department," and the actual dissection would not have been done by the physician himself, but rather by an assistant.

The study of anatomy began to change by the end of the fifteenth century when a new air of freedom invigorated Western thought. Artists began to see the human body as an important subject for oils and marble, and physicians began to hope that by studying anatomic relationships, cures of diseases that had continued to plague Western Europe for centuries could be found. It is not surprising, then, that famous Renaissance painters and sculptors became prominent in the early history of medicine. Clerical leaders who had stifled medical progress by forbidding dissections in the past finally began to allow anatomic studies, partially because some of the artists who were interested in anatomy were the same ones who represented them in painting and sculpture. In 1482, Pope Sixtus IV gave local clergy the opportunity to allow dissections, and in fact one of the early permits was given to a young artist named Michelangelo Buonarroti in Florence, Italy.

RENAISSANCE ART

The first true great anatomic illustrations were by Leonardo da Vinci (1452–1519), who was an acclaimed inventor, engineer, and architect prior to his achieving fame as an artist. He was born illegitimately in Anchiano, a village near the town of Vinci, Italy, and was the son of Caterina and Ser Piero, a peasant and a lawyer. Da Vinci studied anatomy as an art form and had intended to provide his sketches to other artists only for their use as a guide in their work (figures 5–7). He was the first to study fetal membranes, dissect the brain, and he became one of the earliest physiologists with his description of muscles and their function. Da Vinci's work was the first systemic study of the human body and marked a revolutionary departure from Galen's long held doctrines. He sketched on loose leaf, and all his descriptions were written in the margins in mirror writing, a technique that the artist may have employed to prevent unintended use by others. Da Vinci's work in anatomy was the result of thirty carefully performed human dissections, and in fact he was forced to leave the Vatican in order to avoid prosecution.

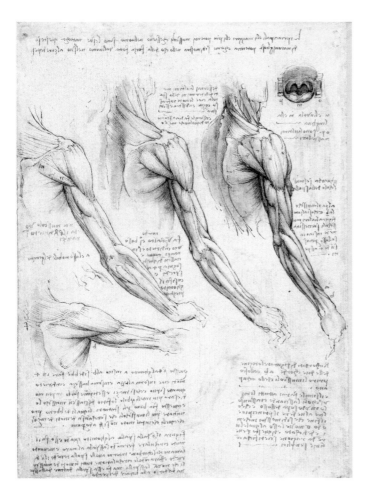

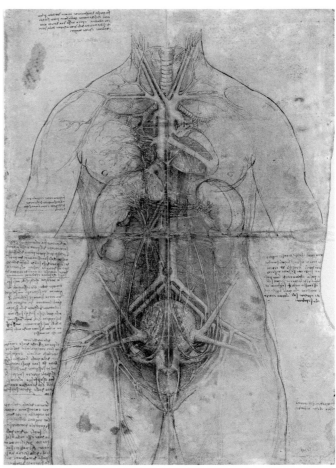

The following passage is taken from one of da Vinci's notebooks and illustrates his dedication to accuracy and scientific clarity as he provided advice (and a warning) to those who would follow after him in the field of anatomic illustration:

> You who say that it is better to watch an anatomical demonstration than to see these drawings, you would be right if it were possible to observe all the details shown in drawings in a single figure, in which with all your cleverness you will not see or acquire knowledge of more than some few veins, while in order to obtain a true and complete knowledge of these, I have dissected more than ten human bodies, destroying all the various members and removing the minutest particles of flesh which surrounded these veins, without causing any effusion of blood other than the imperceptible bleeding of the capillary veins. And as one single body did not suffice for so long a time, it was necessary to proceed by stages with so many bodies as would render my knowledge complete; this I repeated twice in order to discover the differences. And though you should have love for such things you may perhaps be deterred by natural

5. Left. Sketches of muscles of the arm in rotated views by Leonardo da Vinci (ca. 1500)

6. Right. Anatomical studies of the principal organs and arterial system in a female

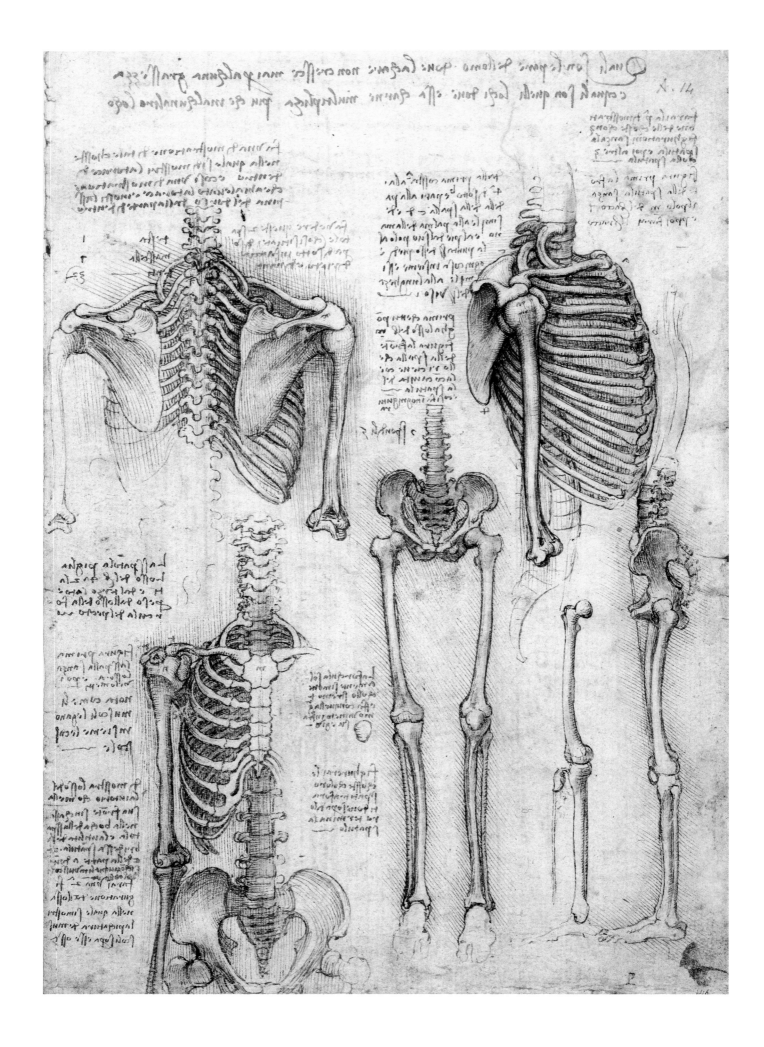

repugnance, and if this does not prevent you, you may perhaps be deterred by fear of passing the night hours in the company of these corpses, quartered and flayed and horrible to behold; and if this does not deter you, then perhaps you may lack the skill in drawing, essential for such representation; and if you had the skill in drawing, it may not be combined with a knowledge of perspective; and if it is so combined you may not understand the methods of geometrical demonstration and the methods of estimating the force and strength of muscles; or perhaps you may be wanting in patience so that you will not be diligent.

The difficulty in obtaining human cadavers for dissection was only one of many obstacles impeding the early study of anatomy, and when a dissection took place, it was frequently a well-publicized and anticipated public event accompanied by a banquet and sometimes a theatrical performance. Venetian surgeon Alessandro Benedetti (1450–1512) described some of the controversies surrounding early dissections in his book *The History of the Human Body*:

Tradition holds that kings themselves, taking counsel for public safety, have accepted criminals from prison and dissected them alive in order that while breath remained they might search out the secrets of nature, how she acts within herself with great ingenuity, and should note carefully the position of the members, their color shape, size, order, progression and recession, many of which are changed in dead bodies. The kings did this carefully and more than piously in order that when wounds had been inflicted it should be understood what was intact and what was damaged. But our religion forbids this procedure, since it is most cruel or full of the horror inspired by an executioner, lest those who are about to die amidst such torture should in wretched despair lose the hope of a future life. Let barbarians of a future rite do such things which they have devised, and of these sacrifices and prodigies. But we, who more mercifully spare the living, shall investigate the inner secrets of nature on the cadavers of criminals.

Early physicians observed that if anyone died of unknown diseases and they dissected cadavers, they might discover the hidden origins of diseases with equal advantage to the living. Galen was not ashamed to do the same thing with his ape when the cause of its death was unknown, just as we have done in the case of the Gallic disease. The pontifical regulations have for a long time permitted this form of dissection; otherwise, it would be regarded as most execrable and abominable or irreligious.

7. Opposite. Sketch of the skeletal system by Leonardo da Vinci (ca. 1500)

Furthermore, ritual purifications of the physicians' souls take place, and we propitiate their offense with prayers. Those who live in prison have sometimes asked to be handed over rather to the colleges of physicians rather than to be killed by the hand of the public executioner. Cadavers of this kind cannot be obtained except by papal consent. Thus by law only unknown and ignoble bodies can be sought for dissection, from distant regions, without injury to neighbors and relatives. Those who have been hanged are selected, of middle age, not thin nor obese, of taller statue, so that there may be available for spectators a more abundant and hence more visible material for dissection. For this a quite cold winter is required to keep the cadavers from rotting immediately. A temporary dissecting theater must be constructed in an ample, airy place with seats placed in a hollow semicircle such as can be seen at Rome and Verona, of such a size as to accommodate the spectators and prevent them from disturbing the masters of the wounds, who are the dissectors. These must be skillful and such as have dissected frequently. A seating order to dignity must be given out. For this purpose there must be an overseer who takes care of all such matters. There must be guards to prevent the eager public from entering. Two treasurers are to be chosen who will buy what is necessary from monies collected. The following are needed: razors, hooks, drills, trepanning instruments, sponges with which to remove blood in dissection, paring knives, and basins. Torches must be also provided for the night. The cadaver is to be placed on a rather high bench in the middle of the theater in a lighted spot handy for the dissectors. A time for attendance is to be established, after which the gathering is dismissed so that the dissection may be completely carried out before the material putrefies.

Despite the fact that the modern study of anatomy began in the sixteenth century, the understanding of physiology and pathology remained primitive, and physicians continued to have limited knowledge regarding the etiology and proper management of most medical conditions. Physicians had hoped that they might find some answers at the dissecting table and that the mysteries of disease would open up before them with the pass of a sharp knife, but that was not to be. Marcello Donato wrote the following in his *De medicina historia mirabile, libri sex* (1586):

Let those who interdict the opening of bodies well understand their errors. When the cause of a disease is obscure, in opposing the dissection of a corpse which must soon become the food of worms, they do no good to the inanimate mass, and they cause a grave damage to the rest of mankind; for they prevent the physicians from acquiring a knowledge which may afford the means of great relief eventually to individuals attacked by a similar disease. No less blame is applicable to those physicians who, from laziness or repugnance, love better to remain in the darkness of ignorance than to scrutinize laboriously the truth, not reflecting that by such conduct they render themselves culpable toward God, themselves, and society at large.

Jacques Cartier (1491–1557), discoverer of the St. Lawrence River, unknowingly described scurvy, a vitamin C deficiency, when he dissected one of his men in search of the cause of his death, and perhaps a cure. (Scurvy was common in the British Navy because sailors often went on long voyages without fresh food. Eventually, they discovered that eating fruit prevented the disease, and many brought limes on board, thus leading to British sailors eventually being called "limeys.") The following is from *The Principall Navigations, Voyages, Traffiques and Discoveries of the English Nation Made by Sea or Over-land to the Remote and Farthest Distant Quarters of the Earth at Any Time Within the Compasse of These 1600 Yeeres* (1589).

And albeit we had driven them from us, the said unknown sicknes began to spread itselfe amongst us after the strangest sort that ever was eyther heard of or seene, insomuch as some did lose all their strength, and could not stand on their feete, then did their legges swell, their sinnowes shrinke as blacke as any cole. Others also had all their skins spotted with spots of blood of a purple coulour: then did it ascend up to their ankles, knees, thighs, shoulders, armes and necke: their mouth became stinking, their gummes so rotten, that all the flesh did fall off, even to the rootes of the teeth, which did also almost all fall out. . . . That day Philip Rougemont, borne in Amboise, died, being 22 yeeres olde, and because the sickenesse was to us unknown, our Captain caused him to be ripped to see if by any meanes possible we might know what it was, and so seeke meanes to save and preserve the rest of the company: he was found to have his heart white, but rotten, and more than a quart of red water about it: his liver was indifferent faire, but his lungs blacke and mortified, his blood was altogether shrunke about the heart, so that when he was opened great quantitie of rotten blood issued out from about his heart: his milt toward the backe was somewhat perished, rough as if it had bene rubbed against a stone. Moreover, because one of his thighs was very blacke without, it was opened, but within it was whole and sound: that done, as well as we could he was buried.

Unfortunately, there remained a great deal of religious resistance to a change in attitudes regarding human dissection and the study of anatomy. Michael Servetus (1509–1553), a Spanish physician and cleric, was the first to describe the pulmonary circulation when he suggested that blood traveled through the lungs rather than through Galen's "pores" in the heart. His theological work, *On the Restitution of Christianity,* was anatomically correct though refuted the sacred teachings of Galen. As a consequence, he upset both Protestants and Catholics, and was buried alive in Geneva (with his own books) by religious reformer John Calvin.

THE FIRST MODERN MEDICAL CLASSIC

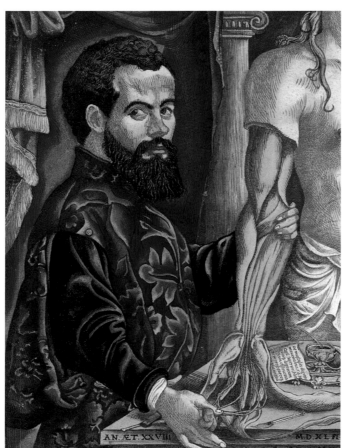

8. Portrait of Andreas Vesalius in *De humani corporis fabrica libri septem* (1543)

9. Opposite. Title page in *De humani corporis fabrica libri septem* (1543)

It was Andreas Vesalius (1514–1564) who brought medicine into the modern era with his monumental work *De humani corporis fabrica libri septem* (1543), now considered one of the greatest books in the history of medicine and science. Vesalius took that first great step away from the dogma that had strangled scientific investigation for centuries when he discarded all of Galen's previously held "truths" and based his anatomic investigations on what he himself observed with his own careful dissections.

Andreas Vesalius was born in Brussels and moved to Paris after studying in Louvain. He was somewhat dissatisfied with his professor, Jacques Dubois (also known as Jacobus Silvius), since his classes were all faithful to the word of Galen. In 1537, Vesalius moved to Padua and joined Jan Stefan van Kalkar who had studied with the famous artist Titian. Kalkar was responsible for the now classic anatomic drawings found in this landmark textbook of anatomy, first printed in 1543 when Vesalius was only twenty-eight years old.

Unfortunately, Vesalius' new discoveries were met with a great deal of hostility. In the first edition, he dispelled highly regarded religious beliefs, including the presence of the bone of Luz (which was supposedly an indestructible bone at the base of the spine that was the seed of resurrection), and he additionally failed to document Adam's missing rib. More importantly, Vesalius departed from concepts based on Galen's animal dissections that had been accepted without question for the previous thirteen centuries. Removed from his pages were the five lobes of the liver found in the hog, the segmented breastbone of the ape, the bicornuate uterus of the dog, and the flared hip bones of the ox. Despite the startling anatomic revelations revealed

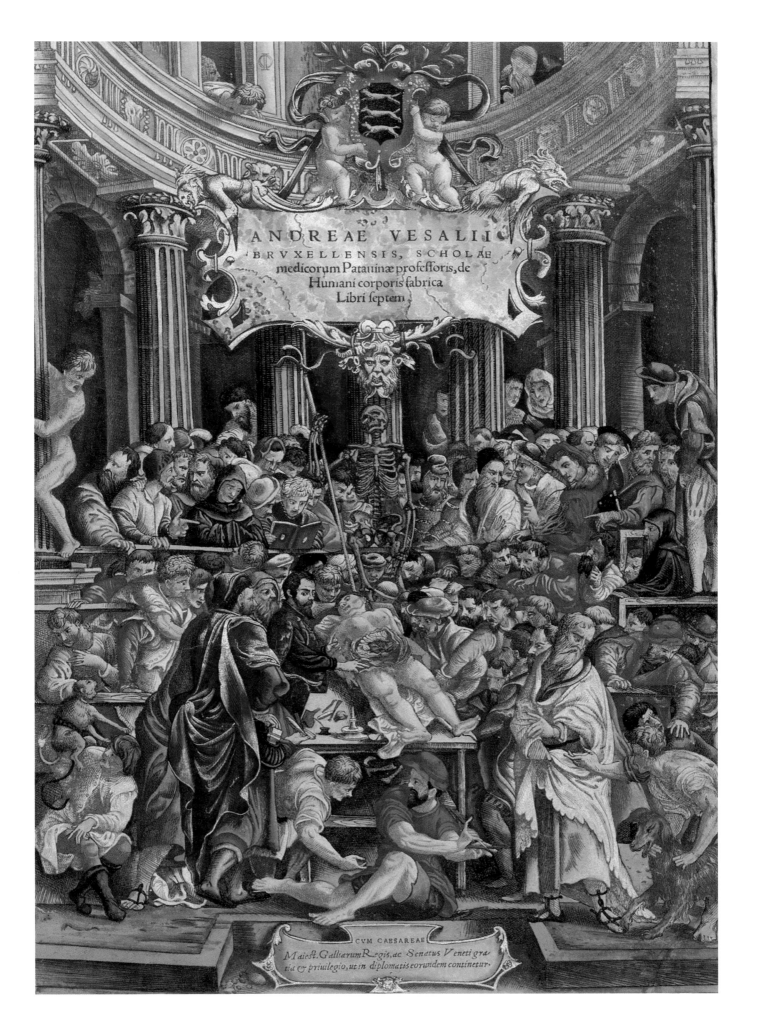

ANDREAE VESALII
BRVXELLENSIS, SCHOLAE
medicorum Patauinæ professoris, de
Humani corporis fabrica
Libri septem

CVM CAESAREAE
Maiest. Galliarum Regis, ac Senatus Veneti gra-
tia & priuilegio, ut in diplomatis eorundem continetur.

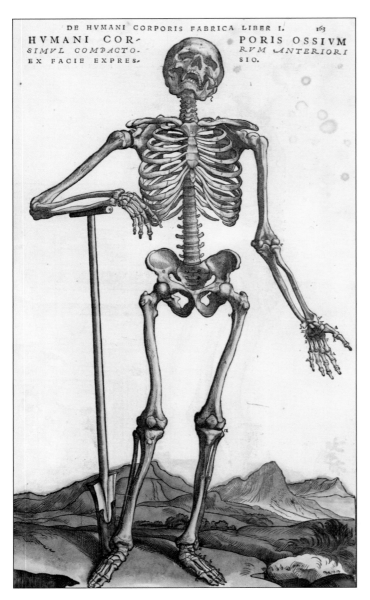

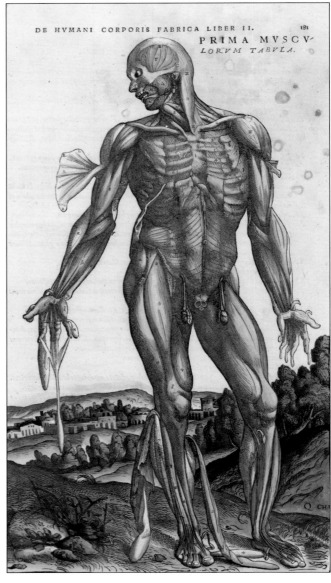

10. Skeletal system in *De humani corporis fabrica libri septem* (1543)

11. Muscular system in *De humani corporis fabrica libri septem* (1543)

in the *Fabrica,* there remained, however, a number of inaccuracies, one of which was the presumption that nasal secretions came directly from the central nervous system (thus giving continued support to those who used snuff to "purge the brain"). In the words of his former professor, Sylvius, Vesalius was "an impious madman who is poisoning the air of all Europe with his vaporings." As a result of the widespread condemnation, Vesalius subsequently burned all his own manuscripts and left Padua for Spain to become the personal physician to the Holy Roman Emperor Charles V.

The unique color illustrations noted here are from an edition that Vesalius had specially made for the emperor himself (figures 8–11). Included is the only colored portrait of Vesalius, and the title page of the *Fabrica* is filled with symbolism as Vesalius himself, rather than an assistant, dissected the mistress of a monk. The animal subjects that Galen had used as the basis of his anatomic descriptions are seen in the lower part of the page. As mentioned earlier, it had been the custom for a physician to sit above these dissections and recite the anatomy of Galen, though in this case there is a skeleton, perhaps representing the end of Galen's views on anatomy. The *Fabrica* marked the beginning of the technique of a progressively layered dissection, and the figures became weaker as muscles were removed, the subjects finally requiring ropes and walls for support. The lush background became more barren as summer turned to winter.

Vesalius never received the credit he was due while he was alive, and the circumstances of his death are somewhat bizarre as recounted in a letter written by Herbert Languer in 1563. According to the story, Vesalius was dissecting a Spanish nobleman and upon opening the chest found the heart still beating. The parents of the nobleman were notified, and they subsequently informed the Spanish Inquisition, accusing Vesalius of murder. The king intervened on behalf of his personal physician and sent the anatomist to the Holy Land for penitence. While away, he received an invitation to resume his former position in Padua, though unfortunately Vesalius never made it back from Jerusalem, dying in a shipwreck near the Greek island of Zante on his return. The original plates from Vesalius' work were kept in Munich where they were used in a facsimile edition as late as 1934, though, unfortunately, they were destroyed in a World War II bombing.

A MISSED OPPORTUNITY

Bartolomaeo Eustachi (1513?–1574) was an Italian physician/anatomist who became a professor of anatomy at the Collegia dalla Sapienza, a position that allowed him to obtain cadavers for dissection from nearby hospitals. His anatomic works were precise and, in many cases, more anatomically correct than those of his contemporary, Andreas Vesalius, though not as artistically advanced. In 1552, Eustachi, with the help of Pier Matteo Pini, produced forty-seven anatomic plates, though he completed the text for only eight that he published in his *Opuscula anatomica*. On Eustachi's death in 1574, the unpublished thirty-nine plates passed on to Pini, and they subsequently found their way into the Vatican Library, where they remained lost for over one hundred fifty years. In the early part of the eighteenth century, Giovanni Maria Lancisi, physician to Pope Clement XI, located the missing plates, completed the text with his own narrative, and released all forty-seven studies under the title *Tabulae anatomicae Bartolomaei Eustachi quas a tenebris tandem vindicates* ("Anatomical Illustrations of Bartolomaeo Eustachi Rescued from Obscurity") (1714) (figure 12). Had his illustrations been published at the time of their initial execution, Eustachi almost certainly would have been recognized with Vesalius as one of the founders of modern anatomy.

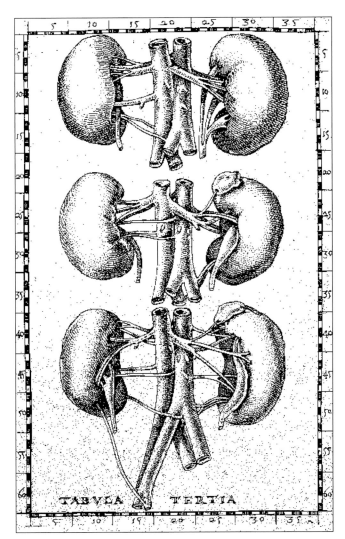

12. Kidneys and adrenal glands in *Tabulae anatomicae Bartolomaei Eustachi quas a tenebris tandem vindicates* (1714) by Bartolomaeo Eustachi

Bartolomaeo Eustachi has been credited with a number of important discoveries related to human anatomy, including the first detailed accounts of the adrenal glands and the kidneys. His most famous discovery, however, was of the tuba auditiva, a connection between the middle ear and the naso-pharynx that retains his namesake, the Eustachian tube. Some historians have surmised that Shakespeare was inspired by the discovery of this connection in his 1602 play *Hamlet*. In act 1, scene 5, Hamlet's uncle, Claudius, killed his brother the king (and Hamlet's father) by pouring the poison henbane (*Hyoscyamus niger*) into his ear:

Sleeping within my orchard,
My custom always of the afternoon,
Upon my secure hour thy uncle stole,
With juice of cursed hebenon in a vial,
And in the porches of my ears did pour
The leperous distillment;
Whose effect
Holds such an enmity with blood of man
That swift as quicksilver it courses through
The natural gates and alleys of the body.
And with a sudden vigour doth posset
And curd, like eager droppings into milk,
The thin and wholesome blood: so did it mine;
And a most instant tetter bark'd about,
Most lazar-like, with vile and loathsome crust,
All my smooth body.
Thus was I, sleeping, by a brother's hand
Of life, of crown, of queen, at once dispatch'd . . . .

LOOKING FOR A SUBJECT AND A PURPOSE

Artists in the sixteenth and seventeenth centuries found the human body to be of great interest, and their representations were not always intended for use by physicians. The role of the artist in medicine remained unclear, and an ongoing dispute was outlined by John Bell, MD, in the preface to his *Engraving of the Bones, Muscles, and Joints* (1804): "Even in the first invention of our best anatomical figures, we see a continual struggle between the anatomist and the painter; one striving for elegant form, the other insisting upon accuracy of representation." Part of the problem was that physicians remained unclear regarding the ability of anatomy to provide clues toward either a diagnosis or a treatment plan. John Locke placed the study of anatomy in an unflattering light when he made the following statement in the mid seventeenth century: "All that anatomy can doe is only to shew us the gross and sensible parts of the body, or the vapid and dead juices all which, after the most diligent search, will be not much able to direct a physician how to cure a disease than how to make a man. . . . If anatomy shew us neither the causes nor cures of most diseases I think it not very likely to bring any great advantages for removeing the pains and maladys of mankind."

Artists represented their subjects in many different ways, some hoping to bring the deceased back to life as they demonstrated their dissected parts. The first seen here was by Charles Estienne (1504–1564) in *De dissectione partium corporis humani* (1545) (figure 13). The anatomist was Estienne de la Rivière, who actually held up the publication of these illustrations because of his lawsuit against the author. Had that not been the case, this work would have predated some of the major innovations introduced by Vesalius in his classic text, and both Estienne and de la Rivière would have held a more significant place in medical history. Note that despite the fact that the brain has been cross-sectioned in this illustration, the figure is able to point out captions in the woodcut.

Dissected figures seemed to delight in playfully showing off their anatomy in the copperplates of Odoardo Fialetti in *Tabulae anatomicae* by Giulio Cesare Casseri (1552–1616) (figure 14). In the latter part of the sixteenth century, Casseri taught anatomy in Padua using dissected specimens under the direction of Fabrizio. The latter developed a great deal of professional hostility toward his associate, and when students favored the teaching of Casseri, Fabrizio restricted his supply of cadavers, and then blocked the publication of his *Tabulae*.

Pierto da Cortona (1596–1669) was one of the most important painters of the Renaissance Italian Baroque period, and his large ceiling frescoes influenced European art for many years after his death. Luca Ciamberlano probably engraved the anatomic plates in Cortona's *Tabulae anatomicae* beginning in about 1618, though they remained unpublished until 1741 (figures 15, 16). Cortona's figures were also anxious to demonstrate their muscles more as an art form than as a guide to physicians. John Browne (1642–1702) produced another copperplate showing a posing nobleman in *A compleat treatise of the muscles, as they appear in the humane body, and arise in dissection* (figure 17). Here the subject appears to be from the upper class though, as noted earlier, the poor were usually the ones whose remains found their way onto dissecting tables for study by artists and physicians.

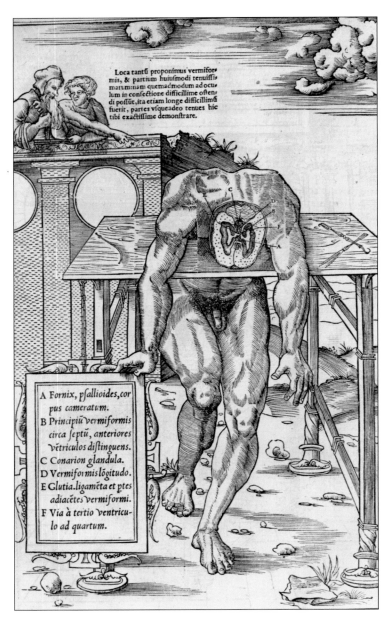

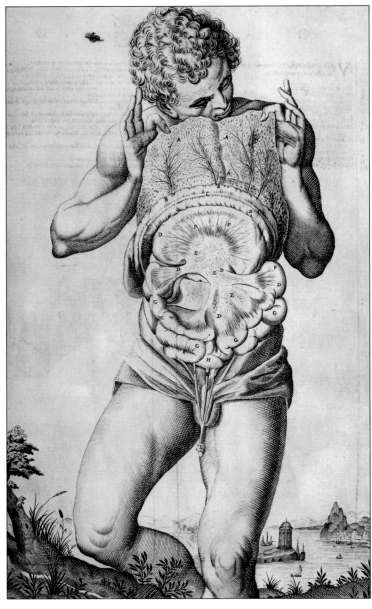

13. Anatomy with cross section of the brain in *La dissection des parties du corps humain* (1546), woodcut by Charles Estienne

14. Anatomy of the internal organs in *Tabulae Anatomicae* (1627), copperplate engraving by Giulio Cesare Casseri

In his etching of the dissection of Tom Nero in *The Reward of Cruelty* (1751), William Hogarth illustrated the criminal source of a great deal of anatomic material (figure 18). Note that the hangman's noose remained tied around the neck of the subject being dissected while his entrails were being fed to a dog, a certain sign of disrespect.

MEDICINE BECOMES A SCIENCE

The next great landmark in the history of medicine, and indeed in all of science, came in 1628 when William Harvey (1578–1657) wrote *Exercitatio Anatomica de Motu Cordis et Sanguinis in Animalibus* (figures 19, 20). Harvey's study of circulatory physiology was another major departure from principles long held by Galen. His use of the scientific method

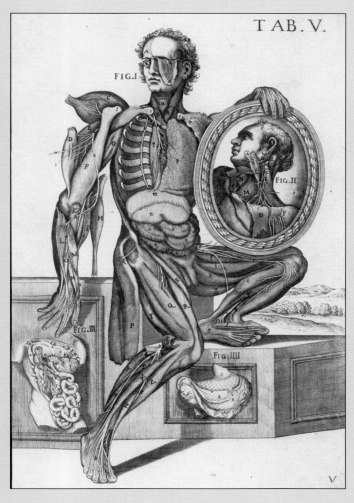

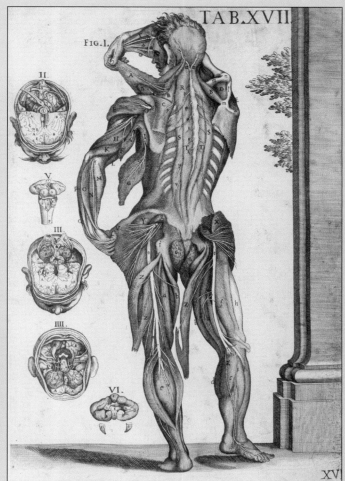

15–16. Above. Demonstration of muscles in *Tabulae anatmicae* (1741) by Pietro da Cortona

17. Muscle anatomy in *A compleat treatise of the muscles, as they appear in the humane body, and arise in dissection* (1681), copperplate engraving by John Browne

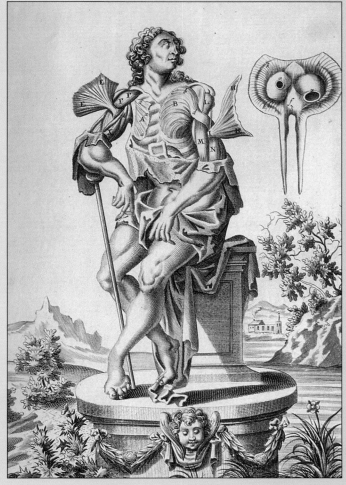

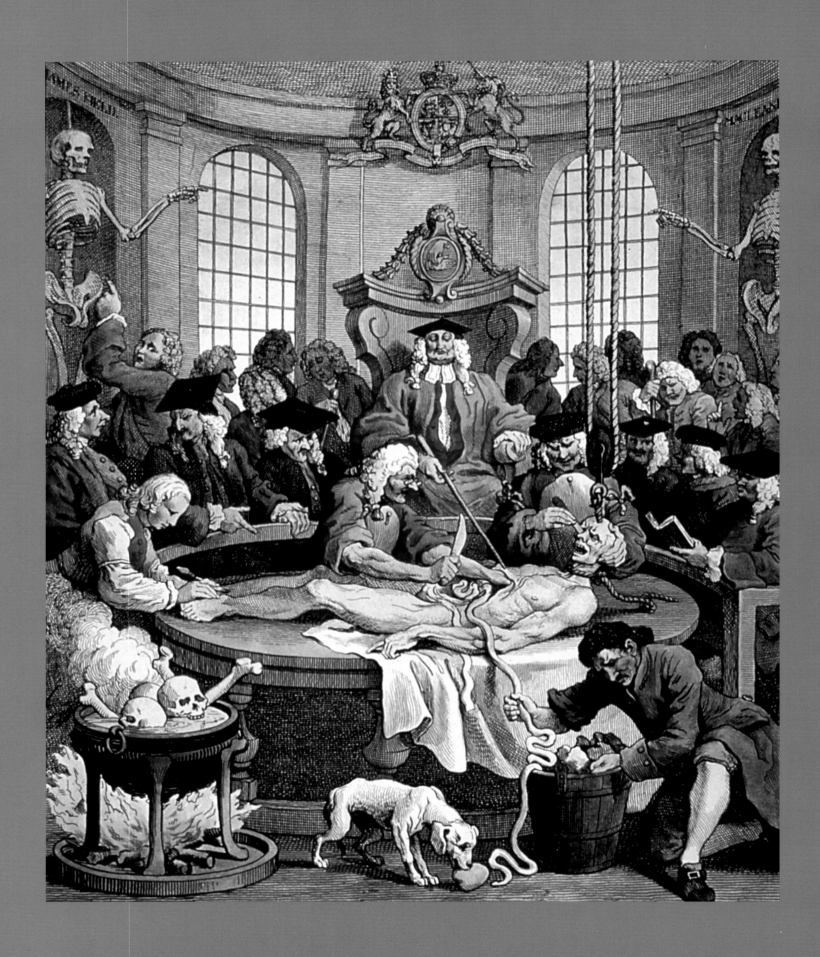

and his application of mathematical measurements to vital phenomena revolutionized medical investigation. The careful observations demonstrated by Vesalius in his *Fabrica* and the impartial investigation in Harvey's *de Motu Cordis* made these the two most important books in the history of medicine. Harvey's first ideas regarding the circulation of the blood may have, in fact, come from Galileo, who was a professor at Padua where Harvey had received his medical degree. Galileo had been working with fluids and pumps, and another of Harvey's professors, Fabrizio, also helped to set the stage with his demonstration of the presence of valves in veins.

The following quote from Harvey's landmark work represents one of the most important in all of scientific investigation:

> And now I may be allowed to give in brief my view of the circulation of the blood, and to prove it for general adoption. Since all things, both argument and ocular demonstration, show that the blood passes through the lungs and heart by the force of the ventricles, and is sent for distribution to all parts of the body, where it makes its way into the veins and porosities of the flesh, and then flows by the veins from the circumference on every side to the centre, from the lesser to the greater veins, and is by them finally discharged into the vena cava and right auricle of the heart, and this in such a quantity or in such a flux and reflux thither by the arteries, hither by the veins, as cannot possibly be supplied by the ingesta, and is much greater than can be required for mere purposes of nutrition; it is absolutely necessary to conclude that the blood in the animal body is impelled in a circle, and is in a state of ceaseless motion; that this is the act or function which the heart performs by means of its pulse; and that it is the sole and only end of the motion and contraction of the heart.

William Osler, MD, put this monumental achievement into perspective at the turn of the twentieth century when he said, "It marks the transition from old tradition to modern thought. We are no longer satisfied with bare observations. Here, for the first time, is an experimental solution of physiological problems, carried out by a man who could evaluate his findings without over valuing them and had the ability to let his conclusions follow naturally from the results. An age of audiences, who merely listened with attention, turned into an age of the eye, in which people were only satisfied with what they could see. But now came the age of the hand—the thinking, advising, planning hand that is the tool of the brain. And this age was introduced by a modest monograph of seventy-two pages, which lays the basis for all experimental medicine!"

18. The dissection of the body of Tom Nero with John Freke presiding in *The Reward of Cruelty* (1751), etching by William Hogarth

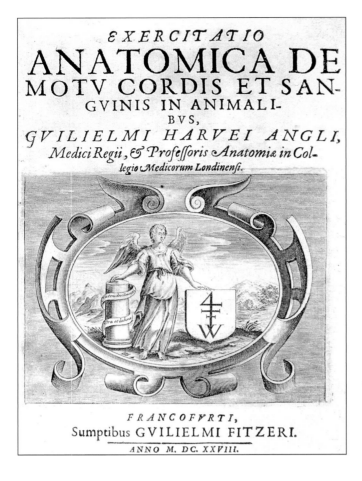

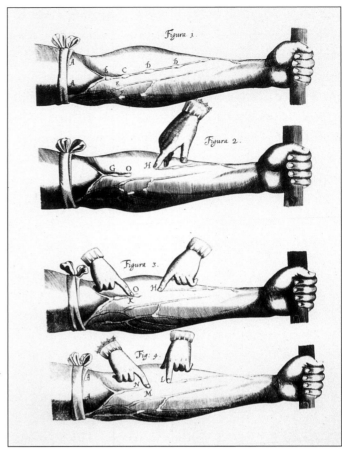

19. Title page of *Exercitatio anatomica de motu cordis* (1628) by William Harvey

20. The circulation and venous valves from *Exercitatio anatomica de motu cordis* (1628) by William Harvey

The first edition of Harvey's work was printed on rather inexpensive paper in Germany since British publishers were afraid to print the book because of some of the negative reaction that was sure to follow. Harvey did his best to ingratiate himself to the king with this introduction: "The King, in like manner, is the foundation of the kingdom, the sun of the world around him, the heart of the republic, the fountain whence all power, all grace doth flow." Unfortunately, it was King Charles I who ultimately faced a tragic future when he was overthrown by the Parliamentarians and beheaded twenty years later.

ART AND PHYSIOLOGY

In 1632, Rembrandt van Rijn (1606–1669) turned his attention to the study of anatomy in his famous *The Anatomy Lesson of Dr. Nicholaes Tulp* (figure 21). The Amsterdam Company of Surgeons had commissioned this work when Rembrandt was only twenty-six years old, and shows Dr. Nicholaes Tulp, a leading Dutch physician at the time, identifying tendons in the arm of a cadaver. It is no coincidence that he was referring to the same tendons highlighted by Andreas Vesalius on the front page of his landmark work, the *Fabrica*, since Tulp had been a disciple of that

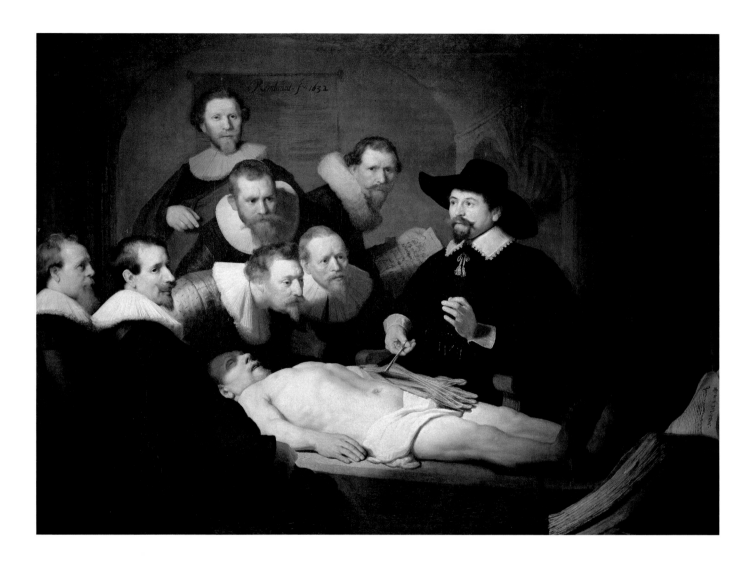

great anatomist. Note that most of the observers were carefully studying the movement of Dr. Tulp's hand as it reproduced the motion of the dissected specimen, rather than its anatomy. He was actually demonstrating the action of tendons that flexed the fingers since his goal was to use functional anatomy as a way to discover the causes of disease. Incidentally, the figure at the far left was added later since he had missed the original sitting for the portrait.

21. *The Anatomy Lesson of Dr. Nicholaes Tulp* (1632), oil on canvas by Rembrandt van Rijn

A SEVENTEENTH-CENTURY CONTROVERSY

The finest anatomic work of the seventeenth century was written by Govert Bidloo in 1685. The *Anatomia humani corporis* included 105 copperplate engravings drawn by Gèrard de Lairesse, and were wonderful examples of contemporary Dutch baroque art (figures 22–24). This publication generated one of the most famous controversies in the history of medicine when Bidloo's figures found their way into William Cowper's *The Anatomy of Humane Bodies*, published later in 1698. Cowper had

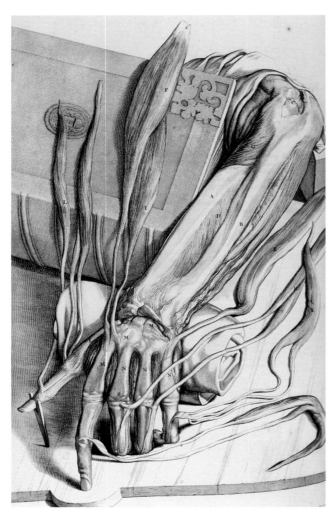

22. Muscles and tendons of the arm in *Anatomia humani corporis* (1685), copperplate engraving by Govard Bidloo

23. Skeletal anatomy in *Anatomia humani corporis* (1685) by Govard Bidloo

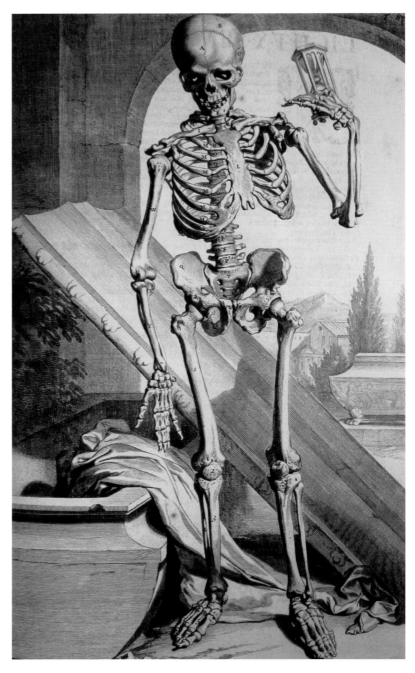

purchased the van Gunst copperplates, and then he reissued the same images under his own name with English text. Cowper did not acknowledge Bidloo anywhere in the book, and he pasted a small printed flap with his own name over that of Bidloo on the engraved title page of the first edition (figure 25). A heated dispute ensued, and Bidloo accused Cowper of plagiarism, calling him a "highwayman" among a number of other epithets. In 1702, William Cowper did provide us with a classic description of aortic insufficiency, and described urethral glands, now referred to as "Cowper's glands." It is ironic, however, that Mery had already discovered those glands in 1684.

STRUCTURE AND FUNCTION

Anatomists and physiologists began to interpret the body in terms of its structure and mechanics, leaving aside questions of religion and the "soul" to clerics. Astronomer and mathematician Giovanni Borelli of Pisa exemplified this approach in his *De Motu Animalium*, published in 1680–1681, when he applied the laws of physics to view the body as a machine that functioned by way of a system of pulleys and levers (figure 26). Dutch physician and anatomist Hermann Boerhaave (1668–1738) also illustrated the body in mechanical terms with his emphasis on the importance of a system of well-balanced bodily fluids in the maintenance of good health. Despite the relatively advanced understanding that physicians had of the anatomy of the nervous system by the beginning of the nineteenth century, an appreciation of physiologic mechanisms was not clear until the work of Charles Bell, whose animal experimentation was presented in six papers to the Royal Society between 1821 and 1829. He found vivisection so repugnant, however, that he depended on his brother-in-law, John Shaw, to do the actual dissections. Bell related his obvious discomfort in this description of an important neurologic finding:

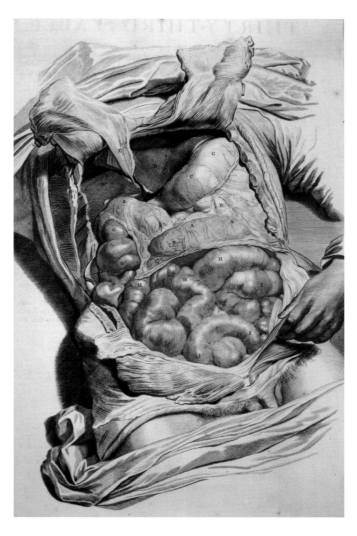

24. Abdominal anatomy in *Anatomia humani corporis* (1685) by Govard Bidloo

After delaying long on account of the unpleasant nature of the operation, I opened the spinal canal of a rabbit and cut the posterior roots of the nerves of the lower extremity; the creature still crawled, but I was deterred from repeating the operation by the protracted cruelty of the dissection. I reflected that an experiment would be satisfactory if done on a animal recently knocked down and insensible; that whilst I experimented on a living animal, there might be trembling or action excited in the muscles by touching a sensitive nerve, which motion it would be difficult to distinguish from that produced more immediately through the influence of the motor nerves. A rabbit was struck behind the ear, so as to deprive it of sensibility by the concussion, and I then exposed the spinal marrow. On irritating the posterior roots of the nerve, at each touch of the forceps there was a corresponding motion of the muscles to which the nerve was distributed. Every touch of the probe or needle on the threads of this root was attended with a muscular motion as distinct as the motion produced by touching the keys of a harpsichord. These experiments

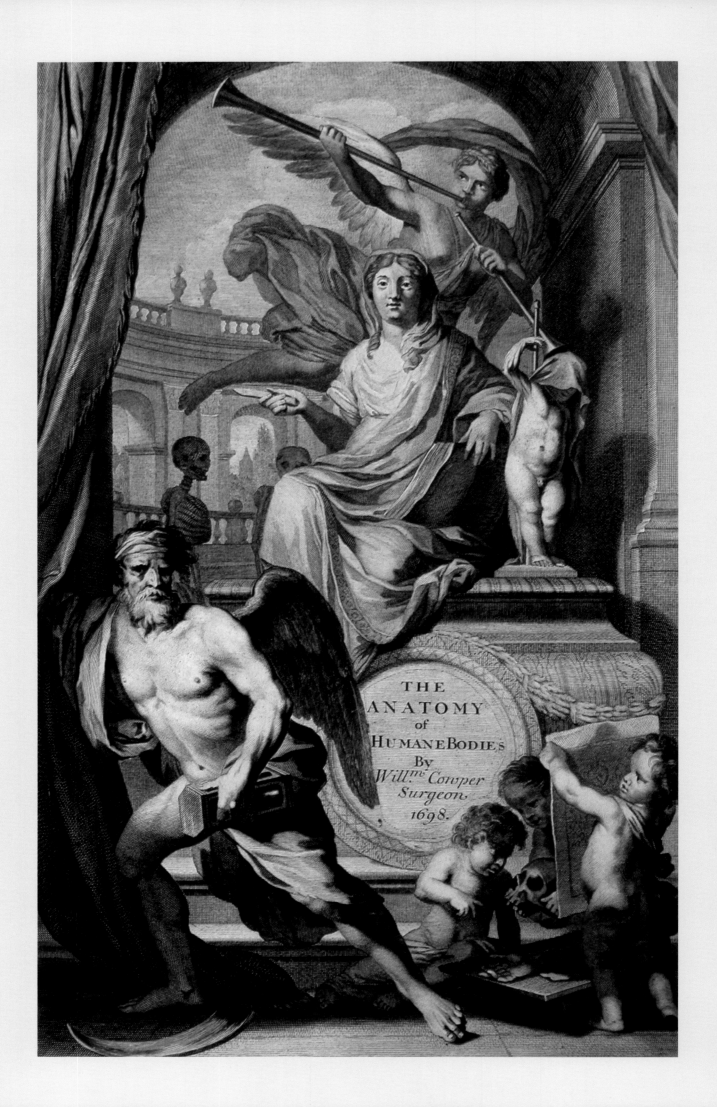

THE
ANATOMY
of
HUMANE BODIES
By
Will.ᵐ Cowper
Surgeon
1698.

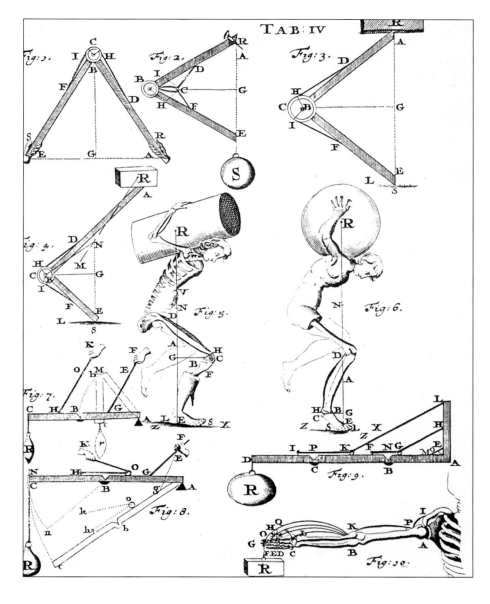

25. Opposite. Title page of *The Anatomy of Humane Bodies* (1698), by William Cowper

26. A demonstration of leg joints in *De motu animalium* (1685) by Giovanni Alfonso Borelli

satisfied me that the different roots and different columns from whence these roots arose were devoted to distinct offices, and that these notions drawn from the anatomy were correct.

WONDERFUL MEDICAL ART

Probably the finest illustrations of the musculoskeletal system produced in the eighteenth century were by William Cheselden in *Osteographia* (1733) (figure 27) and by Bernhardus Siegfried Albinus in his *Tabulae Sceleti e Musculorum Corporis Humani* (1747) (figure 28). In that same century, Jacques Fabien Gautier D'Agoty (1717–1786) gave us perhaps the most magnificent art in the history of medicine. He was the assistant to Jacob Christian Le Blon, inventor of printing in color, and D'Agoty adapted those techniques to his medical illustration by using a four-color

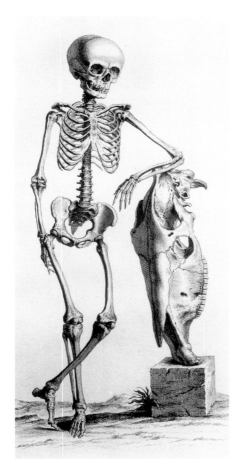

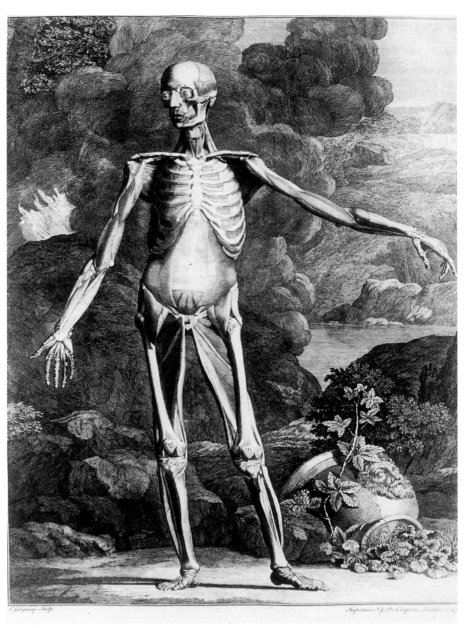

27. Skeletal anatomy in *Ostreographia* (1733) by William Cheselden

28. Right. Muscle man in *Tabulae Sceleti e Musculorum Corporis Humani* (1747), copperplate engraving by Bernhardus Siegfried Albinus

29-30. Opposite, top row. Anatomy in *Anatomie des parties de la génération de l'homme et de la femme* (1773), colored mezzotints by Jacques Fabien Gautier D'Agoty

31. Opposite. Muscular anatomy of the head in *Anatomie de la tête en tableux* (1748) by Jacques Fabien Gautier D'Agoty

32. Opposite. "The Flayed Angel." Female muscles of the back in *Myologie complette en couleur et grandeur naturelle composée de l'essai et de la suite de l'essai d'anatomie* (1746), color mezzotint by Jacques Fabien Gautier D'Agoty

process. He continued the tradition of medical anatomy as an art form in his color mezzotints (figures 29–32).

The art of medical illustration reached another peak in the nineteenth century with the eleven-volume compendium by Bourgery and Claude Bernard with anatomist N.H. Jacob, written between 1866 and 1871. The beauty of the colored illustrations in *Traité complet de l'anatomie de l'homme* has remained unsurpassed (figures 33–37).

Anatomy, Descriptive and Surgical by Henry Gray is the most popular book in the history of medicine. The text remains relevant today, though John W. Parker and Son published the first edition in London in 1858; the engravings were accurately "executed by Messrs. Butterworth and Heath" (figure 38).

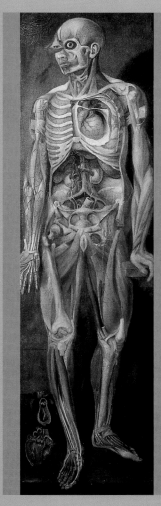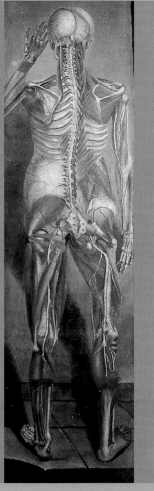

29.

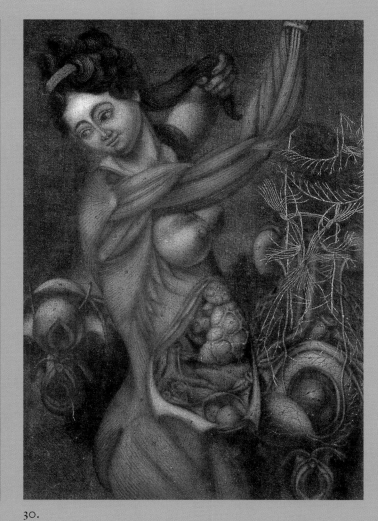

30.

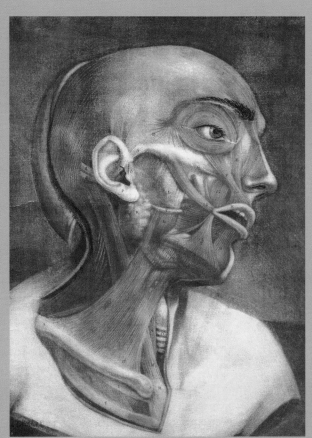

31.

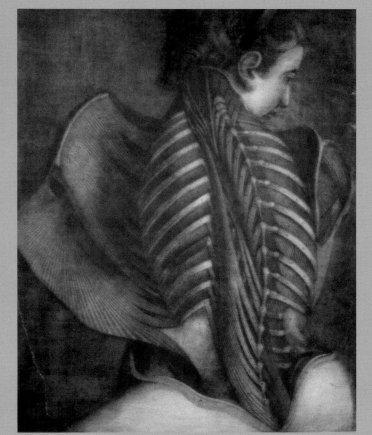

32.

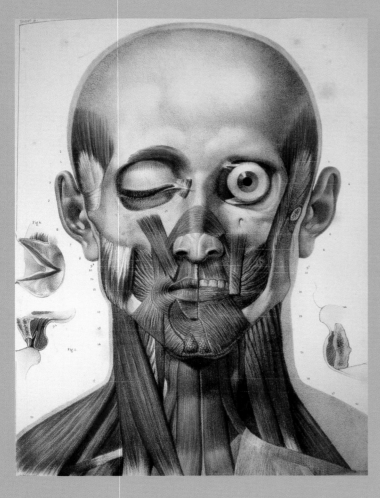

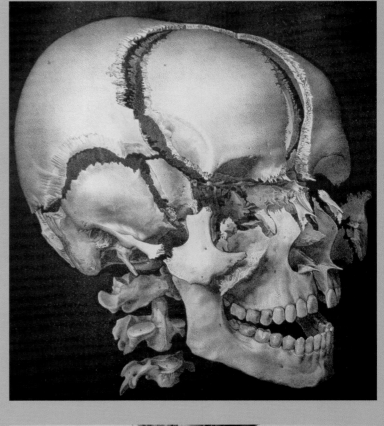

33. Left. Facial muscles in *Traité complet d'anatomie de l'homme*, 2nd ed. (1866–1871) by J.M. Bourgery, Claude Bernard, and N.H. Jacob

34. Above right. Exploded skull in *Traité complet d'anatomie de l'homme*, 2nd ed. (1866–1871) by J.M. Bourgery, Claude Bernard, and N.H. Jacob

35. Back muscles in *Traité complet d'anatomie de l'homme*, 2nd ed. (1866–1871) by J.M. Bourgery, Claude Bernard, and N.H. Jacob

36. Opposite. Venous system of the shoulder and neck in *Traité complet d'anatomie de l'homme*, 2nd ed. (1866–1871) by J.M. Bourgery, Claude Bernard, and N.H. Jacob

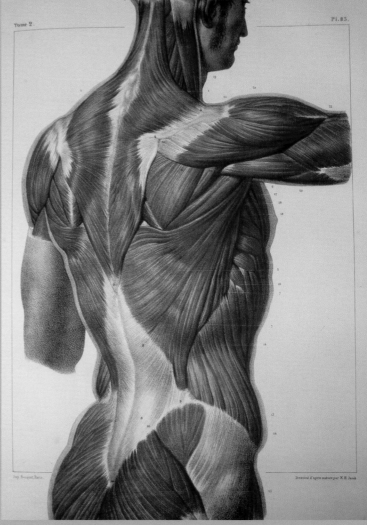

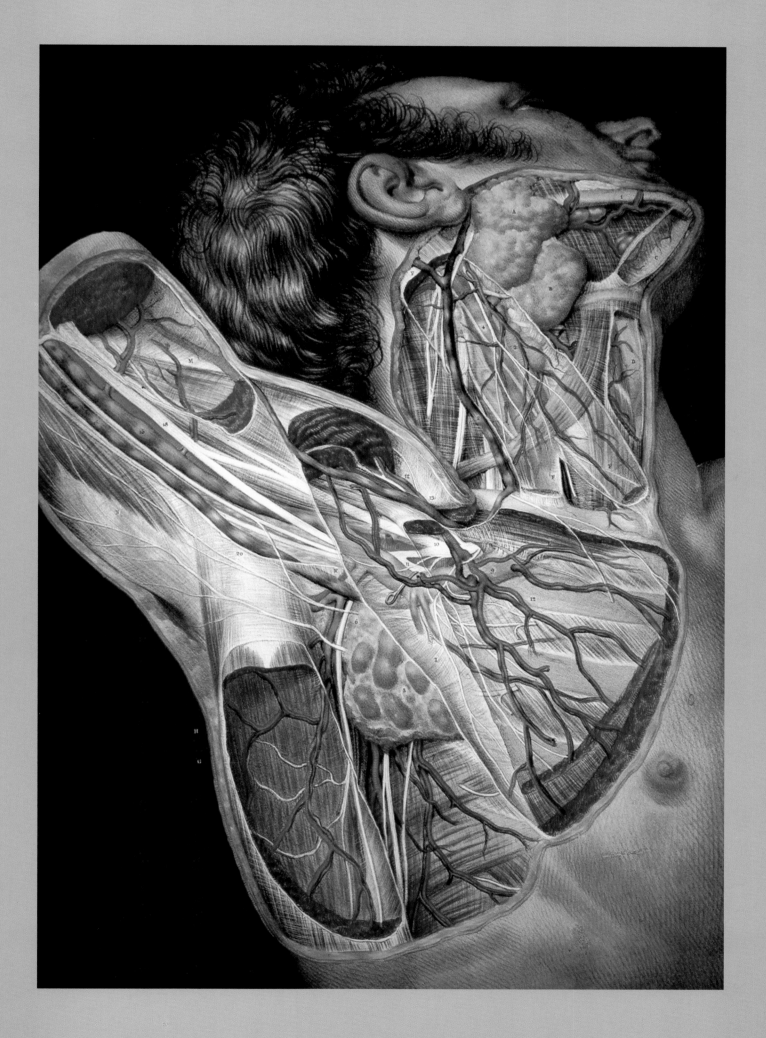

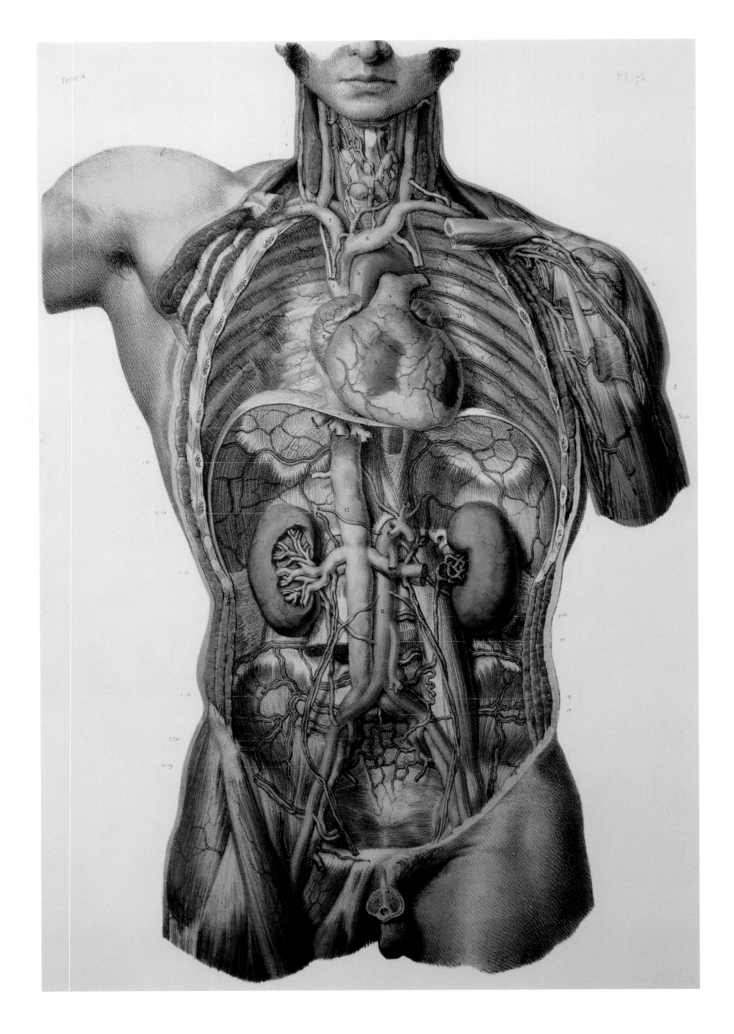

Pl. 75.

ANATOMIC MODELS

Artists who were eager to create representations of the human body employed many different varieties of media, including bronze, ivory, wax, and paper-mache (meaning chewed paper). Écorché statuettes, or flayed anatomic models, were popular during the sixteenth and seventeenth centuries and were often patterned after sketches similar to the pictured copperplate écorchés, one by Bernardino Genga (1620–1690) (figure 39), and another by Flemish baroque painter Peter Paul Rubens (1577–1640) (figure 40). Wonderful anatomic representations were usually made of either bronze or ivory (figure 41) and remained fashionable into the eighteenth century. The ivory manikins were usually between six and seven inches long, and the internal organs sometimes could be taken out for examination (figure 42).

Gaetano Guilo Zumbo was the first to make colored wax models in Bologna during the latter part of the seventeenth century, and Italian craftsmen improved on his techniques the following century, creating some of the finest wax models ever made. Clemente Susini carried on this specialized craft in the eighteenth century, aided by the fine anatomist Paolo Mascagni. The wax figures had to be individually carved, and it took up to two hundred cadavers to make one model because of the lack of adequate preservation. The detailed processes necessary for the production of these intricate wax figures remained the trade secret of each craftsman, though several documents and letters have survived to give us insight into their methods. The dissected specimen was first copied in either chalk or a low-grade wax, reproduced by plaster cast, and then the limbs were added later. An iron frame was constructed, soaked in wax, and then striations of muscle fibers were added followed by the lymphatics and blood vessels. The artisans used wax from Smyrna, China, or Venice with various combinations of paints and turpentine added to simulate a realistic appearance. One if the most guarded secrets was the temperature at which the waxes were melted, and several layers of vegetable and beeswax were sometimes added with soft brushes by hand. The bones were made of finely ground "gilder's chalk," and the fine details were hand painted on the nearly finished models. Artists covered the final product with a film of clear varnish for protection.

In 1771, the Grand Duke of Tuscany was the first to order a collection of these wax models, though it took four years before the exhibit was ready for public viewing, much of the funds for construction coming from the sale of items out of the Medici family. The lower classes "provided they were cleanly clothed" were allowed to visit between eight and ten in the morning, while the "intelligent and well-educated people" were to visit after one in the afternoon. Many of those life-sized works

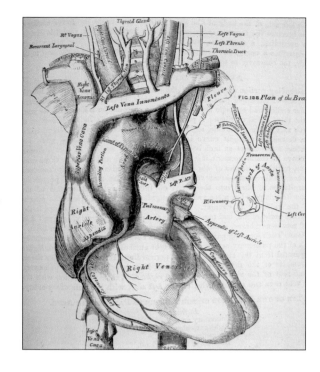

37. Opposite. Chest and abdomen in *Traité complet d'anatomie de l'homme*, 2nd ed. (1866–1871) by J.M. Bourgery, Claude Bernard, and N.H. Jacob

38. Anatomy of the heart in *Anatomy Descriptive and Surgical* (1858) by Henry Gray

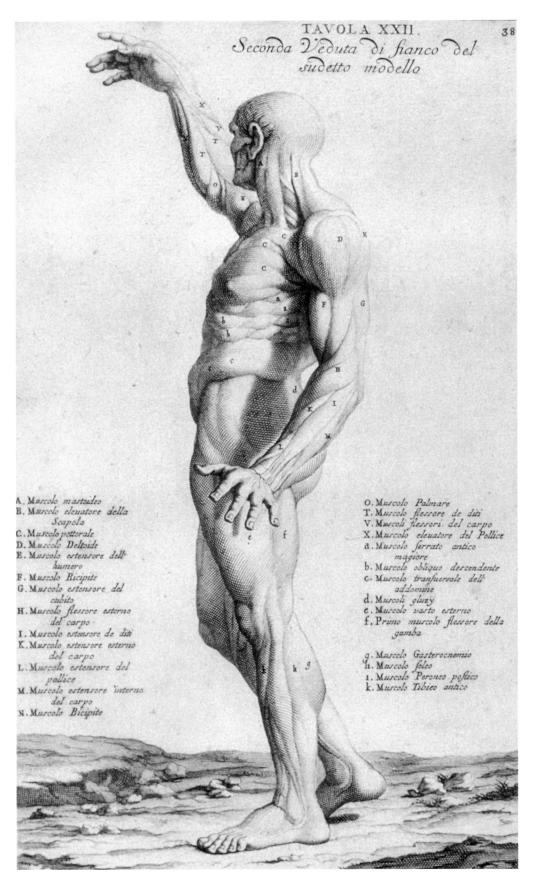

Seconda Veduta di fianco del sudetto modello

A. Muscolo mastoideo
B. Muscolo eleuatore della Scapola
C. Muscolo pettorale
D. Muscolo Deltoide
E. Muscolo estensore dell' humero
F. Muscolo Bicipite
G. Muscolo estensore del cubito
H. Muscolo flessore esterno del carpo
I. Muscolo estensore de diti
K. Muscolo estensore esterno del carpo
L. Muscolo estensore del pollice
M. Muscolo estensore interno del carpo
N. Muscolo Bicipite

O. Muscolo Palmare
T. Muscolo flessore de diti
V. Muscoli flessori del carpo
X. Muscolo eleuatore del Pollice
a. Muscolo serrato antico magiore
b. Muscolo obliquo descendente
c. Muscolo trasuersale dell' addomine
d. Muscoli glutzy
e. Muscolo vasto esterno
f. Primo muscolo flessore della gamba

g. Muscolo Gasterocnemio
h. Muscolo soleo
i. Muscolo Peroneo postico
k. Muscolo Tibieo antico

39. Muscle écorché in *Anatomia per uso et intelligenza del disegno ricercata non solo su gl'ossi* (1691), copperplate by Bernardino Genga

40. Opposite. Muscle écorché, chalk study by Peter Paul Rubens (1577–1640)

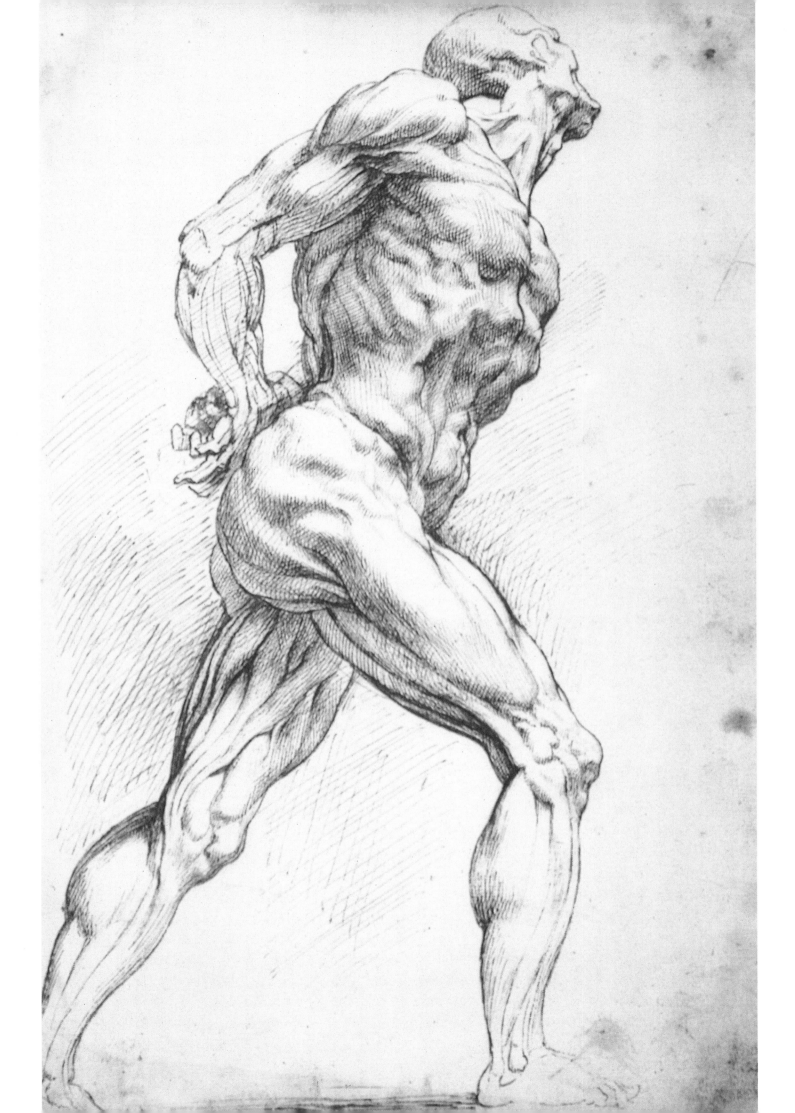

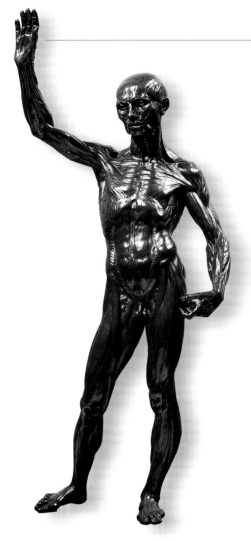

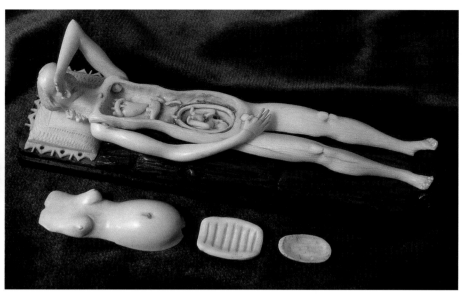

can now be seen on display at the Museo Zoologico dell'Universitá, or *La Specola* (meaning conservatory), at the University of Florence in Italy (figures 43, 44). Throughout the latter part of the nineteenth century, artists also produced fine wax models in Germany and other European cities (figures 45, 46).

Louis Thomas Jerôme Auzoux (1797–1880) addressed the demand for anatomic models in a different way by creating paper-mache representations of body parts, occasionally greater than life-size. Dr. Auzoux was a French medical graduate, though he never practiced medicine, preferring to supply anatomic figures to medical schools in Europe, England, and the United States. He took colored strips of paper and used either hide glue or natural resins to form full figures and anatomic parts for his models. The life-size female model pictured is posing as Venus de Milo, and all the muscles and organs are labeled. It was manufactured in Paris in 1881, just one year after Auzoux's death; the smaller male model currently resides at the Smithsonian Institution in Washington, D.C. (figures 47, 48). Dr. Auzoux is pictured in a nineteenth-century daguerreotype next to a similar male model (figure 49).

By the end of the nineteenth century, topographical anatomy in the style of the early écorché had returned with the invention of photography. This image was taken from *Topographisch-chirurgische anatomie des*

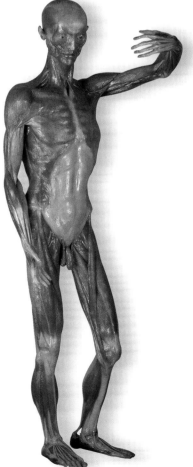

41. Top left. Bronze statuette of a flayed man by Ludovico Cigoli (1559–1613)

42. Above. Ivory female anatomical manikin by Stephan Zwick (seventeenth century)

43. Left. Muscleman (ca. 1780), standing wax model from *La Specola*

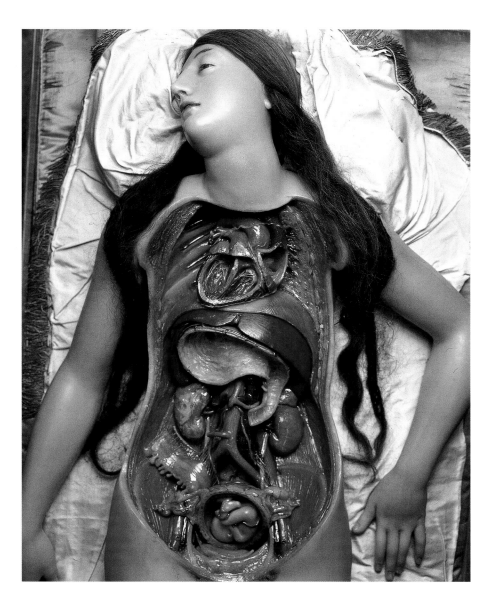

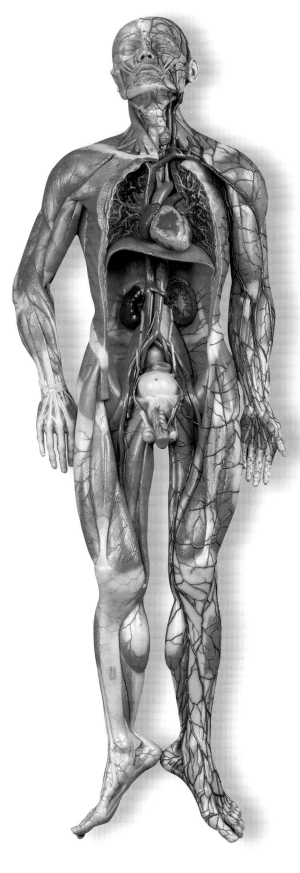

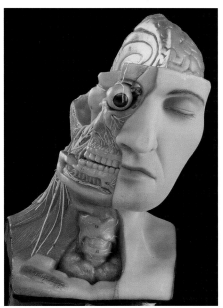

44. Above. Female abdominal anatomy (ca. 1780), wax model from *La Specola*

45. Left. Cranial nerves (ca. 1880), wax model by Emil Kotschi, Leipzig

46. Right. Superficial muscles of the thorax and abdomen (ca. 1880), wax model by G. Zeiller, Dresden

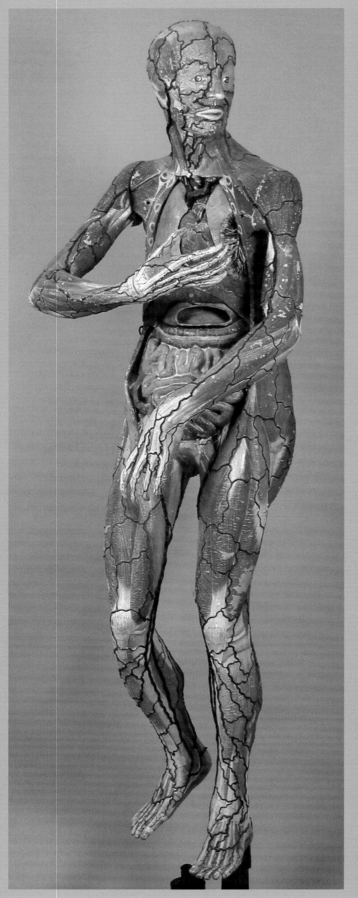 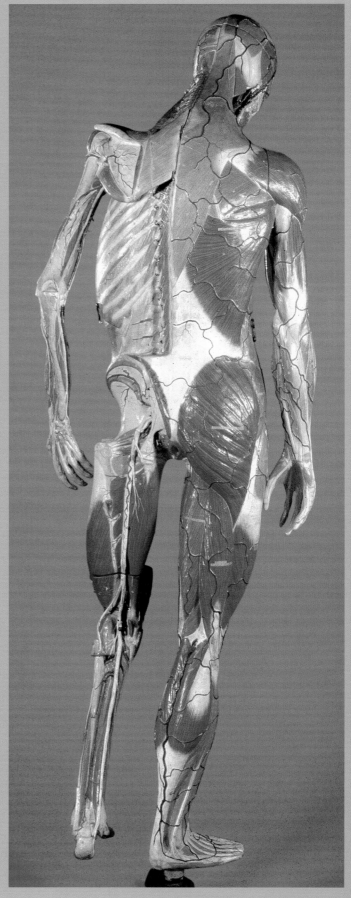

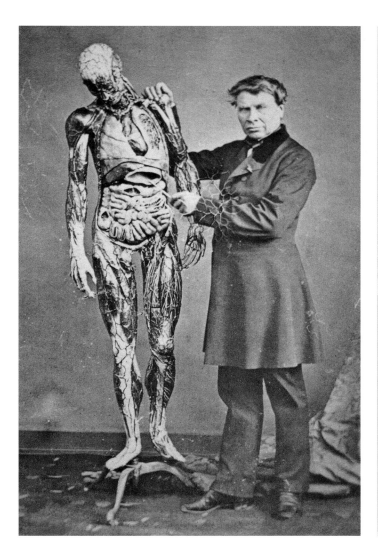

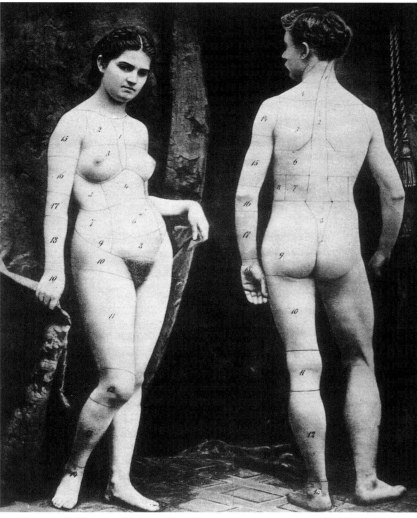

menchen (1873) by Nicolaus Rudinger and was used to point out land-marks for use by surgeons and artists (figure 50).

The population grew rapidly at the beginning of the twentieth century, and the increased need for study materials could only be met through mass production. The artistry of wax and paper-mache figures was lost forever, giving way to "flap" models with the anatomy of each organ revealed as a layer of paper or metal was peeled off from the one above (figure 51).

AT THE DISSECTING TABLE

Anatomy taught by human dissection is an important part of medical training, though public opposition to the use of cadavers continued into the nineteenth century (figure 52). Violence took place in 1788 when a young boy observed a dissection that was being conducted by Dr. Richard Bayle in the laboratory of the Hospital Society in New York. In a playful way, the doctor waved to the boy with the arm of the cadaver, though unfortunately the child became frightened and reported the inci-

47. Opposite left. Female anatomic model (1881), paper-mache model by Dr. Louis T.J. Auzoux

48. Opposite right. Male model (ca. 1880), paper-mache model by Dr. Louis T.J. Auzoux

49. Daguerreotype of Dr. Louis T.J. Auzoux and a paper-mache model (ca. 1860)

50. Male and female figures in *Topographisch- chirurgische anatomie des menschen* (1873), photograph by Dr. Nicolaus Rudinger

51. Flap anatomies (ca. 1880–1910)
(top) *Yaggy's Anatomical Study* by
I.W. Yaggy and J.J. West, *Smith's
American Manikin* by Elias Smith,
MD, *Pilz Anatomical Manikin* by
American Thermo-Wave Co., NY;
(bottom) *Bodyscope* by Ralph Segal,
NY, *Dr. Minder's Anatomical Manikin
of the Human Body* by American
Thermo-Wave Co., NY, *Philip's Model
of the Human Body (Female)* by
George Philip and son, London

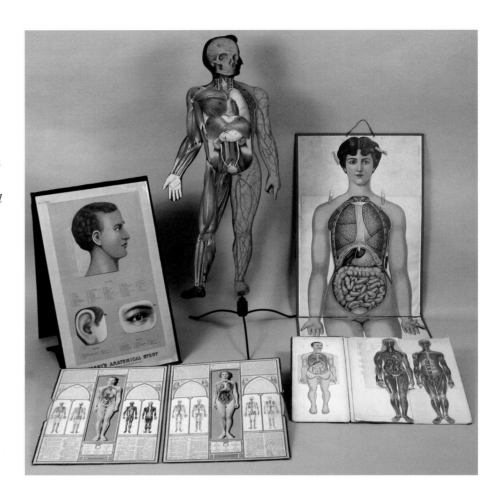

dent. Things quickly got out of hand, and soon the so-called "Doctors'
Mob" gathered outside the building. Angry citizens burned the entire
anatomical collection and forced physicians to withdraw to the city jail
for their own protection. The ensuing riot left seven dead and many
injured, and resulted in a modification of New York State law to allow
persons executed for burglary, arson, and murder to be legally dissected.

Despite the fact that the public perception regarding dissection was
changing, anatomic specimens remained difficult to obtain, and that
scarcity was exacerbated by problems with the preservation of postmortem material. Though criminals often became the object of these
studies, grave robbers, or "resurrectionists," frequently provided specimens to anyone who could pay. Sir Astley Cooper (1768–1841), surgeon
to George IV, suggested that the laws of supply and demand were applicable even in the nineteenth century when he commented: "There is no
person, let his situation in life be what it may, whom if I were disposed
to dissect, I might not obtain. The law only enhances the price, and does
not prevent the exhumation." In response, relatives of the deceased often
hired grave watchers to guarantee the safety of the recently departed.

The stiff penalties imposed upon grave robbers is illustrated by the
story of William Hare and William Burke, who decided to increase their

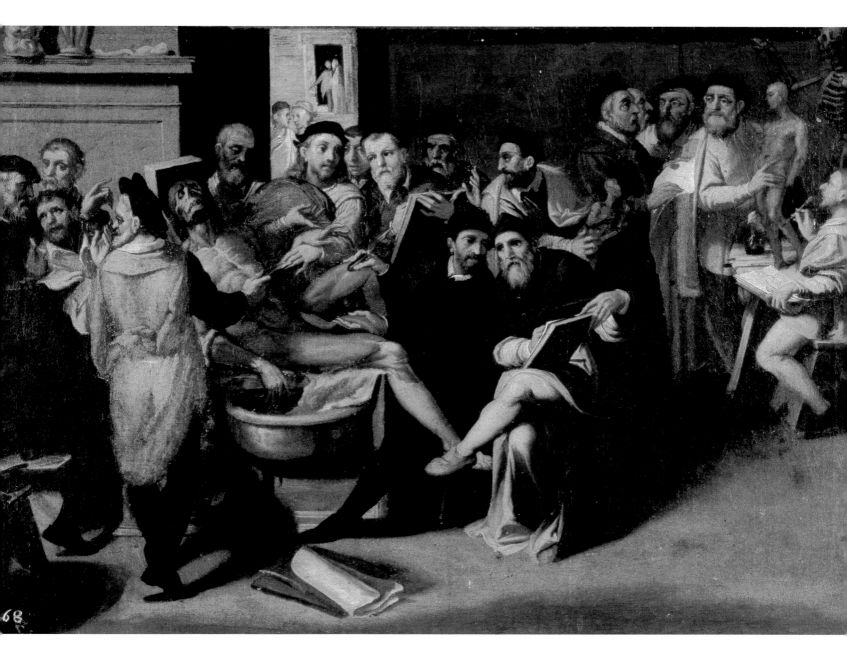

52. *An anatomy lesson given by Michelangelo to other artists* (1529–1592), oil on canvas by Bartolomeo Passarotti

supply of cadavers by murder. In 1828, they sold sixteen cadavers to Robert Knox in Edinburgh, Scotland, all heads having been removed to make identification more difficult. Hare and Burke's methods came to public attention in the case of Abigail Simpson, who was brought to Hare's house by Burke's mistress where she was sedated with liquor and smothered. (As a result, the term "burking" is still in use today to mean suffocation.) Unfortunately, one of Knox's students recognized a prostitute named Mary Patterson with whom he had recently spent some time, and the game was finally up when previously healthy Margery Dougherty was found on the dissecting table. After his arrest, Hare turned in Burke, and the latter was found guilty of murder. They were both prosecuted to the commonly sung tune "Burke's the butcher,

Hare's the thief, Knox the man that buys the beef." The judge ruled that the proper punishment would be for Burke to be hanged, dissected, and his skeleton put on display for all to see. The sentence was carried out on January 28, 1829, in a carnival atmosphere before a large crowd of 20,000, and Burke's skeleton now remains at the Edinburgh Anatomical Museum "so that posterity may remember your repulsive crimes." It is rumored that some of Burke's skin was preserved as covers for several medical-school books in the library, and as a memorial wallet.

In 1847, Oliver Wendell Holmes, MD, was elected Harvard Professor of Anatomy and Physiology at the age of thirty-eight, and he held that position for thirty-five years. His insights and observations made him one of the most famous figures in the history of medicine. One of his assistants, Dr. Chever, described the memorable anatomy lessons taught by this remarkable man:

> He enters, and is greeted with a mighty shout and stamp of applause. Then silence, and there begins a charming hour of description, analysis, simile, anecdote, harmless pun, which clothes the dry bones with poetic imagery, enlivens a hard and fatiguing day with humor, and brightens to the tired listener the details of a difficult though interesting study. We say tired listener because—will it be believed?—the student is now listening to his fifth consecutive lecture that day, beginning at nine o'clock and ending at two; no pause, no rest, no recovery for the dazed senses, which have tried to absorb Materia Medica Chemistry, Practice, Obstetrics, and Anatomy, all in one morning, by five learned professors. One o'clock was always assigned to Dr. Holmes because he alone could hold his exhausted audience's attention.

One example of Holmes' humor was illustrated when he held up a pelvic bone and said, "Gentlemen, this is the triumphal arch under which every candidate for immortality has to pass." Moving to another area of the bone, he continued, "These, gentlemen, are the tuberosities of the ischia, on which man was designed to sit and survey the works of Creation."

POSTMORTEM INSTRUMENTS

Medical students began to look at the human body in a different way when they saw specimens like those depicted by H.W. Cattell in his *Post Mortem Pathology: A Manual of Postmortem Examinations . . .* (1905) (figure 53) and by Charles Landseer in *Chalk Drawing of a Flayed Corpse* (ca. 1815) (figure 54). Instruments specifically manufactured for dissection have been in use for centuries, and one of the earliest illustrations of those instruments was found in Vesalius' *Fabrica* (1543) (figure 55). Cased dissecting sets were made throughout the nineteenth century and were often found along side medical students to be used at a first anatomy lesson (figure 56). Post mortem sets were also quite popular; the small nick in the bowel scissors helps to distinguish these instruments from those found in a surgical set, which may appear similar (figure 57).

MICROSCOPIC ANATOMY

Johannes and Zacharias Jansen of Middleburg, Holland, invented the microscope in 1590. Galileo made several modifications, though the instrument was popularized by Antoni van Leeuwenhoek (1632–1723), a Dutch draper and part-time janitor who ground lenses for his early microscopes in order to count threads (figure 58). He was afforded the time he needed to produce and perfect numerous lenses because of the wealth his family had accumulated in the brewing business. Van

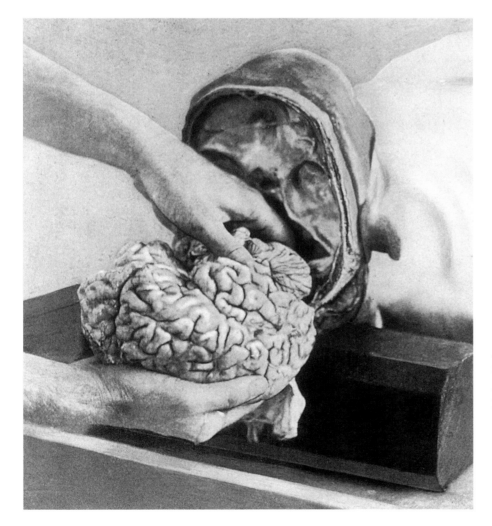

53. Examination of the skull and brain in *Post-Mortem Pathology: A Manual of Postmortem Examinations* (1905) by Henry W. Cattell

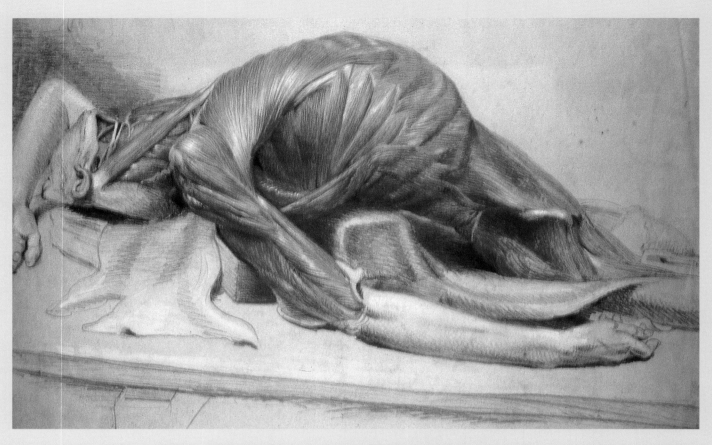

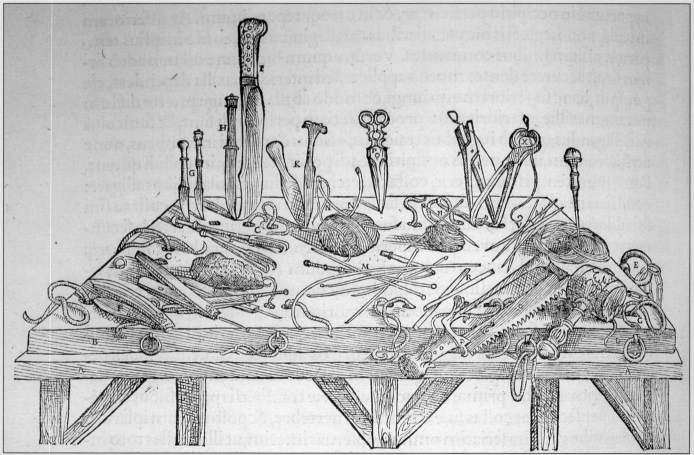

Leeuwenhoek made the microscope an important scientific instrument with the description of his "world of animacules" in 1684, and he was the first to see the capillary network between arteries and veins, red blood cells, muscle tissue, protozoa, and bacteria. He went from being an outcast from the Royal Society of England to such an esteemed position that Queen Mary visited his draper shop in Holland along with fellows of the Royal Society to see the wonders he had discovered through his microscope.

Medical applications for the microscope began in the seventeenth century when Pierre Borel first noted abnormalities in specimens of blood and Athanasius Kircher (1601–1680) first suggested that the organisms he observed could be the cause of disease. Marcello Malpighi (1628–1694) completed Harvey's epic work on the circulation of the blood in 1661 (four years after Harvey's death) when he described the anatomy of capillaries, thus completing the circuit that Harvey had outlined in his *de Motu Cordis*:

> I saw the blood, flowing in minute streams through the arteries, in the manner of a flood, and I might have believed that the blood itself escaped into an empty space and was collected up again by a gaping vessel, but an objection to the view was afforded by the movement of the blood being tortuous and scattered in different directions and by its being united again in a definite path. My doubt was changed to certainty by the dried lung of a frog which to a marked degree had preserved the redness of the blood in very tiny tracts, which were afterwards found to be vessels, where by the help of a glass I saw not scattered points but vessels joined together in a ringlike fashion. And such is the wandering of these vessels as they proceed from the vein on this side and the artery on the other that they do not keep a straight path but appear to form a network joining the two vessels. Thus it was clear that the blood flowed along sinuous vessels and did not empty into spaces, but was always contained within vessels, the paths of which produced its dispersion.

Physicians only began to use microscopes clinically in the middle of the nineteenth century with their early diagnoses of urinary tract infections. The determination of anemia could be made by viewing blood samples under the microscope, and physicians first saw evidence of pneumonia and tuberculosis with this instrument. Microscopes, however, were more a status symbol than a clinically useful tool, and in 1882, Daniel Cathell commented in his book *The Physician Himself*: "If, at your office and elsewhere, you make use of instruments of precision . . . they will not only assist you in diagnosis, etc., but will also aid you

54. Opposite top. A flayed corpse (ca. 1815), chalk drawing by Charles Landseer

55. Opposite bottom. Instruments used for dissection in *De humani corporis fabrica libri septem* (1543) by Andreas Vesalius

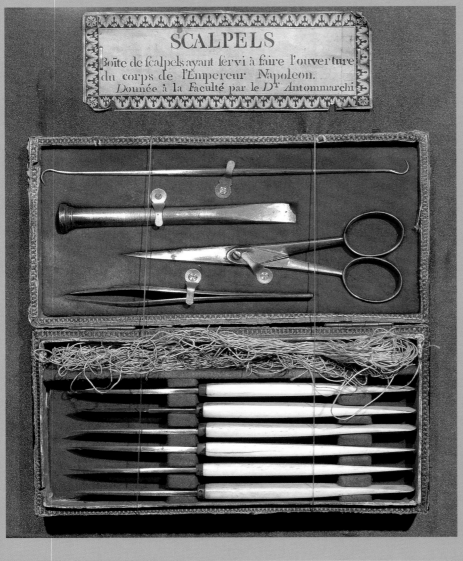

SCALPELS

Boïte de scalpels ayant servi à faire l'ouverture
du corps de l'Empereur Napoléon.
Donnée à la Faculté par le Dr Antommarchi

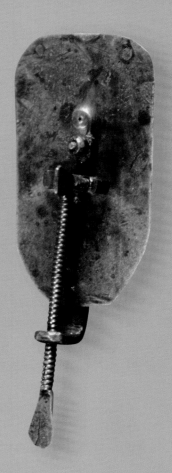

56. Left. Surgical instruments used by
Doctor Antommarchi for the dissection of Emperor Napoléon I
(1769–1821)

57. Below left. Head clamp by
Codman & Shurtleff, postmortem
set by Coxeter, head clamp by John
Weiss & Son; (bottom) headrest by
Savigny & Co. (ca. 1860–1880)

58. Below. First microscope by Antoni
van Leeunwenhoek (ca. 1670)

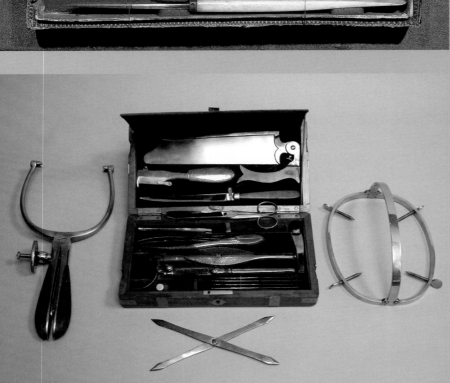

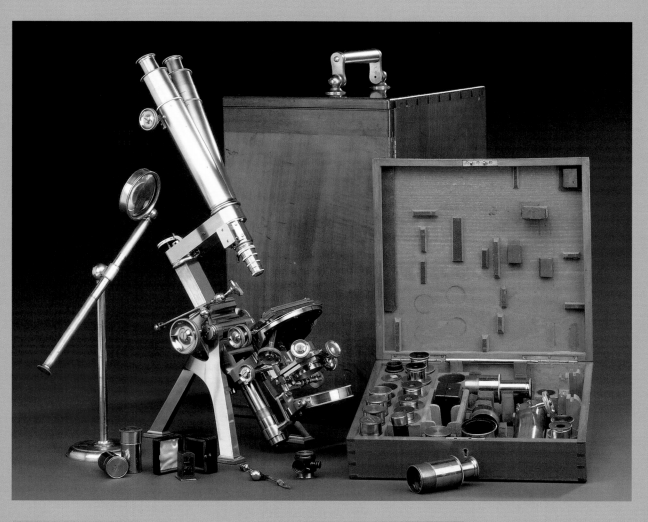

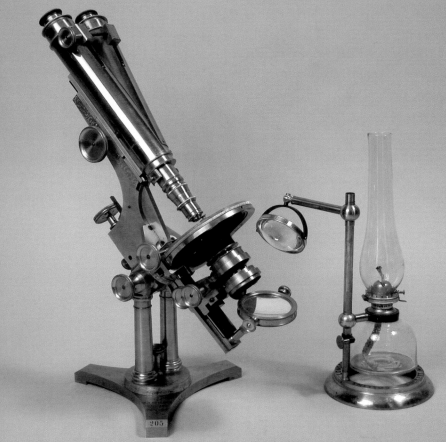

59. Above. Powell and Lealand brass binocular microscope, #1 stand (ca. 1880)

60. Professional Stand No. 1 microscope by Walter Bullock, oil lamp and bull's eye magnifier by Collins (late eighteenth century)

greatly in curing people by heightening their confidence in you and enlisting their co-operation."

The finest early microscopes were made in Europe and in England (figure 59), though American manufacturers Zentmayer and Bulloch eventually caught up and were able to demonstrate comparably fine craftsmanship by the end of the nineteenth century (figure 60).

EMBALMING

Attempts at preserving the deceased date back well before recorded time when the dead were buried in shallow graves in animal skins. Embalming became a science in ancient Egypt where the dry climate of the upper regions made preservation much more successful. Despite the fact that the ceremony was quite religious, entering the body was forbidden and was handled by the *paraschistes*, who were traditionally stoned or driven away after they had made the first incision with a flint knife. The remainder of the preparation was then performed by the *taricheutes*, who were highly respected priests.

The details of the ancient methods of preservation have been lost, but priests likely used the balm of several plants (thus the term *embalming*), the most common being from the genus *Commiphora*. Dehydration by exposure to the sun or to absorbent materials was the first step, followed by the removal of the organs. The brain was felt to be without function and was disposed of after being drawn out through the nostrils with an iron hook, while the heart, lungs, and intestines were preserved in urns containing herbs and alcohol. The cavity was filled with myrrh, cassia, and other spices, and the body was prepared with saltpeter and then wrapped in pretreated cotton bandages for burial. "Mumia" refers to black bituminous materials that were sometimes used in preservation and is the derivation of the term mummification.

There were not many advances until the nineteenth century when a former New York City coroner, Dr. Thomas Holmes, perfected a number of embalming techniques. He is now known as the "Father of Modern Embalming." Holmes' advances were just in time for the Civil War and allowed many families to have their loved ones transported home by train rather than buried on the battlefield, as had been the federal regulation. The first military casualty of American Civil War was Col. Elmer Ellsworth, who was killed in Alexandria, Virginia, on May 24, 1861, when he attempted to remove a Confederate flag from the roof of the Marshall House Hotel. Through the efforts of Secretary of State Seward, Holmes was given permission by President Lincoln to embalm the body.

Embalming during the war was only available to federal soldiers, and the procedure became very competitive with a going price of $25 for an enlisted man and $50 for an officer (later up to $30 and $80 respectively). Not unexpectedly, entrepreneurs invaded the battlefields, and, as armies gathered for a typical huge confrontation, Holmes set up camp nearby. His employees then searched the bodies of casualties for coupons purchased earlier so that the dead could be embalmed and sent back home for burial. The situation got out of hand, and finally in March 1865, the War Department issued regulations governing undertakers: "Hereafter no persons will be permitted to embalm or remove the bodies of deceased officers or soldiers, unless acting under the special license of the Provost Marshal of the Army, Department, or District in which the bodies may be. Provost Marshals will restrict disinterments to seasons when they can be made without endangering the health of the troops. Also license will be granted to those who can furnish proof of skill and ability as embalmers, and a scale of prices will be governed" (figures 61, 62).

Mrs. Lincoln was so impressed with the earlier preparation of Colonel Ellsworth's remains that she asked Henry P. Cattell of the firm of Brown and Alexander, Surgeons and Embalmers, to do the same for her son, Willie, after his death. Following President Lincoln's assassination, Cattell was again hired and made Lincoln the first president to be embalmed. His preserved body made numerous stops for public viewing

61. British embalming pump with multiple attachments (ca. 1840) by Laundy

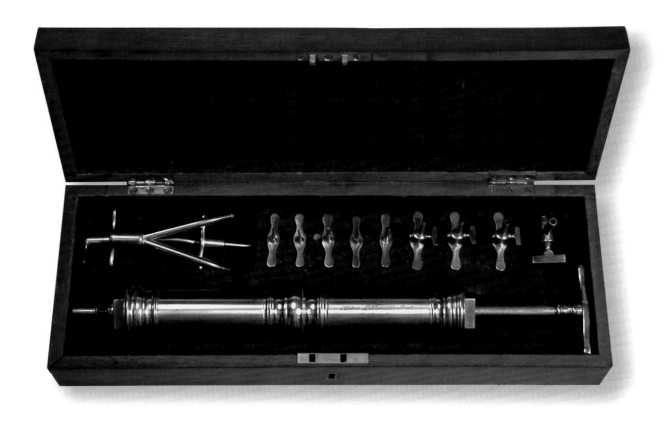

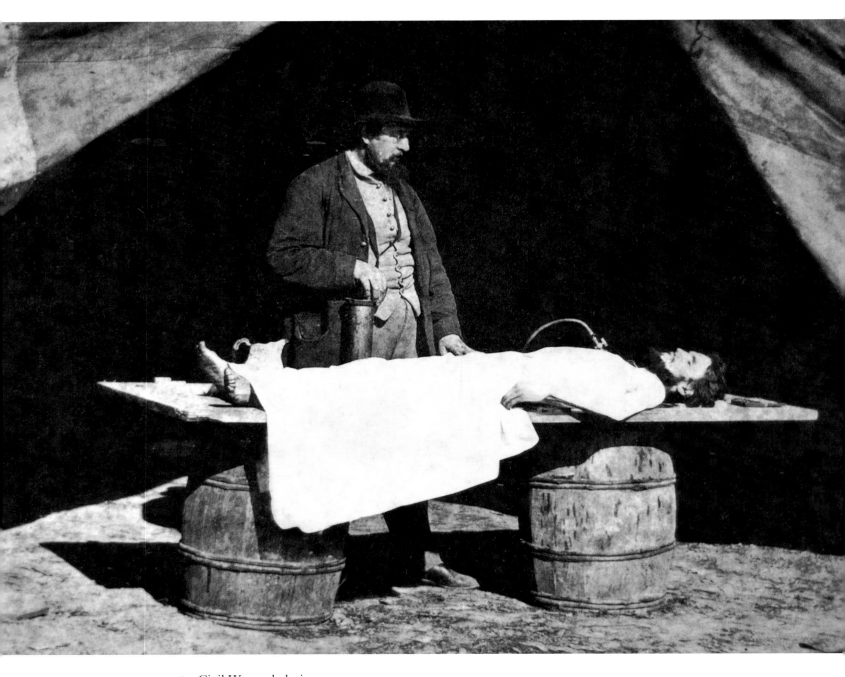

62. Civil War embalming scene
including surgeon Richard Burr
(taken by an associate of Matthew
Brady) (ca. 1864)

on the train ride back to Springfield, Illinois, aboard "The Lincoln Special." Instruments used for embalming have changed little in the last one hundred years, though more attention was paid to the appearance of the departed. According to a nineteenth-century Boston undertaker's advertisement:

For composing the features, $1

For giving the features a look of quiet resignation, $2

For giving the features the appearance of Christian hope and contentment, $5

"And so, from hour to hour, we ripe and ripe,
And then, from hour to hour, we rot and rot;
And thereby hangs a tale."

William Shakespeare, *As You Like It*, Act 2, Scene 7

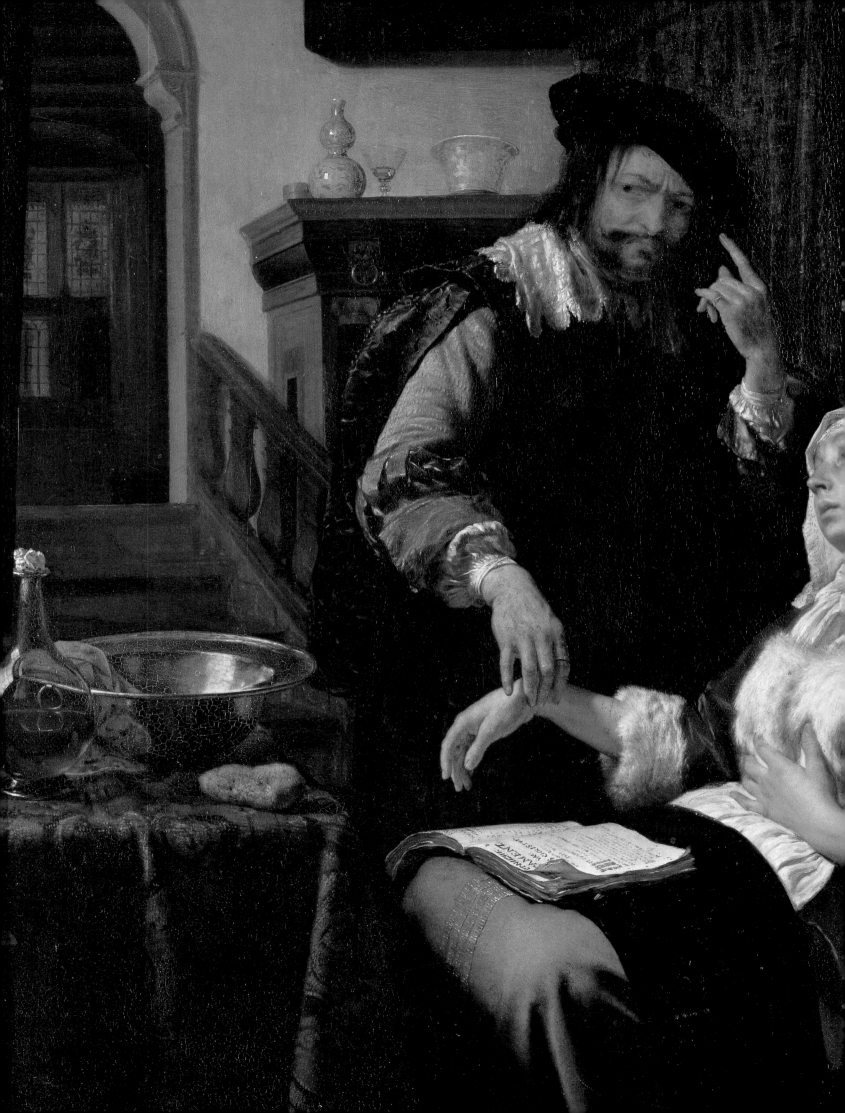

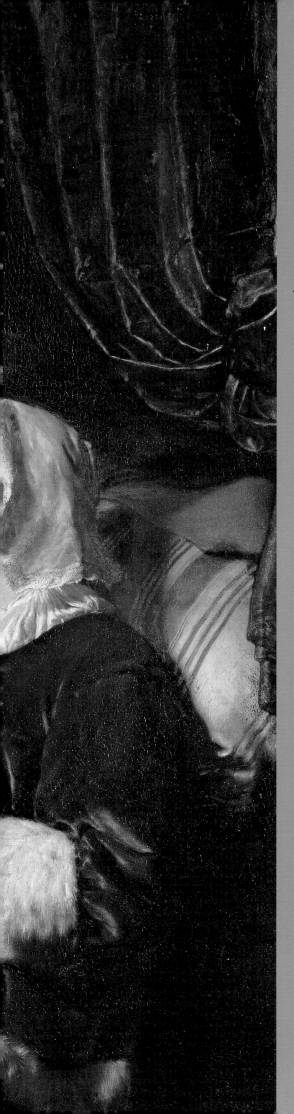

PHYSICAL DIAGNOSIS

Learn to see, learn to hear, learn to feel, learn to smell, and know that by practice alone can you become expert. Medicine is learned by the bedside and not in the classroom. Let not your conceptions of the manifestations of disease come from words heard in the lecture room or read from the book. See, and then reason and compare and control. But see first.

William Osler, MD
Johns Hopkins Hosp. Bull., 1919

Detail, *The Visit of the Physician (The Love Sick)* (1657) by Frans van Mieris the Elder

When physicians had little more to offer their patients than herbs, potions, and minor surgical procedures, the art of physical diagnosis played an important role in the practice of medicine. The liver was felt to be the center of life and the residence of the soul in early Western medicine, so it is not surprising that animal livers were of great interest to priest/physicians as they searched for the causes and treatment of various abnormal conditions (figure 63). Many considered this organ to be an almost magical source of information, and according to the Bible in the Book of Ezekiel (21: 21), "For the King of Babylon stood at the parting of the ways, at the head of the two ways to use divination: he made his arrows bright, he consulted with images, he looked in the liver."

The ability to perform a thorough physical examination evolved over centuries, and reached a high point with the first great modern physician Thomas Sydenham (1624-1684), who considered careful observation a critical step in the determination of an accurate diagnosis.

INSPECTION

The number of differential diagnoses remained limited in many early Eastern cultures, however, partly because of the fact that social customs often prevented physicians from having direct patient contact. The physical examination of women was believed to be inappropriate, and female patients could only point to areas of discomfort on ivory "doctors' ladies" (figure 64). Chinese physicians used what they had available, and therefore carefully noted facial features, body builds, and posture along with the tongue and its coatings, all considered significant elements in evaluating disease processes.

Following are descriptions of the tongue in various abnormal conditions as recorded in early Chinese manuscripts:

> *Purple-red tongue:* acute diseases of heat (infection) or diseases that exhaust body fluids (cancer)
> *Purple-blue tongue:* a stagnation of blood (heart failure)
> *Flabby tongue:* gastrointestinal diseases
> *Stiff tongue:* mental disorders
> *White coating:* dyspepsia
> *White greasy coating:* chronic bronchitis
> *White powderlike coating:* typhoid
> *Yellow coating:* indigestion
> *Greasy yellow coating:* lung abscess
> *Gray coating:* dehydration
> *Peeling coating:* terminal cancer.

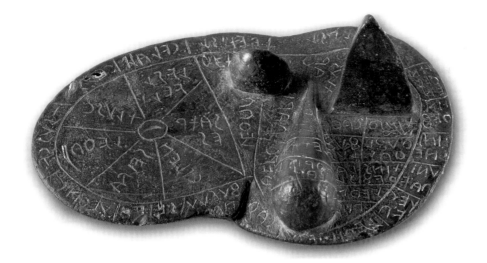

63. Etruscan bronze model of a sheep's liver (third century B.C.)

64. Early twentieth century ivory Chinese doctor's lady

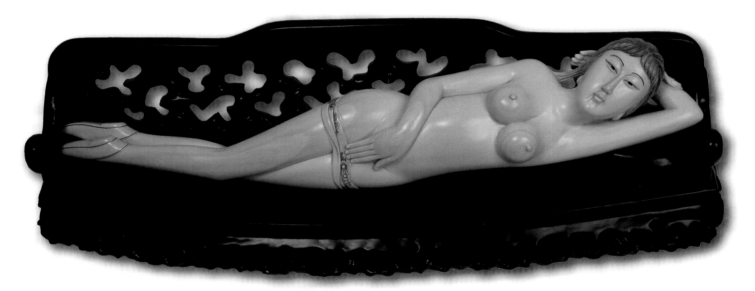

The ancient Indian system of medicine was called Ayurveda, and good health resulted when a balance was reached between the body, the mind, and the consciousness. There were three *doshas*, or bodily humors, that needed to be in equilibrium for health to be maintained: the *vata*, *pitta*, and *kapha*. As in Chinese medicine, the art of tongue diagnosis was an important part of the Indian method of sorting out the relationship between these doshas. Topographical changes in areas of the tongue correlated to pathological conditions affecting corresponding internal organs. For example, the anterior area reflected conditions affecting the heart and lungs, the mid portion the spleen, pancreas and liver, and the proximal portion the kidneys and intestine.

Particular attention regarding the appearance of the tongue continued into the nineteenth century in Western medicine, and according to a Victorian text, "A furred tongue is very common in the case of people who smoke much. When the fur is white, thickish, and tolerably uniform and moist, though the symptoms may possibly be violent, there is little danger of any lurking mischief or a malignant tendency. A yellowish hue of the fur is commonly indicative of a disordered liver. A brown or black tongue is a bad sign, usually indicating a low state of the system and a general condition of depression."

Hippocrates demanded the performance of a careful physical examination employing the senses of observation, palpation, smell, and taste before any consideration of a diagnosis or prognosis could be entertained. Those who practiced under his influence carefully documented their patients' progress and were taught that the specific timing of therapy was of great significance in determining a successful outcome. All began with the observation of the seasons, and in his essay *Airs Waters Place*, Hippocrates wrote, "For knowing the changes of the seasons and the risings and settings of the stars . . . he will have full knowledge of each particular case, will succeed best in securing health, and will achieve triumphs in the practice of his art."

Hippocratic case reports were clear, concise, and an important way of describing each illness since he carefully recorded the symptoms as they developed. For example, this is the case of Erasinus, beginning with his presenting symptoms:

> *Erasinus, who lived near the Canal of Bootes, was seized with fever after supper, passed the night in an agitated state.* During the first day quiet, but in pain at night. On the second, symptoms all exacerbated; at night delirious. On the third, was a painful condition; great incoherence. On the fourth, in a most uncomfortable state; had no sound sleep at night, but dreaming and talking; then all the appearances worse, of a formidable and alarming character; fear, impatience. On the morning of the fifth, was composed, and quite coherent, but long before noon was furiously mad, so that he could not constrain himself; extremities cold, and somewhat livid; urine without sediment; died about sunset. The fever in this case was accompanied by sweats throughout; the hypochondria were in a state of meteorism, with distention and pain; the urine was black, had round substances floating in it, which did not subside; the alvine evacuations were not stopped; thirst throughout not great; much spasms with sweats about the time of death.

Prior to recent advances in medical care, careful observation remained the primary basis on which diagnoses and treatment plans were formulated. Such icons of clinical medicine as Sir Thomas Sydenham and Sir William Osler have always been revered for their deductive skills, amazing medical students and colleagues alike with conclusions based on what appeared to be only a cursory examination. Sydenham has been called the English Hippocrates and stated the following in his *Medical Observations:* "In writing the history of a disease, every philosophical hypothesis whatsoever, that has previously occupied the mind of the author, should lie in abeyance. This being done, the clear and natural phenomena of the disease should be noted—these, and these only. They should be noted accurately, and in all their minuteness; in imitation of the exquisite industry of those painters who represent in their portraits the smallest moles and faintest spots."

Dr. Joseph Bell (1837–1911) was an extraordinarily astute instructor in surgery at the medical school of Edinburgh University. Bell's diagnostic acumen was legendary, one example involving a woman who presented to his clinic with muddy boots and a rash on her right hand. From the color of the mud, Bell immediately knew which road she had taken to get to his office. The woman's accent and the location of the rash led him to correctly conclude that she had worked in a linoleum factory in Fife and that the rash was the result of exposure to some of the chemicals. According to Bell, "In teaching the treatment of disease and accident, all careful teachers have first to show the student how to recognize accurately the case. The recognition depends in great measure on the accurate and rapid appreciation of *small* points in which the diseased differs from the healthy state. In fact, the student must be taught to observe. To interest him in this kind of work we teachers find it useful to show the student how much a trained use of the observation can discover in ordinary matters such as the previous history, nationality and occupation of a patient."

One of Bell's students was a seventeen-year-old lad by the name of Arthur Conan Doyle (1859–1930), who subsequently described his professor as a "thin wiry, dark (man) with a high-nosed acute face, penetrating gray eyes, angular shoulders (who) would sit in his receiving room with a face like a Red Indian, and diagnose the people as they came in, before they even opened their mouths. He would tell them details of their past lives, and hardly would he ever make a mistake." After Doyle successfully completed his studies, he went into the private practice of medicine, though his preferred avocation remained that of writing. Bell's deductive skills had made such an important impression on the young doctor that it was he after whom Arthur Conan Doyle patterned his most famous character and perhaps the most famous sleuth of all time, Sherlock Holmes.

THE PULSE

An early recognition of the pulse is found in the Ebers papyrus: ". . . if a doctor places his hand or fingers on the back of the head, hands, stomach, arms, or feet then he hears the heart. The heart speaks out of every limb." There is no indication that this information was used clinically at the time, though ancient Chinese physicians made pulse diagnosis an important part of traditional Chinese medicine (figure 65). There were twenty-eight different pulse patterns to be determined at eighteen different locations, six on each wrist occupying three different positions. Additionally, there were three levels of palpation pressure, all leading to a great deal of individual interpretation, and thus variation. It took between five and ten years of supervision in order to learn this diagnostic tool, and few "masters" were able to reach the highest levels of proficiency. Pulses were given rather poetic names, like the superficial "Fu" pulse that was light like a piece of wood floating on water, and the deep "Ch'en" pulse similar to a stone thrown into water. Examples of ways to differentiate various pulses included the following: depth (floating or deep), intensity (strong or weak), amplitude (large or small), frequency (fast or slow), rhythm (regular or irregular), length (long or short), type (expanded or deflated), temperature (hot or cold), quantity of energy (large or small), texture (pointed top or round top), and width (wide or thin). Additionally, these categories had subsections of pulse type, and, as noted above, each had to be considered in different locations of the body at three depths. Various pulse characteristics represented different organ systems and diseases, and careful analysis allowed the physician to arrive at a diagnosis, which then led to appropriate therapy.

Although European nurses and physicians were aware of varying pulse rates, they could not be truly accurate until watches were invented with second hands. The examination of the pulse has always been an important physical finding (figure 66), and the following statement by Hippocrates provides an insight into the significance he attributed to the pulse in making a diagnosis (along with his concern regarding the personal appearance of the physician):

> He ought to hold his head humbly and evenly; his hair should not be too much smoothed down nor his beard curled like that of a degenerate youth. He should not use ointment to excess on his hands or the tips of his fingers. He should wear white, or nearly white, garments. He should be lightly clad, and walk evenly without disturbance and not too slowly. Gravity signifies breadth of experience. He should approach the patient with moderate steps, not noisily, gazing calmly at the sick bed. He should endure peacefully the insults of the patient since those suffering from melancholic or frenetic beat by the feeling of the vein. By all means when taking the pulse have your hands warm rather than cold, lest the touch of cold hands upset the warm pulse and make it impossible to determine the true condition.

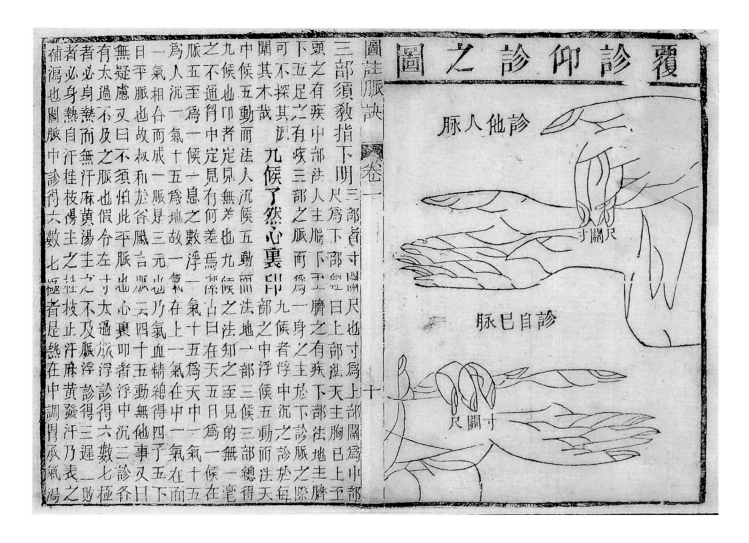

覆診仰診之圖

脉人他診

脉已自診

A rapid pulse was considered a certain sign of severe disease, and slowing the pulse to near shock was often the endpoint of a good bleeding session. Monitoring the pulse was therefore of significant clinical importance and led Santorio Santorio (1561–1636) to invent the pulsilogium. This device represented the pulse rate as the length of a pendulum, and this was first measuring device in medical history. Floyer (1649–1734) adapted a watch for clinical use not long after.

65. A fourth century treatise on the pulse published by Wang Shu-ho

RECORDING THE TEMPERATURE

An abnormal temperature elevation was felt to be the result of imbalanced humors well into the nineteenth century. In fact, many physicians were of the opinion that it was the fever itself that was the primary problem rather than a symptom of another process, and, therefore, fever was often the primary focus of therapy. Phillip Woodman outlined early thoughts regarding the etiology and treatment of an elevated temperature in *Medicus novissimus* (1712):

The cause is from catching cold, that is, when Pores of the Skin

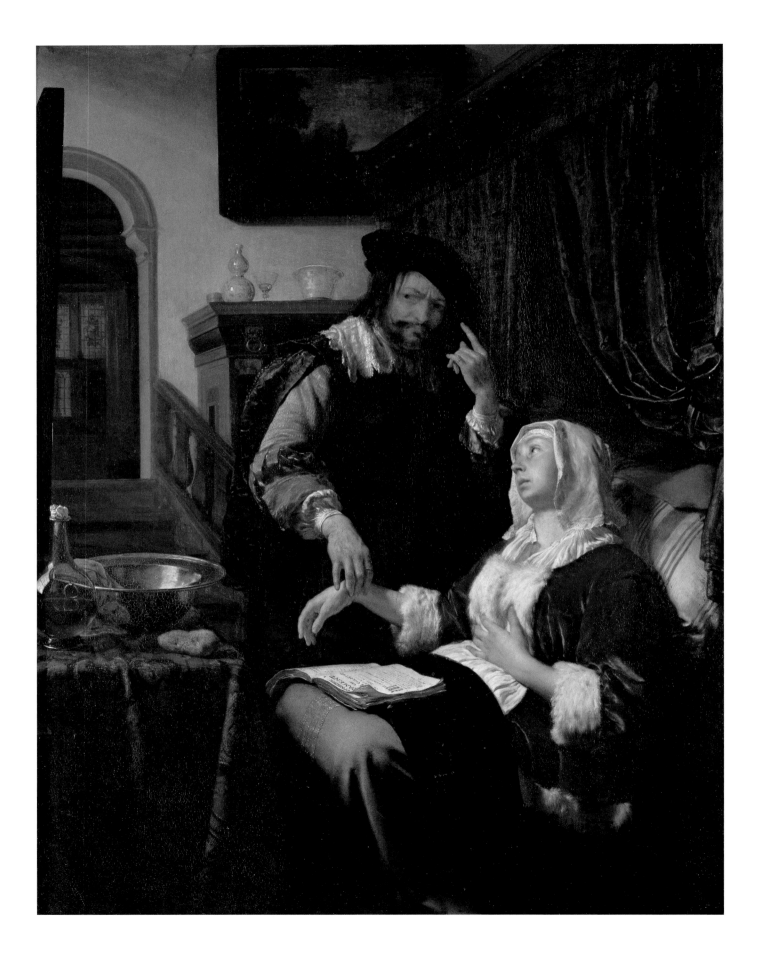

are obstructed by the External Cold Air, whereby the insensible Perspiration is hinder'd, and consequently the Fluids of the Body are increased; and they being thus too long detained in the Body, raises a Febrile or Fermentative Heat . . . if Sweat doth not break out a very great commotion is raised in the Body, and a Fever is produced. . . . Likewise an Inflammation of any part doth often stir up a Fever . . . as also drinking to excess of wine or other Spiritous Liquors. . . . Passions of the mind are often the causes of Fevers, and are seldom cured whilst those Passions last.

The Cure of this Fever must commence with Bleeding, but if the Body has been long Costive, 'tis best to give a laxative or a Clyster first; then whether there be an Inclination to vomit or no, 'tis very proper to give a Vomit within twenty four Hours after Bleeding, to disburden the Stomach of the Vitious Humors, which would otherwise increase the Disorder and feed the Fever. . . .

66. Opposite. *The Visit of the Physician (The Love Sick)* (1657) by Frans van Mieris the Elder

The basic concept of recording a temperature is attributed to Heron of Alexandria (ca. A.D. 75) with his invention of the thermograph. This consisted of a glass column containing a liquid that rose when heated, and it was Galileo who invented the rudimentary water thermometer in 1593. The first clinical use of a thermometer was by Santorio Santorio when he connected a patient's mouth to a vessel filled with water by a graduated capillary glass tube in 1612. Gabriel Fahrenheit invented the mercury thermometer that had a temperature scale in 1714, though it was not given a medical application until 1866 when Thomas Clifford Allbutt invented the clinical mercury thermometer (figure 67). According to his report in *Br Foreign Med-Chir Rev.* (1870),

I have found that the mercurial thermometer is the best for common use. . . . It is a matter of much regret that these instruments are all made by the Fahrenheit scale. . . . It has the . . . disadvantage of making English and foreign observers mutually unintelligible. . . . For patients I always use the axilla. . . . If patients allow of single rectal observation . . . they will certainly rebel against their frequent repetition.

The real credit for the use of the thermometer in clinical medicine belongs to German physician C.A. Wunderlich (1815–1872) who recognized that fever was a symptom of another process rather than a disease in itself. He used a foot-long thermometer placed in the axilla to record one million temperature readings in over 25,000 patients, thus establishing normal values and illustrating important temperature fluctuations

67. Mid to late nineteenth century thermometers. Top: L'Utile, and Faichney in a mother-of-pearl case (likely for use by a nurse), middle: Immisch, bottom: bent and axillary types by Tiemann

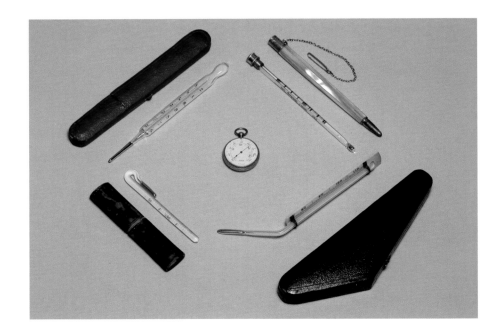

during the progress of various diseases. Wunderlich's clinical chart became a clue to the differential diagnosis of each condition as well as a way in which to judge the efficacy of various forms of medical intervention. Wunderlich made physical diagnosis a science in *On the Temperature in Diseases: A Manual of Medical Thermometry* (1868):

> Whatever the nature of the thermometric observations, if they are to be of any use at all, it is essential that the results obtained should be continuously recorded. This can be best done, and the course of the disease rendered most evident, by indicating it on a chart or ruled map as a continuous curved line. . . . It is convenient to note the frequency of the pulse, and the number of the respirations, in a similar manner, but in different colours. . . . In this way the entire course of the disease, with all its fluctuations, complications, tendencies, and changes can be seen at a single glance. . . . The comparison of many such charts together exhibits the uniformity of the general course of diseases, lets the laws of disease promulgate themselves, so to speak, and exhibits all the variations and irregularities of the malady, and the working of therapeutic agents in so striking a manner, that no unprejudiced mind is able to resist such a method of demonstration.

AUSCULTATION

The discovery of the stethoscope, Greek for "I look into the chest," is credited to René Laënnec (1781–1826), a French physician who invented this instrument after examining a female patient in 1816 (figure 68). In order to listen to her chest and at the same time preserve decorum,

Laënnec rolled up twenty-four sheets of paper and was surprised to find that the sounds were transmitted with more intensity than by simply placing his ear against his patient's chest.

> In 1816 I was consulted by a young woman presenting general symptoms of disease of the heart. Owing to her stoutness little information could be gathered by application of the hand and percussion. The patient's age and sex did not permit me to resort to the kind of examination I have just described (i.e., direct application of the ear to the chest). I recalled a well-known acoustic phenomenon, namely if you place your ear against one end of a wooden beam the scratch of a pin at the other extremity is most distinctly audible. It occurred to me that this physical property might serve a useful purpose in the case with which I was then dealing. Taking a sheaf of paper, I rolled it into a very tight roll, one end of which I placed over the praecordial region, while I put my ear to the other. I was both surprised and gratified at being able to hear the beating of the heart with much greater clearness and distinctness than I had ever done before by direct application of my ear.
>
> I at once saw that this means might become a useful method for studying not only the beating of the heart but likewise all movements capable of producing sound in the thoracic cavity, and that consequently it might serve for the investigation of respiration, the voice, râles, and even possibly the movements of a liquid effused into the pleural cavity of pericardium.

Laënnec described his first stethoscope (figure 69):

> I consequently employ at the present time a wooden cylinder with a tube three lines (2.256 mm) in diameter bored right down its axis; it is divisible into two parts by means of a screw and is thus more portable. One of the parts is hollowed out at its end into a wide funnel-shaped depression one and one half inches deep leading into the central tube. A cylinder made like this is the instrument most suitable for exploring breath sounds and râles. It is converted into a tube of uniform diameter with thick walls all the way, for exploring the voice and the heartbeats, by introducing into the funnel or bell a kind of stopper made of the same wood, fitting it quite closely; this is made fast by means of a small brass tube running through it, entering a certain distance into the tubular space running through the length of the cylinder. This instrument is sufficient for all cases, although, as I have already said, a perfectly solid body might perhaps be better for listening to the beating of the heart.

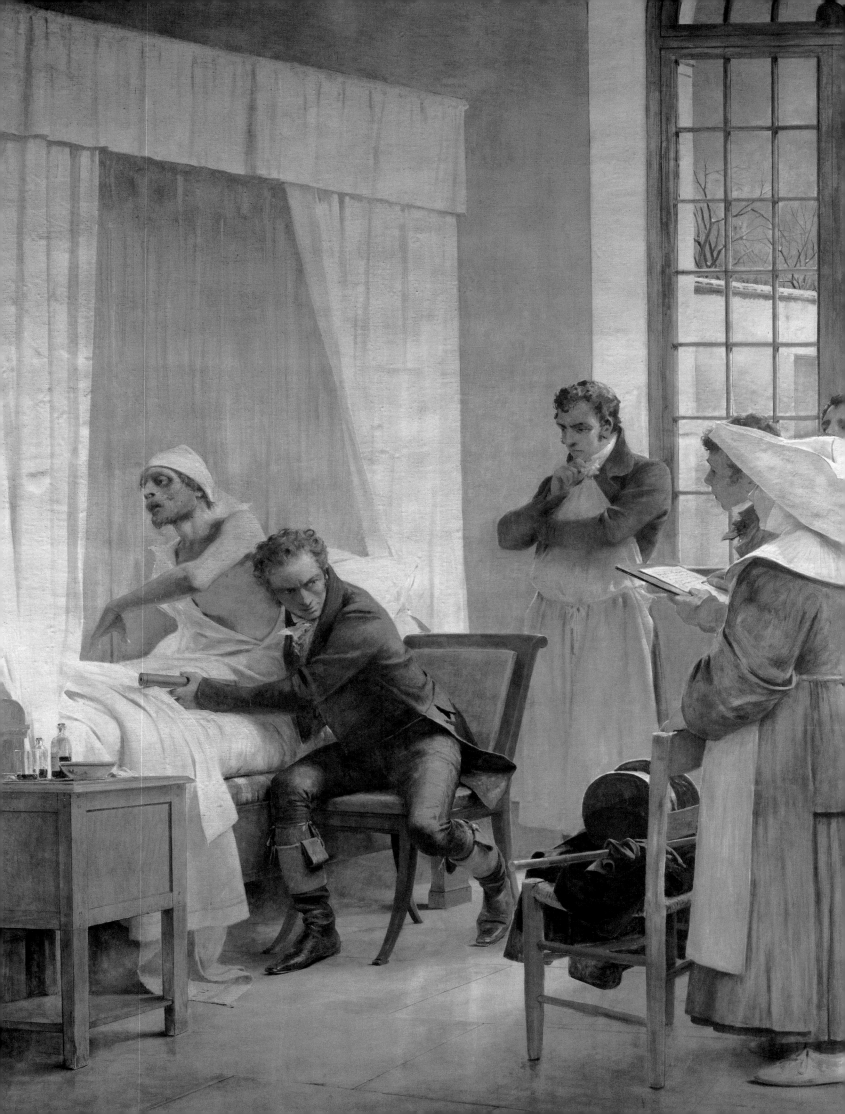

Laënnec published his famous text on auscultation of the chest in 1819, though ironically, he died of consumption (tuberculosis) seven years later. His discovery revolutionized physical diagnosis and was praised by all in the medical community.

Henri Roger placed Laënnec's important discovery in perspective when he said:

> Laënnec in placing his ear on the chest of his patient heard for the first time in the history of human disease the cry of suffering organs. First of all, he learned to know the variations in their cries and the expressive modulations of the air-carrying tubes and the orifices of the heart that indicate the points where all is not well. He was the first to understand and to make others realize the significance of this pathological language, which, until then, had been misunderstood or, rather, scarcely listened to. Henceforth, the practitioner of medicine, endowed with one sense more than before and with his power of investigation materially increased, could read for himself the alterations hidden in the depths of the organism. His ear opened to the mind a new world in medical science.

The great eighteenth-century American clinician Dr. Austin Flint said, "Suffice it to say here that, although during the forty years that have elapsed since the publication of Laënnec's works the application of physical exploration has been considerably extended and rendered more complete in many of its details, the fundamental truths presented by the discoverer of auscultation not only remain as a basis of the new science, but for a large portion of the existing superstructure. Let the student become familiar with all that as now known on this subject, and he will then read the writings of Laënnec with amazement that there remained so little to be altered or added."

Laënnec's stethoscopes were made of turned cedar, boxwood, or ebony, while later monaural stethoscopes were also made of ivory, fruitwood, brass, pewter, aluminum, and a more convenient "flexible" type made of woven silk (figures 70, 71). This last variety is sometimes confused with conversation tubes that were more than eighteen inches in length and had curved rather than straight or flat ear pierces. In 1851, Dr. N.B. Marsh of Cincinnati made the first binaural stethoscope, though his modification was too bulky to be successful. Soon after, Dr. George Cammann of New York developed the prototype for the binaural model with which we are now familiar.

68. Opposite. René Laënnec at the Necker hospital listening to a patient with tuberculosis, mural painting by Theobald Chartran (1849-1907)

69. Wood and brass "Laënnec" stethoscope (ca 1820), owned by Dr. Laënnec

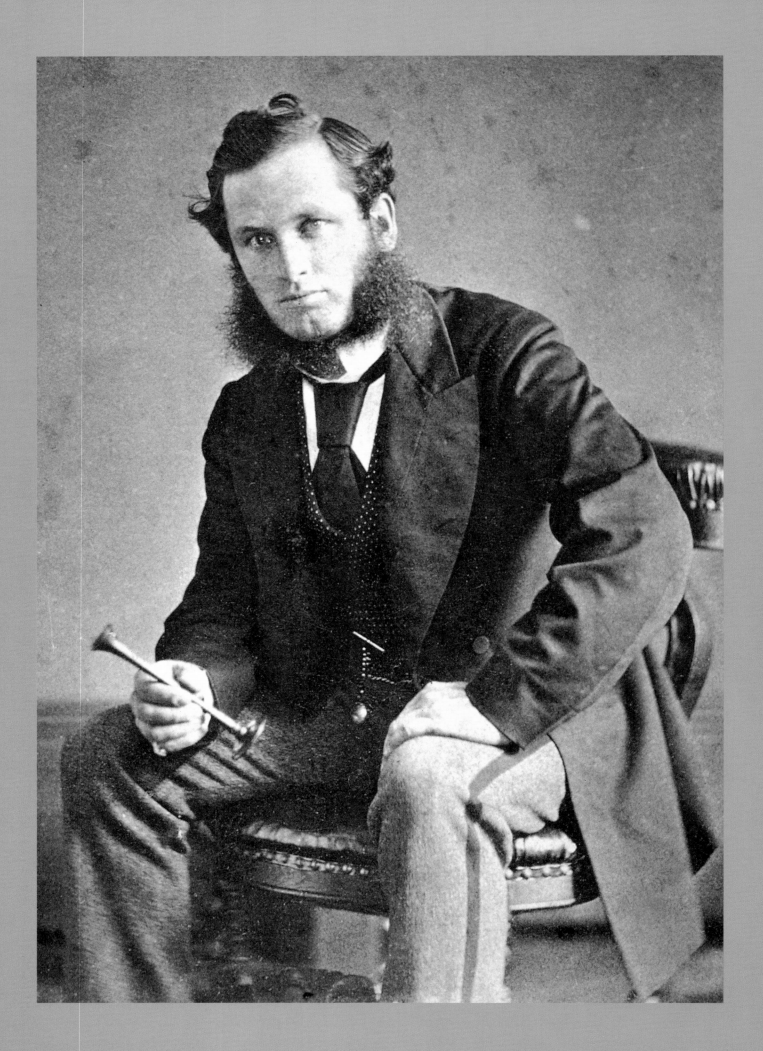

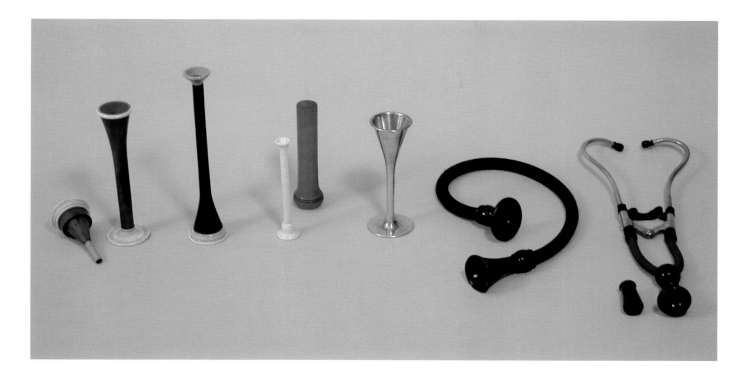

PERCUSSION

Examination of the chest presented a great challenge to physicians prior to the invention of the stethoscope since this was a rigid area not amenable to palpation, though percussion had provided valuable information to physicians for centuries. The first reference to this technique likely was in the Ebers papyrus: ". . . and examine his belly, and knock on the finger . . . place thy hand on the patient and tap."

Leopold Auenbrugger (1722–1809) grew up in Vienna in the middle of the eighteenth century and was the son of an innkeeper who had tapped on barrels to determine the fluid level by noting different pitches as the quantity changed. He played the flute, and, with his ear for sound, Auenbrugger employed this tapping technique to help evaluate respiratory function in his patients. He prefaced his work on percussion in *Inventum novum, ex percussione thoracis humani . . .* (1761):

> I here present to the Reader with a new sign which I have discovered for detecting diseases of the chest. This consists in the percussion of the human thorax, whereby, according to the character of the particular sounds thence elicited, an opinion is formed of the internal state of that cavity. In making public my discoveries respecting this matter, I have been actuated neither by an itch for writing, nor a fondness for speculation, but by the desire of submitting to my brethren the fruits of seven years' observation and reflection. In doing so, I have not been uncon-

70. Opposite. Dageurreotype of a physician with a monaural stethoscope (mid nineteenth century)

71. Evolution of the stethoscope: Cherry and ivory Laennec/Piorry (ca. 1830), ebony and ivory Piorry (ca. 1840), cased ivory monaural stethoscope by Maw (ca. 1860), aluminum stethoscope by Collin (ca. 1900), silk and ebony flexible stethoscope (ca. 1840), Cammann type by Leach and Green (ca. 1860)

scious of the dangers I must encounter since it has always been the fate of those who have illustrated or improved the arts and sciences by their discoveries to be beset by envy, malice, hatred, detraction, and calumny.

Prominent French physician Jean Nicolas Corvisart adopted Auenbrugger's previously unheralded discovery and thirty years later popularized this new form of physical diagnosis throughout France, and indeed the world. It seems that Napoléon Bonaparte had been suffering from a case of bronchitis, and Corvisart was called to his bedside after a number of physicians had failed to provide any relief. Corvisart demonstrated his "new" technique, Napoléon recovered, and Corvisart became the personal physician to the emperor. Percussion then became an important part of the routine physical examination, though Auenbrugger remained a medical footnote, finding later success only after writing an operetta. Pierre-Adolphe Piorry (1794–1879) subsequently developed the pleximeter ("I strike") to aid physicians in their evaluation of fluid levels in the chest by percussion (figure 72).

UROSCOPY

72. Mid to late nineteenth-century percussors and pleximeters: (left) by Hilliard of Edinburgh; (right) combination by Aitken of York

73. Opposite. The twin Saints Cosmas and Damian inspecting urine in *Feldtbüch der Wundartzney* (1517) by Hans von Gersdorff

Uroscopy, or "water casting," was the practice of diagnosing disease through the examination of urine and its varying colors, consistency, smell, and sometimes taste. In ancient Indian medicine, sesame oil was placed in urine with the prognosis more ominous as the oil dropped farther. Uroscopy was taught as early as the second century by Galen and remained an important part of medical diagnosis for the next fifteen hundred years. One of the earliest representations of uroscopy was by Hans von Gersdorff (1456–1517) when he illustrated urine being exam-

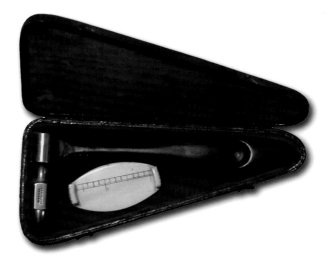

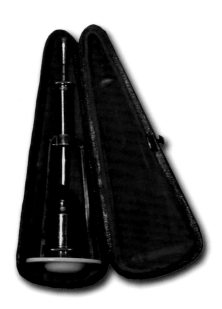

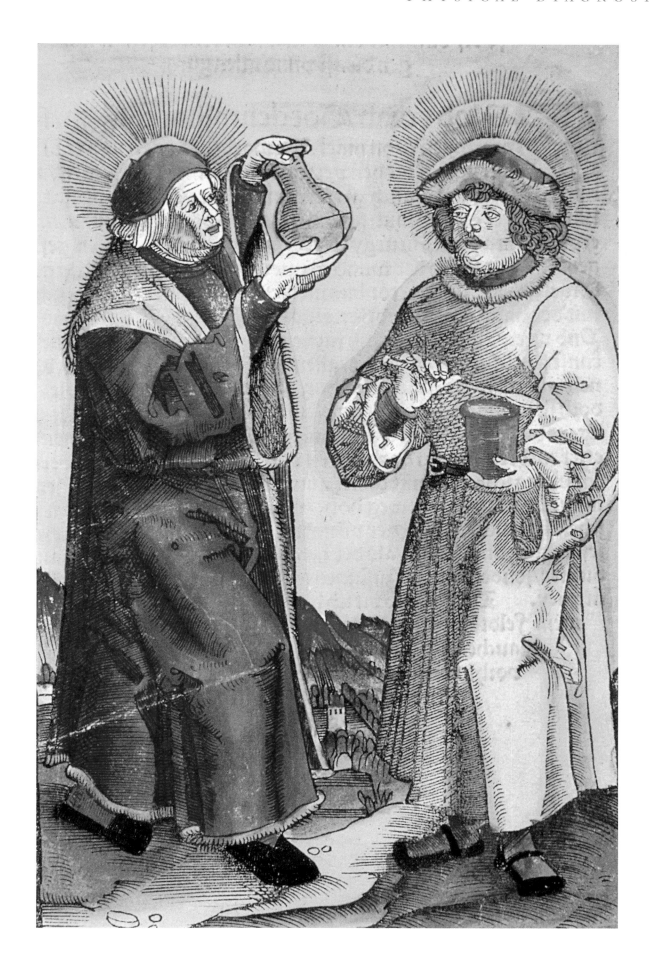

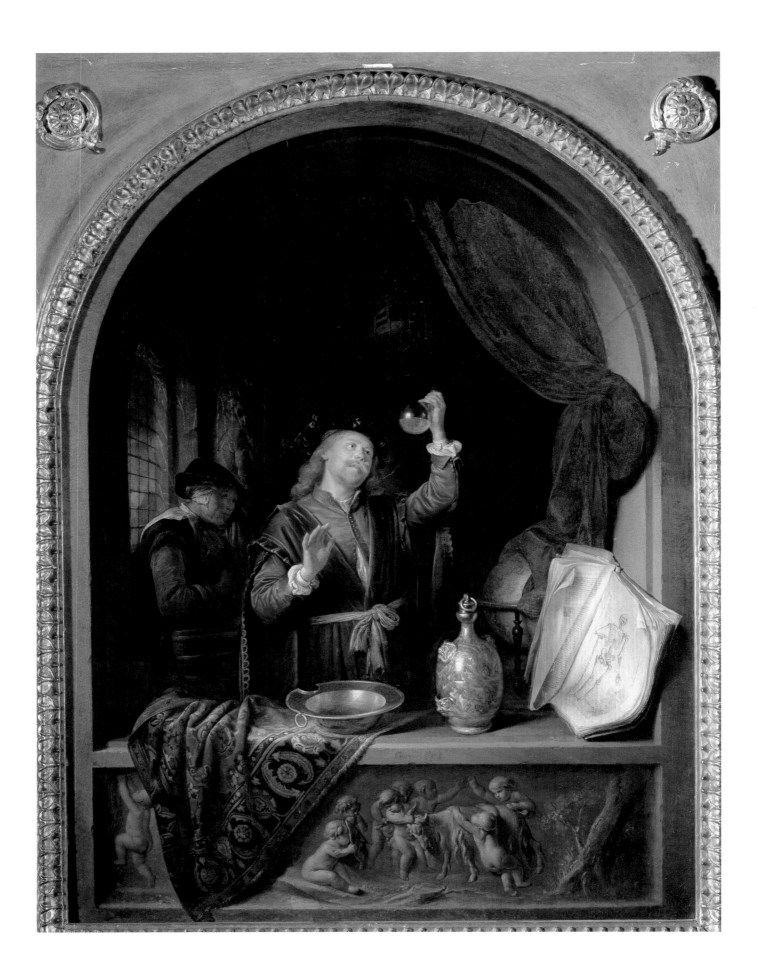

74

ined by twin brothers, the Saints Cosmas and Damian (figure 73). The image of a doctor holding up a flask of urine to the light for evaluation came to represent the practice of medicine, or physic, in medical art from the earliest woodcuts and continued into the eighteenth century (figures 74, 75). Physicians frequently used uroscopy wheels for diagnostic purposes in order to compare the color of urine in various illnesses (figure 76).

Maimonides (Moses ben Maimon) (1138–1204) was a rabbi from Cordova, Spain, who became one of the greatest religious, philosophic, and medical scholars of his age. In 1160, he fled to Morocco with other Jews and subsequently migrated to Cairo, where he began his medical career, rising rapidly to become the physician to sultan Saladin. He provided an important bridge to physicians from the past in that he translated the *Canon* of Avicenna into Hebrew and the aphorisms of Hippocrates and Galen into Arabic. Maimonides wrote ten medical treatises and frequently alluded to characteristics of the urine in making his diagnoses. In chapter six of his *Medical Aphorisms,* he pointed to the kidneys and bladder as an aid in the diagnosis of diabetes mellitus: "Individuals with sweet white humors are very somnolent. Those with an excess of sour white humor are hungry. If an excess of salted white humor prevails, they are extremely thirsty. When the white liquid is neutralized, the thirst disappears."

The practice of uroscopy was widespread, and according to popular medieval thought, "Red Urine signifieth heat of the blood; white, rawness and indigestion in the Stomach; thick, like puddle, excessive labor or sickness; white or red gravel in the bottom threatens the Stone in the Reins (kidneys); black or green, commonly death." As in most superstitions and beliefs, there is some validity to performing uroscopy, and of course, the urinalysis is an important part of a modern physical examination. Sweet-tasting urine was a clue to the diagnosis of diabetes, while patients with liver disease and jaundice will often have brown urine. White urine may signify infection, and foamy or red urine may indicate chronic kidney disease or tumors of the urinary tract. These changes were not overlooked by practitioners of medicine from the earliest times.

Sganarelle was a seventeenth-century physician in French dramatist Molière's (1622–1673) *The Flying Doctor* who referred to a not uncommon way of examining the urine practiced at that time:

74. Opposite. *The Physician* (1653) by Gerrit Dou

75. Eighteenth-century uroscopy flask

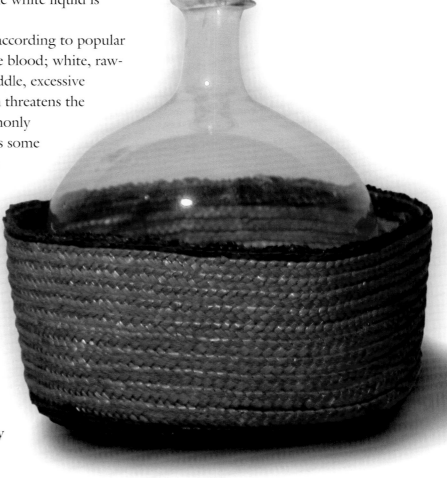

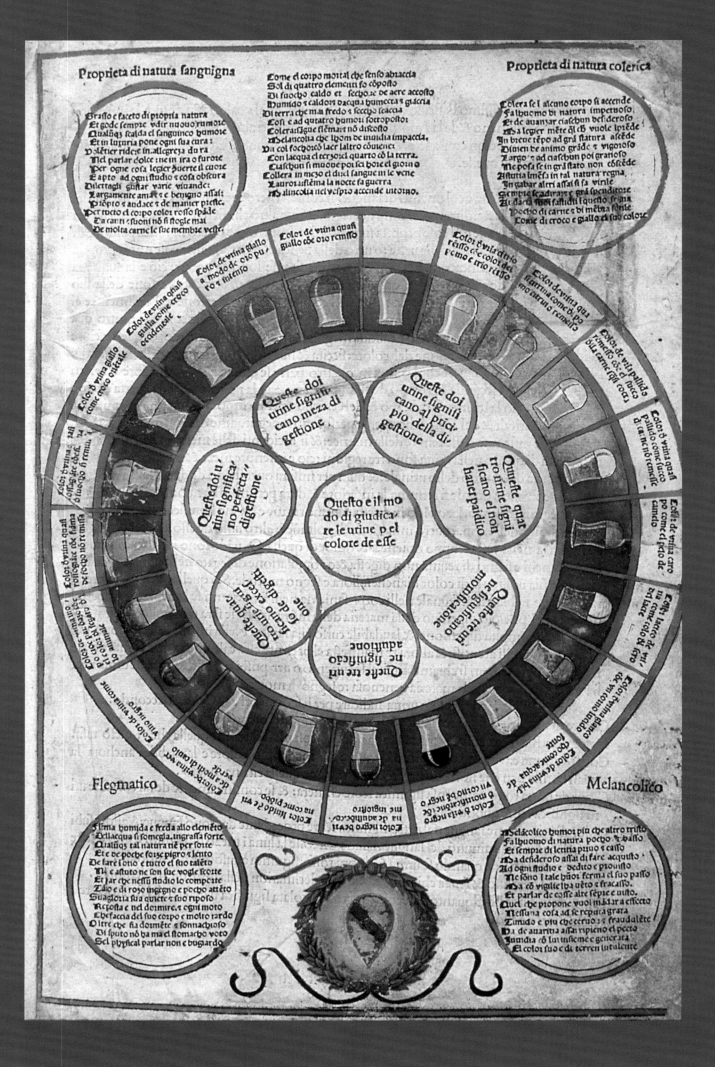

GORGIBUS

> Sabine go have Lucile fill a vial
>
> So that the doctor, here might see her urine.
>
> I fear, Sir, that these ills may be ensuring
>
> That ere too long my daughter will be dead.

SGANARELLE

> Ah! You must keep such notions from her head!
>
> She's not allowed to die in her condition
>
> Without securing, first, the right prescription.
>
> This urine shows heat; an inflammation
>
> The product of a warm preoccupation
>
> A gentle luster; not a bad bouquet. *He drinks the urine.*
>
> You know, it's not so bad. It is okay.

GORGIBUS

> What's that! Oh, my good sir, you haven't swallowed?

SGANARELLE

> Of course! I know some doctors long have followed
>
> The custom that to look at it's enough
>
> And yet, until you've tasted of the stuff,
>
> The patient's state cannot be known for sure.
>
> And yet, I must insist she make some more.
>
> What you provided was to wee a sample, see,
>
> And I must recommend she pee more amply.

As the practice of uroscopy became discredited with medical advances in the seventeenth century, "urine-gazing" came to represent quack medicine.

OBSERVATION: WHEN THE END IS NEAR . . .

A number of predictive guides have appeared in the literature over the centuries, though when death was inevitable, physicians frequently had nothing more to offer than comfort to the patient and his family. One early example of a poor prognosis was given by John of Mirfield in his *Breviarium Bartholomei* (1380–1395): "If the right eye of a sick man sheds tears he will die; in the case of a woman, this applies to the left eye. The sole of a patient's right foot should be anointed with lard, which lard is then thrown to any given dog; if the dog eats it without vomiting, the patient will live, but if the dog returns it or makes no attempt to eat it, the patient will die."

In F. Adams' translation of *The Genuine Works of Hippocrates* (London, 1849, 2 vols., 1:235–236), Hippocrates described the classic physical findings of the terminal patient, or the *facies Hippocratica*:

> . . . first, the countenance of the patient, if it be like those of per-

76. Opposite. Uroscopy wheel in *Fasciculo Medicina* (1493) by Johannes de Ketham

sons in health, and more so, if like itself, for this is the best of all; whereas the most opposite to it is the worst, such as the following: *a sharp nose, hollow eyes, collapsed temples; the ears cold, contracted, and their lobes turned out: the skin about the forehead being rough, distended, and parched; the color of the whole face being green, black, livid, or lead-colored.* If the countenance be such at the commencement of the disease, and if this cannot be accounted for from the other symptoms, inquiry must be made whether the patient has long wanted sleep; whether his bowels have been very loose; and whether he has suffered from want of food; and if any of these causes be confessed to, the danger is to be reckoned so far less; and it becomes obvious, in the course of a day and a night, whether or not the appearance of the countenance proceeded from these causes. But if none of these be said to exist, and if the symptoms do not subside in the aforesaid symptoms, it is to be known for certain that death is at hand. And, also, if the disease be in a more advanced stage either in the third or fourth day, and the countenance be such, the same inquiries as formerly directed are to be made, and the other symptoms are to be noted, those in the whole countenance, those on the body, and those in the eyes; for if they shun the light, or weep involuntarily, or squint, or if the one be less than the other, or if the white of them be red, livid, or has black veins in it; if there be a gum upon the eyes, if they are restless, protruding or are become very hollow; and if the countenance be squalid and dark, or the color of the whole face be changed—all these are to be reckoned bad and fatal symptoms. The physician should also observe the appearance of the eyes from below the eyelids in sleep; for when a portion of the white appears, owing to the eyelids not being closed together, and when this is not connected with diarrhoea or purgation from medicine, or when the patient does not sleep thus from habit, it is to be reckoned an unfavorable and very deadly symptom; but if the eyelid be contracted livid or pale, or also the lip, or nose, along with some of the other symptoms, one may know for certain that death is close at hand. It is a mortal symptom, also when the lips are relaxed, pendant, cold, and blanched.

COMMUNICATING THE DIAGNOSIS

Despite physicians' best efforts, complex medical jargon has often made the communication of physical findings and medical conditions to patients and families problematic. Mark Twain (1835–1910) had numerous adverse encounters with the medical profession. He wrote the following in his satire *Those Extraordinary Twins*:

> Without going too much into detail, madam—for you would probably not understand it anyway—I concede that great care is going to be necessary here; otherwise exudation of the aesophagus is nearly sure to ensue, and this will be followed by ossification and extradition of the maxillaries superioris, which must decompose the granular surfaces of the great infusorial ganglionic system, thus obstructing the action of the posterior varioloid arteries and precipitating compound strangulated sorosis of the valvular tissues, and ending unavoidably in the dispersion and combustion of the marsupial fluxes and the consequent embrocation of the bicuspid populo redax referendum rotulorum.

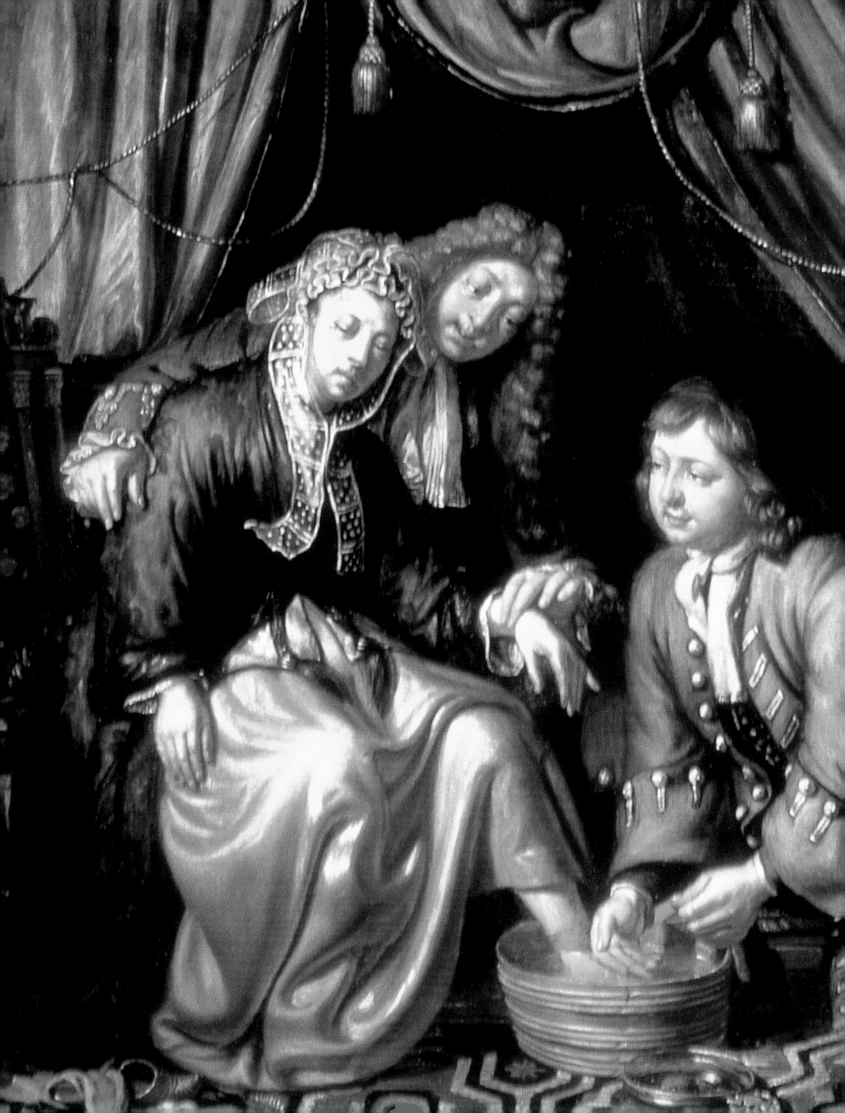

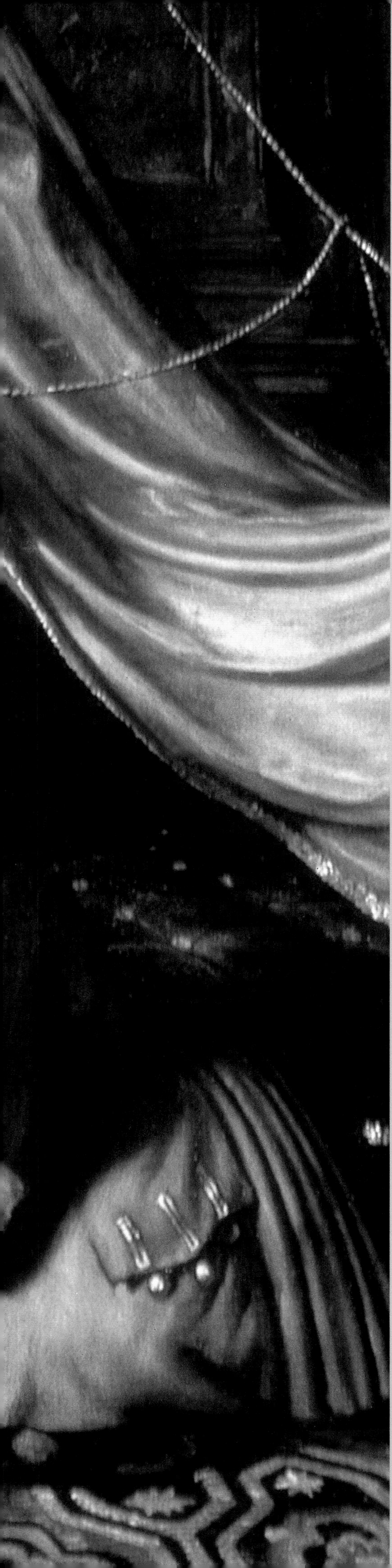

BLEEDING

…daily experience satisfies us that bloodletting has a most salutary effect in many diseases, and is indeed the foremost among all the general remedial means…

Sir William Harvey
Works, 1847

Detail, a female patient having her pulse taken while being bled, oil by Naiveu Matthijs (1647-1726) rior to the beginning of "modern" medicine in the sixteenth century, therapy was not based on sound physiology, and medicine often advanced through trial and error with a great deal of care based on superstition. The mortality was high and the prognosis poor in so many conditions that many could only turn to religious leaders as a last resort for comfort. Not infrequently, those without hope were accused of having angered the gods or of being possessed by demons and then isolated, which was the case in such conditions as leprosy and syphilis.

THE FOUR HUMORS

In the fifth century B.C., Hippocrates established a unified theory regarding the etiology of various diseases, an approach that subsequently influenced medical care for centuries. In his proposed rules of harmony, he taught that all body systems were naturally balanced and that disease was the result of an interruption in those relationships. Hippocrates referred to the four bodily fluids, or humors, that initially had been described by Empedocles of Acragas, in his book *On the Nature of Man* (figure 77):

> The body of man has in itself blood, phlegm, yellow bile, and black bile; these make up the nature of his body, and through these he feels pain or enjoys health. Now he enjoys the most perfect health when these elements are duly proportioned to one another in respect of compounding, power, and bulk and when they are perfectly mingled. Pain is felt when one of these elements is in defect or excess, or is isolated in the body without being compounded with all the others. For when an element is isolated and stands by itself, not only must the place which it left become diseased, but the place where it stands in a flood must, because of the excess, cause pain and distress. In fact, when more of an element flows out of the body than is necessary to get rid of superfluity, the emptying causes pain. If, on the other hand, it be to an inward part that there takes place the emptying, the shifting and the separation from other elements, the man certainly must, according to what has been said, suffer from double pain, one in the place left, and the other in the place flooded.

Galen became the heir to Hippocrates and was similarly concerned with the importance of maintaining a balance between the four bodily fluids. The four humors (blood, phlegm, yellow bile, and black bile) were felt to be related to the four elements, the climate, the four seasons, and specific parts of the body in the following ways: blood ("sanguine," air, hot and wet, spring, head), phlegm ("phlegmatic," water, cold and

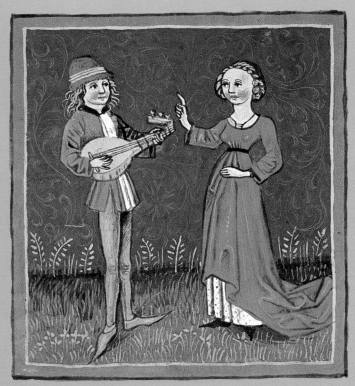

Blood: sanguine or passionate

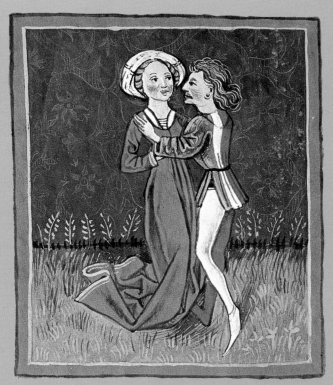

Phlegm: sluggish and dull

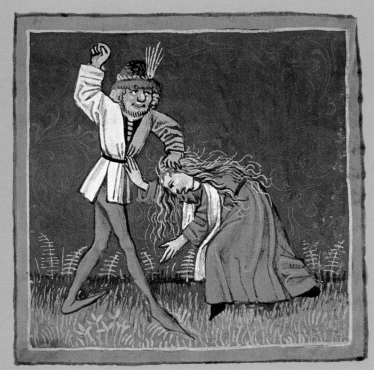

Yellow bile: choleric or quick to anger

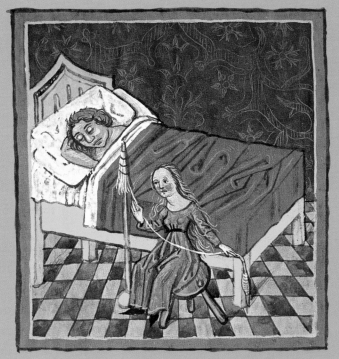

Black bile: melancholic or depressed

77. The four humors of Galen in a thirteenth-century manuscript

wet, winter, lungs), yellow bile ("choleric," fire, hot and dry, summer, gall bladder), and black bile ("melancholic," earth, cold and dry, autumn, spleen). A sanguine individual, for example, might have a rosy personality and was known for laughter, music, and passion, while someone with a phlegmatic personality was obese, sluggish, and dull, often characterized by the respiratory symptoms of a chronic, productive cough. A choleric individual was quick to anger, thin, energetic, arrogant, and intelligent. Lastly, someone who was melancholic was dark, hairy, and had a depressed, gloomy personality (*melos* meaning "black," and *chole* meaning "bile").

After a careful study of these elements and their relationships, physicians felt they could then predict an individual's temperament, disorder, and the most reasonable treatment. Though explanations based on humoral imbalances may appear a bit primitive, a great deal of logic was behind their formulation given the state of knowledge of physicians at the time. For example, one would expect respiratory infections to be increased during a cold, wet winter, and a patient might produce phlegm in an attempt to return to equilibrium. Most people are more active during the summer, and an increase in the amount of yellow bile could explain anger, flushing, sweating, and increased body heat. Spring is a common time to be optimistic, though also a time to experience the fevers and debility related to tertian malaria. The finding of black bile has always carried a poor prognosis in medicine since it suggested the decay of internal organs, and malaria can cause splenic enlargement along with dark urine from hemolysis. The present day expression of someone having an ill or a good humor has evolved from these early diagnostic categories.

Since the treatment of disease depended on the correction of imbalanced humors, therapy often consisted of reducing an excess or by restoring a deficiency (the theory of *contraria contrariis*). Popular ways to keep the system free of excessive poisonous and destructive substances was through the use of emetics, purgatives, diaphoretics, and bloodletting. A cold was considered to be the result of excess phlegm (explaining increased sputum production), and one reasonable treatment was the use of heat. Physicians believed that an overabundance of blood caused fever, so patients were commonly phlebotomized, and given cucumber seeds to lower the temperature (thus the expression "cool as a cucumber"). Later in the nineteenth century, tartar emetic was given to induce emesis, jalap was a popular purgative, and physicians sometimes prescribed toxic doses of calomel (mercury) to elicit salivation. The church supported Galen's expansive edicts regarding the importance of balancing the humors since he invoked internal spirits, or the soul, as affecting the "life force," and he was not seriously questioned as a medical authority until the middle of the sixteenth century.

BLOODLETTING—IT'S GOOD FOR YOU

Bleeding represents the folly, the sorcery, and the misunderstood physiology that we now proudly say marked the dark ages of medicine (figure 78). This procedure appears barbaric, though many patients actually improved after physicians "breathed" a vein, an observation that led to its popularity well into the nineteenth century. The reason is that phlebotomy may in fact be therapeutic in such common conditions as the fluid overload of heart and kidney failure, as well as in polycythemia.

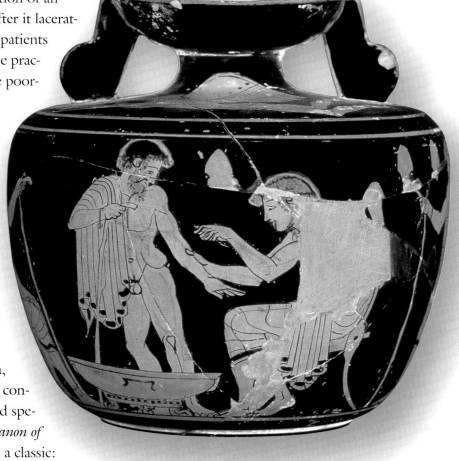

78. Red figure aryballos of a doctor bleeding a patient (fifth century B.C.)

Egyptians first considered the value of withdrawing blood when they observed that the condition of an agitated hippopotamus often improved after it lacerated a vein on a reed. Hippocrates bled his patients to equilibrate imbalanced humors, and the practice continued for hundreds of years since poorly understood pathophysiology did not allow physicians to distinguish between medical conditions that did, and those that did not improve with phlebotomy. Acutely ill patients often presented to their doctor agitated, febrile, flushed and tachycardic. All symptoms appeared to improve following a session of bloodletting as the skin became pale, the pulse diminished, the fever dissipated, and the patient calmed – as blood pressure dropped and shock approached (figure 79)!

Avicenna (abu-Ali al-Husayn ibn-Sina, 980-1037) was the most important Arabic contributor to early medicine, and he outlined specific indications for bloodletting in *The Canon of Medicine* (printed in 1632), which remains a classic:

Bloodletting is only applicable (1) when the blood is so superabundant that a disease is about to develop; (2) when disease is already present. The object in both cases is to remove the superabundant blood, to remove unhealthy blood, or both.

Cases coming under the first category are such as the following: incipient sciatica, podagra, or any arthritic disease due to

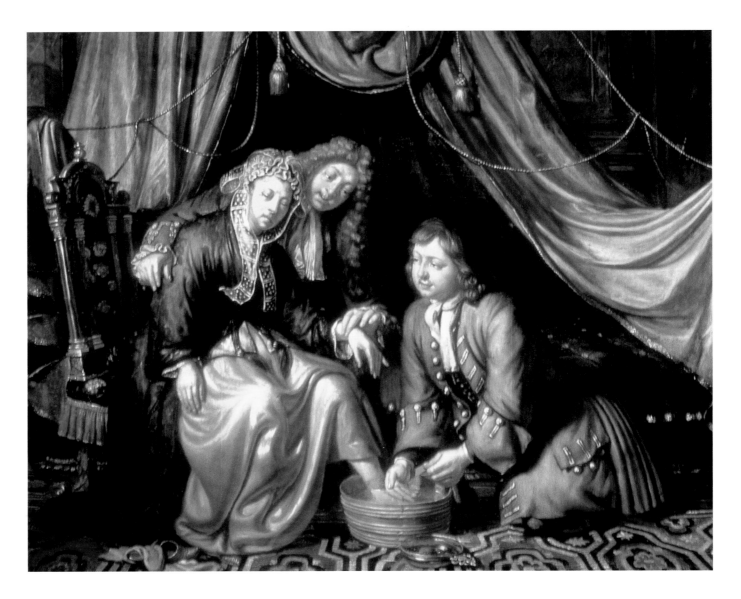

79. A female patient having her pulse taken while being bled, oil by Naiveu Matthijs (1647–1726)

abnormal blood-state; danger of haemoptysis from rupture of a vessel in a rarefied lung, for superabundance of blood then makes the vessel liable to give way; persons on the verge of epilepsy, apoplectic seizure, melancholia with superabundant blood, pharyngotonsillitis, internal inflammatory masses, 'hot' oph-thalmia, persons with piles which generally bleed but now do not; women who fail to menstruate, but do not show the two colours indicative of a need of venesection, because they are so dusky, or pale, or greenish. Persons who suffer weakness from the hot temperament of the interior organs. (In these cases it is best to do the blood-letting in spring.)

Cases of severe blows and falls need bleeding for fear of an inflammatory mass developing (for there is a risk of causing the later to burst before it has matured), provided there is no urgency and not too much blood in that part.

Several hundred years later, Sir William Harvey, who first outlined the circulation of blood in his epic *de Motu Cordis* in 1628, supported the practice of bloodletting even though there remained the unanswered question of how phlebotomy could be helpful in a local condition when the circulation was systemic. Harvey commented in his Works: "…daily experience satisfies us that bloodletting has a most salutary effect in many diseases, and is indeed the foremost among all the general remedial means: vitiated states and plethora of blood, are causes of a whole host of disease; and the timely evacuation of a certain quantity of the fluid frequently delivers patients from very dangerous diseases, and even from imminent death."

Bleeding was performed into the nineteenth century for almost everything, including agitated psychoses (when low blood pressure would have resulted in the desired sedation). Joseph Pancoast wrote his indications for bloodletting in *A Treatise on Operative Surgery* (1844):

> The opening of the superficial vessels for the purpose of extracting blood constitutes one of the most common operations of the practitioner. The principal results, which we effect by it, are 1st. The diminution of the mass of the blood, by which the overloaded capillary or larger vessels of some affected part may be relieved; 2. The modification of the force and frequency of the heart's action; 3. A change in the composition of the blood, rendering it less stimulating; the proportion of serum becoming increased after bleeding, in consequence of its being reproduced with greater facility than the other elements of the blood; 4. The production of syncope, for the purpose of effecting a sudden general relaxation of the system; and, 5. The derivation, or drawing as it is alleged, of the force of the circulation from some of the internal organs, towards the open outlet of the superficial vessel. These indications may be fulfilled by opening either a vein or an artery.

Specific areas to be bled remained an ongoing controversy for hundreds of years. In the eleventh century, Avicenna was one of the first to make specific recommendations regarding this matter (figures 80, 81):

> *The frontal veins.* These are between the two eyebrows. Phlebotomy in this situation benefits heaviness of the head, especially occipital heaviness; heaviness of the eyes; longstanding headache. To make these veins swell, apply fomentations, and also a bandage round the neck, placing a finger over the windpipe to prevent suffocation.
> *The jugular veins.* The instrument to use here is one with a sharp

80. Bloodletting from the head and neck in *Traité complet de l'anatomie de l'homme*, 2nd ed. (1866–1871) by J.M. Bourgery, Claude Bernard, and N.H. Jacob

point. Technique: draw the head to the opposite side until the vein is stretched like a cord. Consider in which direction the vein is likely to slip, and then make the opening accordingly.

Use: at the onset of lepra; in severe angina; in dyspnoea, in "hot" asthma, in hoarseness; in abscess of the lung; in dyspnoea due to superabundance of "hot" blood; in diseases of the spleen and side.

The popliteal vein. This is opened behind the bend of the knee. It is as effective as opening the saphenous vein. For exciting the menstrual flow, however, it is even more efficient, as well as for pain from piles, and pain in the anus.

The proper location for bloodletting became a significant topic of debate later in the sixteenth century when the philosophies of classic Greek medicine clashed with emerging medieval therapeutic approaches based on Moslem teachings. Galen had taught that blood should be withdrawn from a vein near the site of the disease, known as "derivative" bleeding, while later physicians suggested that "revulsive" bleeding from the opposite side of the body might be more effective. The debate became so heated that when Parisian physician Pierre Brissot (1478–1522) publicly supported derivative bleeding, the Paris Faculty of Medicine branded him a heretic, deported him to Spain, and the French Parliament forbad further bleeding anywhere close to the area of a suspected focus of disease.

An unusual and popular reason for phlebotomy was touched upon by an unknown medieval author at the conclusion of the following quote:

> By bleeding, to the marrow commeth heat,
> It maketh cleane your braine, relieves your eye
> It mends your appetite, restoreth sleepe,
> Correcting humours that do waking keepe:
> All inward parts and senses also clearing,
> It mends the voice, touch, smell, & taste, & hearing
> To bleed doth cheer the pensive, and remove
> The raging fires bred by burning love.

The last line is of interest and reflects the origin of some of the aggressive bleeding practices employed by physicians well into the nineteenth century. Early in the middle ages, Christian monks, who were sworn to celibacy, had read in Latin medical texts about the danger of *retentic semenis*, or "withholding the semen." The problem was that sexual relations and masturbation were felt to be sinful, though celibacy, on the other hand, led to an "imbalance of the humors" and thus disease. The perfect solution to this conundrum was bloodletting since the

Pl. 30.

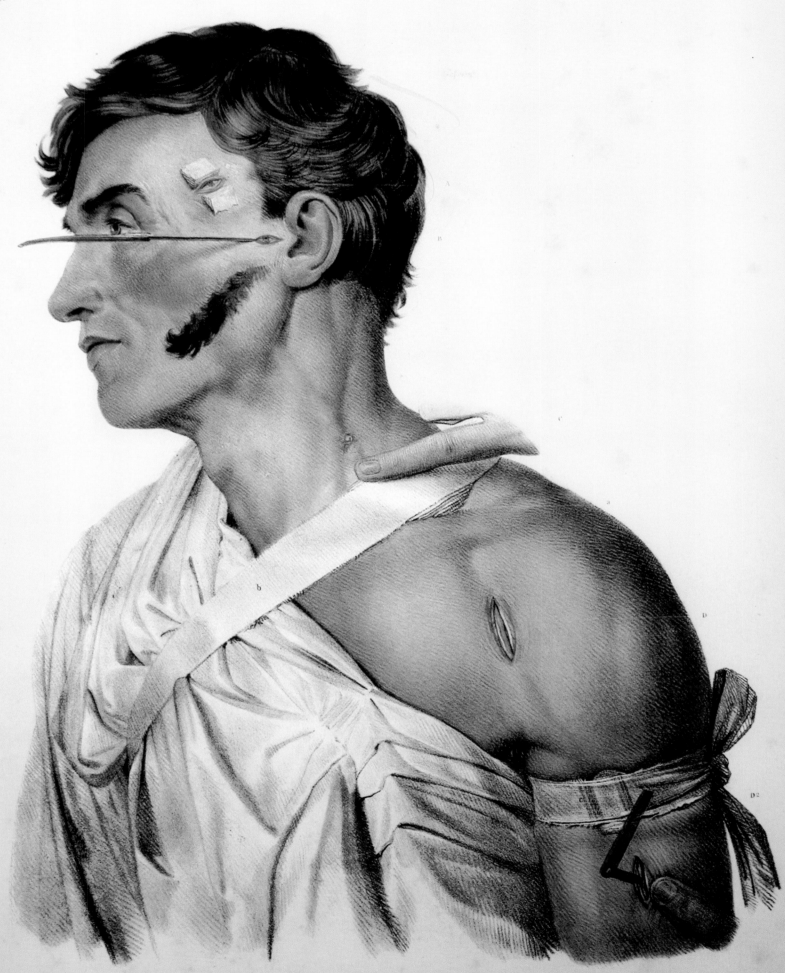

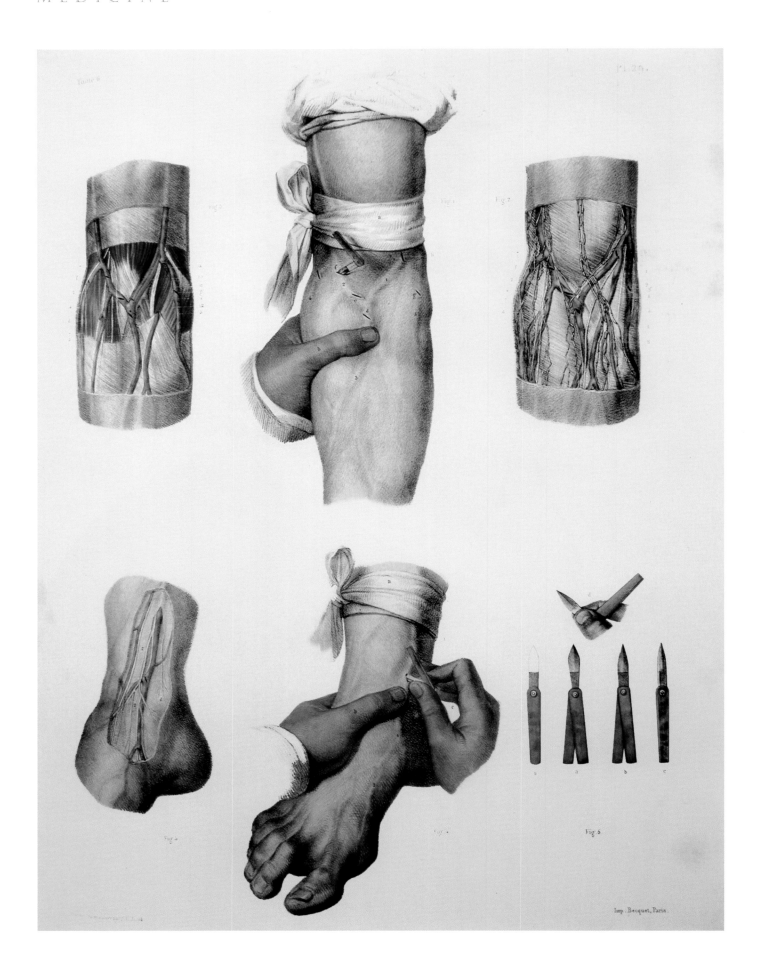

humors could then be balanced while at the same time sexual desires could be quenched. As a result of this thinking, monks bled each other in the monastery on a monthly basis, noting that the monthly menstrual cycle was considered nature's way of normally cleansing and equilibrating the system in women. Eventually, regular phlebotomy spread into the community as a general curative, and patients were sometimes relieved of over half of their entire blood volume at one sitting. When individuals sometimes expired, the blame went to the fact that the bleeding was either too little or too late.

In order to maintain good health, routine bleeding in the spring and fall became a tradition in early nineteenth century England, and, not surprisingly, a journal founded by Thomas Wakeley in 1823 named *The Lancet* remains one of the most important British medical publications. Those donating blood today can get an insight into the symptoms of venesection since the volume of blood removed (about 500 cc, or one pint) is about the same amount customarily taken by a physician at a bloodletting session prior to the twentieth century.

A RISKY PROCEDURE

There were obvious concerns about the dangers of bloodletting, and according to one medieval physician: "Phlebotomy is the beginning of health. It strengthens the mind and memory, purges the bladder, dries out the brain, warms the spinal cord, clears the hearing, restrains tears, relieves anorexia, purifies the stomach, invites digestion, induces sleep, is believed to favor long life, and drives away disease. Phlebotomy should be done with caution, and the amount of blood withdrawn is large or small according to the strength and age of the patient, the time of the year, and the state of his bodily heat. If the blood runs black at first, bleed until it becomes red; if thick or greasy, bleed until it has the consistency of water; but the bleeding should not be allowed to run until the patient is overtaken by lassitude or weakness of the stomach."

The risks of extensive phlebotomy were significant, and included infection, nerve damage, the development of an aneurism, and the loss of consciousness. The standard practice for bloodletters was to "bleed to syncope," and in the early eleventh century, Avicenna alerted the medical community to the dangers of hypotension in his *Cannon of Medicine*:

> Syncope rarely occurs during the flow of blood, unless a great amount is lost. One only bleeds up to syncope in cases of synochal fevers, in incipient apoplexy, in extensive angina or inflammatory swellings, or in cases of severe pain. Even in such cases one would make sure the strength of the patient is adequate.
>
> The persons liable to faint as a result of blood-letting are

81. Opposite. Bloodletting from the upper and lower extremities in *Traité complet de l'anatomie de l'homme,* 2nd ed. (1866–1871) by J.M. Bourgery, Claude Bernard, and N.H. Jacob

those of hot temperament, and with lean and flabby bodies. Those with equable temperament, and with firm flesh, are not likely to faint unless a large amount of blood is withdrawn. Watch the pulse.

The first blood-letting may by accompanied by syncope if it is carried out quickly on a person not accustomed to it; therefore emesis should first be procured to guard against that, and it may be repeated at the time of blood-letting.

If an artery was accidentally severed, hemostasis sometimes became a challenge, and according to Avicenna: "One must quickly put rabbit-hair into the wound, with a little powdered frankincense and dragon's blood, and aloes and myrrh, and a little zinc sulphate. Apply a cold compress and bandage tightly. If this arrests the bleeding, keep it so for three days, and even then be very cautious about loosening the bandage. Apply a styptic plaster instead. When the artery is hit deep down, the flesh may close over it and stop the bleeding. But usually death from haemorrhage will result. Some have died of the great pain produced by a ligature sufficiently tight to arrest the bleeding, or from the mortification of the limb produced by the tight bandage."

Maimonides (1138–1204) adhered to Galen's theory of the four humors, and also practiced medicine with attention to the importance of maintaining a balance in diet and behavior. He believed in therapeutic bleeding despite a number of specific concerns:

Referring to what I said about the advisability of blood-letting to the point of a fainting fit I think it helps in mitigating the heat of a chronic fever, occasioned by the unsettled digestion, and soothing the inflammation. In most cases, however, (blood-letting) causes no small harm, namely when it is administered at the wrong time or in the wrong proportions.

I know of two cases in which death occurred after fainting fits occasioned by the intervention of physicians, I am told, after blood-letting. The patients succumbed on the spot. Other cases did not die at once, but after some time, of progressive weakening. On the other hand, febrile cases where blood-letting stopped short of total invalidation, stayed alive. Again, others suffered long from grave diseases because their strength ebbed away from excessive loss of blood. Others suffered a change in their normal constitution and acquired a life-long cold disposition which no remedy could improve. All this caused by excessive blood-letting. This change of constitution causes in some people a change in appearance or a lowering of their stamina so that they easily fall ill on the slightest occasion. Eventually they become critically asthenic, their liver and stomach functioning fails them, some fall into lethargy, suffer loss of strength and show paralytic symptoms.

Though Maimonides was an advocate of bleeding, he took into account the unique psychological and environmental factors of each case, and treated patients in a holistic manner. Maimonides stated what may be the defining feature of the way in which medicine should be practiced when he said: *"quoniam medicus non curabat speciem aegritudinis sed individuum ipsius"* ("the physician should not treat the disease but the patient who is suffering from it").

Probably the most egregious abuse of bloodletting and other forms of contemporary medical care took place following a seizure suffered by King Charles II on February 2, 1685. Sir Charles Scarburgh, the king's chief physician, kept a detailed account of the king's treatment that began with the sixteen ounces of blood that was let by Dr. Edmund King before Scarburgh arrived, followed by the eight ounces he then withdrew himself. In a valiant effort to stabilize the king's "disrupted humors," his fourteen royal physicians then exposed his highness to multiple bloodletting sessions, emetics, purgatives, and enemas. They "flocked quickly to the King's assistance; and after they had held a consultation together, they strenuously endeavoured to afford timely succour to His Majesty in his dangerous state." The king's head was shaved and mustard plasters were applied which contained the urinary tract irritant (and aphrodisiac) cantharis, or Spanish Fly, followed by *Veratrum album* blown up the king's nose to induce sneezing (and thereby balance his white phlegm). More phlebotomy followed, and Charles was given a substance made from the crushed skull of an "innocent man" in order to cure his convulsions. He was again bled, and finally when at wit's end, the royal physicians gave him "an antidote which contained extracts of all the herbs and animals of the kingdom." This was followed by the administration of a bezoar from the stomach of an East Indian goat, and perhaps thankfully by that time, King Charles slipped into a coma and died, having suffered several days of the finest modern medical care available in the seventeenth century. Ironically, it is almost a certainty that any of the king's subjects would have received better care, and might have had a better chance of survival – since they would have not been exposed to such nonsense.

Dr. Laurence Heister graphically described other risks awaiting the patient about to be bled in his *General System of Surgery* (1743):

Nor is the Operation in many Cases practicable with so much Ease and Safety as is commonly imagin'd; for though in some Patients the Veins lie so open and conspicuous that even a Novice will find no Difficulty in making their Apertion, yet in others they are either so small or deeply situated that the most expert Surgeon is sometimes at a Loss, and may by Accident miscarry. Add to this, that as the Arteries, Nerves, and Tendons, are frequently very nearly seated to the Veins, 'tis no uneasy Matter to injure one or other of them with the Instrument used in Bleeding, which is quickly follow'd either with a profuse or fatal Haemorrhage, and Aneurism, violent Pains, Inflammation, Fever, Mortification, or even Death. Phlebotomy therefore should be performed with no less Judgment and Caution than the other important Operations in Surgery; especially as the Reputation of a young Surgeon may suffer as much by Neglect or Accidents in this Way as in many of the older less usual and seemingly more difficult Operations.

A good Phlebotomist should have a steady, nimble and active Hand, with a sharp Eye and undaunted Mind, without which he may either be liable to miss the Vein, or commit some Accident that may be injurious or fatal to the Patient and his own Character. For these Reasons it is that Venesection is less readily practiced by the Surgeon as he advances in Years; because old Age is generally accompanied with a weak Eye and a trembling Hand.

LEECHES

The word *leech* is derived from the Old English word *laece,* which means "doctor," and Syrian physicians reportedly first used leeches for bleeding as early as 100 B.C. This was a painless and efficient way of drawing blood because the leech excretes several hormones including one to anesthetize the bite, one to dilate vessels to insure flow, and a third, hirudin, to act as an anticoagulant. *Hirudo Medicinalis,* or the European leech, was plentiful in swamps, and thousands were imported into the United States from Europe following the work of French physician Joseph Victor Broussais (1772–1832), who advocated the use of this little parasite to restore imbalanced humors in almost every imaginable disease, both physical and mental. Leeches were transported in pewter or silver carriers, placed on various predetermined areas of the body, and were often directed toward difficult to reach places such as the mouth, larynx, ear, conjunctiva, rectum, and vagina by way of small glass leech tubes (figure 82). The ability to use leeches in confined areas made this a preferred form of venesection in many circumstances. In fact, in 1833, British physician Jonathan Osborne suggested passing a thread through the tail of leeches so that they could be used in the anus without being lost. After drinking their fill, the leeches would drop off and were stored in glass jars or decorative ceramic jars (figures 83, 84). The technique for

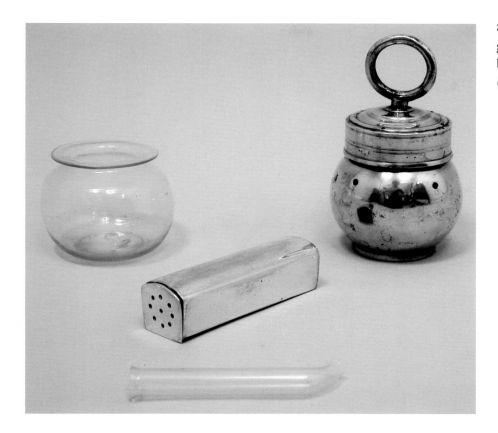

82. Leech carriers: (top left to right) glass, silver, and pewter *pot a sansues* by Niolas Bolceroise (1790–1810); (bottom) small glass leech tube

the application of leeches was described by Dr. Laurence Heister in *A General System of Surgery* (1743):

> Leeches, or *Sanguifugae*, are a Species of aquatic Worms or Insects . . . which being applied to any Part of the Body, bite through the Skin and extract Blood from the small Veins, which frequently conduces much to the Health and Recovery of the Patient; for which Reason they have been used from the most early Times by the ancient Greek and Roman Physicians, as may be seen in Galen's professed Dissertation on this Insect, commented on by Sebezius. As there are Leeches of different Kinds and Natures, it will first be proper to distinguish and make a due Choice of the best, which are always found in clear Brooks or Rivulets, whereas those taken from Lakes, Fish-ponds, and stagnant Waters, generally have something malignant in their Bite, insomuch as sometimes to excite great Pain, Inflammation, and Tumour in the Part, and Uneasiness in the whole Body. It is also an Observation made by some of the most expert Surgeons, that the best Leeches have slender and pointed Heads, with greenish and yellow Lines or Streaks on their Backs, and their Bellies of a reddish yellow; whereas those are the worst, or most malignant, which having a thick and obtuse Head, incline from a dark blue to a black Colour on the Back and Sides. But you ought to

83. Leech jars: pedestal type Staffordshire ceramic leech jar (ca. 1830); blown glass leech container; Staffordshire ceramic leech jar by Samuel Alcock and Co. (ca. 1840)

84. Mid nineteenth-century ceramic leech jar

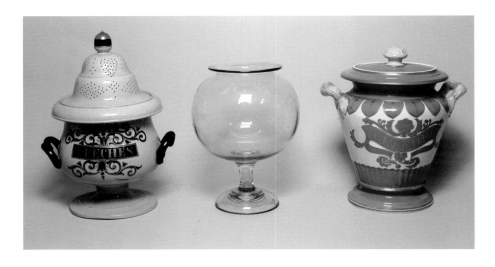

observe it as a necessary Caution, never to apply Leeches which have been lately catched in Rivers or foul Waters, before they have been kept some time in a Glass full of clean Water, to be often shifted, that they may cleanse themselves from what Filth or Venom they may have imbibed; and when they have been thus kept for a few Months, they may be afterwards safely used, without incurring any bad accident.

Before the Leech is applied to the Skin, it should be taken out of the Water to stand an Hour in an empty Cup, or other Vessel, to drain it self, that being thus rendered thirsty and empty, it may both adhere more firmly to the Part, and draw off a larger Quantity of Blood. As for the Part to which they may be applied, that may be on the Temples or behind the Ears, when the Disorder lies in the Head or Eyes, and especially when the Patient is delirious in a Fever, or over-charged with Blood: but sometimes they may be commodiously enough applied to the Veins of the *Rectum*, in Disorders proceeding from an Obstruction of the wonted Evacuation this Way, or in the blind and painful Piles; and by Way of Revulsion they will be here usefully applied in profuse Haemorrhages of the Nose, and spitting or vomiting of Blood; in which Cases they are of incredible Service, especially when the Disorder arises from Obstructions of the haemorrhoidal Flux. But before you apply the Leech, the Skin of the Part must first be rubbed till it becomes hot and red; which done, you take hold of the Leech by its Tail with a dry Cloth, or you may place it leaning half way over the Edge of a

Cup, and so apply it that it may creep out upon the Part, which they are no sooner fixed upon but they generally bite and draw the Blood very eagerly. When several Leeches are to be used, you must apply each of them to the Part in this manner successively; and if they should refuse to bite or adhere to the Skin, as they sometimes do, you may in that Case put a little Blood of a Pigeon, Chicken, &c. upon the Skin; and if that will not allure them, you must apply fresh Leeches in their stead. The Application of Leeches to the Caruncle in the greater of inner Canthus of the Eye, is found to be extremely useful in all inflammatory Disorders of that Organ, after a Phlebotomy has been first premised.

When the Leeches are distended with Blood, they generally separate from the Skin, and leave the Part of themselves; but if it be necessary to draw still a larger Quantity of Blood, you must either apply fresh Leeches, or else cut off the Tails of those which are drawing with a Pair of Scissors, by which means the Blood will run through them, and they will draw almost as long as you please. If the Leeches do not separate spontaneously after a sufficient Quantity of Blood has been evacuated, upon sprinkling a little Salt or Ashes upon the Part, they usually leave it presently; which Method should be the rather taken, because forcing or pulling them away often occasions a Tumour and Inflammation of the Part. The Operation being thus finished, those Leeches which are whole may be returned into the Glass again, and reserved for future Uses; but those die which have had their Tails cut off. The Wound made by this Insect may be first washed with warm Wine or Water, and then dressed with some vulnerary Plaster; though there is seldom any occasion for the latter, as it generally heals up fast enough of itself.

NURSING RESPONSIBILITIES

Leeches remained an important part of the medical armamentarium throughout the nineteenth century, and nurses played a significant role in their use. Percy Lewis, MD, described the duties of the nurse in his book *The Theory & Practice of Nursing* (1892):

Leeches are much more used in some hospitals than others, and there are several details in applying them which it is necessary to know. The part to which they are to be applied is to be well washed first. The leeches are to be handled as little as possible. They are best placed in a wine-glass, which is then inverted over the spot where they are wanted to bite. . . . A nurse may be frightened of a leech herself—if so, she should not let the patient notice it, as fright is catching—but familiarity, especially with a leech, breeds contempt. Nurses frequently have great difficulty in knowing which is the head end of the animal. The head is the more pointed end, which a nurse may find out by letting him 'walk.' A leech always moves head first. When replete they drop off of themselves, but should they be tardy in doing so, it is only necessary to sprinkle on them a little salt. A leech must never be pulled off, or their teeth will be left in the wound, and the patient will be hurt. After the leeches have dropped off, it is as a rule only necessary to apply a little absorbent wool to stop the bleeding; a very vigilant watch must, however, be kept on the punctures for some hours after, for they sometimes bleed profusely.

INSTRUMENTATION

Following the application of a tourniquet, physicians withdrew blood using a number of instruments, including a thumb lancet that might be carried in a small case (figure 85), a single-bladed, spring-loaded lancet, or perhaps a multiple-bladed scarificator (figure 86). Fleams were knives containing blades of varying size, one of which was held over a vein and then struck with a fleam stick, a method preferred by veterinarians. Blood was collected in bleeding/barbers bowls, that sometimes had rings to measure the amount of blood withdrawn in ounces (a distinguishing feature from rather common nineteenth-century porringers) (figure 87). The "Helmet of Mambrino" worn by Don Quixote in the book by the same name was such a bowl. Author Miguel de Cervantes (1547–1616) was the son of a surgeon and may have gotten the idea of using a bleeding bowl in his famous character's costume from the time he spent with his father.

The use of leeches was obviously objectionable to many, so with the technological advances of the nineteenth century came the invention of the mechanical or "artificial" leech. An argument in favor of this device was presented by one of its inventors, Andrew Smith, in the 1869–1870 edition of the *Medical Record*: "In the first place the appearance of the animal is repulsive and disgusting, and delicate and sensitive persons find it difficult to overcome their repugnance to contact with the cold slimy reptile. This is especially the case when it is a question of their application about or within the mouth. Then again, their disposition to crawl into cavities or passages results sometimes in very annoying accidents. Another source of annoyance is that they are often unwilling to bite—the patience of all concerned being exhausted in fruitless efforts

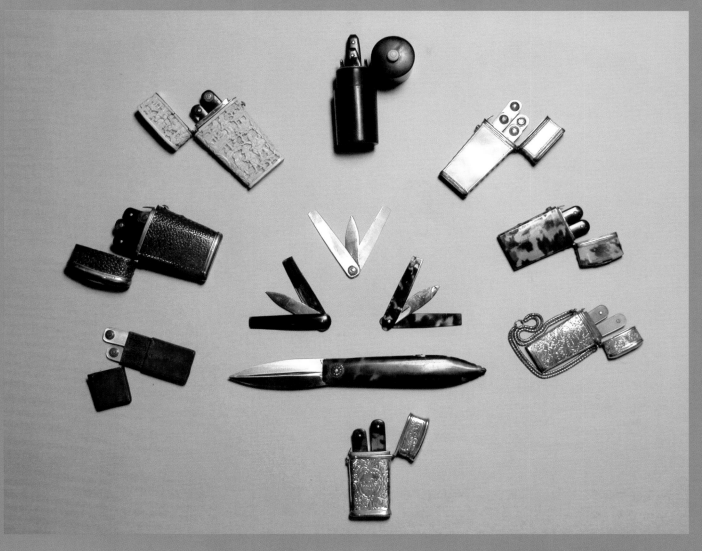

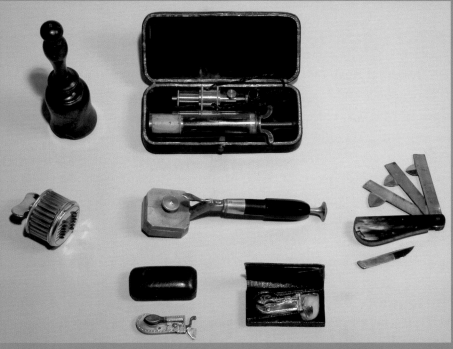

85. Portable cased thumb lancet sets: (from left clockwise) leather, shagreen (fish skin), ivory, ebony, mother of pearl, tortoiseshell, gold, and silver

86. Nineteenth century bloodletting instruments, Top: Bleeding stick (to be used with the folding fleam), Heurteloup's mechanical leech, Middle: French multi-bladed scarificator by Collin, Tiemann's scarificator, folding fleam with horn shield, Bottom: cased brass spring lancet, silver spring lancet of Samuel Jackson, presented by H. Brooke, MD to Dr. Worthington.

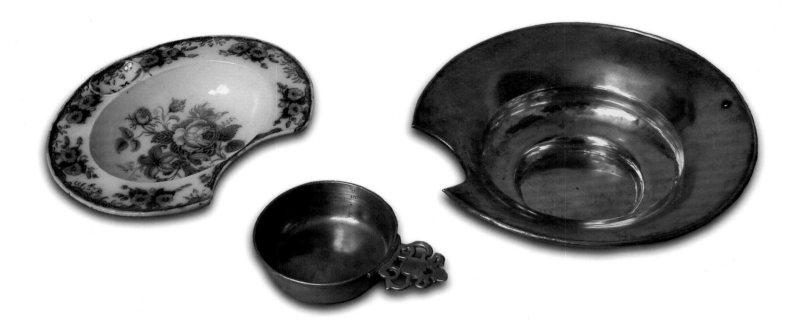

87. Top: mid nineteenth century barber/bleeding bowels, ceramic (left), brass (right), middle: eighteenth century pewter bleeding bowl with measured rings

to induce them to take hold. . . . The expense, too, of a considerable number is by no means trifling."

Bloodletting was popular for thousands of years, and certainly into the nineteenth century (figure 88). Barber-surgeons asked their patients to squeeze a pole during phlebotomy in order to improve the flow of blood. The poles were subsequently stained red and, when not in use, they were hung outside the door with the white linen tourniquet wrapped around. The familiar red and white pole outside of barbershops today remains a vestige of those early bloodletting sessions by barber-surgeons.

THE BLEEDING OF GEORGE WASHINGTON

Dr. Benjamin Rush (1746–1813) was a signer of the Declaration of Independence and had a major influence on the practice of medicine in colonial America. He was an important proponent of bleeding, though he mistakenly thought that the body held twelve quarts instead of six. Shortly before his death, George Washington was bled an astonishing four-and-one-half quarts of blood in a twenty-four hour period for an infected throat (figure 89).

The story of the first president's final hours began on December 12, 1799, when George Washington, then sixty-seven years old and two years out of office, was exposed to "rain, hail, and snow falling alternately, with a cold wind" during a horseback ride on his Mt. Vernon estate. The first to arrive was Washington's family physician, Dr. James Craik, who had served with Washington in every major battle of the Revolutionary

War. Two other physicians attended the president during the next several hours, Dr. Gustavus Brown from Port Tobacco, Maryland, just across the Potomac River, and Dr. Elisha Cullen Dick, a nearby resident of Alexandria.

The president's sore throat progressed despite the best efforts of his physicians, and George Washington died within twenty-four hours. According to the *Times* of Alexandria, the cause of death was *Cynanche trachealis*, one of a number of upper airway infections that might have been described today as acute epiglottitis perhaps caused by *Haemophilas influenzae*. Craik and Dick made the following statement regarding the president's final moments:

> Some time in the night of Friday, the 13th inst., having been exposed to rain on the preceding day, General Washington was attacked with an inflammatory affection of the upper part of the windpipe, called in technical language, *cynanche trachealis*. The disease commenced with a violent ague, accompanied with some pain in the upper and fore part of the throat, a sense of stricture in the same part, a cough, and a difficult rather than painful deglutition, which were soon succeeded by fever and a quick and laborious respiration. The necessity of blood-letting suggesting itself to the General, he procured a bleeder in the neighborhood, who took from the arm in the night, twelve or fourteen ounces of blood; he would not by any means be prevailed upon by the family to send for the attending physician till the following morning, who arrived at Mt. Vernon at eleven o'clock on Saturday morning. Discovering the case to be highly alarming, and foreseeing the fatal tendency of the disease, two consulting physicians were immediately sent for, who arrived, one at half past three and the other at four in the afternoon. In the interim were employed two copious bleedings; a blister was applied to the part affected, two moderate doses of calomel were given, an injection was administered which operated on the lower intestines, but all without any perceptible advantage, the respiration becoming still more difficult and distressing.

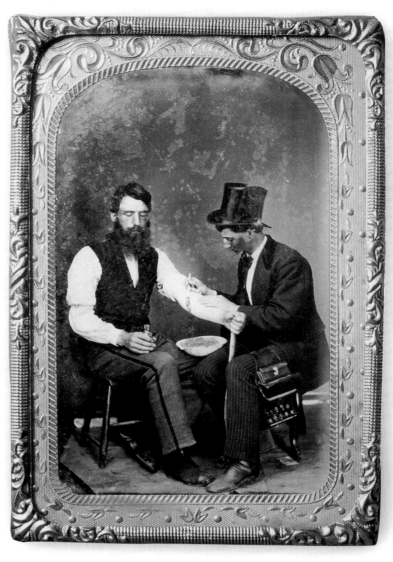

88. Daguerreotype of a patient being bled (ca 1859)

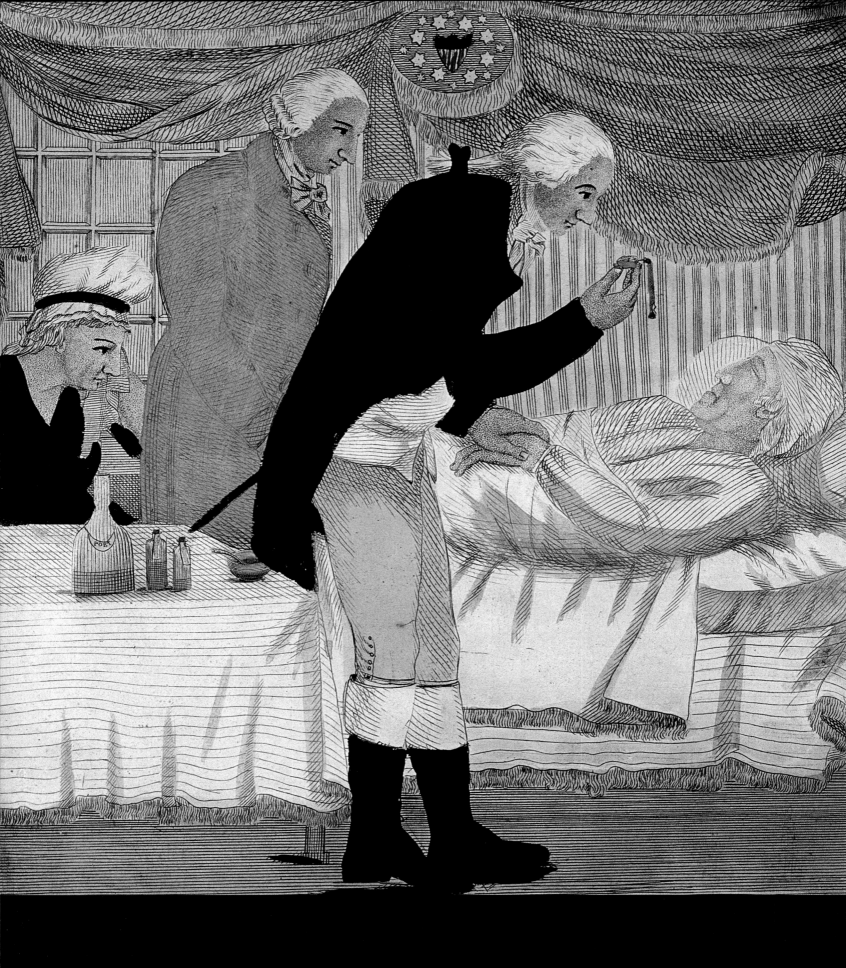

Upon the arrival of the first of the consulting physicians, it was agreed, as there were yet no signs of accumulation in the bronchial vessels of the lungs, to try the result of another bleeding, when about thirty-two ounces were drawn, without the smallest apparent alleviation of the disease. Vapours of vinegar and water were frequently inhaled, ten grains of calomel were given, succeeded by repeated doses of emetic tartar, amounting in all to five or six grains, with no other effect than a copious discharge from the bowels. The powers of life seemed now manifestly yielding to the force of the disorder. Blisters were applied to the extremities, together with a cataplasm of bran and vinegar to the throat. Speaking, which was painful from the beginning, now became almost impracticable, respiration grew more and more contracted and imperfect, till half after eleven o'clock on Saturday night, when, retaining the full possession of his intellect, he expired without a struggle.

Perhaps recognizing the incompetence of his physicians, Washington's final words reflected his fear of being buried alive: "Have me decently buried, but do not let my body be put into a vault in less than two days after I am dead. . . . Tis well."

The care provided to President Washington was controversial, and the youngest of his three physicians, Dr. Elisha Dick, had recommended that a tracheotomy be performed. This was not a common procedure at the time, and, unfortunately, his perhaps life-saving suggestion was denied by the other two physicians. Dr. Gustavus Brown summarized his findings to the medical community: "In their treatment of Washington his doctors followed the accepted rules laid down by the best authorities of that day. As bleeding was then practiced, the amount of blood withdrawn was not unusual. From the nature of the illness death was a foregone conclusion. The vigorous therapy resorted to by his physicians may have hastened Washington's death, but it could in no way have caused it." That statement, of course, remains a topic of debate to this day.

TRANSFUSION

Early transfusions were based on the notion that receiving blood was yet another way in which to help balance the humors. Blood had also been revered by the medical community for its curative and sometimes magical power, though some seventeenth-century physicians had other goals in mind for its use based on the concept of "vitalism," which was the theory that an individual's or animal's personality could perhaps be transferred by way of its blood. The possibility that one could pass on a

89. Opposite. *George Washington in his last illness* (ca 1800) attended by Doctors Craik and Brown, engraving by a unknown artist

lion's courage or a lamb's passivity to another by transfusion encouraged physicians to experiment for hundreds of years (figure 90). The first recorded "transfusion" was in 1492 in Rome, and the purpose was to rejuvenate Pope Innocent VIII through the transfusion of blood from three healthy boys. Unfortunately, the three boys succumbed as did the Pope, followed by the rapid departure of the attending physician, Giacomo di San Genesio.

Christopher Wren and Richard Lower performed the first successful procedure when they transferred blood from one dog to another in 1665. After reports regarding transfusion reached France, members of the Montmort Academy appointed two physicians, Jean-Baptiste Denis (the physician to King Louis XIV) and surgeon Paul Emmerez, to investigate further. Denis experimented with calves and dogs, and performed the first interspecies transfusion on June 15, 1667, when he gave about twelve ounces of lamb's blood to a drowsy fifteen year old who "rapidly recovered from his lethargy, grew fatter and was an object of surprise and astonishment to all who knew him." After that apparent success, the two physicians were encouraged enough to continue their experimentation. Their next procedure was a successful transfusion from a sheep to a forty-five-year-old gentleman, and then they gave the blood of a calf to a Swedish nobleman. Their subject tolerated the first procedure, though unfortunately he died during the second attempt.

Dr. Denis' fourth subject was a psychotic named Antoine Mauroy whose bizarre behavior included disrobing and setting fires throughout the town. It therefore made sense to Denis that the blood from a tranquil calf might confer those characteristics to this disturbed individual, and thus improve his agitated state. The first transfusion from a calf seemed to be successful in sedating the man, though the second resulted in some discomfort (with probable hemolysis since his urine turned black). He survived the procedure, though Denis was reluctant to go any further. However, the patient's wife, Madame Mauroy, approached him to attempt a third transfusion. Denis set it up though did not complete the procedure, and was later surprised to find out that the patient had died the following day. He was angered at the attempted extortion of Madame Mauroy after the death of her husband and reacted by taking the woman to court in order to forestall her efforts at slander. In the trial that followed, Madame Mauroy was discovered to have been responsible for her husband's death by having added arsenic to his soup on a regular basis. Denis was exonerated, though the trial essentially marked the end of his experimentation with transfusion. Denis had been reporting his results in the *Journal of the Royal Society of London*, publicity that had angered physicians in the French Academy. Prompted in some degree by jealously, they took the position that transfusion was unethical and, in

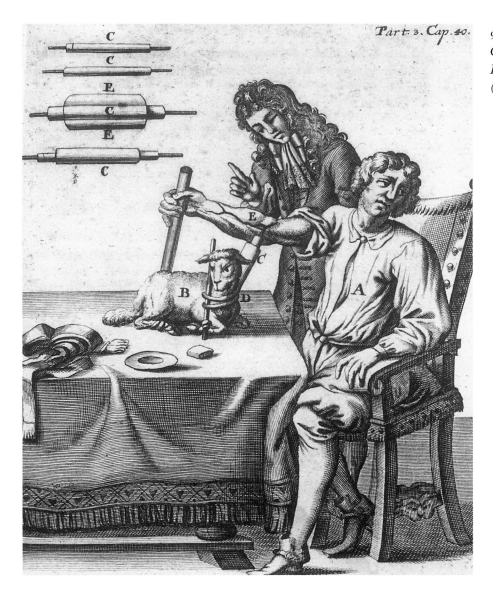

90. Transfusion from lamb to man in *Grosser und gantz neugewundener Lorbeer-Krantz, oder Wund Artzney* (1705) by Matthäus Purmann

fact, sinful. Unfortunately, this was the same group of physicians to whom the court had assigned an oversight responsibility, and no further transfusions were performed for over a century, having been outlawed not only in France, but in England and Italy as well.

Matthäus Purmann described the technique for interspecies blood transfusion in his *Chirurgia Curiosa* (1694):

> Chirurgical *Transfusion* was also for some time in great vogue and reputation; but since it could not be always practiced, and that Patients were unwilling to submit to it, it soon grew out of use; but I am of the opinion if Dr. Major, Etmuller, Eltzholtz, Dr. Wren and Clark had lived somewhat longer, it might have been further advanced in the World; but they dying the Operation began to be neglected and dyed soon after them.
>
> I tried it on a Merchant's Son at Berlin who for severall years

was afflicted with a Leprosie; I gradually drew out a great quantity of Blood, and put into his Veins the Blood of a Lamb; by which means the patient was happily cured, to the admiration of several ingenious Persons.

Transfusion is performed in this manner. Generally the Legs or Arms are chosen for this Purpose; in the Arm the *Vena Mediana*, and in the Leg the *Vena Cruralis*; from which you must take as much Blood as the Strength of the Patient will permit. The Arm or the Leg, where the Vein is to be opened, must be tyed fast below the opening with a strong Fillet. Then you must have in readiness an Instrument which is a kind of a *Tube*, surrounded with a Linen Cover, in which Cover you must put some warm Water to hinder the blood from coagulating or congealing, which passes through the *Tube*. This *Tube* must have on each side a fine *Silver Pipe*, one of which must be put into the Vein of the Man and the other into the Vein of the Beast, from whom Blood must be transfused, the Hair or Wool of whose Neck must be cut away and a Fillet bound about its Neck, and the Creature tyed so fast that it cannot move one way or other; then the Vein being opened both in the Man and the Beast, the Blood of the Beast will rise into the *Tube* and empty it self into the Vein of the *Arm*; and so much for this Operation.

In 1818, British obstetrician James Blundell resurrected the procedure in humans when he successfully transfused blood from a husband to his wife (figures 91, 92). Because of blood incompatibility, only one half of his next ten transfusions were successful; the use of blood transfusions on a regular basis awaited the discovery of blood typing by Karl Landsteiner in 1900.

OTHER USES FOR BLOOD

Well before anyone considered the direct transfusion of blood therapeutically, it was employed in any number of other ways for the provision of health care. Paul of Aegina (A.D. 625–690) summarized several early uses in *Pauli Aeginetae de re medica libri septem, graece* (printed in 1528):

Sanguis, *Blood*: no kind of it is of a cold nature, but that of swine is liquid and less hot, being very like the human in temperament. That of common pigeons, the wood pigeons, and the turtle, being of a moderate temperament if injected hot, removes extravasated blood about the eyes from a blow; and when poured upon the dura mater, in cases of trephining, it is anti-inflammatory. That of the owl, when drunk with wine or water,

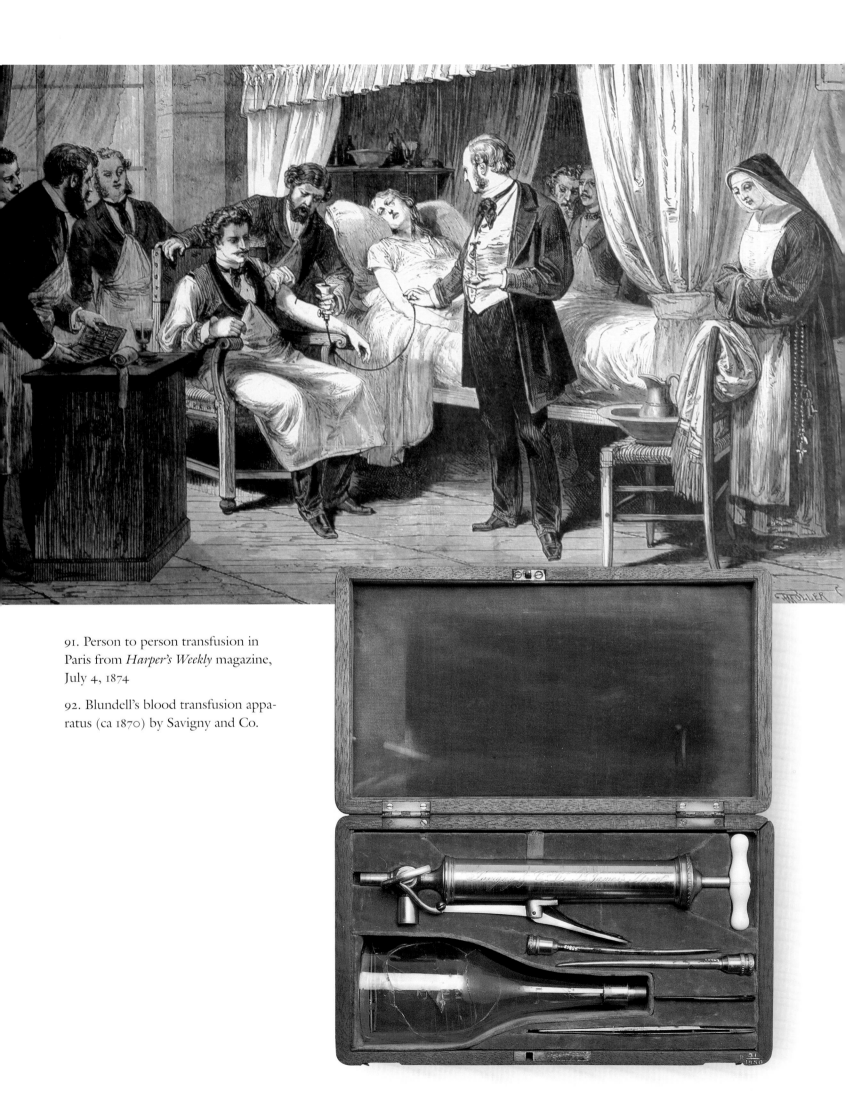

91. Person to person transfusion in Paris from *Harper's Weekly* magazine, July 4, 1874

92. Blundell's blood transfusion apparatus (ca 1870) by Savigny and Co.

relieves dyspnoea. The blood of bats, it is said, is a preservative to the breasts of virgins, and, if rubbed in, it keeps the hair from growing; and in like manner also that of frogs, and the blood of the chamaeleon and the dog-tick. But Galen, having made trial of all these remedies, says that they disappointed him. But that of goats, owing to its dryness, if drunk with milk, is beneficial in cases of dropsy, and breaks down stones in the kidneys. That of domestic fowls stops hemorrhages of the membranes of the brain, and that of lambs cures epilepsies. The recently coagulated blood of kids, if drunk with an equal quantity of vinegar, to the amount of half a hemina, cures vomiting of blood from the chest. The blood of bears, of wild goats, of buck goats, and of bulls, is said to ripen apostemes. That of the land crocodile produces acuteness of vision. The blood of stallions is mixed with septic medicines. The antidote from bloods is given for deadly poisons, and contains the blood of the duck, of the stag, and of the goose.

COUNTERIRRITATION AND CUPPING

Physicians were rarely able to address internal problems surgically, so in addition to bleeding and purging, counterirritation and cupping became popular in the seventeenth and eighteenth centuries to readjust the internal environment and presumably stabilize imbalanced humors. In *Mitchell's Therapeutics* (1857), counterirritation was defined as "the setting up of a new action in the neighborhood of a diseased spot with the view of transferring it from its original seat, as in the use of blisters for the relief of pleurisy." Glasgow surgeon John Burns said, ". . . if the internal parts be inflamed, the action of the surface is diminished; and, by increasing this action, we can lessen or remove the disease below." In 1838, A.B. Granville, MD, FRS, wrote in *Counter-Irritation, Its Principles and Practice*:

1. The term Counter-irritation, now very generally used in ordinary language, as referable to the treatment of disease, is of a comparatively recent adoption, and succeeded to the more expressive, though antiquated word, "Revulsion."

2. The history of the origin of the term itself contains the most comprehensive explanation of its etymology. When certain disorders, according to the views of some prevailing systems of medicine, are supposed to depend on *irritation*—meaning that peculiar action which certain physical agents are known to exert on particular organs, and which consists in *irritating* those organs;—and when it

is found that the excitement of a somewhat similar *irritating* action, on another part of the body, by artificial means, cures the original disease dependent on *irritation*;—the action by which the disorder is removed receives the name of Counter-irritation.

3. This origin of the word, it is contended, fully explains its meaning. A familiar example will make the thing still clearer. When a degree of internal pain exists in some part of the chest, denoting a low grade of inflammation, it is considered that the part is in a state of irritation. A common blister being applied externally to the pained part, relief is soon obtained, and at last a complete removal of the pain is the result. The blister, at the same time, has produced considerable irritation, and its concomitant, pain on the part to which it was applied. It is therefore fair to conclude, that it is through that very artificial *irritation* that the original irritation or disease was removed; and hence such a sanative agency has been deemed entitled to the distinguishing appellative of Counter-irritation.

According to Granville, the following "may be expected to take place in the part morbidly affected":

a. Increase of circulation in the part.
b. Greater influx of humors towards it, which will partially remain and dilate the vessels.
c. Extrication of heat.
d. Redness of the skin.
e. Pain.
f. Progressive inflammation.
g. Vesication or ustion, or destruction of the skin, and sometimes of the tissues under it.
h. Serous or purulent secretion from the part, and sometimes sloughing.

A common form of counterirritation was the use of blisters and caustics to promote a continuous area of drainage for internal toxins. A number of substances were used, including cantharides, or Spanish Fly. The treating physician prepared a plaster of crushed and dried beetles and placed it over the diseased organ, causing blistering. When the blisters broke, the diseased serum was released, and more powder was deposited on the area. Acetic acid was also used to blister the skin on occasion, and other irritating agents, including "rubefacients," were employed by physicians over the years to redden the skin without injury. Physicians used "issues," or potassium hydroxide (caustic potash), to produce superficial ulcers for the treatment of liver, lung, and joint disease. According to one physician, "When the stomach, intestines, or kidney have been very irritable, I have known a sinapism (mustard plaster) to act like a charm." Moxas, or pieces of cotton wool wet with a flammable substance, were burned on the skin to form scars in treating a number of internal conditions, and some physicians recommended the simpler method of creating "healing" blisters with boiling water.

Granville described an interesting use of counterirritation in case twenty-three of his text:

> A young woman was presented in 1837 to Professor Esquirol, at the Salpétriére Hospital for Female Lunatics, near Paris, during my visits to that establishment, who had for some years been suffering from epileptic fits every four weeks, at particular periods, and who had been treated for them by some of the first medical men in the metropolis. Esquirol had at this time under his care, in the above-named asylum, a whole ward of epileptic patients, on whom he used to make cautious and proper trials of every species of treatment, which the faculty, whether national or foreign, recommended from time to time,—such as that by nitrate of silver, tartar emetic, and sulphate of zinc. But as he had not hitherto obtained any appreciable good result, he determined on managing the present case differently. For this determination he considered himself warranted, by the repeated observations he had made, in cases where the patients had died as a consequence of severe paroxysms of epilepsy, and in most, if not all of whom, he had found the superior portion of the spinal cord in a softened condition, and of a gray or rosy colour. Such a state of things induced him to believe that the employment of counter-irritation in the shape of the moxa, applied several times over the vertebrae, might afford a better chance of recovery. He therefore acted on that principle, and he was not long in discovering the correctness of his reasoning, by the success of his treatment. The paroxysms of the disease in the course of the first few months became less frequent, and of much shorter duration, until at last they ceased altogether.
>
> Professor Esquirol recorded this case in a memoir which he read in 1917, before the *Société de la Faculté de Médecine,* in Paris, on which occasion I had the honour of being present as a member; and he has since adopted the same method in more instances than one, with equal success.

Another method of counterirritation was by cupping, a procedure which remained popular into the latter part of nineteenth century. The indications for cupping were similar to those for venesection, and were reviewed by Thomas Mapleson, professional cupper at Westminster Hospital in *A Treatise on the Art of Cupping* (1813): "Apoplexy, angina pectoris, asthma, spitting blood, bruises, cough, catarrh, consumption, contusion, convulsions, cramps, diseases of the hip and knee joints, deafness, delirium, dropsy, epilepsy, erysipelas, giddiness, gout, whooping cough, hydrocephalus, head ache, inflammation of the lungs, intoxication, lethargy, lunacy, lumbago, measles, numbness of the limbs, obstructions, ophthalmia, pleurisy, palsy, defective perspiration, peripneumony, rheumatism, to procure rest, sciatica, shortness of breath, sore throat, pains of the side and chest."

The procedure began when a barber-surgeon heated a cupping glass with an alcohol lamp and then placed it on the skin, usually over a diseased internal organ (figure 93). As the cup cooled, it created a vacuum that brought blood to the surface to act as a counterirritant; many patients did indeed notice pain relief as discomfort was produced in one place to reduce the awareness of pain in another. The earliest cupping vessels were made of hollowed out animal horns and, later in the twelfth century, Persian physicians cupped with "spouted glasses" as they removed air through a side channel. Beautiful "wet" cupping sets were manufactured with syringes to draw out blood after scarificators had made their multiple incisions, while "dry" cupping sets were only meant to bring blood to the surface (figure 94). Laurence Heister described the practice of cupping in his textbook of medicine:

Scarification and Cupping was an Operation frequently performed by the most ancient Surgeons and Physicians, notwithstanding the Moderns have by their Pride or Neglect turned the Business over to those who attended the Baths and Hot-houses: Yet, as it makes none of the least Operations in Surgery, we shall here briefly consider and explain the same. The Operation of Cupping is indeed vague and not confined to any particular Member of the Body; but when ever the Cupping-glass is apply'd, 'tis fixed upon the Skin, either entire or scarify'd; and hence we have a two-fold Distinction of Cupping into *dry* and *gorey*. . . . In dry Cupping the Glass adheres to the Skin by expelling or rarifying its included Air by lighted Flax or the Flame of a burning Candle within it, so that the Glass is pressed upon the Part with a considerable Force by the external Air in which Artifice our ordinary Cuppers are sufficiently well versed. The Use of this dry Cupping is two-fold, either to make a *Revulsion* of the Blood from some particular Parts affected, or else to cause a *Derivation* of it into the affected Part upon which the Glass is applied. Hence we have a Reason why Hippocrates orders a large Cupping-glass to be apply'd under the Breasts of Women who have a too profuse Discharge of their Menses, intending thereby to cause a Revulsion of the Blood upwards from the Uterus. And upon the same Principle I have myself successfully cured a profuse Haemorrhage at the Nose, and an Haemorrhage or Spitting of Blood from the Lungs, by applying Cupping-glasses to the Legs and Feet, particularly about the Ancles and Knees. Scultetus gives us a remarkable Instance . . . of a Woman who by the repeated Application of six Cupping-glasses (without Scarification) to her Thighs was not only relieved of the troublesome Symptoms caused by an Obstruction of her Menses, but was also thereby freed from the Obstruction itself. Dry Cupping is also used with Success to make a Revulsion by applying the Glasses to the Temples, behind the Ears, or to the Neck and Shoulders, for the Removal of Pains, Vertigos, and other Disorders of the Head; they are also apply'd to the upper and lower Limbs to derive Blood and Spirits into them when they are paralytic; and lastly, to remove the Sciatica and other Pains of the Joints. The Operation is in these Cases to be repeated upon the Part 'till it looks very red, and becomes painful.

Of course, there were risks to cupping, and Avicenna described several in *The Canon of Medicine* (printed in 1632):

There is a danger of transmitting forgetfulness, for as some say, the posterior part of the brain has to do with the preservation of memory, and the cupping enfeebles this faculty, and the off-spring will suffer. Some say that cupping over the occiput and top of the head is beneficial for insanity, vertigo, and for preventing the hair from going grey. But we must take it that this effect on the hair applies only to feeble-minded people and not to other types of person, for in most cases the use of cupping in this situation brings premature greyness, and also dulls the intellect. But it is beneficial for eye-diseases, and indeed this is its chief value, namely for pustular keratitis and staphyloma. But cupping in this situation is harmful for cataract, unless the proper moment is chosen. It impairs the activity of the intellect, making the offspring dull and forgetful, with poor reasoning powers, and permanent infirmity.

Not unexpectedly, competition arose between "professional cuppers" and others performing this service. In the nineteenth century, bathhouse attendants, or Bagnio men, cupped their clients during sessions in

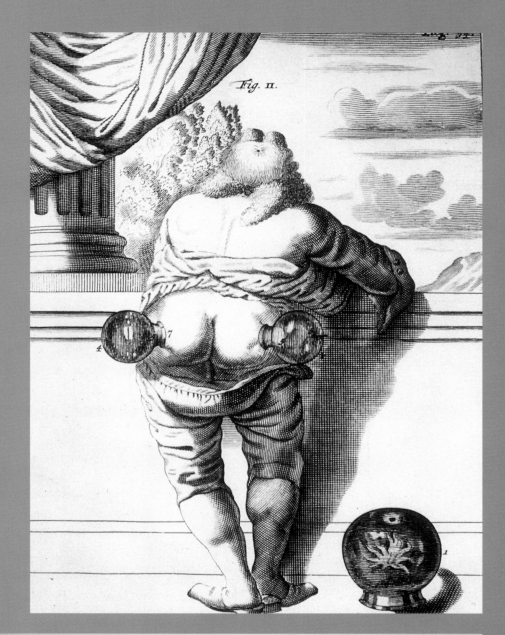

93. Cupping glasses in *Exercitationes practicae* (1694) by Frederik Dekkers

94. Nineteenth century cupping sets, top: by Arnold and Sons (left), and Charrière and Collin (right), bottom: silver teapot burner, twelfth century Persian spouted cupping glass, two cupping glasses, and a cupping tin

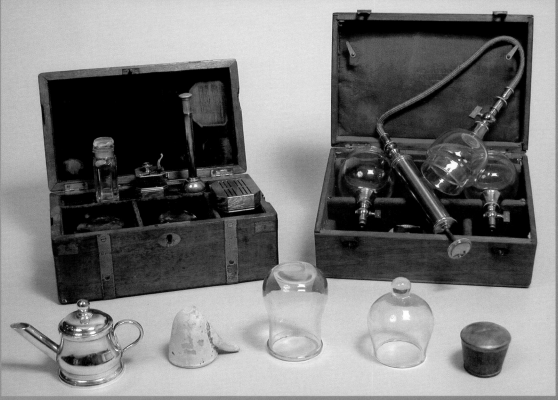

steam rooms and frequently left personalized attractive scars. Thomas Mapleson summarized the cuppers' response, "The custom which appears to have become prevalent of resorting to these Bagnios, or Haumaums, to be bathed and cupped, appears to have superseded the practice of this operation by the regular surgeons. Falling into the hands of mere hirelings, who practiced without knowledge, and without any other principle than one merely mercenary, the operation appears to have fallen into contempt, to have been neglected by Physicians, because patients had recourse to it without previous advice, and disparaged by regular Surgeons, because, being performed by others, it diminished the profits of their professions."

At the end of the nineteenth century in France, Victor-Théodore Junod (1809–1881) extended the application of dry cupping to whole extremities so that blood was temporarily removed from the circulation, sometimes to the point of the patient fainting. This "temporary bleeding" was reversible, though according to Junod, it was an effective derivative method of treatment.

In 1908, Willy Meyer, MD, and Prof. Dr. Victor Schmieden wrote *Bier's Hyperemic Treatment*, which expanded Junod's treatment with suction devices. These physicians logically proposed a form of treatment that, unfortunately, was based on erroneous physiology, and therefore was not therapeutic. Their (correct) conclusion was that the best way to cure infection was to increase circulation to diseased tissue. To reach that end, they advocated either the placement of a tourniquet above the affected parts to cause reddening or the use of suction devices to increase blood to those areas of the body. "Hitherto it was considered the physician's first duty to fight every kind of inflammation, since inflammations were looked upon as detrimental. Bier teaches just the opposite; namely, to artificially increase the redness, swelling and heat, three of the four cardinal symptoms of acute inflammation. . . ." Medical science took thousands of years to understand the pathophysiology of inflammation; Bier was almost there, but not quite (figures 95, 96).

THE SETON

Another form of counterirritation involved the use of the seton needle, which was a lancet inserted under the skin usually behind the neck and left there to form a draining tract. The purpose was to reduce internal inflammations and poisons by their external discharge, the area kept open to drain pus by a silk or cotton thread, and sometimes by the use of a hot cautery (figures 97, 98). A good description for the use of the seton needle was supplied by Laurence Heister in 1743:

A Seton is a few horse-hairs, small Threads, or a larger

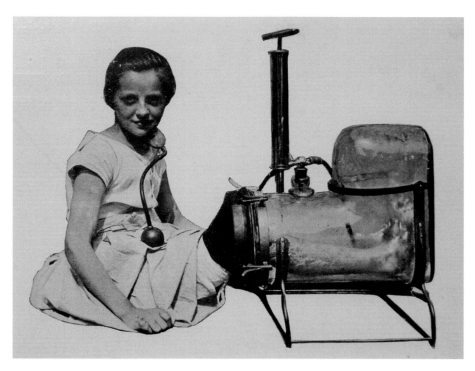

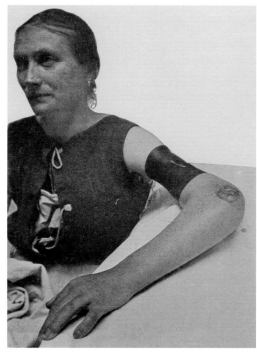

Packthread, drawn through the Skin, with a View to restore or preserve Health . . . by taking up the Skin in the lower Part of the Neck, while an Assistant draws it tight about an Inch above, then the Surgeon passes through the Skin a large and crooked Needle armed with Silk or Thread, either twisted together into a large String, or in 20 or 30 small and loose Threads, which being drawn through the Skin are to be left in the Neck after the Needle has been removed. The Wound is then dressed with some digestive Ointment, and covered with a Piece of Plaster, perforated on each Side for the Ligature to pass through, and thus the Seton is decently compleated. The Name seems to be derived from *Seti Equini*, or Horse-hairs; which were by the Ancients used instead of Thread: But our modern Surgeons changed them for Thread of Silk or Flax, which are much more easy to the Patient. The Ligature is to be shifted or drawn through the Wound a little every Day, and the Matter is to be wiped off every Morning and Night as in Issues; by which Means it will degenerate into an Ulcer with a double Orifice, making a copious Discharge daily, and when one Ligature is become foul and unfit for Use, a fresh one may by introduced by fastening it to the End of the old, which may be then drawn out. . . .

There are many Physicians and Surgeons who esteem Setons to be of little Consequence in the Cure of Disorders . . . whereas others, on the contrary, propose it to be one of the best Means

95. Foot and neck therapy for tuberculosis in *Bier's hyperemic treatment* (1908) by Willy Meyer MD, and Prof. Dr. Victor Schmieden

96. Bier's hyperemic treatment for tuberculosis of the elbow in *Bier's Hyperemic Treatment* (1908) by Willy Meyer MD, and Prof. Dr. Victor Schmieden

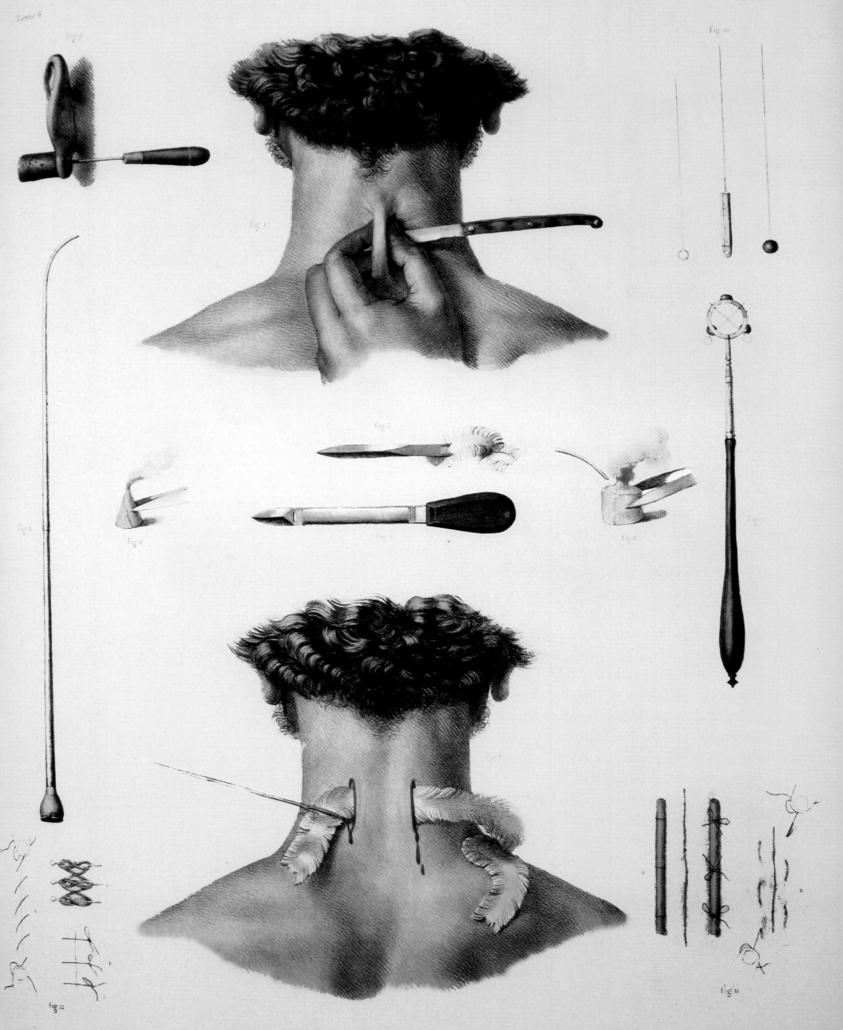

Pl. 22.

of relieving many chronical and obstinate Disorders, particularly those of the Head; such as Drowsiness, Head-achs, Epilepsy, and Disorders of the Eyes: And as it is certain many superfluous and pernicious Humours may be drawn from the Parts affected, and be this Way discharged, we need not wonder that a Seton should be preferred by many Physicians as more effectual than a Pair of Issues. We also find by Experience, that they are very useful in the Hydrocephalus, Catarrhs, Inflammation, and other Disorders of the Eyes, Gutta Serena, Cataract, and incipient Suffusion to which we may add intense Head-achs, with Stupidity, Drowsiness, Epilepsies, and even the Apoplexy itself: But as Setons are usually attended with much Uneasiness and Trouble, their good Effects are but seldom experienced by Patients in those Disorders.

A LIFE AWAKENER

The Bauncheidt Lebenswecker was an ebony device containing multiple spring-loaded needles that was popular during the latter art of the nineteenth century (figure 99). The physician made several punctures after he prepared the skin with a coat of special oil, or "Oleum." The device was intended for use as a counterirritant and was "discovered" in the nineteenth century by a German mechanic, Charles Baunscheidt. He was once bitten on the hand by a gnat and noted that his "rheumatism" improved over the next few hours. He incorporated this finding with the pain relief noted by those using Chinese acupuncture and Perkins Tractors, and came up with the new field of "Baunscheidtism." After Baunscheidt's death, the torch was passed on to John Linden in the United States, who became the Practical Baunscheidtist of Cleveland, Ohio. The Lebenswecker, German for "life awakener," was renamed the "Resuscitator" and was fully described by Linden in his book *Baunscheidtism, or a New Exanthematic Method of Cure* (1874). According to Linden, "This bold instrument is really nothing but a collection of very keenly-pointed needles, designed, by puncturing the skin, (*an almost painless operation*), to create artificial pores, through which all health-destroying morbid matter, accumulated in the afflicted portions of the body in consequence of the arrested activity of the skin, may escape (*by perspiration*) in a natural and simple manner."

Linden began his argument for the use of the Resuscitator in the preface to his book:

Of the old method, in which cupping, bleeding, and the application of leeches, poultices and fomentations, and too often the

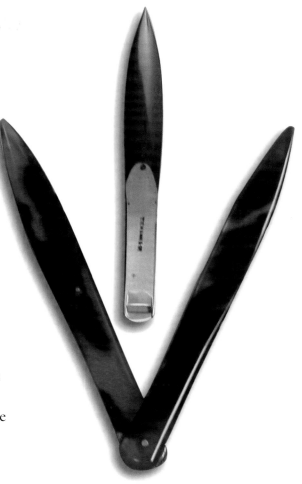

97. Above. Tiemann seton needle (ca 1860)

98. Opposite. Use of the seton needle in *Traité complet de l'anatomie de l'homme* second edition (1866-1871) by JM Bourgery, Claude Bernard, and NH Jacob

frequently poisonous and injurious internal purgatives are the standard remedies, which only scatter, but cannot expel the morbid matter from the system, and too often lay the foundation for the development of new forms of disease, the world is becoming more and more disgusted, since 'Baunscheidtism' offers them the most rational, most simple, and most natural method for the expulsion of morbid matter, in a mechanical manner, from the system. . . . Thousands of the physicians of the old-school could say the same to-day, if they were impelled by nothing but purpose to say the truth; but they take good care not to say it—they continue the 'doctoring,' now as formerly, for this is the most congenial, and pays best.

This remarkable device was promoted as a curative for some of the most devastating diseases of the nineteenth century, including whooping cough, jaundice, epilepsy, paralysis, cholera, pneumonia, cancer, consumption, smallpox, rheumatism, fever, and even "apparent death." Linden went on: "And here especially, does the Resuscitator justify his beautiful name. . . . We remark in a general way, therefore, that in cases of fainting, suffocation, and drowning, the applications must be made over the region of the heart, along the spine, and on the calves of the legs. As soon as it commences to operate, the patient is saved, and although but a single spark of vitality remained in the body, the Resuscitator is sure to fan it into a flame once again."

Without a scientific way to establish death, many people feared inadvertently being buried alive. Linden had the answer with his "life awakener":

And here a remark is in place, which, I trust, will be generally heeded. It relates to the burial of those apparently dead, which barbarity the respective Boards have recently endeavored to prevent, by authoritative orders, that, deceased persons shall not be submitted for burial before three days are past from the hour of their decease . . . let us imagine the unspeakable horror, the indescribable torture and agony of one prematurely buried, and waking into life and consciousness assures him that all efforts to break through his horrid prison are utterly in vain. Although the air contained in the coffin may be sufficient to support life only for two hours, yet the agonies of the poor victim, for whom perhaps dear ones are weeping, but who is kept firmly in his tight coffin and beneath the pressure of more than one thousand pounds of earth, are enough, even during this short time, to outweigh the concentrated sorrows of a lifetime. The invaluable and unsurpassed remedy for preventing, for once and always, the occurrence of this terrible accident, the *Resuscitator* now holds

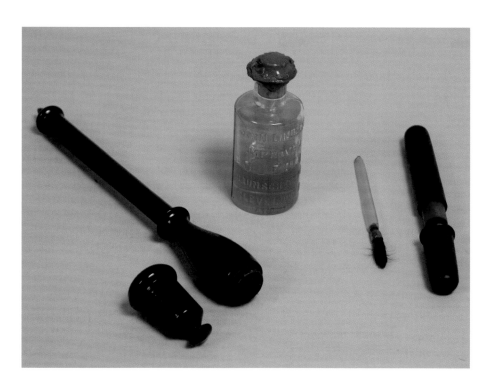

99. Bauncheidt Lebenswecker with oleum and application brush (ca 1870)

forth to mankind . . . if the feeblest spark of life is still lingering, it will be waked-up by the operations, and fanned to a bright flame . . . each citizen in easy circumstances, will, for the reasons already advanced, be unwilling to do without an instrument, that secures him the constant assurance that in no event shall he be buried alive.

It is not surprising that Linden eventually found himself at odds with the medical community. He was portrayed as a huckster selling a worthless cure; the cost for his Resuscitator with Oleum was a rather steep $8. At the same time, Linden's product was copied by others and, ironically, he issued the following warning at the beginning of his text:

> Certain unprincipled persons professing to be agents, representatives, dealers, importers, &c., for the long since deceased C. Baunscheidt, have announced to the public that they have been thus constituted to guard against imposition. But the truth is, that in most cases they deal only in a spurious article (Oleum sealed with a counterfeit signet of C. Baunscheidt,) which they offer and sell for Genuine Oleum; and inasmuch as those parties have had the impudence to copy or imitate my circulars, bills, superscriptions, vignette, directions, &c., and in those very copies or imitations have craftily cautioned the public against me, I am necessitated to state, that the only object those persons have in view, is, to basely deceive the people and prejudice them against me in a most malicious manner. The method of

healing, so benevolent in its results, is brought into disrepute by these representatives and humbugs, and the so frequent complaint of ineffectiveness of the articles sold by them, is disheartening to the suffering and prevents them from making any further trial. I would, therefore, again earnestly warn the public against these humbugs.

The testimonial is an advertising technique still very much in use today, and Linden included many in his text. He attributed amazing results to his device, though certainly more than a few therapeutic successes were secondary to spontaneous recovery and placebo effect:

Big Prairie, Wayne Co., O., Jan 11, 1864

My Dear Mr. J. Linden: — I deem it both a duty and a privilege, to report to you the benefit I received in my own person and family, during a two-years' trial, from the Resuscitator and oil.

Over two years ago, I had a stroke of palsy, which paralyzed my entire left side; my power of speech was so injured, and I could speak only with difficulty. My family physician, from Wooster, Ohio, did all he could for me, but my wretchedness continued to increase. At last, a good friend who was acquainted with the virtues of the Resuscitator, upon hearing of my condition, wrote to me that he believed if he had me in hand, he could help me. I had myself conveyed to him; he applied the Resuscitator thoroughly; and on the fifth day following, I already felt signs of returning vitality to the paralyzed parts. I continued for several months, and am now perfectly cured of my paralysis. Since then I have applied the Resuscitator on several others for similar disorders, and in every case with happy results. I have used it in my family, for deafness, croup, colic, dysentery, diphtheria, &c., with the best success. Toothache and neuralgia have in all cases obediently yielded to the Resuscitator. So highly do I regard this little instrument, that I would not do without it for ten times the cost.

Respectfully yours, &c.,
G. F. Spreng
St. Louis, Mo., December 25, 1873

Dear Mr. Linden: — Having used your Resuscitator already for six months in my family, with good success in different diseases, I will recommend it and you everywhere.

My wife suffered for a whole year from chills and fever, and by the aid of doctors she was almost sent to her grave. The first application was made by Mrs. Pale, and the subsequent ones by me, and, thank God, she is by the help of the instrument, quite well. The application has done myself some good, too, in stopping the spitting of blood and congestion of the brain, with which I am frequently afflicted, every time I apply the instrument to my back and the calves of the leg. The urine takes on a greenish color after each application, and during the night I have twitching in my limbs.

I wish you would instruct me about further treatment of my troubles, and let me know the charges, when I will remit the amount.

Respectfully,
Jacob Jud, Machinist,
No. 1836 N. Second Street, 2nd Floor

"Experience must, indeed, as Hippocrates says in his first aphorism, be fallacious if we decide that a means of treatment, sanctioned by the use of between two and three thousand years, and upheld by the authority of the ablest men of past times, is finally and forever given up. This seems to me to be the most interesting and important question in connection with this subject. Is the relinquishment of bleeding final? or shall we see by and by, or will our successors see, a resumption of the practice? This, I take it, is a very difficult question to answer; and he would be a very bold man who, after looking carefully through the history of the past, would venture to assert that bleeding will not be profitably employed any more."

W. Mitchell Clarke
The British Medical Journal, July 1875

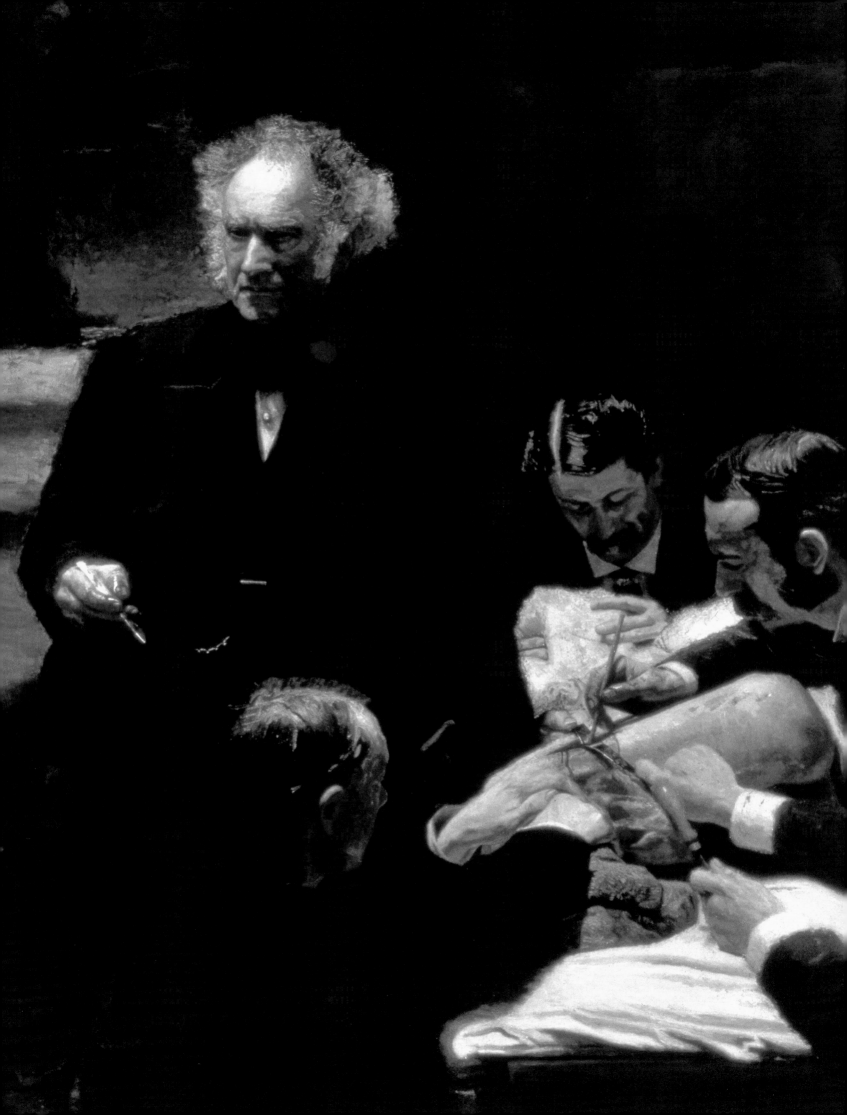

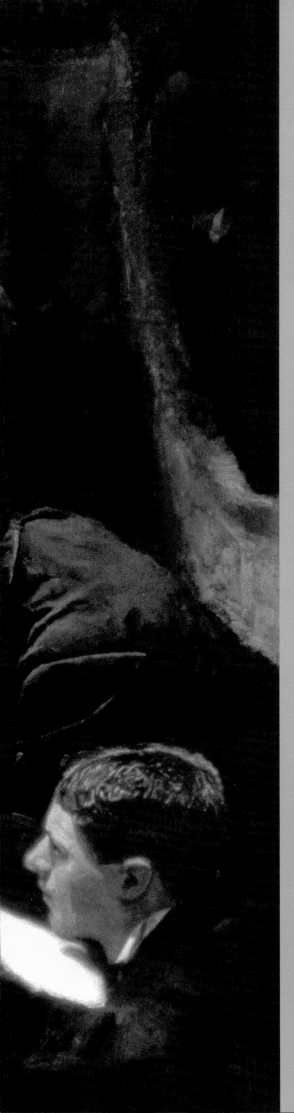

"*He must begin first in youth with good learning and exercise in thys noble arte, he also must be clenly, nimble handed, sharpe sighted, pregnant witted, bolde spirited, clenly apparailed, piteful harted, but not womenly affecionated to wepe or trimble, when he seeth broken bones or bloodies woundes, neither muste he geve place to the cries of his sore patiente, for soft chyrurgians maketh fowle sores. Of the other syde, he maie not plaie the partes of a butcher to cutte, rende or teare the bodie of mannekynde. For although it be fraile, sore, and weake, yet it is the pleasure of God, to cal it his Temple, his instrument, and dwelyng place.*"

William Bullein in *Bullein's Bulwarke Of Defence Againste All Sicknes, Sores, And Woundes* (1579)

Detail, *The Gross Clinic* (1875) by
Thomas Eakins

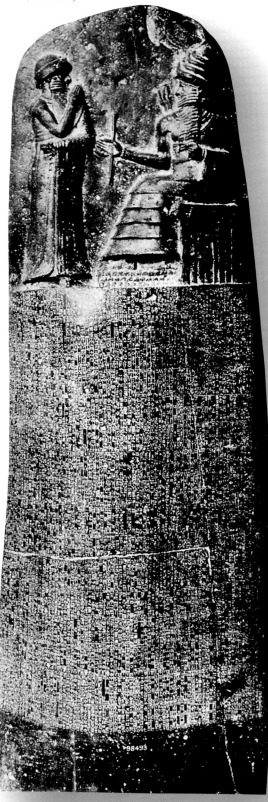

100. The Code of Hammurabi inscribed on black diorite rock (ca. 1780 B.C.)

For thousands of years, those who practiced surgery were perceived more as craftsmen than as professionals, and it was not until the last few hundred years that surgeons were considered "physicians." Western surgical technique had its inception in an area now called Mesopotamia, or the so-called "fertile crescent" between the Tigris and Euphrates rivers, and according to the first written language, cuneiform, priest/physicians were the first to provide medical care in about 3500 B.C.. Hammurabi ruled the Mesopotamian civilization of Babylon from 1792 to 1750 B.C. and was responsible for formulating the first recorded code related to medicine. This now famous Code of Hammurabi is housed at the Louvre in Paris and represents an early effort to form a social structure based on law (figure 100). It comes as no surprise that the first documented referral to medicine in history was written by lawyers, and that the malpractice penalties were quite harsh. They were based on "lex talionis," or the law of retaliation, which included "an eye for an eye, a tooth for a tooth.":

> If a physician shall cause on anyone a severe operation with a bronze operating-knife and cure him, or if he shall open a tumor with a bronze operating-knife and save the eye, he shall have ten shekels of silver; if it is a slave, his owner shall pay two shekels of silver to the physician.
>
> If a physician shall make a severe wound with the bronze operating-knife and kill him, or shall open a growth with a bronze operating-knife and destroy his eye, his hands shall be cut off.
>
> If a physician shall make a severe wound with a bronze operating-knife on the slave of a freed man and kill him, he shall replace the slave with another slave. If he shall open an abscess with a bronze operating-knife and destroy the eye, he shall pay the half of the value of the slave.
>
> If a physician shall heal a broken bone or cure diseased bowels, he shall receive five shekels of silver; if it is a matter of a freed slave, he shall pay three shekels of silver; but if a slave, then the master of the slave shall give to the physician two shekels of silver.

SURGERY IN ANCIENT EGYPT

The earliest written representation of surgery is that found in Egyptian ruins and early papyri. A number of minor procedures are noted there, including the practice of circumcision, which is the first operation ever illustrated and the only surgical procedure mentioned in the Bible (Exodus 4:25) as Moses' wife, Zipporah, "took a sharp stone and cut off

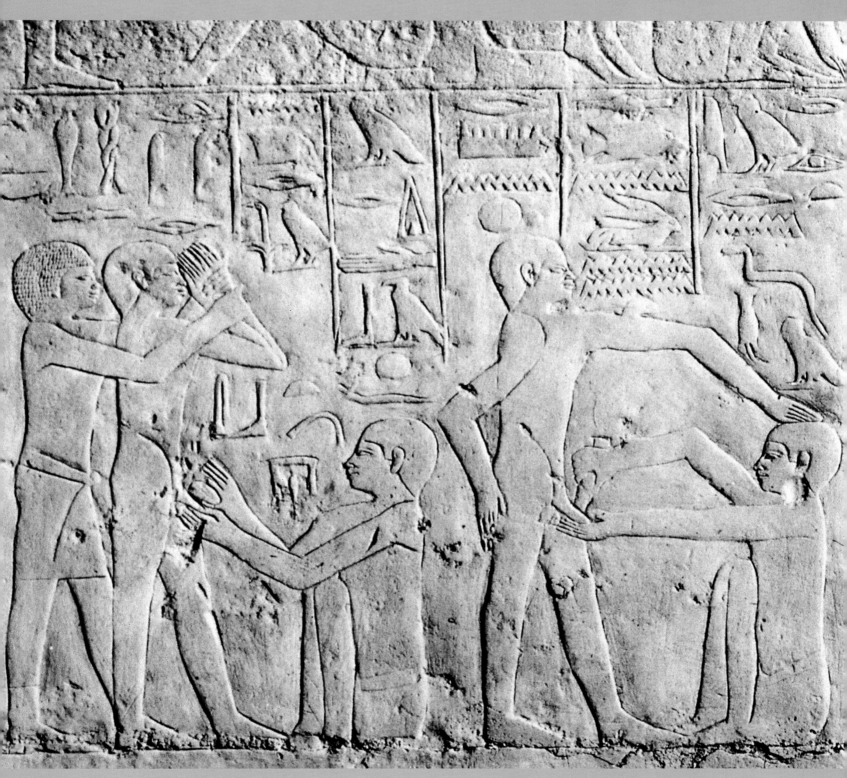

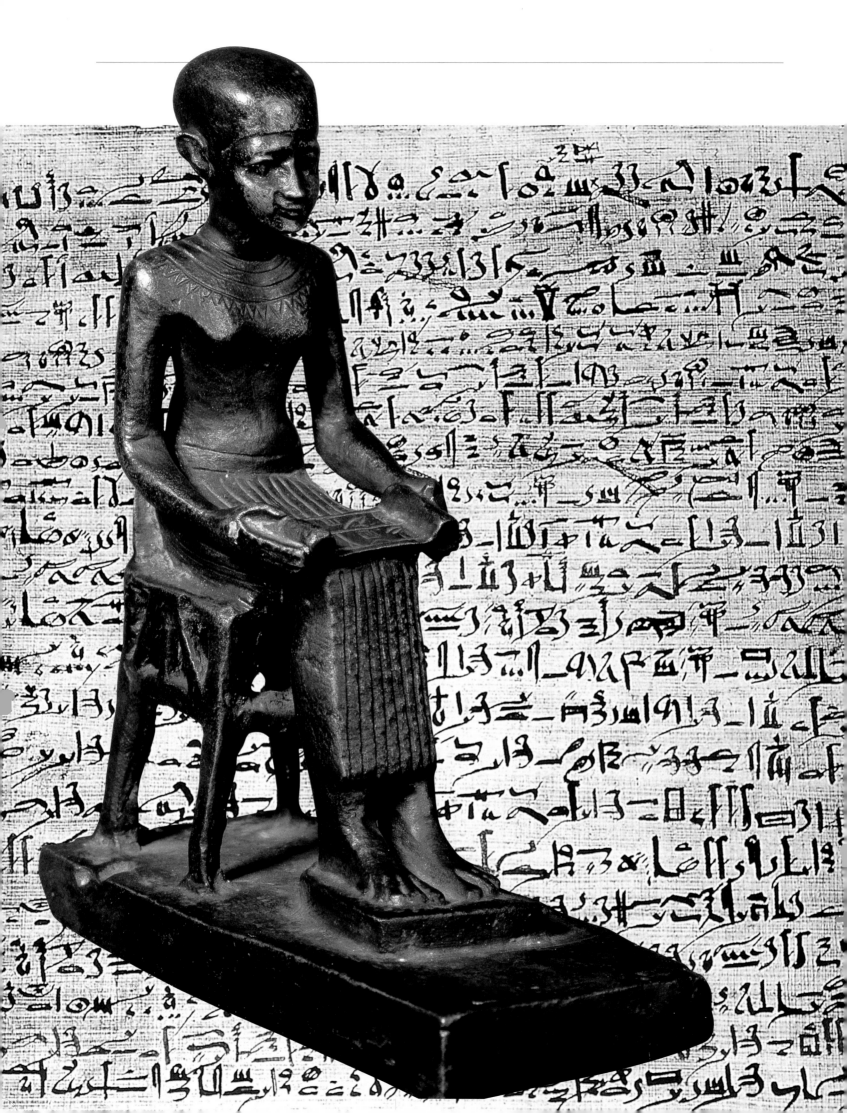

the foreskin of her son" (figure 101). This relief was found in a cemetery in Memphis at the home of Imhotep, grand vizier to King Zoser (2980–2900 B.C.).

Imhotep ("the one who comes in peace") was, according to Sir William Osler, ". . . the first figure of a physician to stand out clearly from the mists of antiquity" (figure 102). In addition to being a physician, Imhotep was a great astronomer, and the architect of the first pyramid, the step pyramid of Saqqara. His influence was enormous and he was worshipped throughout all of Egypt, subsequently being elevated to the status of a god. Imhotep's fame grew so great that he ultimately became the prototype for the Greek and later Roman god of medicine, Aesculapius.

The level of care available to the common Egyptian is unclear, though certainly the elite received specialized medical attention. According to Greek historian Herodotus (fifth century B.C.): "The art of medicine is thus divided among them: Each physician applies himself to one disease only, and not more. All places abound in physicians; some physicians are for the eyes, others for the head, others for the teeth, others for the intestines, and others for internal disorders." For example, the chief physician for a pharaoh of the Sixth Dynasty (2625–2475 B.C.) was Iry, and from his tombstone we learn that he bore the titles of the "palace doctor, superintendent of the court of physicians, palace eye physician, palace physician of the belly and one who understands the internal fluids and who is guardian of the anus."

Several papyri have survived, though the most important from a medical standpoint are those discovered by Smith and Ebers, which were written between the seventeenth and sixteenth centuries B.C.. Georg Ebers (1837–1898) was a German professor of history whose discovery is the oldest yet found and dates to approximately 1550 B.C.. In addition to the description of surgical procedures and medical conditions, it describes diseases of the eye, skin, and conditions particular to women. The religious and supernatural were important components of Egyptian medical care, and a physician discussed not only the diagnosis and treatment of each case, but he also included a prognosis. The outlook was good if the physician "will treat" it, the condition uncertain if he "will combat" it, and hopeless if he "will not treat" it:

> When thou comest upon a tumor of the flesh in any part of the
> body of a person and thou dost find it like skin on his flesh; it is

102. (Overprint) Twenty-sixth dynasty bronze statuette of Imhotep, Egyptian god of medicine (664–525 B.C.)

103. (Overprint) Edwin Smith surgical papyrus (ca. 1600 B.C.), cases 9–12

104. Relief of Egyptian surgical instruments inscribed on the wall of the outer corridor of the Temple of Sobek and Horus built by Ptolemy VII, Kom Ombo, Egypt (181–146 B.C.).

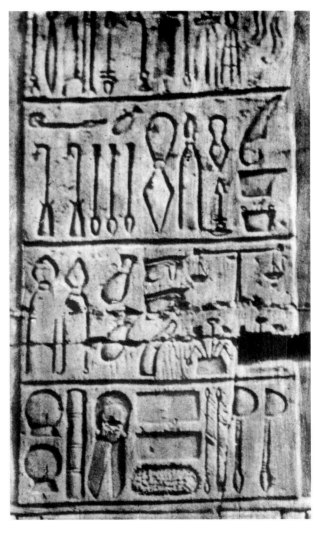

moist; it moves under thy fingers save when thy fingers are held still, then its movement is caused by thy fingers. So shalt thou say 'It is a tumor of the flesh, I will treat the disease since I will try to cure it with fire, as the metal-worker cures.'

When thou findest a purulent swelling with the apex elevated, sharpley defined and of a rounded form, then sayest thou, 'It is a purulent tumor which is growing in the flesh. I must treat the disease with a knife.'

When thou meetest a large tumor of the God Xensu in any part of the limb of a person, it is loathsome and suffers many pustules to come forth; something arises therein as though wind were in it, causing irritation. The tumor calls with a loud voice to thee: 'Is it not like the most loathsome of pustules?' It mottles the skin and makes figures. All the limbs are like those which are affected. Then say thou: 'It is a tumor of the God Xensu. Do thou nothing there against.'

In 1862, American Egyptologist Edwin Smith (1822–1906) discovered probably the most important Egyptian medical document yet found. The Smith papyrus was written in about 1600 B.C. and reflects medicine as practiced as far back as the thirtieth century B.C. (figure 103).

105. Aeneas (between Venus and Ascanius) being treated by a physician, first-century fresco from the Casa di Sirico, Pompeii

106. Second-century Roman surgical instruments: scoops, probes, scalpel, and tweezers

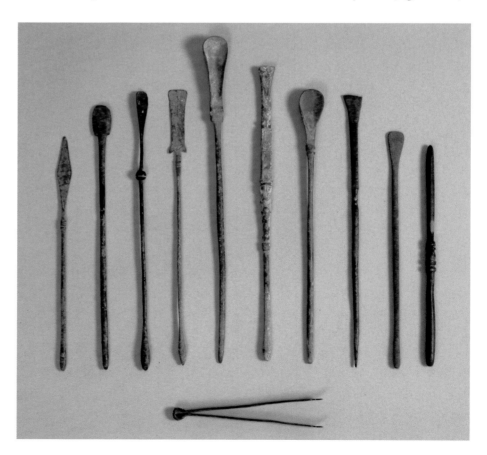

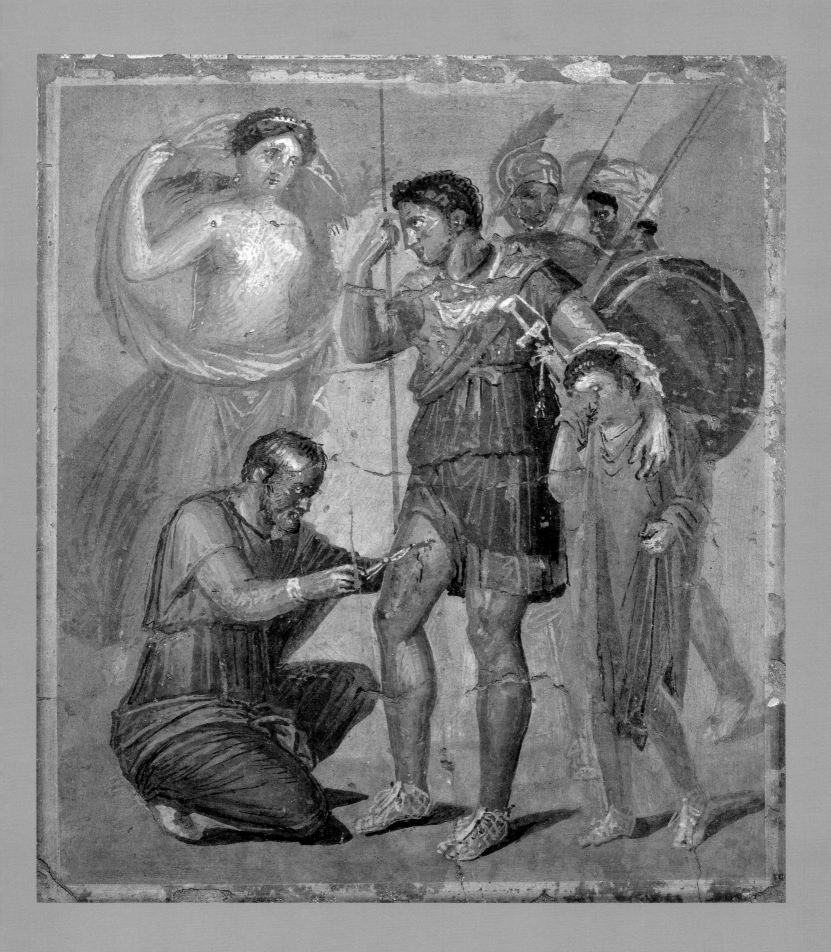

107. Below. Roman bronze scalpel (ca. 200 B.C.)

108. Surgical instruments in *Altasrif* (thirteenth-century Latin translation) by Albucasis

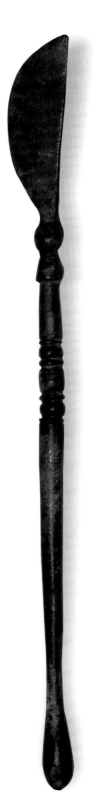

Smith discovered the manuscript in Thebes in 1862, and J.H. Breasted translated it in 1930. The papyrus contains text on both sides of a fifteen-foot roll and is made up of forty-eight individual surgical cases describing examinations, diagnoses, and methods of therapy. Some postulate the author to be Imhotep, and the treatment recounted was both conservative and thoughtful. Reliefs of instruments used by ancient Egyptians can currently be seen inscribed at Kom Ombo, Egypt (figure 104).

ROME

There is little information available regarding surgery during the high point of the Roman Empire. Initial distain for Greek physicians gave way to admiration and, by the end of the third century B.C., Greek physicians were at the center of Roman medical care both in the aristocracy and on the battlefield (figure 105). Though many Greeks were slaves, Julius Caesar offered citizenship to all "free born" Greek physicians and surgeons. The same craftsmen who made armor for soldiers in battle produced surgical instruments to treat their wounds, though as medical care spread to wealthier sectors of the population, more refined instruments were made of bronze and silver (figures 106–107).

Galen (A.D. 120–200) was the most important and influential physician of the Greco-Roman period, and his writings remained popular into the seventeenth century. His interest spanned the breadth of medicine and pharmacology, though the first printed edition of his works did not appear until 1525. Galen gave us insight into the types of procedures available to him when he defined the scope of surgical intervention: "All the operations in surgery fall under two heads, separation and approximation. Approximation has to do with the reduction and dressing of fractures, reduction of dislocation of the joints, reductions of prolapsed intestines, uterus, or rectum, sutures of the abdomen and restoration of tissue deficiencies, as in the nose, lips, and ears. Division is concerned with simple incisions, circumcisions, elevations of the skin, scalping, excisions of veins, amputation, cauterization, scraping, smoothing, excisions with the saw."

As the Roman Empire declined, so did progress in medicine and surgery. Unfortunately, surgical intervention of any kind was accompanied by a significant risk to the patient, so physicians sometimes required guarantees of safety (for themselves) before providing their services. This was certainly necessary in the sixth century since Theodoric (A.D. 454–526), king of the Ostrogoths, allowed the surviving relatives of those patients experiencing a bad outcome the right to determine the fate of the treating physician. In A.D. 580, Gutram, the king of Burgandy, had two surgeons executed on the tomb of his queen after their unsuccessful operation on her plague sores and, in 1464, the pun-

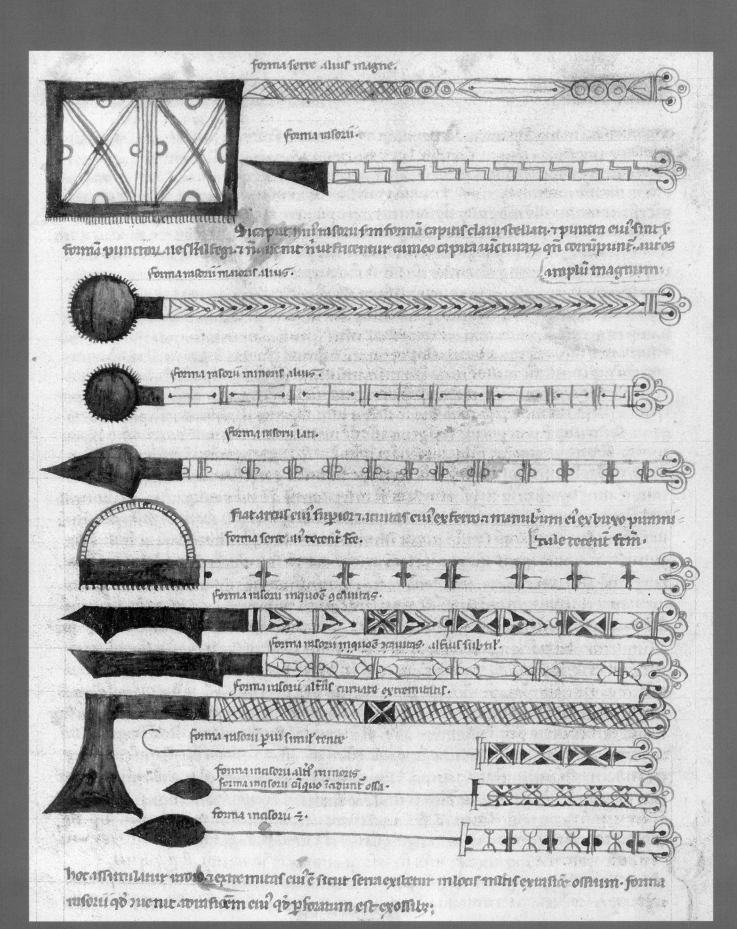

forma serre alius magne.

forma rasoru.

forma rasoru minoris alius.

forma rasoru minoris alius.

forma rasoru lati.

forma serre ut recenti fee.

forma rasoru inquot gechutas.

forma rasoru inquot acuitas. altius subtil.

forma rasoru altius curuate extremitas.

forma rasoru pui simil rente

forma rasoru altii minoris.
forma rasoru aliquo radunt ossa.

forma rasoru 4.

ishment was death to the surgeon who was unable to remove an arrow from the king of Hungary. Pope John XII burned an unsuccessful surgeon in Florence and, following the pope's death, the surgeon who failed to keep him alive was whipped.

MIDDLE EASTERN SURGERY

The center of all knowledge in the ancient world was at the library in Alexandria, Egypt. With its destruction in A.D. 640, Arab clerics became the guardians of medical thinking, retaining that responsibility for centuries. Greek medicine was translated into Arabic and Hebrew, and few medical advances were made in the Christian Roman Empire for hundreds of years because of recurrent barbarian invasions and rigid religious control. Ibn Sina (Avicenna) (980–1037) practiced in Baghdad and wrote what became the basis of medical care for six centuries, the *Canon of Medicine*. His *Canon* was a summary of Galen's approach to medicine with concerns regarding church dogma impeding a more scientific approach to learning by observation. Surgeons remained separated from the fraternity of physicians for many centuries and were not considered to be a part of mainstream medicine until barber-surgeons were readmitted to the medical community in the sixteenth century.

Al-Zahrawi (Albucasis) (936–1013) was a surgeon of Spanish and Arab descent, and became a major figure in the history of medicine with his comprehensive and systematic review of surgery, the *Altasrif*. It was referred to by physicians for hundreds of years and was translated into Latin, providing the basis for all future European surgical writings. Albucasis carefully and thoughtfully described more than fifty surgical procedures, including bloodletting, urinary diversion into the rectum, reduction mammoplasty, tracheotomy, craniotomy, and lithotomy. The *Altasrif* contained early instruction in midwifery along with the first illustrations of surgical instruments in printed form (figure 108).

FROM BARBER-SURGEONS TO PATRON SAINTS

Cosmas and Damian were prominent Arab twins who converted to Christianity and traveled about Persia, freely giving their medical services to the needy. The brothers were, however, tortured and beheaded during the reign of Emperor Diocletian (A.D. 303), though they subsequently became the patron saints of barber-surgeons as the legends of their medical and surgical accomplishments grew in time. They became famous following their legendary transplantation of the leg of a Moor (figure 109). It seems that a Christian Roman deacon, Justinian, had a malignant growth on his leg and fell asleep while praying for a cure in the

109. Saints Cosmas and Damian performing the miraculous transplantation of a leg (late sixteenth century) by Ambrosius Francken

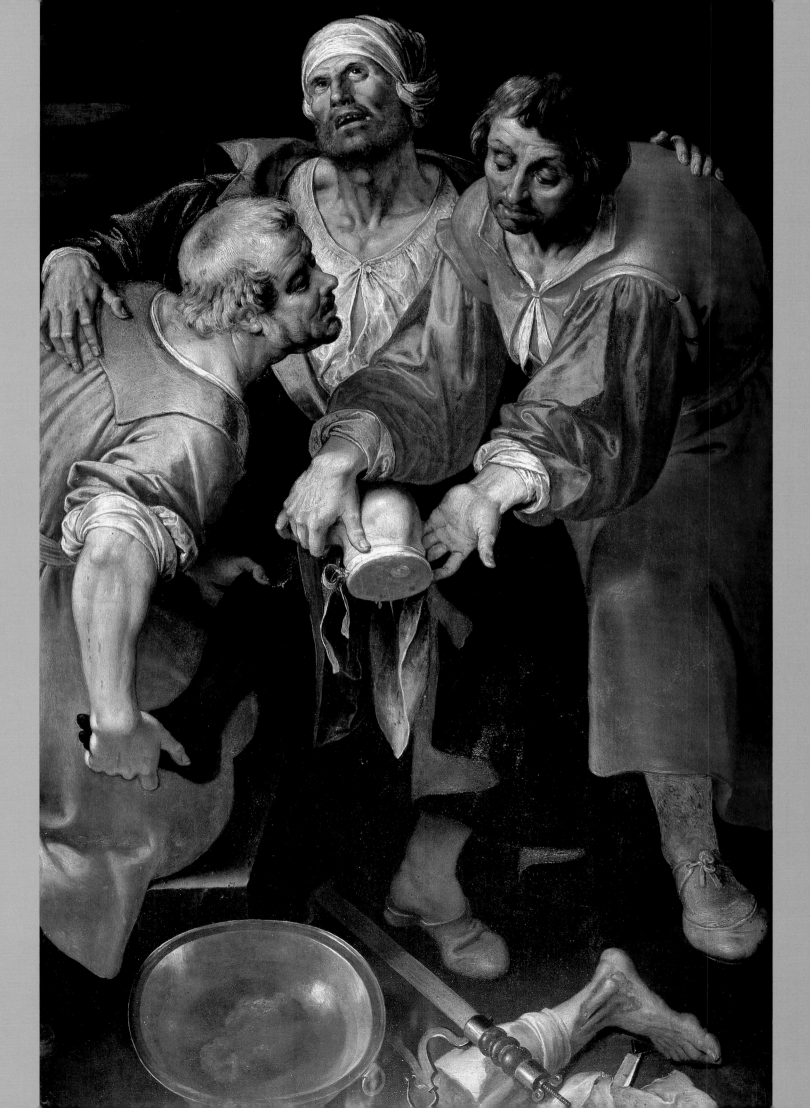

Church of Cosmas and Damian in Rome. In his dreams, the saints amputated the diseased limb and transplanted the leg of a Moor who had been brought to the church for burial. The patient awoke and gratefully observed a now healthy leg, though black in color.

Animism, the belief that evil spirits are the cause of disease and a punishment for sinful behavior, was popular for centuries. Early medical care, therefore, frequently took place in a religious setting, and prayer was an important part of any treatment. Monks and others in monasteries offered various forms of therapy, though gratefully delegated minor surgical procedures to barbers who visited to trim their beards (since monks were required to be clean-shaven after the decree of 1092). Eventually, barbers became responsible for such procedures as dental extraction, lancing boils, fracture repair, and occasionally the removal of bladder stones (figure 110). They were looked down on as only technicians and not part of the medical community. Over the years, friction developed between barber-surgeons, physicians who prescribed medications, and those who did more extensive surgery including amputations. In 1210, the first guild of surgeons was organized in Paris containing the "surgeons of the long robe" composed of trained barber-surgeons and "surgeons of the short robe" who performed only minor procedures. In 1255, Jean Pitard founded the Confraternity of Sts. Cosmas and Damian, an organization in Paris that drew together all French surgeons in order to protect them from the increasing activities of Parisian barbers, who traditionally performed shaving, haircutting, bleeding, cupping, the lancing of boils, and tooth extraction. Members of the Confraternity of St. Côme competed with barber-surgeons throughout the fourteenth century, Philip IV allowing members of the Confraternity to become "masters of surgery" only after having passed an examination. In 1372, Charles V authorized a special charter for barber-surgeons (with encouragement to do so by his personal barber).

The two organizations clashed for the next two hundred years, the real prize coveted by both groups being recognition by the faculty of the University of Paris. Since the faculty felt more threatened by the self-importance of the Confraternity, members contracted with the barber-surgeons in 1505 for the promise of annual dues, along with a limit on the extent of their procedures to only minor surgery under faculty supervision. The next shot was fired by the Confraternity when Francis I granted them university privileges in 1544, and they were allowed to become "surgeons of the long robe." This competition was ultimately counterproductive regarding surgical progress in France since the surgeons of St. Côme refused to document their surgical procedures for fear that this might be of assistance to their rivals, the barber-surgeons. A status symbol revered by both groups of physicians was the type of shaving/bleeding bowl that hung on the physician's door; the barber-surgeon had one of pewter, while that of the surgeon was brass.

A letter written by Guy Patin (1601–1672), dean of the Paris medical faculty, summed up his view of the bitter controversy between medical groups in the seventeenth century, which he felt was largely economic:

> We are now at odds with our barber-surgeons who wish to unite with the surgeons of St. Cosmas, our ancient enemies. Those of St. Cosmas are miserable rascals, nearly all tooth-pullers and very ignorant who have attached the barber-surgeons to their string, by making them share their halls and their pretended privileges. . . . (These surgeons of St. Cosmas) would produce for us doctors ignorant of Latin who would not know even how to read and write. We do not attempt to obstruct their being surgeons of St. Cosmas or that others unite with them. But we would only have a company of barber-surgeons, as we have had until now, which would be dependent on our Faculty, and would take every year an oath of fidelity in our schools before the Dean . . . and pay us every year a certain sum for the rights which we have in their functions. . . .

Fistula-in-ano, or a connection between the rectum and bladder, was a painful condition long suffered by French King Louis XIV which resulted in the uncontrollable discharge of stool and urine. There were several causes for this common condition, including the extended time many spent on horseback, the prolonged labor experienced by many women during delivery, and in the king's case, the frequent enemas ordered by royalty and members of the court. A special knife was constructed for the royal surgery and, in 1686, Louis XIV's surgeon, Charles-François Fèlix, cured him of this condition (after practicing on anuses of the peasantry, unfortunately with a number of fatalities). Only one month after surgery, the king proudly displayed the success of his operation by marching about his palace at Versailles. Louis XIV rewarded Fèlix with 300,000 livres, an estate, and political power, which the physician then used to unify the French surgical community, finally elevating it to a legitimate branch of medicine. France subsequently became a center for surgery with the establishment of the Academié Royale de Chirurgie in 1731.

In London, surgery was also looked on as an unfit profession for a gentleman, though with the spread of untrained surgeons, "barbers exercising the faculty of surgery" were first admitted to the Guild of Surgeons in London in 1368. The Guild of Barbers had existed since the early fourteenth century, and while some barbers were allowed to perform surgical procedures, surgeons could not be barbers. Surgery was also regarded as a trade there, and the first act to regulate the perform-

110 . Following page. *The Surgeon*, oil painting on canvas by David Teniers the Younger (1610–1690)

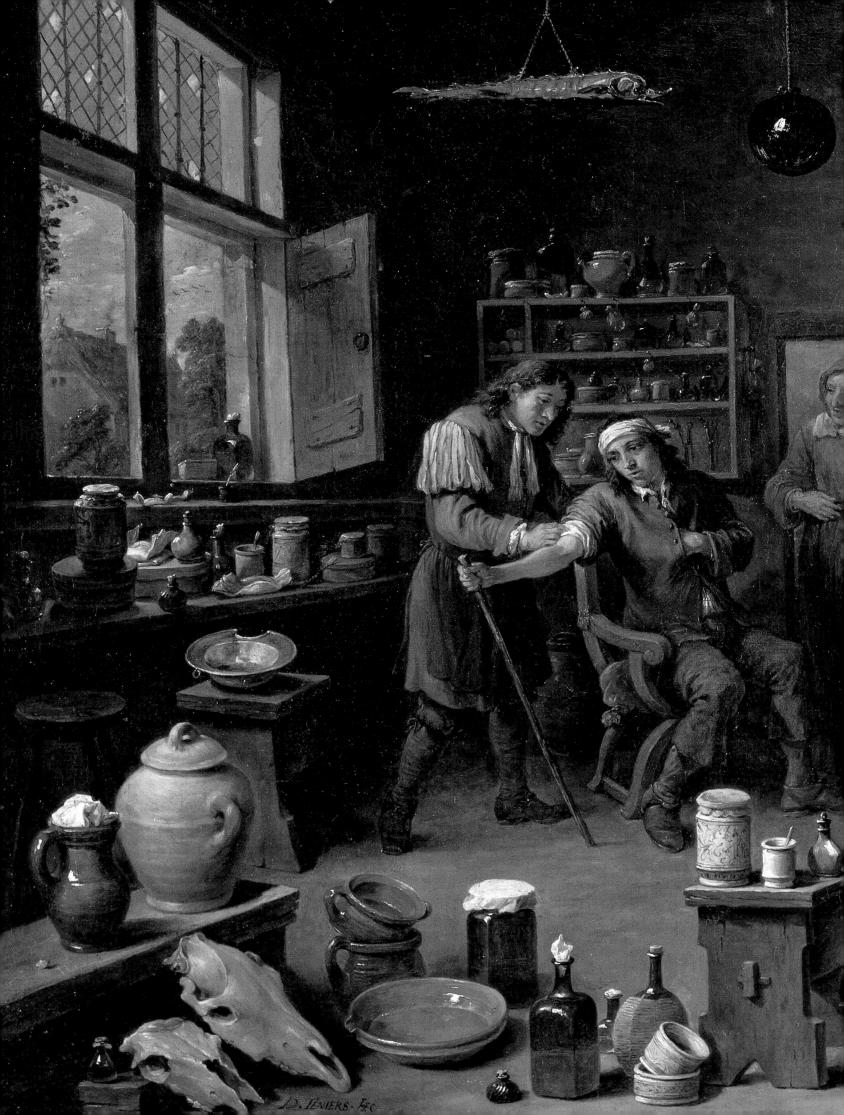

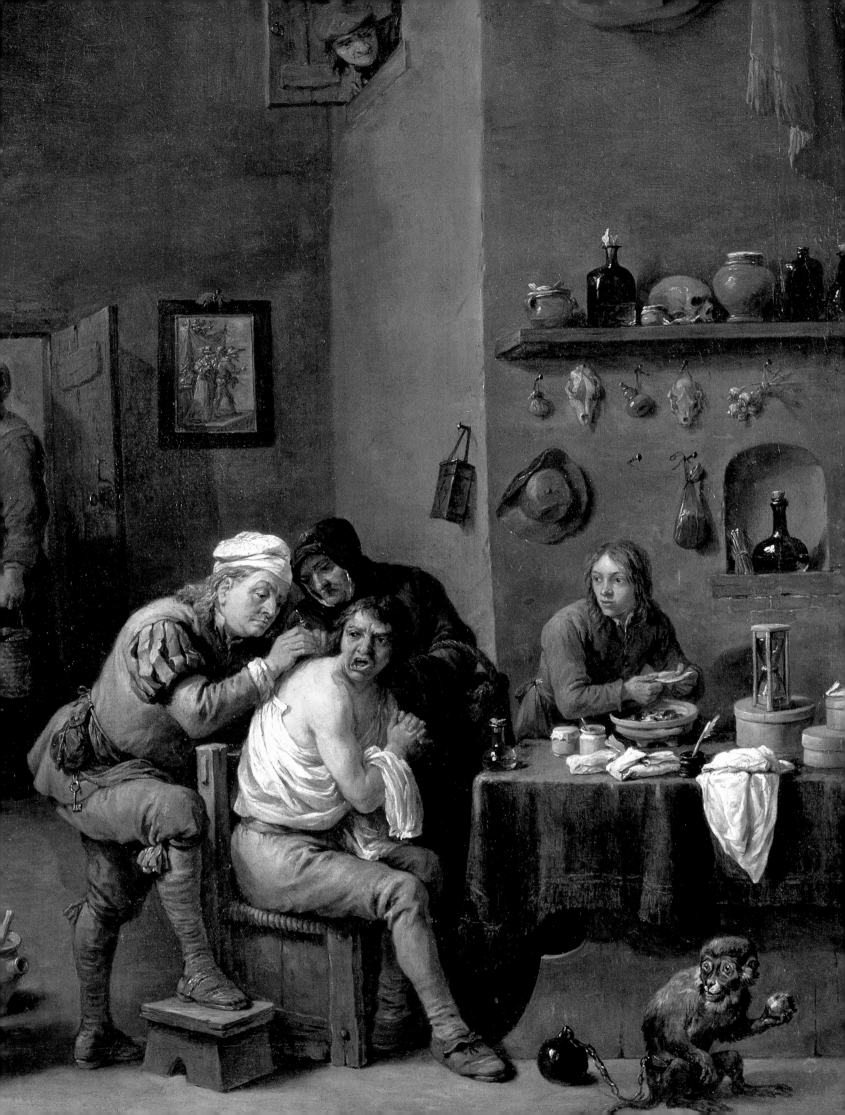

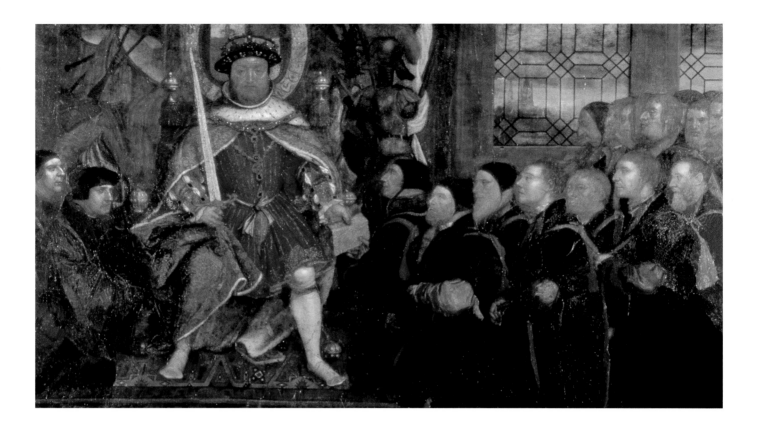

III. Henry VIII handing the *Act of Union* to Thomas Vicary, uniting barbers and surgeons, oil painting by Hans Holbein the Younger (1541)

ance of procedures was passed in 1421 (with no women allowed). An act of Parliament in 1512 required that those practicing medicine within a seven-mile radius of London had to pass an examination given by the Bishop of London or the Dean of St. Paul's Church. The line between medicine and surgery was sometimes blurred, though in London in 1519, a court petition by the warden of the Guild of Surgeons provided clarification: "In manuall application of medicines: in staunching of blod, serchying of woundes with irons and with other instruments, in cutting of the sculle in due proporcyon to the pellicules of the brayne with instruments of iron, cowchyng of catharactes, takyng owt bonys, sowyng of the flesshe, launchung of bocchis, cuttyng of apostumes, burnyng of cankers and other lyke, settyng in of joyntes and byndyng of theym with ligatures, lettyng of blod, drawyng of tethe. . . ."

Licensed physicians became more and more concerned about the increased activity of "untrained" barber-surgeons as well as the growing number of quacks practicing surgery. As in France, physicians wore long robes and left minor procedures to short-robed surgeons who often traveled from one county to the next, performing fracture repair, bleeding, dental extraction, and occasionally the removal of bladder stones. Throughout the early part of the sixteenth century, the situation remained more confusing since licensing authorities in London included the Guilds of Military Surgeons and Barber-Surgeons, universities, and the bishop.

In 1540, Henry VIII united the two guilds, allowing barbers to add only dental surgery to their usual trade. Hans Holbein the Younger memorialized the union between the barbers and surgeons of London the following year as Henry VIII is seen handing the proclamation declaring that union to Thomas Vicary, who himself had been "a meane practiser in Maidstone until the King advanced him for curing his sore legge" (figure 111). The situation largely remained unresolved, however, and several years later William Clowes (1540–1604) of St. Bartholomew's Hospital, a surgeon who practiced under Elizabeth I, remarked: "Nowadays it is apparent to see how tinkers, tooth-drawers, pedlars, ostlers, carters, porters, horse-gelders and horse-leeches, idiots, apple-squires, broom-men, bawds, witches, conjurers, sooth-sayers and sow-gelders, rogues, rat-catchers, runagates, and proctors of spital-houses, with such rotten and stinking weeds, which do in town and country, without order, honesty and skill daily abuse both Physic and Chirurgery, having no more perseverance, reason or knowledge in this art than hath a goose."

British surgeons continued to suffer prejudice for another century, and, in 1745, the Company of Surgeons separated from the barbers. The continuing controversy is alluded to by an act passed by the Royal College of Physicians of Edinburgh on May 17, 1765—"An act was passed declaring that for the future no person should be admitted to be one of the Fellows, 'whose common business it is either to practice Surgery in general, or Midwifery, Lithotomy, Inoculation, or any other branch of it in particular; and further, that if any Member of the College shall, after his being received as a Fellow, practise any of these lower acts in the manner above-mentioned, and shall thereof be lawfully convicted, he shall be degraded from the honor conferred a Fellow, and his name shall be struck out of the Roll." To this day, British physicians are addressed as "doctor," though after they have received further specialized training in surgery are once again, ironically, referred to as "mister" as a sign of distinction.

The Royal College of Surgery was established in 1800, finally bringing order to the profession after hundreds of years of bickering.

SURGERY BECOMES A PROFESSION

Ambroise Paré (1510–1590) is considered by many to be the first great modern surgeon, and he was responsible for raising his profession in France from a level of scorn and ridicule to one of admiration and esteem. He was the son of a barber-surgeon and was thereby exposed at an early age to minor surgical procedures performed by those without a formal medical background. Paré gives us an insight into his early training (and to his sensitive nature) with this story: "I entered a stable, thinking to lodge my horse and that of my man, where I found four dead soldiers and three who were propped against the wall, their faces wholly disfigured, and they neither saw, nor heard, nor spoke, and their clothes yet flaming from the gunpowder, which had burnt them. Beholding them with pity, there came an old soldier who asked me if there was any way of curing them. I told him no. At once he approached them and cut their throats gently and without anger. Seeing this great cruelty, I said to him that he was an evil man. He answered me that he prayed to God that when he should be in such a case, he might find some one who would do the same for him, to the end that he might not languish miserably."

Despite the fact that barber-surgeons were making political advances at the time, they were still looked down on by the community of university-trained physicians. As a result of his keen power of observation and unusual deductive reasoning, Paré developed a practical approach to surgery and became the surgeon to four kings (Henri II, Francis II, Charles IX, and Henri III). His technique was "hands on" and was illustrated in this response to critical remarks made by one of his professors, Etienne Gourmélon: "How dare you teach me surgery, you who have done nothing all your life but look at books! Surgery is learnt with the hand and the eye. And you—mon petit maître—all you know is how to talk your head off, sitting comfortably in your chair." On another occasion, Paré reiterated the importance of experience when he said (in an early translation): "Thou shalt fare more easily and happily attaine to the knowledge of these things by long use and much exercise, than by much reading of Bookes, or daily hearing of Teachers. For speech how perspicuous and elegant soever it be, cannot so vively express any thing, as that which is subjected to the faithfull eyes and hands."

Ambroise Paré gained a wealth of experience and was able to try new surgical techniques because of his service with the French military. In the introduction to his surgical writings, Paré gave his view on the role of a surgeon: "Chyrurgerie is an Art, which teacheth the way by reason, how by the operation of the hand we may cure, prevent, and mitigate disease, which accidentally happen to us. Others have thought good to describe it otherwise, as that; it is the part of Physicke which undertaketh the cure of diseases by the sole industry of the hand; as by cutting, burning, sawing off, uniting fractures, restoring dislocations, and performing other workes, of which we shall hereafter treate." Paré's famous response to a soldier after having saved his life also appears on Paré's tombstone as "Je le pansay. Dieu le guérit" or "I treated him, God healed him."

John Hunter (1728–1793) was a British anatomist and pathophysiologist, and became the leading surgeon of the eighteenth century. John Abernathy, one of Hunter's pupils, remarked: "Those who far precede others must remain alone; and their actions often appear unaccountable, nay, even extravagant, to their distant followers, who know not the causes that give rise to them, or the effects that they were designed to produce. In such a situation stood John Hunter in relation to his contemporaries. It was a comfortless precedence, for it deprived him of sympathy and social cooperation." Hunter was not merely interested in surgical technique, but he transformed surgery into a science, establishing the discipline of surgical experimentation. With his innovations, John Hunter placed surgery on an equal footing with all other branches of medicine.

AMPUTATION

Prior to the aseptic era, by far the most commonly performed major surgical procedure was an amputation, which was also one of the earliest operations depicted in medical literature. Even with great speed and precision on the part of the surgeon, however, the operative mortality was up to forty percent, and much higher with underlying infection.

Famous German surgeon Hans von Gersdorff (ca. 1480–1540) gave this advice to physicians prior to an amputation: "You should advise the patient above all to go to confession and receive the Holy Sacrament. . . ." Once a limb became infected, physicians were relatively helpless short of amputation, though some relied on a bizarre concoction of ingredients, such as those found in the seventeenth-century "wound salve" of Sir Kenelm Digby: earth worms, pig brain, and powdered mummy. To be effective, however, the salve had to be applied to the wound and to the weapon that caused it.

In the illustration by von Gersdorff, note that the physician was using his left hand as a tourniquet to both reduce bleeding and to compress the nerves for pain control (figure 112). The man on the right of the illustration was wearing a "T", which likely indicates that he suffered from St. Anthony's Fire, a Group A streptococcal infection common at the time. Throughout the Middle Ages, St. Anthony's Fire was often confused with ergotism, a condition that resulted from eating rye infected with the fungus *Claviceps purpurea*. The resultant peripheral vasoconstriction caused a syndrome similar to erysipelas that included vomiting, diarrhea, itching, rash, and sometimes gangrene with a loss of life should one not remove the affected limb. This disorder also had religious connotations because of a similarity between Hell and the burning symptoms it caused. St. Anthony (A.D. 251–356) had lived as a hermit in Egypt until he was fifty-four years old when he founded a monastery. About two hundred years after his death, St. Anthony's bones were retrieved and sent to France where they were purportedly effective in curing patients with ergotism.

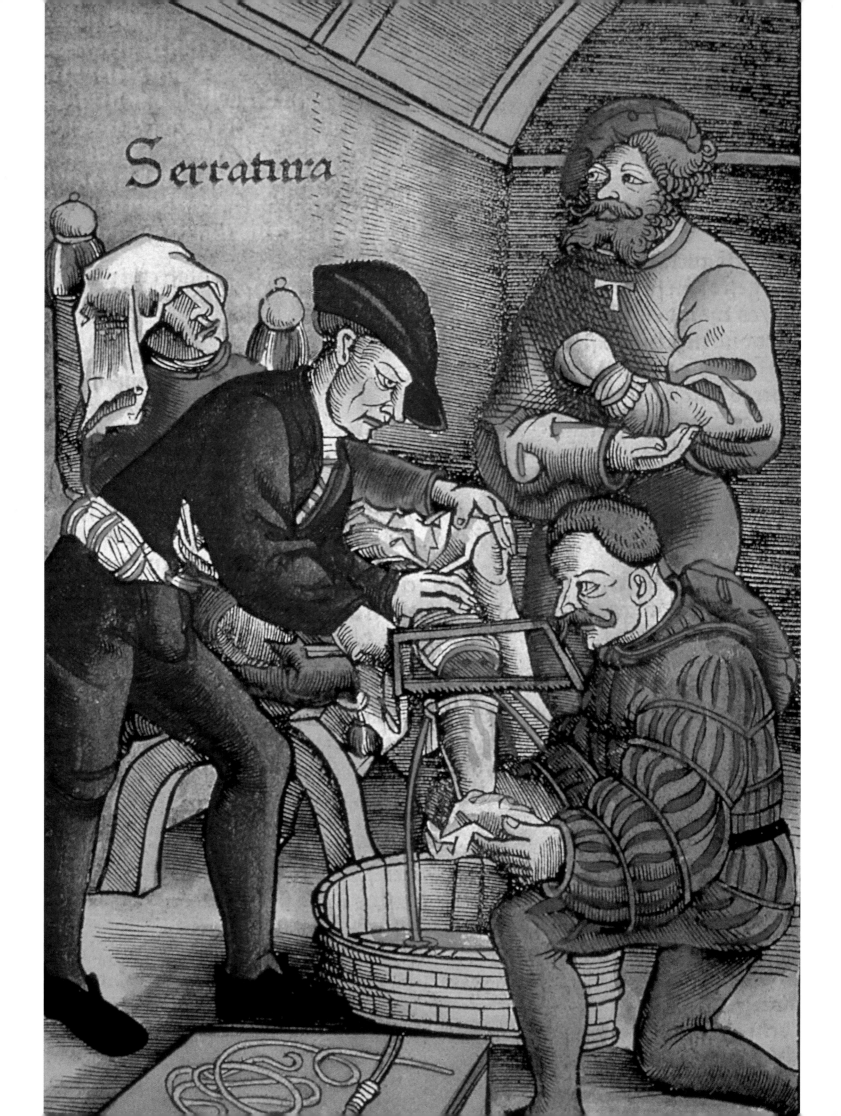

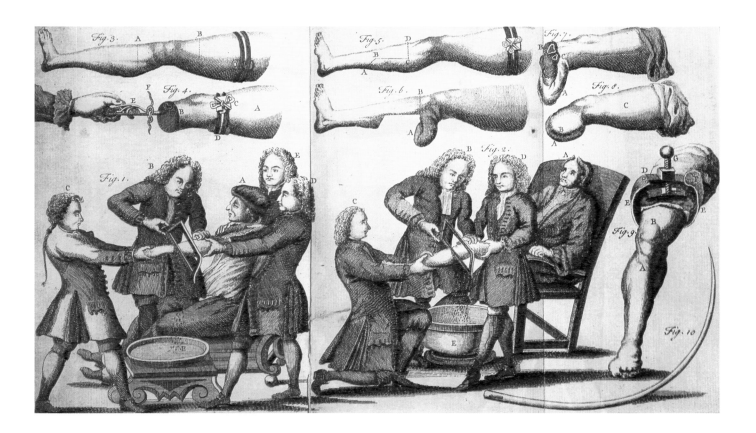

Ambroise Paré described the signs that justified amputation, along with an early description of phantom pain, in his *Apologie Et Voyages* (1585):

You shall certainly know that a Gangrene is turned into a Sphacell, or mortification, and that the part is wholly and thoroughly dead, if it looke of a blacke colour, and bee colder than stone to your touch, the cause of which coldnesse is not occasioned by the frigiditie of the aire; if there bee a great softnesse of the part, so that if you presse it with your finger it rises not againe, but retaines the print of the impression. If the skinne come from the flesh lying under it; if so great and strong a smell exhale (especially in an ulcerated Sphacell) that the standers by cannot endure or suffer it; if a sanious moisture, viscide, greene or blackish flow from thence; if it bee quite destitute of sense and motion, whether it be pulled, beaten, crushed, pricked, burnt, or cut off. Here I must admonish the young Chirurgion, that hee be not deceived concerning the losse or privation of the sense of the part.

For I know very many deceived as thus; the patients pricked on that part would say they feel much paine there. But that feeling is often deceiptful, as that which proceeds rather from the strong apprehension of great paine which formerly reigned in the part, than from any facultie of feeling as yet remaining. A

112. Opposite. Amputation in *Feldbüch der Wundartzney* (1497) by Hans von Gersdorff

113. Amputation in *A General System of Surgery* (1743) by Laurence Heister

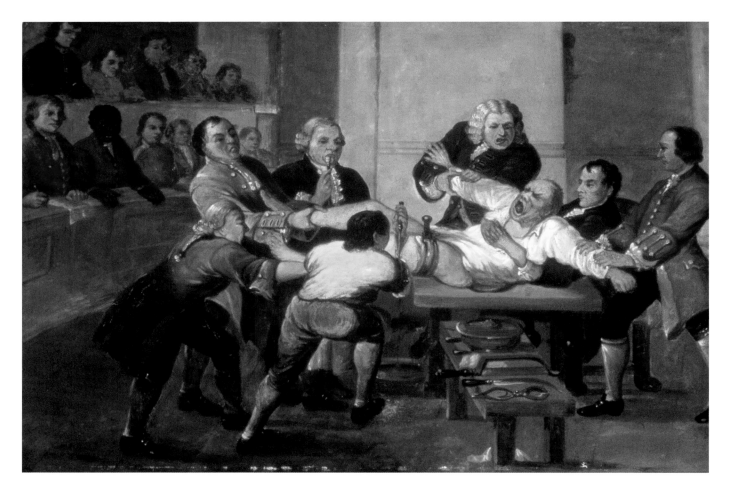

114. Mid nineteenth-century amputation, oil on board by an unknown artist

most cleare and manifest argument of this false and deceitful sense appears after the amputation of the member; for a long while after they will complaine of the part which is cut away.

Verily it is a thing wondrous strange and prodigious, and which will scarse be credited, unlesse by such as have seene with their eyes, and heard with their eares the patients who have many moneths after the cutting away of the Legge, grievously complained that they yet felt exceeding great paine of that Leg so cut off. Wherefore have a speciall care least this hinder your intended amputation; a thing pittifull, yet absolutely necessary for to preserve the life of the patient and all the rest of his body, by cutting away of that member which hath all the signes of a Sphacell and perfect mortification; for otherwise the neglected fire will in a moment spread over all the body, and take away all hope of remedy. . . .

The removal of a limb was the last surgical resort, and the most dramatic surgical procedure prior to the discovery of anesthesia in the middle of the nineteenth century (figures 113, 114). The pain and fear must have been beyond description, and patients often had to be held down by several assistants. There were two ways to perform an amputation, the earliest technique being the circular variety first described by Aulus Cornelius Celsus (25 B.C.–A.D. 50):

> When the malady gets the better of our medications the limb must be amputated . . . but one remedy, expediency and not safety, is the paramount consideration. We are therefore to make an incision with a knife between the sound and morbid parts down to the bone, with this qualification, that we are never to cut opposite a joint and always to include some of the sound part rather than leave any of that which is diseased. When we come to the bone the sound flesh must be retracted so as in some measure to denude it; then it must be divided with the saw close up to the sound flesh. The end of the bone is then to be smoothed where the saw has left any asperity and the integuments brought over it, which in this operation, ought to be left loose enough to cover the entire stump as far as possible.

Dutch physician Hermann Boerhaave (1668–1738) gave a later and more complete description how to perform a circular amputation in *Boerhaave's Aphorisms Concerning the Knowledge and Cure of Diseases* (1715): The preparation is accomplished

1. By a Compression of the large blood Arteries, by means of pyramidal Bolsters, and by twisting the Ligature to be placed over them on the Sound part near the Diseased.

2. By drawing the Muscles of the Part strongly and equally by means of a Leather Bandage, made with Loops and Strings to pull by.

3. By keeping the whole body of the Patient, and the part to be amputated very steady.

4. Bending gently the part, that the Muscles may hang loose, and may not be cut beyond the place of Extirpation.

5. Giving a cordial sleeping Draught to the Patient sometime before the Operation.

The Operation is perform'd after this foregoing Preparation.

1. With a sharp, strong, crooked Knife, obtuse on the Back, well temper'd, which is thrust under the Leg, and remounting by the Inside till it comes to the place where the Operator began, which makes a circular Incision, cutting all the Flesh to the very Bones, not forgetting the Periosteum; which is soon done if the Operator cuts with all his strength, and equally.

2. If there be two Bones in the Part, instead of the Knife, the Surgeon takes the Penknife to cut the Flesh betwixt the Bones exactly, and even repasseth the said Penknife around the Tibia to cut the Periosteum, if not already well separated.

3. The separated parts ought to be drawn from each other by some Servents, or by means of some Linnen put between the Lips of the Wounds, to make the more room for the Saw, that the same may not touch the Flesh.

4. Then is the Bone divided with a sharp, fine, strong, and strait Saw; which is to be moved first gently, till the Saw be fixed in, but then strongly and equally, and always perpendicularly; beginning to saw the smaller Bone first, and afterwards the biggest (when there are two) for fear that otherways the weakest shou'd fly out into Splinters by the falling of the Saw upon it.

5. During all the time of Sawing, some Servants ought to bend the Bones to make more way for the Saw.

The chief Symptom which follows after this Operation is the Loss of Blood, which requireth immediate Help.

1. *The Vessels*, whose situation is discovered by the streaming of the Blood upon the slacking of the Ligature, must be taken hold of with Pincers that have a Spring, or are held by a Servant, and being pull'd out towards the Knee-pan, are secured by running a Thread through them, and tying them close with it, *if large*, Or else we shut the Vessels up, by means of a Thread run in at both Sides of 'em, and threaded in two crooked Needles.

2. The Hemorragie may also be stopp'd by applying red hot Irons to the Vessels, which makes 'em shrink.

3. Or with Bolsters impregnated with Vitriol to the Parts; as also other adstringent and adsorbing Medicines outwardly applied.

4. The Muscles and Parts which were drawn back and kept asunder are loosen'd and pull'd over the Bone as far as they can go to cover the same.

5. The Stump well lay'd over with two Stopples and charg'd with Adstringents is forced into a Bladder slit on purpose for that end, and also furnish'd with adstringent Pouders.

6. Then is a very firm Ligature lay'd all over this.

7. The Patient ought to be kept quiet, well Dieted, and have Sleep procured him by proper Means.

115. Opposite. Circular amputation technique in *Traité complet d'anatomie de l'homme,* 2nd ed. (1866–1871) by J.M. Bourgery, Claude Bernard, and N.H. Jacob

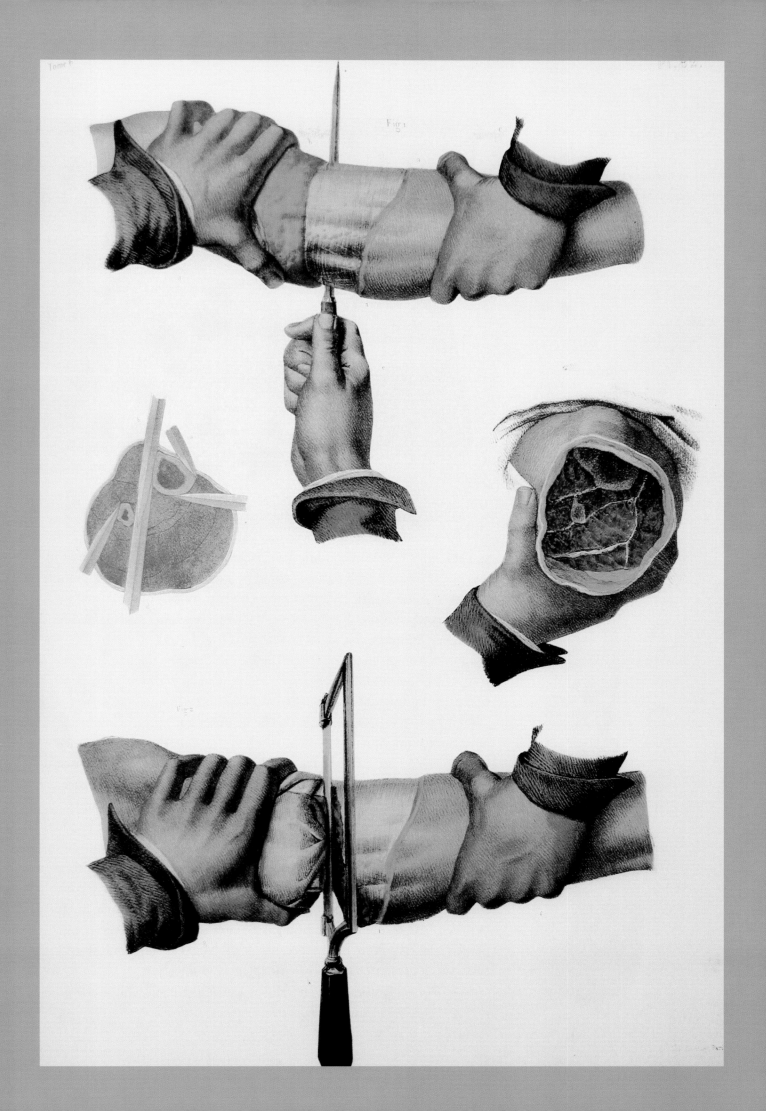

116. Amputation set (ca. 1770) by Savigny

117. Eighteenth-century circular amputation knife by Price

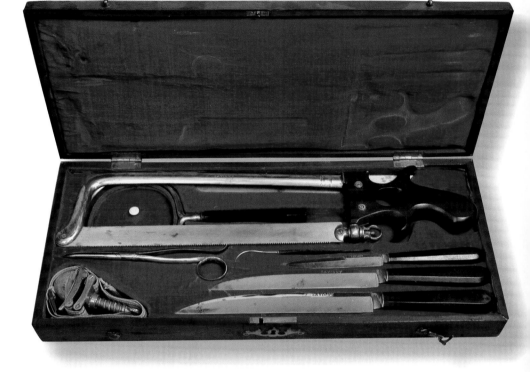

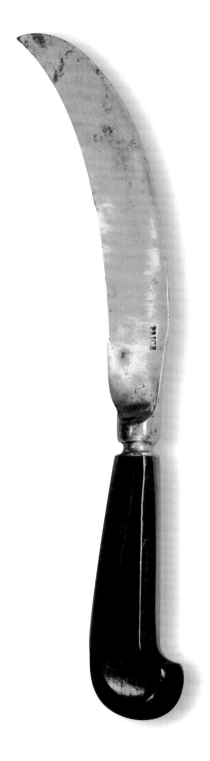

Military surgeons preferred the circular technique because the wound healed quickly, and there was less soft tissue to be exposed to the possibility of infection. Additionally, this type of amputation resulted in less operative pain, and patients could be transported with fewer complications (figures 115, 116). Amputation knives from this period usually were curved with the sharp edge on the concave surface, best suited for a rapid pass around the limb to be removed (figure 117).

James Yonge (1646–1721) was the first to describe the flap amputation, a later method that was faster and associated with less postoperative pain (figures 118–120). Yonge reviewed his technique in *Currus Triumphalis, E Terebintho* (1679): "The ligatures and gripe being made after the common manner you are with your catlin, or some long incision-knife, to raise a flap of the membranous flesh covering the muscles of the calf, beginning below the place where you intend to make excision and raising it thitherward of length enough to cover the stump. Having so done turn it back under the hand of him that gripes; and as soon as you have severed the member, bring this flap of cutaneous flesh over the stump and fasten it to the edges thereof by four or five strong stitches and, having so done, clap a dossil of lint into the inferior part, that one passage may be open for any blood or matter than may lodge between." Although this method left a better stump for the surviving patient, the risks were higher because of the larger wound, and thus there was a greater chance for hemorrhage and infection.

Dr. Robert Liston (1794–1847) was a prominent surgeon in the nine-

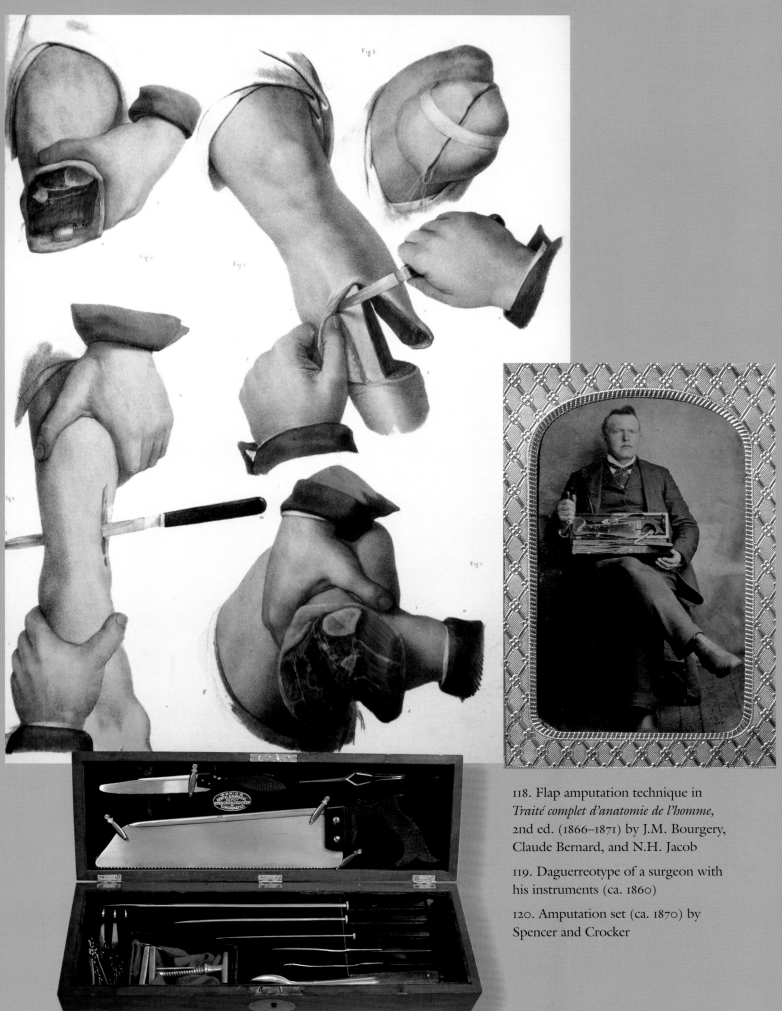

118. Flap amputation technique in *Traité complet d'anatomie de l'homme,* 2nd ed. (1866–1871) by J.M. Bourgery, Claude Bernard, and N.H. Jacob

119. Daguerreotype of a surgeon with his instruments (ca. 1860)

120. Amputation set (ca. 1870) by Spencer and Crocker

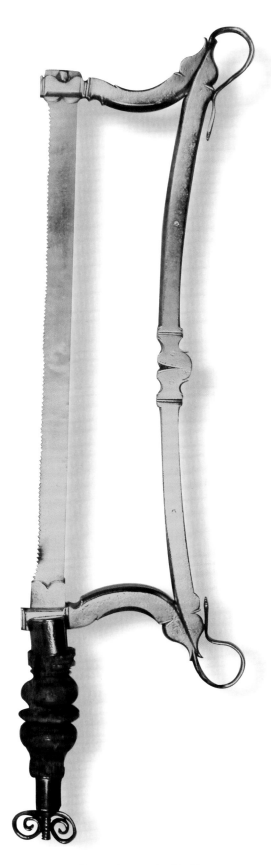

121. Large (24 1/2-inch) German
amputation saw (ca. 1540)

teenth century, and it was he who popularized the flap amputation.
Liston was a professor of surgery at the University College Hospital in
London and, on December 21, 1846, he was the first to perform surgery
(an amputation) under anesthesia in Europe, commenting, "This Yankee
dodge beats mesmerism hollow." He invented a number of surgical techniques still used today and many of the instruments in his surgical sets
were named after him. Liston was a large man who cut a broad figure in
the operating room and was proud of his reputation as a fast surgeon, an
attribute that was well respected in this preanesthetic era for obvious reasons. He was a legend in the operating room, and stories regarding his
surgical technique were numerous, including the carved notches he
made on his amputation knife following each procedure. He held a
major artery with his large left hand while making one great cutting pass
with his right. With the knife held in his teeth, he then sutured the limb,
the whole procedure lasting only a few minutes. On one occasion, while
he was trying to break his speed record for a leg amputation, Liston accidentally amputated both of his patient's testicles, and on another, he cut
off his assistant's fingers, the poor fellow succumbing to gangrene. The
mortality in that procedure rose to three since not only did the patient
and Liston's assistant expire, but so did a surgical colleague who died of
freight after Liston had ripped through the poor man's coattails while he
was observing the operation.

The sight alone of the amputation saw must have been shocking to
those about to undergo surgery (figures 121–123). John Ashhurst, MD,
related the horrors of a preanesthetic amputation encountered by a
physician/patient in a letter written to his friend Sir James Simpson and
reprinted in *The Boston Medical and Surgical Journal* (1896):

I at once agreed to submit to the operation but asked a week to
prepare for it, not with the slightest expectation that the disease
would take a favorable turn in the interval, or that the anticipated horrors of the operation would become less appalling by
reflection upon them, but simply because it was so probable that
the operation would be followed by a fatal issue, that I wished to
prepare for death and what lies beyond it, whilst my faculties
were clear and my emotions were comparatively undisturbed. . . .
The week, so slow, and yet so swift in its passage, at length came
to an end, and the morning of the operation arrived. . . . The
operation was a more tedious one than some which involve
much greater mutilation. It necessitated cruel cutting through
inflamed and horribly sensitive parts, and could not be dis-
patched by a few strokes of the knife. . . . Suffering so great as I
underwent cannot be expressed in words, and thus fortunately

cannot be recalled. The particular pangs are now forgotten; but the blank whirlwind of emotion, the horror or great darkness, and the sense of desertion by God and man bordering close upon despair, which swept through my mind and overwhelmed my heart, I can never forget, however gladly would I do so. Only the wish to save others some of my sufferings makes me deliberately recall and confess the anguish and humiliation of such a personal experience; nor can I find language more sober or familiar than that I have used, to express feelings which, happily for us all, are too rare as matters to general experience to have been shaped into household words. . . . During the operation, in spite of the pain it occasioned, my senses were preternaturally acute, as I have been told they generally are in patients under such circumstances. I watched all that the surgeon did with a fascinated intensity. I still recall with unwelcome vividness the spreading out of the instruments, the twisting of the tourniquet, the first incision, the fingering of the sawed bone, the sponge pressed on the flap, the tying of the blood-vessels, the stitching of the skin, and the bloody dismembered limb lying on the floor. Those are not pleasant remembrances. For a long time they haunted me, and even now they are easily resuscitated; and though they cannot bring back the suffering attending the events which gave them a place in my memory, they can occasion a suffering of their own, and be the cause of a disquiet which favors neither mental nor bodily health.

Obviously amputation was a last resort, though a less invasive procedure was devised in the middle of the nineteenth century for severely abscessed or injured limbs in an attempt to save as much bone (and

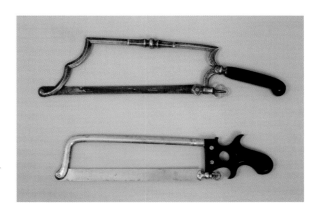

122. (Top) Perrot saw (ca. 1770) by Spear & Sagnson; (bottom) Otto's bow saw (ca. 1780) by Savigny

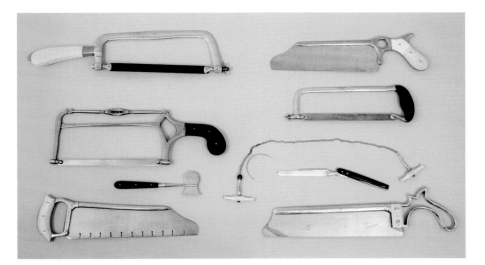

123. Mid to late eighteenth-century amputation saws: (top left column) exhibition bow saw by Aubry, (Richard) Butcher's bow saw by Evans & Co., Hey's saw by Down, serrated Parker's Capital saw by Tiemann; (top right column) Sattertlee's saw by Tiemann, Rust's bow saw by Tiemann, chain saw with carrier by Aubry, lifting-back metacarpal saw with universal handle by Tiemann; Tenon saw by Evans & Wormull

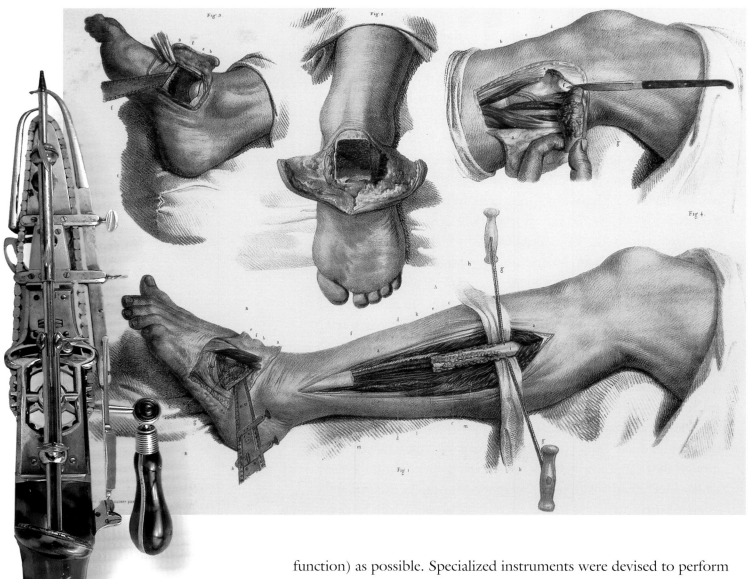

124. Bone-excision procedure in *Traité complet d'anatomie de l'homme*, 2nd ed. (1866–1871) by J.M. Bourgery, Claude Bernard, and N.H. Jacob

125. Heine's osteotome by Tiemann (ca. 1870)

function) as possible. Specialized instruments were devised to perform this "excision" procedure, which was especially popular in the American Civil War (figures 124–128). Surgeons removed joints and sections of bone to hopefully retain at least some function in the remaining part of the limb, though unfortunately few patients actually benefited.

The decision of whether or not to proceed to amputation was always a difficult one, and the high mortality and morbidity of surgical intervention severely strained patient/physician relationships. Irish playwright and social critic George Bernard Shaw (1856–1950) was faced with amputation after a long battle with leg ulcers. Shaw's contempt for physicians and the possible conflicts of interest in that profession led to early efforts at socialized medicine in Great Britain: "It is simply unscientific to allege or believe that doctors do not under existing circumstances perform unnecessary operations and manufacture and prolong lucrative diseases." Shaw was certainly not alone in his suspicions regarding economic motives that may have been influenced some physicians in the past:

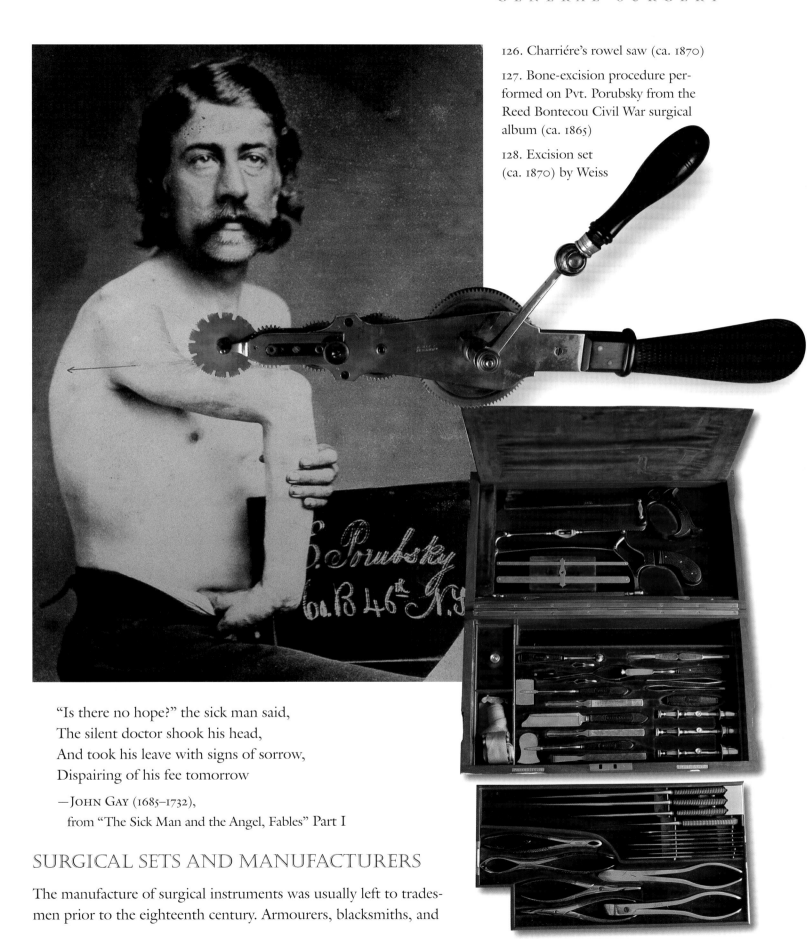

126. Charriére's rowel saw (ca. 1870)

127. Bone-excision procedure performed on Pvt. Porubsky from the Reed Bontecou Civil War surgical album (ca. 1865)

128. Excision set (ca. 1870) by Weiss

"Is there no hope?" the sick man said,
The silent doctor shook his head,
And took his leave with signs of sorrow,
Dispairing of his fee tomorrow

—JOHN GAY (1685–1732),
from "The Sick Man and the Angel, Fables" Part I

SURGICAL SETS AND MANUFACTURERS

The manufacture of surgical instruments was usually left to tradesmen prior to the eighteenth century. Armourers, blacksmiths, and

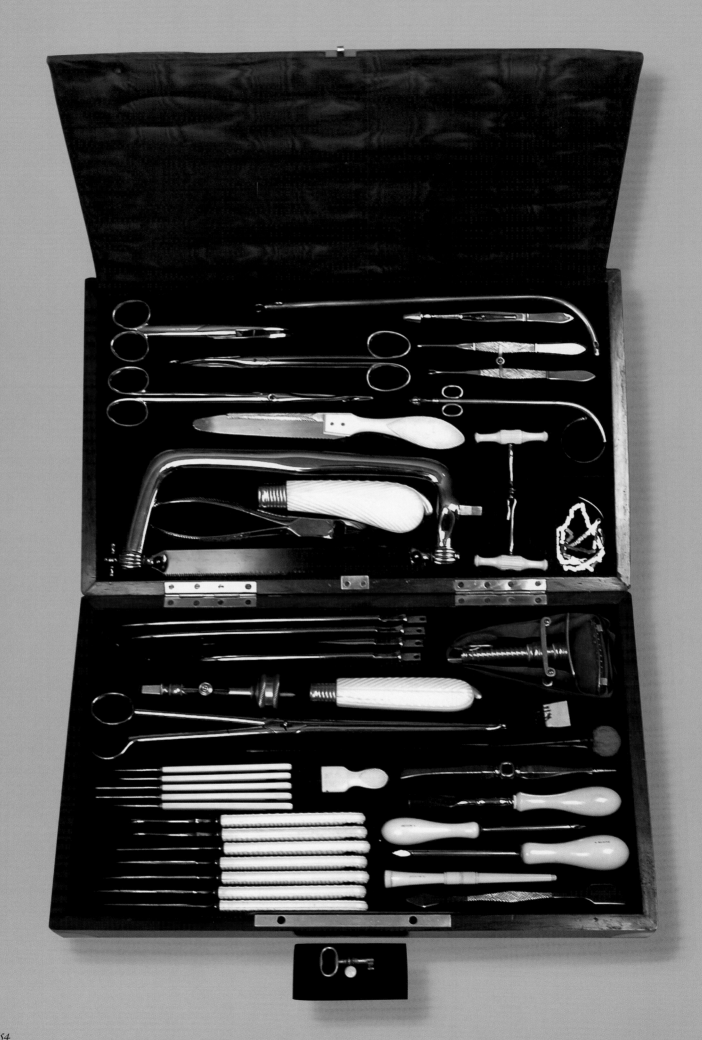

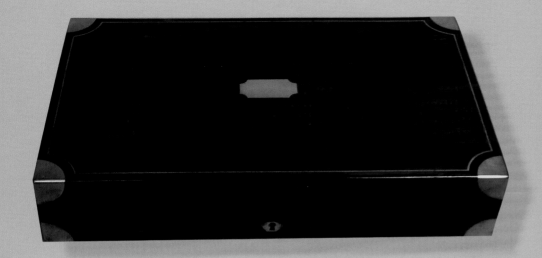

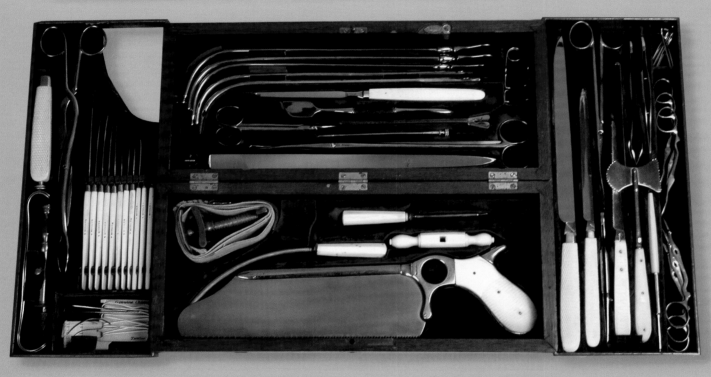

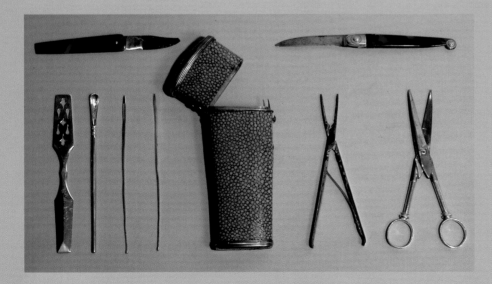

129. Opposite. Exhibition ivory general surgery set (ca. 1880) by A. Aubry

130. Top. Rosewood brass-bound case for the A. Aubry exhibition surgical set (ca. 1880)

131. Late eighteenth-century Parker's surgical set by Tiemann

132. Left. Surgical etui with folding thumb lancet and scalpel (ca. 1750): (from left) tongue blade, ear scoop, probes, shagreen case, tweezers, and scissors, all probably by Savigny

cutlers made instruments that were designed for crude surgery, and later, silversmiths were responsible for finer work. A dramatic increase in the complexity of surgical procedures occurred in the nineteenth century as the development of technology provided physicians with a new class of diagnostic and therapeutic instrumentation. These advances contributed to the development of specialties in surgery, the first being ophthalmology after the invention of the ophthalmoscope. The discovery of anesthesia at about the same time allowed surgeons the time to perform procedures never before imagined, and with the use of aseptic techniques, patients were willing to submit to new operations since surgery was no longer a death sentence.

There was no standardization of equipment, and, in fact, it was an honored practice for a physician to invent a new instrument that remained a namesake. There were no regulatory bodies, and the act of patenting new instruments was felt to be improper. According to the Code of Ethics of the American Medical Association in 1847, "equally derogatory to professional character is it, for a physician to hold a patent for any surgical instrument or medicine." This point continues to be debated today, and early on was a disincentive to the discovery of new devices. Large military contracts and later regulations tended to provide standardization in the manufacture of surgical instrumentation.

The finest instruments in the nineteenth century were made in France by Aubry, Charriére, Collin, Grangeret, and Mathieu, and in England by Arnold, Coxeter, Down, Evans, Pepys, Maw, Savigny, and Weiss. High tariffs, however, hindered their import into the United States, thus providing an incentive for recent immigrants to establish manufacturing bases in Boston, Philadelphia, and New York. Names that became important in America were Kern, Gemrig, Snowden, and Kolbe (Philadelphia); Codman—Shurtleff (Boston); Otto, Chevalier, and Shepard & Dudley (New York); Leach & Green (Boston); Wocher (Cincinnati); Sharp & Smith (Chicago); and Aloe (St. Louis). The most prominent of all was George Tiemann (1795–1868), a German immigrant who settled in New York and provided extraordinary instruments for military and civilian physicians into the twentieth century. Many physicians went out of their way to purchase and display the finest surgical armamentarium, presumably in order to earn the respect and admiration of their patients, despite the irony of the destruction that some of these large surgical sets caused (figures 129–131).

Monson Hills was a British cupper who, on the other hand, argued in support of the use of small folding surgical sets in the nineteenth century in the *Boston Medical and Surgical Journal* (1834). Many early obstetricians agreed with his point of view and hid their instruments from expectant mothers: "A person about to be cupped, is often needlessly alarmed by the arrival of his operator, with a capacious box of instruments; and he measures the severity of the pain he is about to undergo, by the seeming multitude of instruments required to inflect it. If, on the contrary, the few implements used are carried in the pocket, and produced when about to be used, unobserved by the patient, this evil is easily avoided" (figures 132, 133).

By the turn of the century, materials such as English cast steel with fancy ebony or ivory handles were replaced by one piece alloy steel that could be massively produced and easily sterilized (figures 134–135). An instrument must be heated to 150–160 degrees centigrade in order to be sterilized, a temperature that destroyed many of the materials that had allowed instrument making to be an art. According to Brooklyn surgeon H. Beeckman Delatour in the *Brooklyn Medical Journal* (1890): "You cannot bake instruments with cemented handles. . . . The bone handles, even if riveted, appear to become brittle if heated too high, and possibly at times, on account of the repetition of baking, even when the degree of heat is not very high. I have found practically that I dare not run my thermometer higher than about 130°C, which is about 266°F. Once my oven, being neglected, ran up so high that the instruments had reached about 150°C. . . . This does not take the temper out, but it makes them look not so pretty."

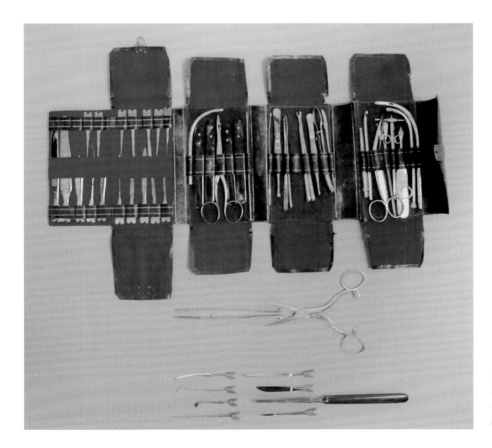

133. Large pocket surgical set with various forceps and scalpel blades fitting universal handles (ca. 1870) by Tiemann

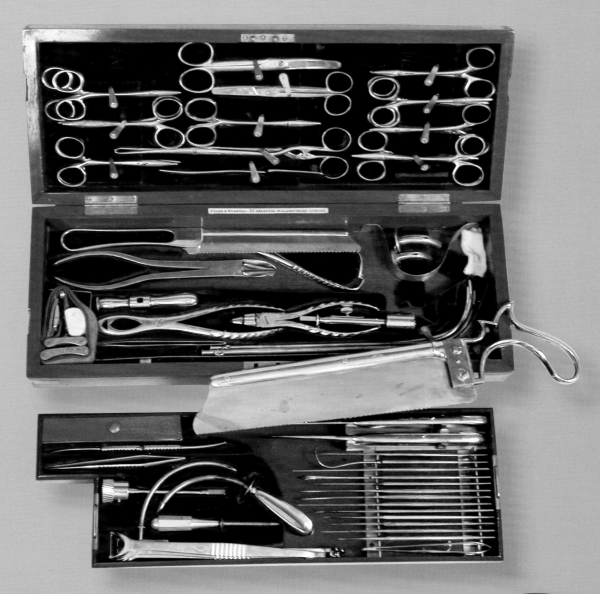

134. All-metal general operating set
(ca. 1900) by Evans & Wormull

135. Metal pocket surgical set (ca.
1900) by George Frye

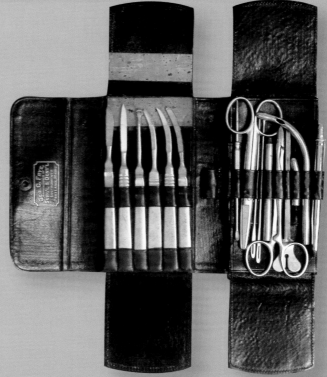

THE CONTROL OF BLEEDING

The most dangerous perioperative complication related to amputation
was the uncontrolled loss of blood, and Monfalcon wrote in the 1896
edition of the *Boston Medical and Surgical Journal*:

> Who can read without a kind of horror the account of those
> frightful operations which were then practiced? And yet the time
> is not yet very far distant from ours when they lopped off a limb
> by striking it violently with a heavy knife; that time when they
> knew neither how to stop nor how to prevent hemorrhage but by
> burning the part whence the blood jetted with boiling oil or the
> red-hot iron; that time when surgeons armed themselves at every
> moment with pincers, with burning cauteries, and with a thou-
> sand instruments the representations even of which cause terror.

Hemostasis has always been a challenging problem, and there were a
number of inventive ways in which surgeons attempted to control
bleeding. This advice was found in the Saxon *Leech Book of Bald*, the earliest know herbal of British origin (ca. A.D. 950):

> If thou wilt stop blood running in an incision, take kettle root,
> rub it to dust, shed it on the wound. Again, take rye and barley
> balm, burn it to dust; if thou may not staunch a blood-letting
> wound, take a new horses turd, dry it in the sun or by the fire,
> rub it into dust thoroughly well, lay the dust very thick on a
> linen cloth and tie up for a night. If thou may not staunch a
> gushing vein, take that same blood which runneth out, dry it on
> a hot stone and rub it to dust, lay the dust on a vein and tie up
> strong. If in blood-letting a man cut upon a sinew, mingle
> together wax and pitch and sheeps grease, lay on a cloth and on
> the cut.

Galen recommended the use of spider webs, and, in fact, little boxes
containing spider webs were part of every soldier's field equipment at
the battle of Crecy in 1346. There is a pertinent reference in William
Shakespeare's *A Midsummer Night's Dream* (act 3, scene 1), where
Bottom says:

> I shall desire you of
> more acquaintance,
> good Master Cobweb:
> If I cut my finger I shall make bold with you. . . .

C. LeClerc recommended additional ingredients in order to provide
adequate hemostasis in *The Compleat Surgeon* (1696): "To this Purpose

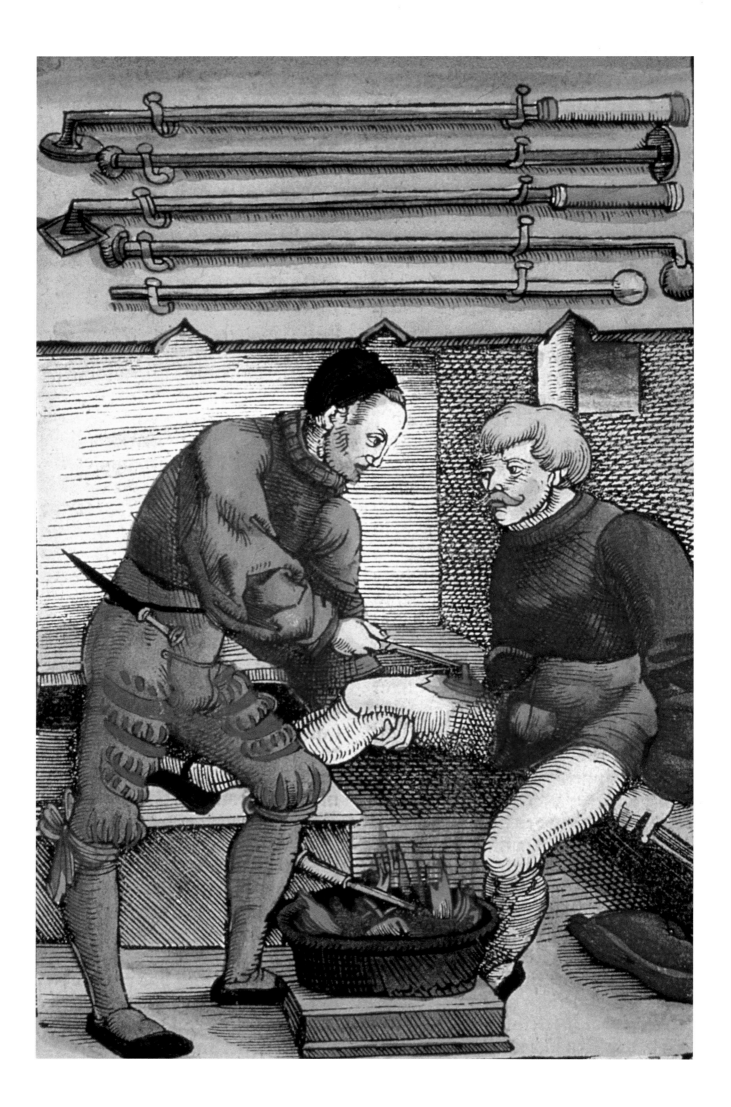

you may also make use of Cobwebs, Mill-Dust, and the Powder of Worm-eaten Oak; or else take Oven-Soot mixt with the Juice of the Dung of an Ass or Ox, adding only thereto the White of an Egg."

Later in the sixteenth century, von Gersdorff controlled bleeding with a styptic containing lime, vitriol, alum, aloe, gallnuts, colophony, white hair of the belly of a hare, or deer chopped up and mixed with egg whites. "And afterwards, take a bladder of a bull or ox or hog, which should be strong, and cut off the top widely enough so that it will go over the stump and the dressing. The bladder should be moistened, but not too soft and draw it over and bind it firmly with a cord, then you need not worry that it will bleed."

The Cautery

One of the earliest and most feared devices employed by surgeons to control bleeding was the cautery (figures 136, 137). Though very effective in hemostasis, this simple piece of metal made significant and unappreciated contributions to asepsis (and thus survival), thus leading to its faithful use by physicians throughout the ages. However, according to William Clowes, surgeon to Queen Elizabeth: "The yron is most excellent but that it is offensive to the eye and bringeth the patient to great sorrowe and dread of the burning and smart."

In addition to hemostasis, surgeons used the cautery in other ways. Hippocrates said, "What cannot be cured with medicaments is cured by the knife, what the knife cannot cure is cured with the searing iron, and whatever this cannot cure must be considered incurable." The horror of preanesthetic surgery with the cautery is understandable after reviewing Hippocrates' description of its use in rectal surgery: ". . . force out the anus as much as possible with the fingers, and make the irons red-hot, and burn the pile until it be dried up, and so as that no part may be left behind. . . . You will recognize the hemorrhoids without difficulty, for they project on the inside of the gut like dark-coloured grapes, and when the anus is forced out they spirt blood. When the cautery is applied the patient's head and hands should be held so that he may not stir, but he himself should cry out, for this will make the rectum project the more. . . ."

Abul Qasim (Albucasis) (936–1013) also discussed a surgical use for the cautery in his landmark tenth-century text *Altasrif* as part of his treatment for hernea: "When a rupture occurs in the groin, and part of the intestine and omentum comes down into the scrotum . . . bid him hold his breath till the intestine or omentum comes out. Then heat the cautery . . . when it is white hot and emits sparks then return the intestine or omentum into his abdominal cavity, and have an assistant put his hand over the place to prevent the exit of the intestine. . . . Then apply the cautery to the mark . . . and hold it until it reaches the bone. . . . You

136. Use of the cautery in *Feldtbüch der Wundartzney* (1517) by Hans von Gersdorff

137. Mid eighteenth century cauteries: (right) cased set by Mariaud; (below) bullet cautery (ca. 1860)

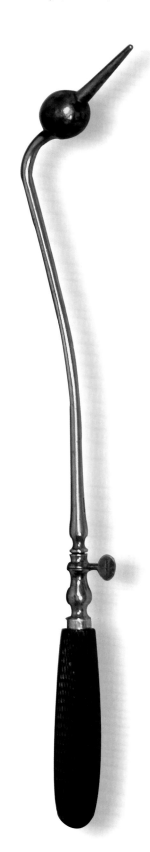

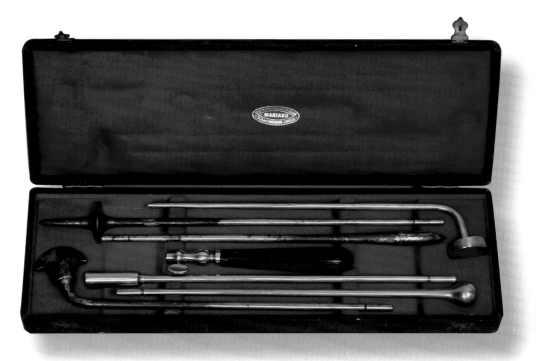

must take the greatest care that the intestine does not come out while you are cauterizing, lest you burn it and it result in death or grave injury. . . . The patient should lie on his back for forty days so that the wound may cicatrize."

Laurence Heister (1683–1758) was the preeminent surgeon of the eighteenth century and described the use of the cautery in his famous text, *A General System of Surgery, in Three Parts* (1718):

If this method should also fail you must have recourse to the *actual Cautery*: The Orifices of the Vessels being burned, a Crust is formed over them, and this method is so effectual, that it is scarce possible for an Haemorrhage to happen in Wounds of the external Parts, but what may be stopped by it, you should in this case always have two Cauteries ready, that if one should be extinguished before the Operation is finished, you may be prepared with another. Cauteries are made of very different shapes and sizes, according to the Parts to which the are to be applied. . . . There are two Inconveniences which generally attend the use of the Cautery, and sometimes force us to neglect it; for first, not only the Patient is usually wonderfully terrified at the apprehension of it, but Mankind in general look upon it as a piece of Barbarity to advise the use of it; when, to say truth, it does not occasion such violent Pains as are usually apprehended from it, and what Pain there is in the Operation, is instantly over. But it is also attended with another Inconvenience of greater

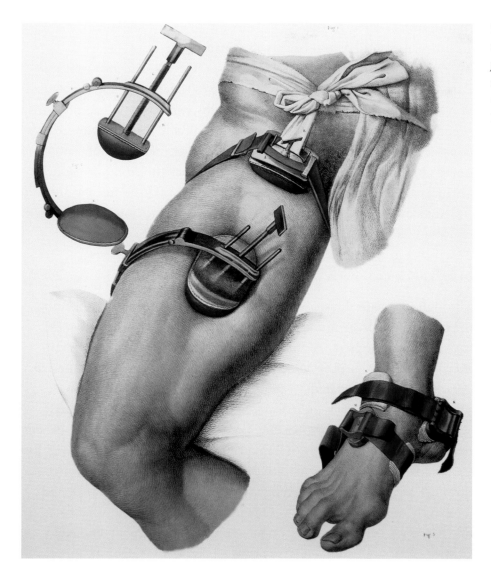

138. Use of the tourniquet in *Traité complet d'anatomie de l'homme comprenant l'anatomie chirurgical et la médicine opératoire*, 2nd ed. (1866–1871) by J.M. Bourgery, Claude Bernard, and N.H. Jacob

Consequence, that is, the Eschar which is brought on by the Cautery, frequently falls off in two or three days, from whence a fresh Haemorrhage succeeds, and most likely a deadly one. To prevent this, two things are to be observed, first to handle the Wounds tenderly at the time of dressing; and secondly, to be provided always with a fresh Cautery, to repeat the Operation if necessary.

The Tourniquet

Certainly no device in the history of medicine has been more popular for the control of bleeding than the tourniquet. The application of pressure to control blood loss is a natural reaction, though it was not until 1674 that Morell reported the use of a field tourniquet when he attached a cord to a wooden rod and twisted it to achieve hemostasis. Jean-Louis Petit devised a metal screw device in 1718 and named it a "tourniquet" (figure 138). Obviously, this devise remains an important part of the surgical armamentarium, and likely will remain so.

Another of the many contributions by the great sixteenth-century French surgeon Ambroise Paré was his use of the ligature for the control of bleeding, a discovery much appreciated by patients who had previously endured caustics and the hot cautery. Catgut and thread sutures were popular in the nineteenth century, though earlier methods were sometimes a bit unusual, including the use by the ancient Hindu surgeon Susruta of the heads of red ants, which were cut off just after the ant had closed its mouth on the tissue to be sutured. This method was later used by Albucasis and remained popular into the nineteenth century.

SURGICAL ASEPSIS

Throughout medical history, there have been many theories explaining the progressive decay noted in untreated wounds. Possible etiologies have included the anger of the gods, punishments for sinning, imbalanced humors, unhealthy air sent from misaligned planets, and internal organs that were "irritated." The role of microorganisms in causing superficial infection was only discovered within the last few hundred years, and without that knowledge, there was no reason to expect proper treatment. In fact, methods of wound care have changed and evolved for thousands of years and, even with our present understanding of infectious disease, "appropriate therapy" remains mysterious, debated, and frequently modified to this day. One must, however, begin with an accurate diagnosis before deciding on an appropriate treatment, and Aulus Cornelius Celsus (25 B.C.–A.D. 50) gave us that correct description of inflammation over two thousands years ago. His observation regarding superficial infection remains relevant today and is one of the classic descriptions of medicine: *calor, rubor, dolor,* and *tumor* (heat, redness, pain, and swelling).

The treatment of wounds has never been standardized, and many different formulae remain available for the care of traumatized tissue. The ancient Egyptians may have unknowingly been the first to use an antibiotic (penicillin) when they packed wounds with moldy bread. They also treated superficial lesions with coagulated milk and honey wrapped in a muslin dressing. Honey was later used as an antibacterial in wound healing by such diverse cultures as the Romans in Europe, African tribesman, Indians, and Native Americans. Sugar is a well-known preservative and may be bactericidal because of the high osmotic gradient it creates. Additionally, honey contains chemicals that may be helpful in wound-healing, such as hydrogen peroxide, formic acid, vitamins, and trace metals. The Greeks seemed to understand infectious disease when they dipped surgical dressings in wine and vinegar, and antibacterial agents used by others have included alcohol, creosote, ferric chloride, zinc chloride, and nitric acid.

Ancient Hebrews were the first to pay attention to good hygiene as a way of controlling the spread of communicable disease. The following passages are from the Bible (Leviticus 15):

> 1—The Lord also spoke to Moses and to Aaron, saying, Speak to the sons of Israel, and say to them, When any man has a discharge from his body, his discharge is unclean.
> 7—Also whoever touches the person with the discharge shall wash his clothes and bathe in water and be unclean until evening.
> 10—Whoever then touches any of the things which were under him shall be unclean until evening, and he who carries them shall wash his clothes and bathe in water and be unclean until evening.
> 13—Now when the man with the discharge becomes cleansed from his discharge, then he shall count off for himself seven days for his cleansing; he shall then wash his clothes and bathe his body in running water and will become clean.

One of the earliest written surgical texts was in manuscript form and the author, Heinrich von Pfolspeundt, seemed to have had an understanding of contagion well before his techniques were widely accepted. The following is from his *Buch der Bündth-Ertznei* (1460):

> Item, firstly I advise anyone who wishes to work in this art and to heal, that he should not go to a wounded or sick person in the early morning or treat him before he has heard Mass, so far as is possible, unless there is great need, but he shall pray to the good Lord to bless the wounds, to say a pater noster and an Ave Maria and confess his faith, so that strength and wisdom be given him to heal the people whom he has under his hands.
> And he should guard himself against drunkenness when he is to treat patients, for because of it they may easily be neglected, and the doctor would be guilty of that and be punished by God. And especially, he should guard himself, if he has eaten onions or peas, or slept the previous night with an unclean woman, in the morning, against breathing into anyone's wound. Also, he should bind with clean white cloths, for if they are not clean, harm results. He should also wash his hands before he treats anyone. Also he should love healing for the sake of God, if he is able: also if the doctor knows himself to be unclean, he should not look actively into the wounds, nor should any other unclean person, else mischief and harm arises, and may even cause death

of the patient. And keep people protected, or you will have to do penance before God, if you are to blame.

Early physicians believed gunpowder to be poisonous, so the accepted treatment for gunshot wounds included the use of boiling oil (though members of the British Navy commonly treated amputations by exploding gunpowder on the fresh stump). Many important medical advances are serendipitous, which was certainly the case with Ambroise Paré's discovery of an alternative to boiling oil in Turin in 1537, as recounted in his *Oeuvres complètes d'Ambroise Paré*:

> Now all the soldiers at the Chateau, seeing our men coming with a great fury, did all they could to defend themselves and killed and wounded a great number of our soldiers with pikes, arquebuses, and stones, where the surgeons had much work cut out for them. Now I was at the time an untried soldier; I had not yet seen wounds made by gunshot at the first dressing. It is true that I had read in Jean di Vigo, first book, *Of Wounds in General*, chapter eight, that wounds made by firearms were poisoned wounds, because of the powder, and for their cure he commands to cauterize them with oil of elder, scalding hot, in which should be mixed a little theriac; and in order not to err before using the said oil, knowing that such a thing would bring great pain to the patient, I wished to know first, how the other surgeons did for the first dressing, which was to apply said oil as hot as possible, into the wounds, of whom I took courage to so as they did. At last my oil lacked and I was constrained to apply in its place a digestive made of the yolks of eggs, oil of roses, and turpentine. That night I could not sleep at my ease, fearing by lack of cauterization that I should find the wounded on whom I had failed to put the said oil dead or empoisoned, which made me rise early to visit them, where beyond my hope I found those upon whom I had put the digestive medicament feeling little pain, and their wounds without inflammation or swelling, having rested fairly well throughout the night; the others to who I had applied the said boiling oil, I found feverish, with great pain and swelling about their wounds. Then I resolved with myself never more to burn thus cruelly poor men wounded with gunshot.

Paré was able to obtain the formula for a secret balsam from a surgeon in Turin, but only after a great deal of effort (and promises not to reveal the ingredients to anyone). In his *Apologie*, Paré gives us an interesting insight not only into the vexing problem of the treatment of gunshot wounds but also into the politics of sixteenth-century medicine in this early translation:

When wee first came to *Turin*, there was there a Cirurgion farre more famous than all the rest in artificially and happily curing wounds made by Gun-shot; wherefore I laboured with all diligence for two yeeres time to gaine his favour and love, that so at the length, I might learne of him, what kinde of Medicine that was, which he honoured with the glorious title of Balsame, which was so highly esteemed by him, and so happily and successfull to his patients; yet could I not obtaine it. It fell out a small while after that the Marshall of *Montejan* the Kings Leiftenant, Generall there in *Piedmont* dyed, wherefore I went unto my Chirurgion, and told him that I could take no pleasure in living there, the favourer and *Macenas* of my studies being taken away; and that I intended forthwith to returne to *Paris*, and that it would neither hinder, nor discredit him to teach his remedy to me, who should be so farre remote from him. When he heard this, he made no delay, but presently wished mee to provide two Whelpes, 1 pound of earth-wormes, 2 pounds of oyle of Lillyes, six ounces of Venice Turpentine, and one ounce of *Aqua vitae*. In my presence he boyled the Whelpes put alive into that oyle, until the flesh came from the bones, then presently he put in the Wormes, which he had first killed in white wine, that they might so be clensed from the earthy drosse wherewith they are usually repleate, and then hee boyled them in the same oyle so long, till they became dry, and had spent all their juyce therein: then hee strayned it through a towell without much pressing; and added the Turpentine to it, and lastly the *aqua vitae*. Calling God to witnesse, that he had no other Balsame, wherewith to cure wounds made with Gunshot, and bring them to suppuration. Thus he sent me away as rewarded with a most precious gift, requesting me to keepe it as a great secret, and not to reveale it to any.

The primary ingredient, however, was the earthworm found in the ancient formula of Dioscorides, the modifications being the substitution of puppies' fat for goose grease, and the addition of oil of lilies, turpentine, and aqua vitae. Several hundred years later in the nineteenth century, earthworms remained a part of English therapeutics and were found in John Quincy's *Dispensatory of the Royal College of Physicians in London*, and in William Lewis' *Materia Medica*.

Professor Samuel Gross was one of the most prominent surgeons of the nineteenth century and was the chairman of surgery at the Jefferson Medical College from 1856 to 1882 (figure 139). He was an extremely important American surgeon, author, and medical teacher, and his two-volume *System of Surgery* (1859) provided a basis for surgical techniques

139. Admission card to the class of Dr. Samuel Gross, Jefferson Medical College

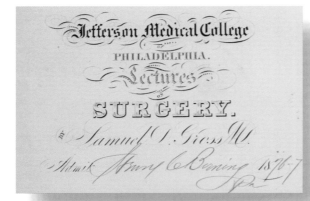

used during the American Civil War. His text went on to six editions and was translated into several foreign languages. Unfortunately, Gross remained one of the last major medical figures of the nineteenth century to be unconvinced by the monumental discoveries earlier that century regarding asepsis. Gross' view of "inflammation," which was the Victorian term for infection, provides us with a window to the misunderstood pathophysiology of that period:

Inflammation may be defined to be a perverted action of the capillary vessels of a part, attended with discoloration, pain, heat, swelling, and disordered function, with a tendency to effusion, deposits, or new products. In addition to these changes, there is also an altered condition of the blood and nervous fluid as an important element of the morbid process. In what inflammation essentially consists, it would be idle to inquire, since it would be just as impossible to unravel its true nature as it would be to explain the intimate character of attraction, repulsion, gravitation, or cohesion. Hence, in studying its history, all that we can do is to examine its causes, symptoms, and effects, or, more properly speaking, to institute a rigid analysis of its appreciable phenomena. If we endeavor to step beyond this, we shall, like our predecessors, lose ourselves in the mazes of conjecture and hypothesis, those quicksands upon which so many of the noblest minds of the profession have, in all ages, since the origin of medicine and surgery, been wrecked and stranded, as if to warn us of their folly and the impossibility of further progress.

Gross was seventy years old when he was approached by thirty-one-year-old Thomas Eakins to approve a portrait that represented American surgical excellence at the upcoming Philadelphia Centennial Exposition (figure 140). The 1875 painting became one of the most superb examples of American portrait art, though the selection committee for the Centennial's art exhibition rejected it since it was criticized as being too graphic and not appropriate for display. Ironically, a *New York Tribune* reporter complained that the painting was too lifelike when he said, "It is a picture that even strong men find it difficult to look at long, if they can look at it at all; and as for people with nerves and stomachs, the scene is so real that they might as well go to a dissecting room and have done with it." The scene in this famous painting was the surgical amphitheater of the Jefferson Medical Hall as Gross demonstrated the removal of a section of bone from a patient with osteomyelitis. Gross' son, Samuel W. Gross, also a surgeon, is the figure at the right in the

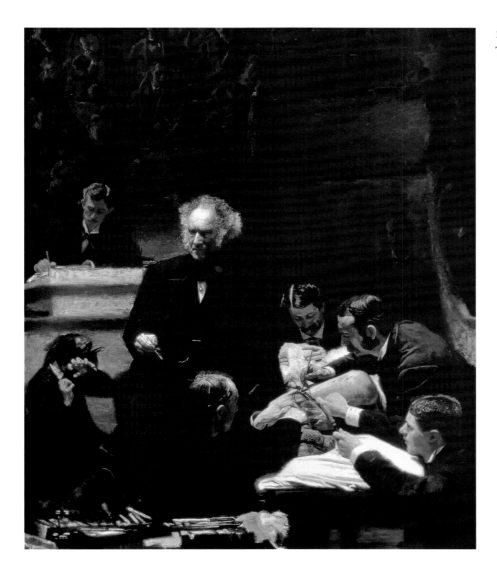

140. *The Gross Clinic* (1875) by Thomas Eakins

tunnel, and Thomas Eakins' is seen in a self-portrait as he sits sketching at the left. The patient's mother is seated at the lower left of the portrait and is obviously overcome by the surgery; family members sometimes attended these procedures at the surgeon's request for medicolegal purposes. Note that Gross is dressed in a business suit and is making no effort at sterile technique.

Many other surgeons also remained reluctant to accept the "theory" of asepsis in the nineteenth century, and conditions in the operating room played a large role in a high perioperative mortality. Lawson Tait (1845–1899) was a pioneer of the appendectomy and made the following observations:

> Through the folding doors what a difference. Everywhere hurry and untidiness . . . but much dirt. . . . The wards stank. The operating table was of wood and of fabulous age. . . . The only correct garb of a surgeon was a frock coat (the oldest and shabbiest in his wardrobe) which was kept in the surgeon's room and

never renewed or cleaned during his twenty years of operating work. . . . The surgeons came direct from the dissecting room to operate. . . . Ligatures were used, which had already been soiled by handling with blood stained fingers, to bind up wounds in a second case. And at Edinburgh these ligatures were always worn ostentatiously by the House Surgeon, like a badge of knighthood, in the button hole of a coat, which often rivaled that of his chief for dirt.

Eminent surgeon John Bell described the all too common fate of patients who succumbed to unchecked sepsis in his 1802 *The Principles of Surgery*, ". . . the wan visage, the pale and flabby flesh, the hollow eyes and prominent cheekbones, the staring and squalid hair, the long bony fingers and crooked nails, the quick, short breathing, and piping voice, declare the last stage of hectic debility! . . . the pain is dreadful; the cries of the sufferers are the same in the night as in the day-time; they are exhausted in the course of the week, and die: or if they survive, and the ulcers continue to eat down and disjoin the muscles, the great vessels are at last exposed and eroded, and they bleed to death."

Joseph Lister (1827–1912) had made a number of observations regarding the transmissibility of certain diseases clinically relevant to the surgeon, and his use of disinfectants significantly reduced the rate of morbidity and mortality in the operating room. That fact, along with the discovery of anesthesia and advances pertaining to the control of bleeding in the nineteenth century, established surgery as a true medical specialty, giving surgeons the ability to develop techniques with which to enter areas of the body never before thought possible. On August 12, 1865, Lister performed the first case of aseptic surgery when he operated on an eleven-year-old boy, James Greenlees. According to Lister:

My house surgeon, Dr. MacFee, acting under my instructions, laid a piece of lint dipped in liquid carbolic acid upon the wound, and applied lateral pasteboard splints padded with cotton wood, the limb resting on its outer side, with the knee bent. It was left undisturbed for four days, when, the boy complaining of some uneasiness, I removed the inner splint and examined the wound. It showed no signs of suppuration, but the skin in its immediate vicinity had a slight blush of redness. I now dressed the sore with lint soaked with water having a small portion of carbolic acid diffused through it, and this was continued for five days, during which the uneasiness and the redness of the skin disappeared, the sore meanwhile furnishing no pus.

Though Lister and others had initially believed in the theory of "miasma," or the transmissibility of wound infections through the air, they later abandoned carbolic sprays in favor of the topical application of disinfectants.

Gross remained unconvinced and wrote, "Little if any faith is placed by any enlightened or experienced surgeon on this side of the Atlantic in the so-called carbolic acid treatment of Professor Lister." Other prominent physicians agreed, including the famous obstetrician Sir James Simpson. Surgeon Berkeley Moynihan illustrated the painful transition to sterile technique when he described this scene in 1888:

> The surgeon arrived, doffed his coat lest he should soil it with blood or pus, rolled up his shirt-sleeves and took down from the cupboard in the passage leading to the theatre an old coat, as a rule a frock coat of antique design which bore many marks of usage, and was stiff here, there, and everywhere with blood. One at least of the coats was worn with special pride, indeed with a certain jauntiness, for it had been inherited from a retiring member of the staff. The cuffs were rolled back a little, just above the wrists, and the hands were washed in a basin. The hands, when clean in a social sense, were soaked in a solution of carbolic acid. The instruments were taken from the cupboard, whose shelves were lined with green baize, and placed in a tray of 1 in 20 carbolic acid, about half an hour before the operation. When all was ready the spray was turned on, and a fine mist of steam, odorous with carbolic acid, soon bathed all engaged in the operation (figures 141, 142).

In 1883, Frank Emory Bunts described aseptic technique as practiced by Dr. Gustav Weber at the Marine Hospital in Cleveland:

> We could not enter the amphitheater until carbolic acid atomizers had been playing along enough to fill the room with a haze of steam. The patient was brought in and the field of operation was scrubbed with soap and water and a stiff brush, and then washed with bichloride of mercury, and then surrounded with towels wrung out of the same solution. Before beginning the operation, Dr. Weber would carefully spray his luxuriant beard with 5% carbolic acid and, as soon as the operation began, two atomizers spraying from opposite sides kept the wound continually bathed in carbolic acid mist. The making of the carbolic solutions was usually left to the hospital interns, and frequently the acid was so poorly mixed that large globules floated in the solutions in which we bathed our hands or immersed our instruments. The result was minor burns of the fingers and distinct numbing of the sense of touch. At this time iodoform was first becoming popular because of its anesthetic effect upon open wounds, and its supposed antiseptic properties. I think it was

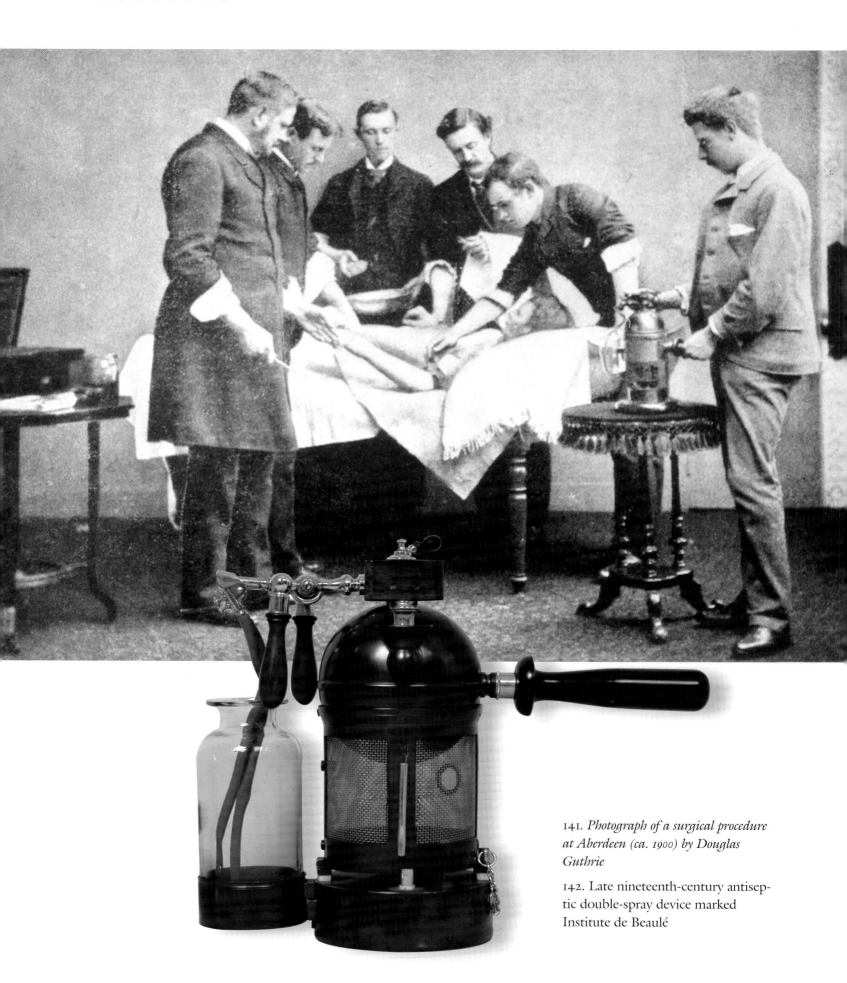

141. *Photograph of a surgical procedure at Aberdeen (ca. 1900) by Douglas Guthrie*

142. Late nineteenth-century antiseptic double-spray device marked Institute de Beaulé

due chiefly to the free use of iodoform and carbolic acid, whose disagreeable odor clung to ones clothes and hair and became particularly noticeable when in a warm room, that I contracted a habit of not going to church.

William Stewart Halsted (1852–1922) popularized the use of surgical gloves with which we now attribute the most careful aseptic technique. One of the most famous surgeons in the twentieth century, he was a founding father of the Johns Hopkins University Medical School, and he established many ways of teaching bedside medicine that are still in use today. While in the operating room, his chief nurse (and the future Mrs. Halsted) had complained of the caustic effect that carbolic acid had on her hands. She recommended the use of gloves and that they be scrubbed directly with the carbolic acid. The nurse's hands healed quite nicely with this new technique, and Halsted followed suit, reportedly commenting, "What's good for the geese should be good for the ganders." The custom quickly spread worldwide and became a standard of surgical care.

A Johns Hopkins University graduate once questioned a visiting obstetrics professor regarding whether or not he wore gloves for home delivery. The response was, "Well, if I get there in time, I take them off!"

ANESTHESIA

The control of pain had been a major barrier to the development of more complex types of surgical intervention, and the discovery of anesthesia thus became one of the greatest discoveries in the history of medicine (figure 143). Opium was a popular early analgesic, and an account of its use is found in the Ebers papyrus: "The great Sun-God Ra called on the Goddess Tefnut to cure the terrible pains he endured. Beautiful Tefnut was not skilled in the art of medicine and the concoction she gave her master produced a terrible headache. But pitying Isis brought juice from the 'berry-of-the-poppy plant' and Ra was instantly cured." Without adequate pain control, the chest and abdomen could not be entered, leaving physicians with only noninterventional forms of therapy for what are now easily addressed surgical conditions.

Despite the fact that Greeks were responsible for a great deal of early progress in the practice of medicine, it was a Roman, Aulus Cornelius Celsus (25 B.C.–A.D. 50), who wrote one of the most important medical treatises from the time of Hippocrates to the Renaissance. In his handbook for laymen, *De Medicina* (A.D. 40, published in 1478), Celsus clearly recognized the significance of pain control in the provision of medical care: "A surgeon ought to be in early manhood, or at any rate not much older; have a swift and steady, never faltering hand, and no less skill in

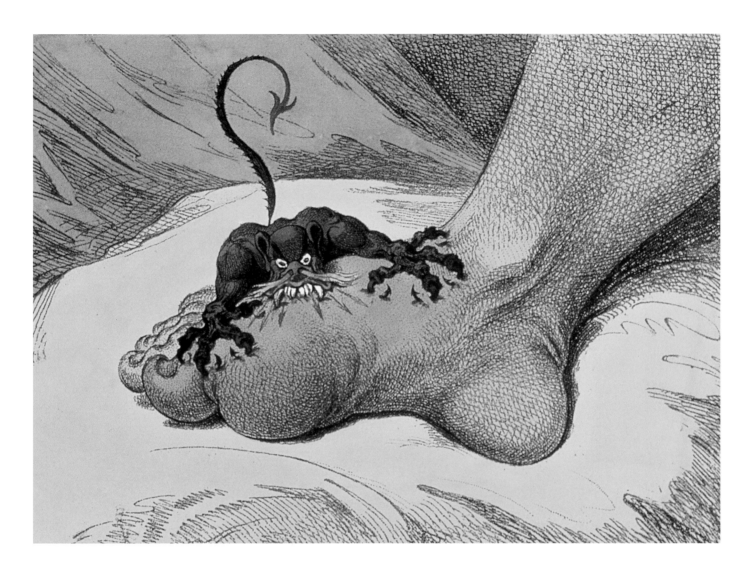

143. The pain of gout (1799), soft-ground etching and aquatint with watercolor by James Gillray

the left hand than the right hand; have sharp and clear eyesight; appear undistressed, and compassionate inasmuch as he wishes to heal those whom he treats, but does not allow their cries to hurry him more than the circumstances require, or to cut less than is necessary, and permits the patient's groaning to make not the slightest impression on him in anything he does."

Physicians provided pain relief throughout the ages in many ways. Extracts from the mandrake plant, for instance, were used as an anesthetic agent from the time of the earliest recorded medical texts. Because of its hallucinogenic properties, mandragora (*Mandragora officiarum*) was a standard ingredient in medieval "witches' brew" though it was also used as a sedative, purgative, emetic, and as an ointment to treat local ulcers. Because the roots are forked, the mandrake plant resembles the human form, and many believed that the plant cried out when pulled from the ground, causing death or insanity to anyone listening. According to a medieval text, the proper way to harvest the mandrake was the following: "Stuff the ears with good bees' wax. Sift the earth around the mandrake and then attach a long piece of string to a dog's tail. See that the dog is either ailing or at the most very small and worthless. Then tie the other end of the string to the mandrake, give a sharp kick in the wretched cur's loins. As the creature jumps forward, the root will give its dreadful cry and the dog instead of a man will go mad or drop dead." Juliet referred to this plant in Shakespeare's *Romeo and Juliet* (act 4, scene 3):

> And shrieks like mandrakes' torn of the earth,
> That living mortals, hearing them, run mad.

Of course, the effects of the plant were significantly enhanced of it had grown over a grave, especially if that grave had belonged to an executed criminal.

Throughout the ages, many other options were available to those interested in providing pain relief, like hashish in India and opium in China. In 1805, Friedrich Wilhelm Sertürner modified opium to produce the useful analgesic morphine, which he named after Morpheus, the Greek god of dreams. Inca priests in South America achieved pain control by spitting into wounds after chewing coca leaves, and, of course, the anesthetic properties of alcohol have been well-known for centuries.

In the eighteenth century prior to the advent of general anesthesia, Laurence Heister felt that surgeons were required to address pain management before patients could be operated on:

> . . . every thing should now be carefully provided which is necessary for Incision, Dressing, or any other Action, before the Operation be entered upon; but this Apparatus of Instruments and Dressings should never be got ready in your Patient's Chamber, or in his Sight, lest they should strike him with a sudden Fear, and bring on fainting Fits and other Accidents, which would very much disturb the Operation. For the same reason a crowd of useless Spectators should never be admitted into the Room, because, besides the Disturbance that they create to the Patient, it is to be feared they will very much annoy the Operator, by intercepting the Light, and filling up the Room: Besides, should any one rudely press upon him, whilst he is performing any nice Operation, it might be of the utmost ill Consequence.
>
> When the Surgeon is entering upon the Operation, he ought to use his utmost Endeavours to encourage the Patient, by promising him in the softest Terms to treat him tenderly, and to finish with the utmost Expedition; and indeed he should use Expedition but not Hurry, and should be very careful to give no unnecessary Pain, but at the same time to leave no Mischief unremedied; if he observes these Rules, he will be sure to gain credit with the standers by.

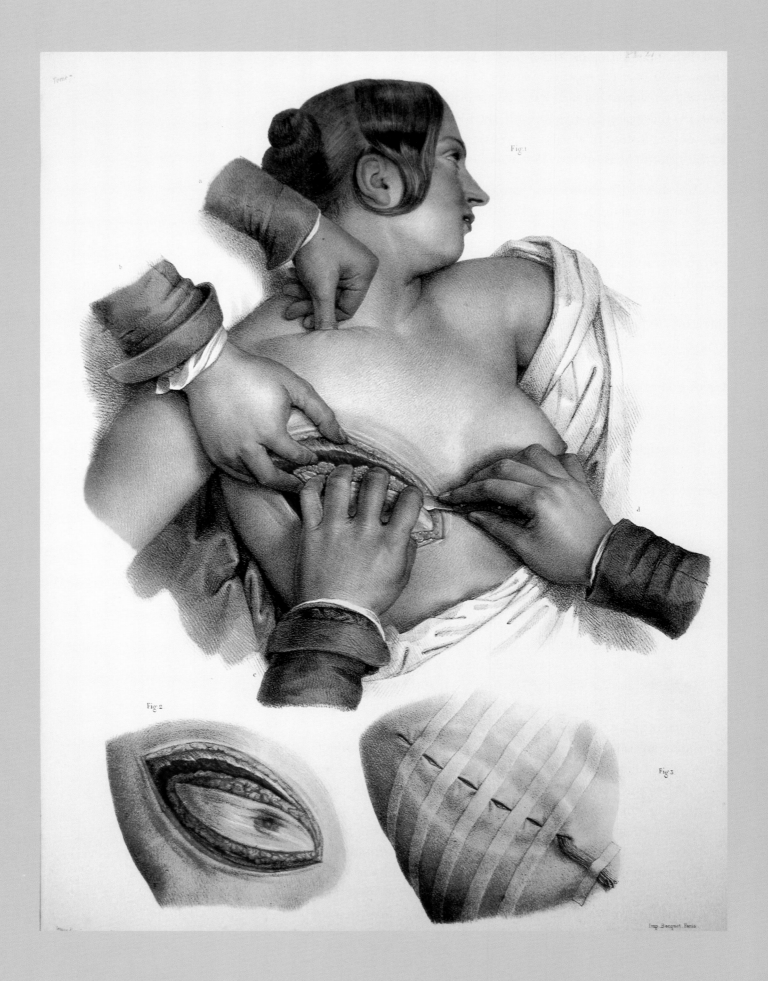

Fig. 1

Fig. 2

Fig. 3

From a patient's perspective, however, surgery without anesthesia was terrifying. (figures 144, 145). In her "journals and letters," Fanny Burney gave us a personal account of her September 30, 1811, mastectomy performed by the famous French surgeon to Napoléon, Dominique-Jean Larrey. In order to spare her from excess anxiety, she was given little notice of the procedure:

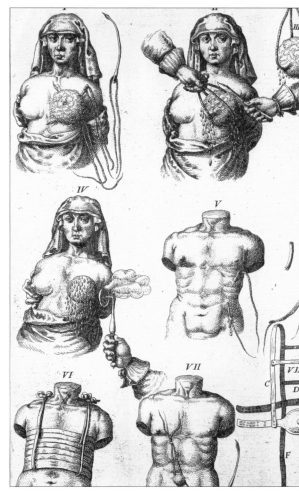

> M. Dubois acted as commander in Chief. Dr. Larrey kept out of sight; M. Dubois ordered a Bed stead into the middle of the room. Astonished, I turned to Dr. Larrey, who had promised that an Arm Chair would suffice; but he hung his head, & would not look at me. . . . I stood suspended, for a moment, whether I should not abruptly escape—I looked at the door, the windows—I felt desperate—but it was only for a moment, my reason then took the command, & my fears & feelings struggled vainly against it. . . . I knew not, positively, then, the immediate danger, but every thing convinced me danger was hovering about me . . . & M. Dubois placed me upon the mattress, & spread a cambric handkerchief upon my face.
>
> It was transparent, however, & I saw through it that the Bedstead was instantly surrounded by the 7 men and my nurse, I refused to be held; but when, Bright through the cambric, I saw the glitter of polished Steel—I closed my Eyes. I would not trust to convulsive fear the sight of the terrible incision. . . .
>
> Yet—when the dreadful steel was plunged into the breast—cutting through veins—arteries—flesh—nerves—I needed no injunctions not to restrain my cries. I began a scream that lasted uninterruptedly during the whole time of the incision—& I almost marvel that it rings not in my Ears still! So excruciating was the agony. When the wound was made, & the instrument was withdrawn, the pain seemed undiminished, for the air that suddenly rushed into those delicate parts felt like a mass of minute but sharp & forked poniards, that were tearing the edges of the wound,—but when again I felt the instrument—describing a curve—cutting against the grain, if I may so say, while the flesh resisted in a manner so forcible as to oppose & tire the hand of the operator, who was forced to change from the right to the left—then, indeed, I thought I must have expired.
>
> I attempted no more to open my Eyes,—they felt as if hermetically shut. . . . The instrument this second time withdrawn, I concluded the operation was over—Oh no! presently the terrible

144. Mastectomy in *Traité complet d'anatomie de l'homme,* 2nd ed. (1866–1871) by J.M. Bourgery, Claude Bernard, and N.H. Jacob

145. Mastectomy in *Armamentarium Chiruigicum* (1655) by Joannis Scultetus

cutting was renewed—& worse than ever, to separate the bottom, the foundation of this dreadful gland from the parts to which it adhered . . . yet again all was not over. . . . I then felt the Knife tackling against the breast bone—scraping it!—This performed while I yet remained in utterly speechless torture. . . .

When all was done, & they lifted me up that I might be put to bed, my strength was so totally annihilated, that I was obliged to be carried, & could not even sustain my hands and arms, which hung as if I had been lifeless; while my face, as the Nurse has told me, was utterly colourless. This removal made me open my Eyes—& I then saw my good Dr. Larrey, pale nearly as myself, his face streaked with blood, its expression depicting grief, apprehension, & almost horror.

Charles Darwin had attended medical school in Edinburgh and was similarly horrified by surgical practices in the early nineteenth century. Had anesthesia been invented just a few years earlier, one of the greatest books in the history of man might not have been written. In his autobiography Darwin stated, "I attended on two occasions, the operating theatre in the hospital at Edinburgh, and saw two very bad operations, one on a child, but I rushed away before they were completed. Nor did I ever again for hardly any inducement would have been strong enough to make me do so; this being long before the blessed days of chloroform. The two cases fairly haunted me for many a long year."

Laughing Gas

The story of modern anesthesia began with the discovery of nitrous oxide, or "laughing gas," by Joseph Priestly in 1772. The anesthesia that this chemical produced was first recognized by Bristol physician Thomas Beddoes and his assistant Sir Humphry Davy (1778–1829). It was Davy who first reported his exposure to this agent and the potential use that it had in surgery when he wrote in 1799, "To ascertain with certainty whether the more extensive action of nitrous oxide compatible with life was capable of producing debility, I resolved to breathe the gas for such a time, and in such quantities, as to produce excitement equal in duration and superior in intensity to that occasioned by high intoxication from opium and alcohol. . . . A thrilling extending from the chest to the extremities was almost immediately produced. I felt a sense of tangible extension highly pleasurable in every limb; my visible impressions were dazzling, and apparently magnified, I heard every sound in the room, and was perfectly aware of my situation. . . ." The following year, Davy came to an extraordinary conclusion in *Researches, Chemical and Philosophical, Chiefly Concerning Nitrous Oxide* while suffering from severe dental pain:

"On the day when the inflammation was most troublesome, I breathed three large doses of nitrous oxide. The pain always diminished after the first four or five inspirations, the thrilling came on as usual, and uneasiness was for a few minutes swallowing up in pleasure. As the former state of mind, however, returned, the state of the organ returned with it; and I once imagined that the pain was more severe after the experiment than before. . . . As nitrous oxide in its extensive operation seems capable of destroying physical pain, it may probably be used with advantage during surgical operations. . . ." Unfortunately, Davy never took that next step to clinical relevance, and almost half a century passed before anyone benefited from his observation.

Throughout the nineteenth century, the effects of nitrous oxide were well known, though the gas was primarily used for entertainment at exhibitions. The following advertisement appeared in the *Hartford Courant* in 1884:

☞A GREAT EXHIBITION

of the effects of inhaling

NITROUS OXIDE, LAUGHING GAS!

FOURTY GALLONS

of this gas will be produced and given to everyone

in the auditorium who wishes to breathe it.

EIGHT STRONG MEN

have been engaged and will be in the front row to protect those

who may injure themselves or others under the gas's influence.

This is a safety measure, since surely no danger exists

– probably no one will try to fight.

THE GAS'S POWER

is to release the urge to laugh, sing, dance, make speeches, or

fight, depending on individual nature.

NOTE:

gas will only be made available to gentlemen of the highest

respectability!

English poet Samuel Taylor Coleridge (also addicted to opium) attended one of the many public demonstrations of nitrous oxide: "I experienced the most voluptuous sensations. The outer world grew dim and I had the most entrancing visions. For three and a half minutes I lived in a new world of sensations." Others who experimented with nitrous oxide at these events were William Wordsworth, James Watt, and a dentist by the name of Horace Wells (1815–1848).

One of the early contenders in the race for the discovery of anesthesia was that same Connecticut dentist, Dr. Horace Wells, who had attended a demonstration of nitrous oxide on December 11, 1844, given by "professor of science" (and medical school dropout) Gardner Quincey Colton. Sam Cooley was a drugstore clerk who commented after having bloodied his knees and legs during that frenzied event: "If a man would be restrained, he could undergo a severe surgical operation without feeling any pain at the time." The following day, Wells asked Colton and one of his associates, Dr. John Riggs, to administer him nitrous oxide in order to remove one of his molars . . . and there was no pain! After several additional successful trials, Wells returned to Boston to ask his former partner, Dr. William Morton, to help arrange a public demonstration at the Massachusetts General Hospital specifically for the Dental Society of Boston. Unfortunately, the proper dose had been calculated incorrectly, and Wells had used too little. According to an observer, "What started next was pandemonium—the patient started yelling his head off and gesticulating wildly, nearly knocking Dr. Wells on the floor. The two dentists tried vainly to restrain him, but he was too strong for them, and pushing aside the chair and instruments scattered on the floor, he went for Wells, bent on revenge for the hoax that had been played on him. And the audience followed suit. 'Humbug, swindle,' they shouted, 'throw him out. This is a university and not a circus.'" The first public demonstration of anesthesia was a dismal failure, and the humiliated Wells returned to Hartford, apparently having lost his chance to claim credit for the discovery.

Ether

Ether was another important anesthetic agent that gained popularity by the middle of the nineteenth century. Spanish chemist Raymundus Lillius discovered "sweet vitriol" in 1275, though its hypnotic properties remained unknown until they were recognized by physician and alchemist Paracelsus in the sixteenth century. In 1730, German scientist W.G. Frobenius adopted the name "ether," and in 1794 English physicians Richard Peterson and Thomas Beddoes used ether in the treatment of bladder calculi, scurvy, and tuberculosis. None of these gentlemen had recognized the enormous medical significance of this agent, and the discovery of ether did not become clinically relevant until it was picked up by a surgeon in Georgia, Dr. Crawford Long (1815–1878). Dr. Long attended an "ether frolic" and noted that other participants had felt no pain from their bumps and bruises. He came to the appropriate conclusion and used ether as an anesthetic agent during the removal of a tumor from the neck of James Venables on March 30, 1842, in Danielsville, Georgia—$2 for the operation and 25 cents for the ether. According to Long, "the patient continued to inhale ether during the time of the operation and when informed it was over seemed incredulous. He assured me that he did not experience the slightest degree of pain from its performance." By the end of 1846, Long had used ether during seven more procedures, though unfortunately he failed to properly report his findings to the medical community, and thus he had lost his opportunity to be recognized as the discoverer of anesthesia. As Long and others subsequently found out, there are three prerequisites in order to achieve recognition for any new discovery. One must 1) discover something not known, 2) be aware of the significance of that finding, and 3) communicate it to others.

On September 30, 1846, Dr. William Morton, having been impressed by Wells' work, visited physician/chemist Charles T. Jackson (1805–1880) to learn more about nitrous oxide, and to obtain a sample. Jackson previously had given a chemistry lecture in Boston when he accidentally burned his throat with spilled chlorine gas. He also inhaled ether and ammonia, and subsequently noted the immediate absence of pain. This accident probably led him to suggest to Morton that he consider using ether as a more effective anesthetic than nitrous oxide. The evening after Morton's encounter with Jackson, Eben Frost visited Morton with a severe toothache. Using ether, Morton painlessly removed his patient's bicuspid. Frost later testified, "This is to certify that I applied to Dr. Morton at 9 o'clock this evening suffering under the most violent toothache; that Dr. Morton took out his pocket handkerchief, saturated with a preparation of his, from which I breathed for about half a minute, and then was lost in sleep. In an instant more, I awoke and saw my tooth lying upon the floor. I did not experience the slightest pain whatever. I remained 20 minutes in his office afterward, and felt no unpleasant effects from the operation." Dr. William Morton thereby established his claim to fame as having performed the first documented surgical procedure under anesthesia.

Dr. Jacob Bigelow was aware of Morton's work, and provided an important link in the story when he introduced Morton to the well-known professor of surgery, Dr. John Collins Warren of the Harvard Medical School, in order to demonstrate "his" amazing new discovery. Morton's wife documented the feelings that she experienced just prior to

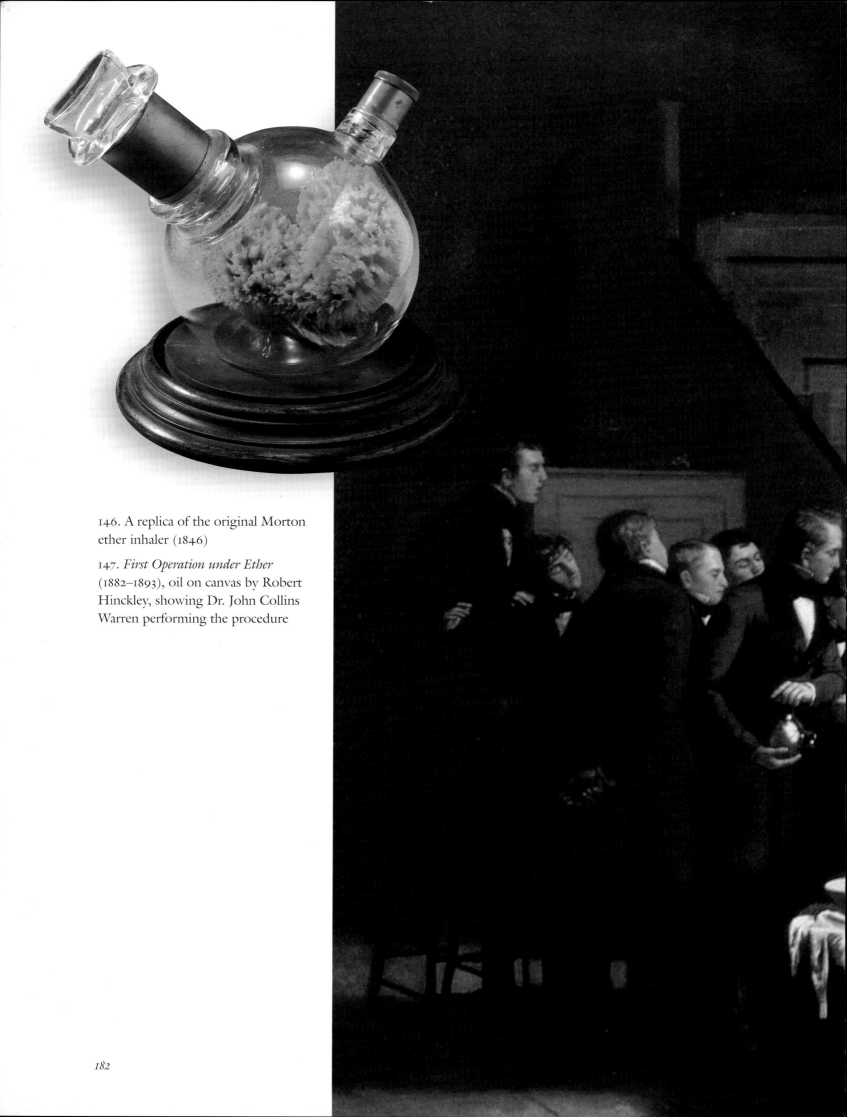

146. A replica of the original Morton ether inhaler (1846)

147. *First Operation under Ether* (1882–1893), oil on canvas by Robert Hinckley, showing Dr. John Collins Warren performing the procedure

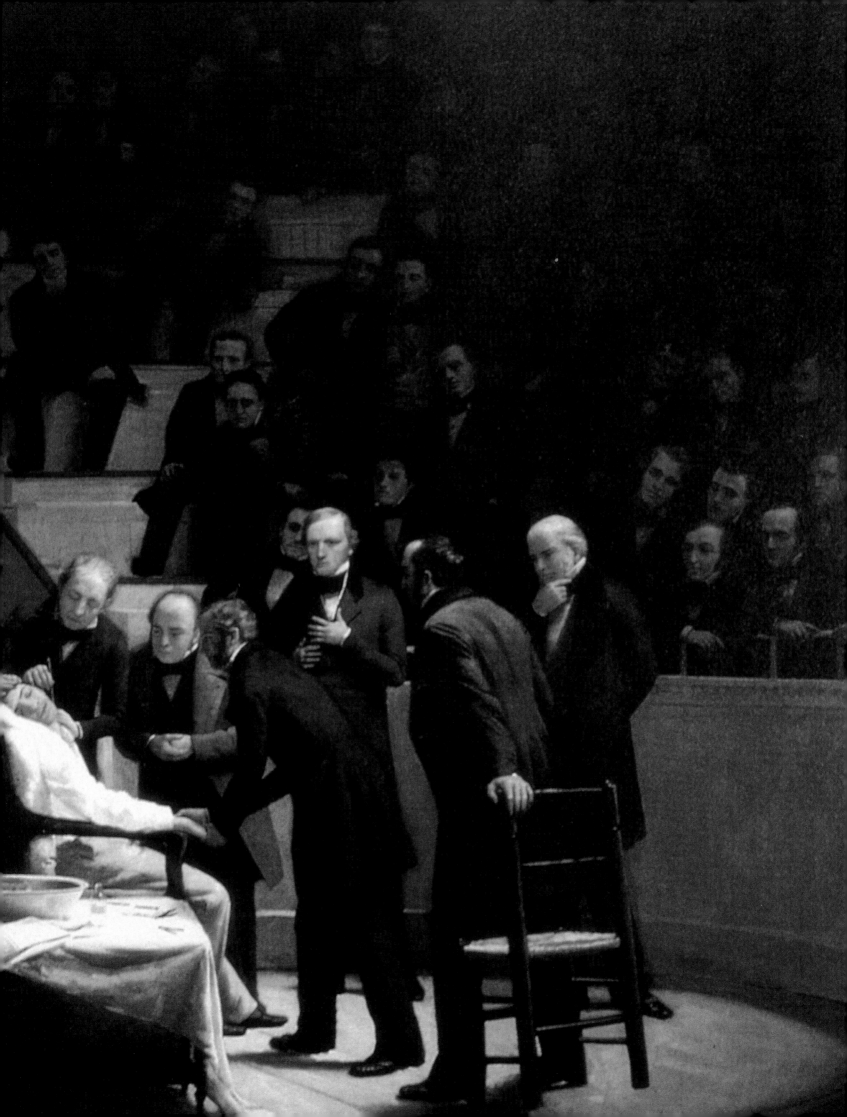

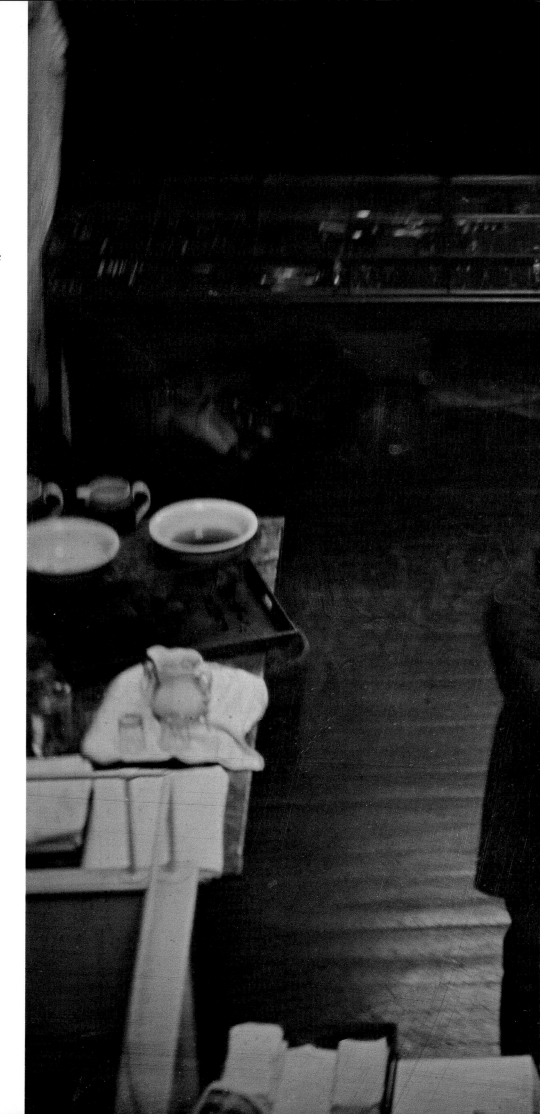

148. Operation using ether for anesthesia in the operating room of the Massachusetts General Hospital in Boston, daguerreotype probably by Josiah Johnson Hawes. This scene depicts Dr. John Collins Warren standing with his hands on the patient's thighs during his last lecture at the MGH in the spring 1847. To Warren's right is Dr. Solomon Townsend, who actually performed the procedure.

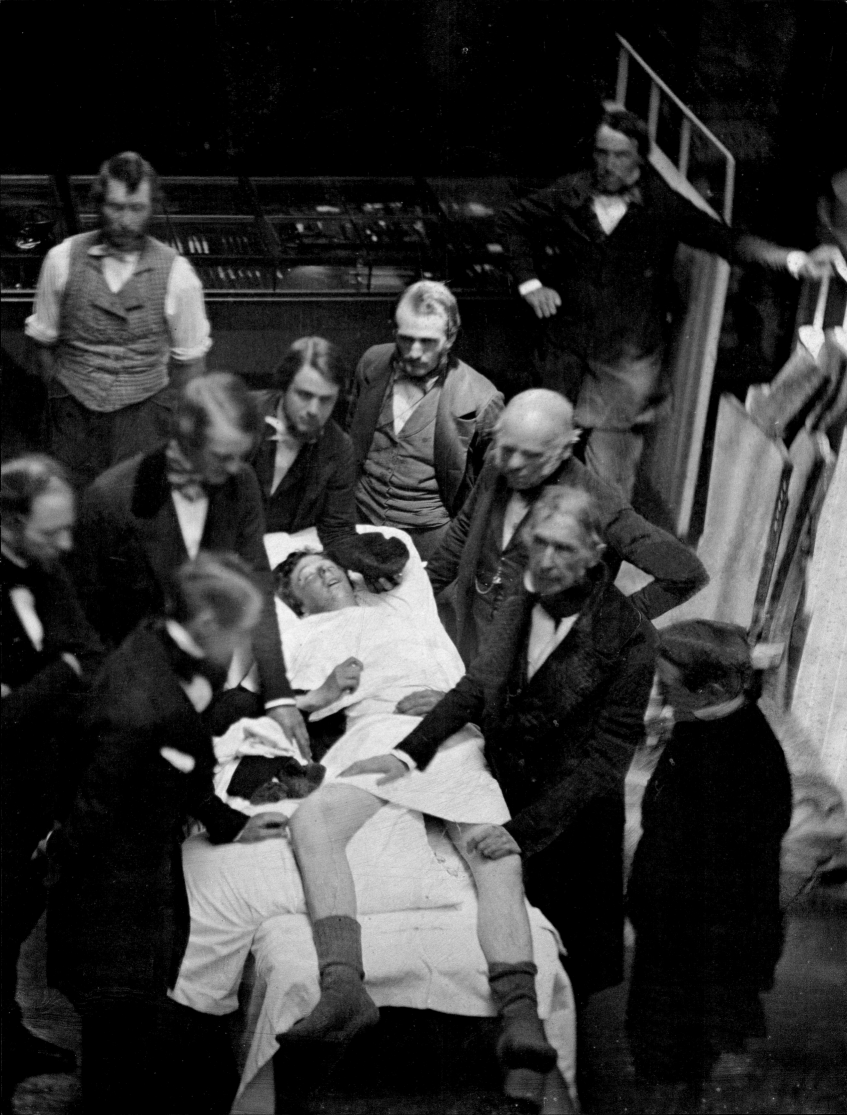

this landmark demonstration, concerns probably shared by all families of those stepping into unchartered scientific territory: "The night before the operation my husband worked until 1 or 2 o'clock in the morning upon his inhaler. I assisted him, nearly beside myself with anxiety, for the strongest influences had been brought to bear upon me to dissuade him from making this attempt. I had been told that one of two things was sure to happen; either the test would fail and my husband would be ruined by the world's ridicule, or he would kill the patient and be tried for manslaughter. Thus I was drawn in two ways; for while I had bounded confidence in my husband, it did not seem possible that so young a man could be wiser than the learned and scientific men before who he proposed to make his demonstration."

The introduction of anesthesia to the medical community took place on October 16, 1846, at the Massachusetts General Hospital amphitheater, now known as the "ether dome" (figures 146–148). The surgeon was Dr. John Collins Warren (1778–1856), and he was a bit distressed by the tardy arrival of Morton who was making some final adjustments to his ether device. Collins, not used to being detained, commented to the prestigious audience, "As Dr. Morton has not arrived, I presume he is otherwise engaged." Morton soon appeared and, after having prepared the patient, responded, "*Your* patient is ready, doctor." During a twenty-five-minute procedure, Collins removed a benign vascular tumor from Gilbert Abbott's neck.

Following the operation, Dr. Warren expressed his approval with the now famous comment, "Gentlemen, this is no humbug." A major turning point in the history of medicine, it was described in the *Boston Medical and Surgical Journal*, November 18, 1846, under the title "Insensibility during Surgical Operations Produced by Inhalation." Warren supplied a firsthand account in a later December 9 edition:

> About five weeks since, Dr. Morton, dentist of this city, informed me that he had invented an apparatus for the inhalation of a vapor, the effect of which was to produce a state of total insensibility to pain and that he had employed it successfully in a sufficient number of cases in his practice to justify him in a belief of its efficacy. He wished for an opportunity to test its power in surgical operations, and I agreed to give him such an opportunity as soon as practicable.
>
> Being at the time in attendance as Surgeon of the Massachusetts General Hospital, a patient presented himself in that valuable institution a few days after my conversation with Dr. Morton, who required an operation for a tumor of the neck, and agreeably to my promise I requested the attendance of Dr. M.
>
> On October 16th, the patient being prepared for the operation,

the apparatus was applied to his mouth by Dr. Morton for about three minutes at the end of which time he sank into a state of insensibility. I immediately made an incision about three inches long through the skin of the neck, and began a dissection among important nerves and blood-vessels without any expression of pain on the part of the patient. Soon after he began to speak incoherently, and appeared to be in an agitated state during the remainder of the operation. Being asked immediately afterwards whether he had suffered much, he said that he had felt as if his neck had been scratched; but subsequently, when inquired of by me, his statement was that he did not experience pain at the time, although aware that the operation was proceeding.

In a more personal description of the events of the day, Mrs. Morton later wrote, "The patient lay silent, with eyes closed as if in sleep; but everyone present fully expected to hear a shriek of agony ring out as the knife struck down into the sensitive nerves, but the stroke came with no accompanying cry. Then another and another, and still the patient lay silent, sleeping while the blood from the severed artery spurted forth. The surgeon was doing his work, and the patient was free from pain."

Harvard's soon-to-be professor of anatomy and physiology, Dr. Oliver Wendell Holmes (and father of the Supreme Court chief justice by the same name), subsequently coined the term "anesthesia," Greek for insensitivity. He pointed out the importance of this discovery when he said, "Nature herself is working out the primal curse which doomed the tenderest of her creatures to the sharpest of her trials, but the fierce extremity of suffering has been steeped in the waters of forgetfulness, and the deepest furrow in the knotted brow of agony has been smoothed for ever."

The controversy regarding credit for the discovery of anesthesia was intense, and began with Long, Wells, Morton, and, Jackson each claiming it for themselves. Following is a brief and sad history of their claims to fame (and to the $100,000 award offered by Congress—later withdrawn):

CRAWFORD LONG, MD
Dr. Long was the first to successfully anesthetize a patient during a procedure with his use of ether in March, 1842, though he did not publish that finding until 1849, and thus was not recognized as the discoverer of anesthesia. He began to use ether in obstetrical cases and died on June 16, 1878 at the bedside of a woman who had just given birth.

HORACE WELLS, DDS
Dr. Wells successfully had his own tooth extracted with nitrous

oxide, but his subsequent public demonstration of anesthesia failed. Wells later withdrew from his practice after the death of one of his patients during a demonstration of nitrous oxide. He began experimenting with chloroform as an alternate anesthetic agent, though became hopelessly addicted. On one occasion, Wells was recovering from the effects of a self-administration when he was imprisoned after throwing sulfuric acid at two prostitutes on Broadway. By one account: "It was not long before Wells was seen as a vagrant tramp, roaming the dark streets of New York. The only companions he could find were the prostitutes of the city, the beggars and the drunkards of the obscure underworld. Soon even these began to shun him which, of course, made matters worse. Horace Wells was toppled head over heels into the realm of madness. One day, believing the whole world was against him, particularly the despicable outcasts and prostitutes, Wells bought a bottle of vitriol and threw it upon two girls who happened to pass by. Amidst the screams of pain and agony, a great multitude assembled, and it was a wonder that Wells was not lynched there and then; the police managed to rescue him with great effort."

While in jail, Wells attended church services, wrote to his family, and then again gained possession of more chloroform. Perhaps still under the influence, that evening he committed suicide by slashing a femoral artery. In the final letter he had earlier written to his family, Wells said: "May God forgive me! Oh! my dear wife and child, whom I leave destitute of the means of support—I would still live and work for you. But I cannot—for were I to live on, I should become a maniac. I feel that I am but little better than one already. . . ." Tragically for Dr. Horace Wells, he was not aware that in the mail at the time of his suicide was a letter sent from the French Academy of Medicine in Paris crediting him with the discovery of anesthesia. To follow were similar accolades by The American Dental Society in 1864, and the American Medical Association in 1870. Wells' finding proved to be a seminal event in nineteenth century health care, and was one of the most important discoveries in the history of medicine!

WILLIAM THOMAS GREEN MORTON, DDS

Dr. Morton was the former partner of Horace Wells, and administered ether at the first successful public demonstration. He tried to patent ether under the name "Letheon" which was a term derived from the river Lethe found in Virgil's *The Aeneid* from which the dead drank to forget their past lives. Morton retired early from the practice of dentistry and unsuccessfully attempted to privately market rights for the use of his anesthetic agent. He entered another business that failed, and subsequently died in poverty of a cerebral hemorrhage in Central Park in July of 1868. He was on his way to file one of his many lawsuits related to the discovery of anesthesia, this one against *The Atlantic Monthly*. The following is on Morton's epitaph:

WILLIAM T. G. MORTON
Inventor and Revealer of Anesthetic Inhalation.
By whom pain in surgery was averted and annulled.
Before whom in all time surgery was agony.
Since whom science has control of pain.

PROFESSOR CHARLES JACKSON
Dr. Jackson had suggested to his pupil, William Morton, that ether could be used as an anesthetic agent. In later testimony, he claimed: "I determined, therefore, to make a more thorough trial of ether vapor, and for that purpose went into my laboratory, which adjoins my house in Somerset Street, and made the experiment from which the discovery of anesthesia was deduced."

As a result of the struggle over the credit for the discovery of anesthesia, Jackson later mentally deteriorated, and, after reading the epitaph on Morton's grave, "uttered a piercing cry and flung himself onto the statue, trying with his fingers to tear it to pieces. Soon an assembly gathered round, staring at the unusual sight of the raving maniac." Jackson was admitted to the McLean Asylum, which was a department in the Massachusetts General Hospital, diagnosed there as a psychotic. Ironically, he spent the last seven years of his life at the same institution where the landmark demonstration of the first use of anesthesia had taken place twenty-seven years earlier.

In fact, this was not the first time that Jackson had alleged his participation in a major discovery. After meeting Samuel Morse on an ocean voyage in 1839, Jackson had claimed responsibility for Morse's invention, and it took Morse "seven years and half of his wealth to clear his name and get the well-deserved priority of being the inventor of the telegraph."

In 1946, Victor Robinson poignantly summed up the relationship between those caught up in the intense rivalry for credit over the discovery of anesthesia: "The four men did not meet in a tavern and pledge eternal brotherhood as the world rejoiced in the Victory over Pain. Alone they drank the wine of bitterness, and tasted the lees of hatred. There was limitless glory for all, but not one would grant a share to another."

Chloroform

Another early anesthetic agent was chloroform, which was discovered by both Dr. Samuel Guthrie in New York and by Eugene Soubeiran in France in 1831. The champion of this anesthetic was Sir James Young Simpson (1811–1870), a renowned obstetrician who first noted its effects after experimenting on himself. Simpson's neighbor, Professor James Miller, reported the rather bizarre events surrounding this great discovery in *The Principles of Surgery* (1852):

> Late one evening—it was the 4th of November, 1847—on returning home after a weary day's labor, Dr. Simpson, with his two friends and assistants, Drs Keith and Matthew Duncan, sat down to their somewhat hazardous work in Dr. Simpson's dining room. Having inhaled several substances, but without much effect, it occurred to Dr. Simpson to try a ponderous material, which he had formerly set aside on a lumber table, and which, on account of its great weight, he had hitherto regarded as of no likelihood whatever. That happened to be a small bottle of chloroform. It was searched for, and recovered from beneath a heap of waste paper. And with each tumbler newly charged, the inhalers resumed their vocation. Immediately an unwonted hilarity seized the party; they became bright-eyed, very happy and very loquacious—expatiating on the delicious aroma of the new fluid. The conversation was of unusual intelligence, and quite charmed the listeners—some ladies of the family and a naval officer, brother-in-law of Dr. Simpson.
>
> But suddenly there was talk of sounds being heard like those of a cotton mill, louder and louder; a moment more, then all was quiet, and then—a crash. On awakening, Dr. Simpson's first perception was mental—'This is far stronger and better than ether', said he to himself. His second was to note that he was prostrate on the floor. . . ."

Dr. Simpson gained international attention following the birth of Wilhelmina Garstairs, the first child to be delivered with the aid of chloroform anesthesia. Simpson reported his discovery to the Medico-Chirurgical Society of Edinburgh on November 10, 1847:

> The lady to whom it was first exhibited during parturition had been previously delivered in the country by perforation of the head of the infant, after a labour of three days' duration. In this, her second confinement, pains supervened a fortnight before the full time. Three hours and a half after they commenced, and ere the first stage of the labour was completed, I placed her under

the influence of the chloroform, by moistening, with half a tea-
spoonful of the liquid, a pocket handkerchief, rolled up into a
funnel shape, and with the broad or open end of the funnel
placed over her mouth and nostrils. In consequence of the evap-
oration of the fluid, it was once more renewed in about ten or
twelve minutes. The child was expelled in about twenty-five minutes after the inhalation was begun. The mother subsequently
remained longer soporose than commonly happens after ether.
The squalling of the child did not, as usual, rouse her; and some
minutes elapsed after the placenta was expelled, and after the
child was removed by the nurse into another room, before the
patient awoke. She then turned round and observed to me that
she had 'enjoyed a very comfortable sleep, and indeed required
it, as she was so tired but would now be more able for the work
before her. . . .' In a little time she again remarked that she was
afraid her 'sleep had stopped the pains.' Shortly afterwards, her
infant was brought in by the nurse from the adjoining room, and
it was a matter of no small difficulty to convince the astonished
mother that the labour was entirely over, and that the child presented to her was really her 'own living baby.'

Chloroform immediately became a popular choice over ether by
physicians, though each anesthetic agent had its drawbacks. Ether was
slow acting, had an unpleasant odor, and the vapor was explosive. It
stimulated the secretion of mucous which increased the cough reflex,
and often resulted in the need for attendants to restrain a struggling
patient. On the other hand, chloroform was more potent and had a
sweet pleasant smell. It was more rapid acting, and it was neither explosive nor flammable. Most changed to the use of chloroform from ether
after its introduction by Dr. James Simpson in 1847, though chloroform
was banned in the United States following a number of related sudden
deaths that occurred over the next few years. The first and most famous
fatality was that of Hannah Greener on January 28, 1848, only ten weeks
after the first use of chloroform. Hannah was a healthy fifteen year old
who had been admitted for the removal of a toenail. Her case was widely read in *The London Medical Gazette* (1848): "At the termination of the
semi-lunar incision, she gave a kick or twitch, which caused me to think
the chloroform had not sufficient effect. I was proceeding to apply more
to the handkerchief, when her lips, which had been previously of a good
colour, became suddenly blanched, and she spluttered at the mouth, as if
in epilepsy. . . . I threw down the handkerchief, dashed cold water in her
face, gave her some internally, followed by brandy, without, however,
the least effect. . . . We laid her on the floor, opened a vein in her arm,

and the jugular vein, but no blood flowed. The whole process of inhalation, operation, venesection, and death, could not, I should say, have occupied more than two minutes." Other reports of death with chloroform followed, and, by 1870, ether and nitrous oxide had replaced chloroform as the anesthetic agents of choice.

An Immediate Controversy

The discovery of anesthesia was not immediately embraced by members of the medical community, and part of the reason was an eighteenth-century attitude toward suffering described by F. Cartwright in 1952: "Behind the decent, civilized Georgian facade, there lies a callousness, a brutality almost unparalleled in history. Pain and suffering were held to be of no account; what mattered was not the degree of pain inflicted, but the fortitude with which it was borne. To such a mentality, anesthesia would have seemed not the greatest single boon ever vouchsafed to suffering humanity, but a matter of very minor importance."

Childbirth is a common and painful part of life, so without surprise it was in the field of obstetrical care that the controversy regarding the use of anesthetic agents first came to the public's attention. A German obstetrician described the ordeal of "natural" childbirth in *Remarks on the Superinduction of Anaesthesia in Natural and Morbid Parturition* (1847): "The bearing down becomes more continued, and there is not unfrequently vomiting. The patient quivers and trembles all over. Her face is flushed, and, with the rest of the body, is bathed in perspiration. Her looks are staring and wild; the features alter so much that they can scarcely be recognized. Her impatience rises to a maximum with loud crying and wailing, and frequently expressions which, even with sensible, high principled women, border close upon insanity."

A great number of obstetricians and religious leaders initially opposed the use of anesthetics, and, in fact, Eufame Macalyane had been burned at the stake in Edinburgh after asking for relief during childbirth. The Presbyterian Church in Scotland relied on the Bible to support their position, and many quoted a passage from Genesis 3:16: "Unto the woman he said, I will greatly multiply thy sorrow and thy conception; in sorrow thy shalt bring forth children; and thy desire shall be to thy husband, and he shall rule over thee." J.F. Meigs, a professor of obstetrics at the Jefferson Medical College in Philadelphia, commented in a June 1848 article in the *Lancet*: "I have always regarded a labour-pain as a most desirable, salutary, and conservative manifestation of life-force. I have found that women, provided they were sustained by cheering counsel and promises, and carefully freed from the distressing element of terror, could in general be made to endure, without great complaint, those labor pains which the friends of anaesthesia desire so earnestly to abolish and nullify for all the fair daughters of Eve." And if he were to lose a patient to anesthesia, "I should feel disposed to clothe myself in sack-cloth, and cast ashes on my head for the remainder of my days. What sufficient motive have I to risk the life or the death of one in a thousand, in a questionable attempt to abrogate one of the general conditions of man?"

At the center of the controversy was a frustrated and angry Dr. James Simpson, who became the chief advocate for the use of chloroform during delivery. In 1847, Simpson sharply responded to religious concerns in his *Answers to the Religious Objection against the Employment of Anesthetic Agents in Midwifery and Surgery*:

> Besides, those who urge, on a kind of religious ground, that an artificial or anesthetic state of unconsciousness should not be induced merely to save frail humanity from the miseries and tortures of bodily pain, forget that we have the greatest of all examples set before us for following out this very principle of practice. I allude to that most singular description of the preliminaries and details of the first surgical operation ever performed on man which is contained in *Gen* II:21, 'And the Lord God caused a deep sleep to fall upon Adam, and he slept; and he took one of his ribs, and closed up the flesh instead thereof.' In this remarkable verse the whole process of a surgical operation is briefly detailed. But the passage is principally striking as affording evidence of our Creator himself using means to save poor human nature from unnecessary endurance of physical pain.

That same year, Simpson issued a plea to his fellow physicians regarding the use of chloroform:

> Medical men will, no doubt, earnestly argue that their established medical opinions and medical practices should not be harshly interfered with by any violent innovations of doctrine regarding the non-necessity and non-propriety of maternal suffering. They will insist on mothers continuing to endure, in all their primitive intensity, all the agonies of childbirth, as a proper sacrifice to the conservatism of the doctrine of the desirability of pain. They will perhaps attempt to frighten their patients into the medical propriety of this sacrifice of their feelings; and some may be found who will unscrupulously ascribe to the new agency any misadventures, from any causes whatever, that may happen to occur in practice. But husbands will scarcely permit the sufferings of their wives to be perpetuated, merely in order that the tranquility of this or that medical dogma be not rudely disturbed. Women themselves will betimes rebel against enduring the usual tortures and miseries of childbirth, merely to sub-

serve the caprice of their medical attendants. And I more than doubt if any physician is justified, on any grounds, medical or moral, in deliberately desiring and asking his patients to shriek and writhe on in their agonies for a few months or a few years longer—in order that, by doing so, they may defer to his professional apathy, or pander to his professional prejudices.

Simpson's struggle to make the use of anesthesia a part of routine medical care dramatically improved in April 1853 when Queen Victoria's physician, Dr. John Snow, administered chloroform for the birth of her seventh child, Prince Leopold. Simpson was subsequently knighted, and the Queen commented, "Dr. Snow gave me the blessed chloroform and the effect was mild, calming, and beautiful beyond bounds." The Queen's acceptance of anesthesia had a profoundly positive effect on the use of chloroform in England and America.

Significant resistance to the use of anesthesia by physicians remained, however, and included Dr. William Coulson, a lithotomist who stated the following in his address to the Medical Society of London regarding the removal of a bladder stone, as reported in the *Lancet* (1855):

> Yet when the nature of this delicate operation is considered, carried on, as it were, in the dark, and when it is further borne in mind that the operator should be fully aware of every step he is taking; in an organ completely removed from his sight, it cannot be expedient to render the patient insensible, and thus lose the aid which his feelings afford. . . . A case in point occurred in a public hospital before the introduction of crushing, at a time when the perforator alone was employed. Notwithstanding the cries of the patient, the surgeon went on using the perforator in a most industrious manner. The bystanders feared something wrong, but the surgeon appealed to the sound of the metallic body striking against stone, as a proof that the calculus was actually seized, and undergoing the process of perforation. In a few seconds the cries of the patient became more violent; blood issued abundantly from the urethra. The bystanders now interfered, and pointed out to the surgeon, that the noise which he had heard was produced by the external end of the perforator striking against the seals of his watch-chain. The operation was suspended, and the life of the patient was saved; but had he been insensible, there is no saying what mischief might not have been inflicted, for the calculus was not between the blades of the instrument.

William Atkinson, the first president of the American Dental Association, once said:

I think anesthesia is of the devil,
and I cannot give my sanction. . . .
I wish there were no such thing as
anesthesia! I do not think man
should be prevented from passing
through what God intended them to
endure.

In the latter part of the twentieth century, more physicians used anesthetic agents in surgery, and more favorable papers were to be found. For example, in 1896, Dr. Valentine Mott argued in the *Boston Med and Surgical Journal* that the use of anesthesia reduced surgical complications by keeping the patient still during the procedure: "How often when operating in some deep, dark wound, along the course of some great vein, with thin walls, alternately distended and flaccid with the vital current—how often have I dreaded that some unfortunate struggle of the patient would deviate the knife a little from its proper course, and that I, who fain would be the deliverer, should involuntarily become the executioner, seeing my patient perish in my hands by the most appalling form of death! Had he been insensible, I should have felt no alarm." Another favorable statement came from F.J. Grant in the *Lancet* (1872): "The old operators—ignorant of anatomy, and always of pathology—are described as 'agitated trembling, miserable, hesitating in the midst of difficulties, turning round to their friends for that support which should come from within, feeling in the wound for things which they did not understand, holding consultations amid the cries of the patient, or even retiring to consult about his case, while he lay bleeding, in great pain and awful expectation.' Nowadays, this picture is commonly reversed: witness the calm composure of the surgeon and the placid sleep of the patient."

German physician Johann Friedrich Dieffenbach (1795–1847), the first to perform practical plastic surgery on a regular basis, immediately recognized the significance of this landmark discovery. He said, "The wonderful dream that pain has been taken away from us has become a reality. Pain, the highest consciousness of our earthy existence, the most distinct sensation of the imperfection of our body, must bow before the power of the human mind, before the power of ether vapor."

By the end of the nineteenth century, a number of different devices were available to the growing number of surgeons who had decided to use anesthetic agents during their procedures (figure 149). Physicians could now develop interventional procedures never before possible, allowing them to treat conditions that had previously considered fatal. The great irony of the history of anesthesia remains the pain suffered by those who participated in its descovery.

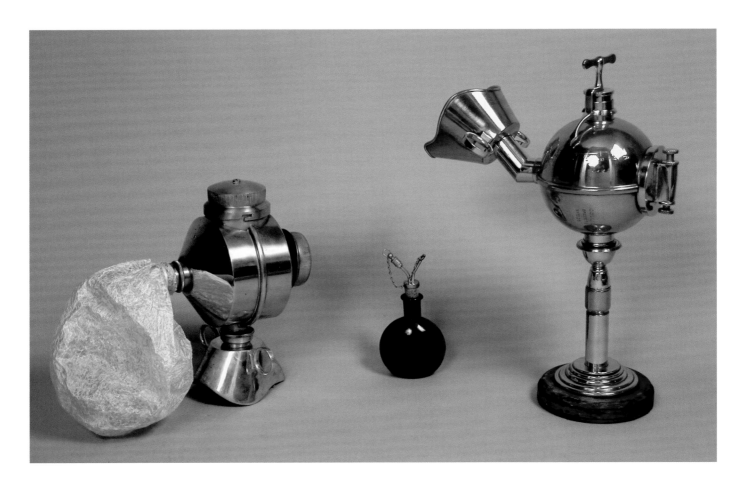

149. Late nineteenth-century ether apparatuses: Ombredanne with animal bladder by Drapier, ether drip bottle, mounted ether inhaler by Collin

Local Anesthesia

Another narcotic "discovered" in the nineteenth century was cocaine, an effective extract from the Peruvian coca plant that had been used as an anesthetic agent for centuries in South America. Somewhat surprisingly, the first to recommend the local use of cocaine for anesthesia was Dr. Sigmund Freud, though he never received credit in medical circles for making that important discovery. Cocaine was legal at the time and could be found in many over-the-counter preparations; Freud, along with many others, took cocaine as an antidepressant and stimulant, a habit that left him with a strong addiction. One of the reasons that Freud got involved in research with cocaine was in the hope that he could somehow use the drug to help his friend Ernst von Fleischl-Marxow withdraw from a morphine addiction. Freud was unsuccessful, however, and his friend soon died even more addicted to cocaine.

The discovery of the anesthetic properties of cocaine began with the abdominal pain of an associate for which Freud recommended a five per-cent cocaine solution for relief. The drug was effective, though his friend complained of numbness around his lips and tongue. Dr. Carl Koller became aware of the incident and went on to demonstrate the effective-ness of cocaine hydrochloride as a topical anesthetic for surgery on the eye, ear, nose, and throat. Cocaine quickly became popular worldwide as a local anesthetic, though Freud received no credit. This is Freud's account of the incident:

> In 1884, a side but deep interest made me have the Merck Company supply me with an alkaloid quite little known at the time, to study its physiological effects. While engrossed in this research, the opportunity for me then occurred to make a trip to see my fiancée, whom I had not seen for almost two years. I then quickly completed my investigation on cocaine and, in the short text I published, I included the notice that other uses of the substance will soon be revealed too. At the same time, I made an instant recommendation to my friend L. Konigstein, an eye doctor, to check on the extent to which the anesthetic qualities of cocaine might also be used with sore eyes. On my return, I found that it was not him but another friend of mine, Carl Koller (now in New York), who, after hearing me talking about cocaine, had in fact made the decisive experiments on animals' eyes and had presented his findings at the Ophthalmology Congress in Heidelberg. That is why Koller has been rightfully considered as the discoverer of cocaine-based local anesthesia, which has become so important in minor surgery. . . .

Freud was thus overlooked regarding one of the most important discoveries of the nineteenth century as the two loves of his life drew him away from his research, his fiancée Martha Bernays and his cocaine. In a letter to Ms Bernays on June 2, 1884, Freud wrote, "In my last serious depression I took cocaine again and a small dose lifted me to the heights in a wonderful fashion. I am just now collecting the literature for a song of praise to this magical substance."

Dr. William Halsted remarked on the momentous progress that had taken place in surgery during the nineteenth century in his essay to a graduating class from Yale University in *The Training of a Surgeon*: "Pain, hemorrhage, infection, the three great evils which had always embittered the practice of surgery and checked its progress, were, in a moment, in a quarter of a century (1846–1873) robbed of their terrors. A new era had dawned; and in the 30 years which have elapsed since the graduation of the class of 1874 from Yale, probably more has been accomplished to place surgery on a truly scientific basis than in all the centuries which had proceeded this wondrous period."

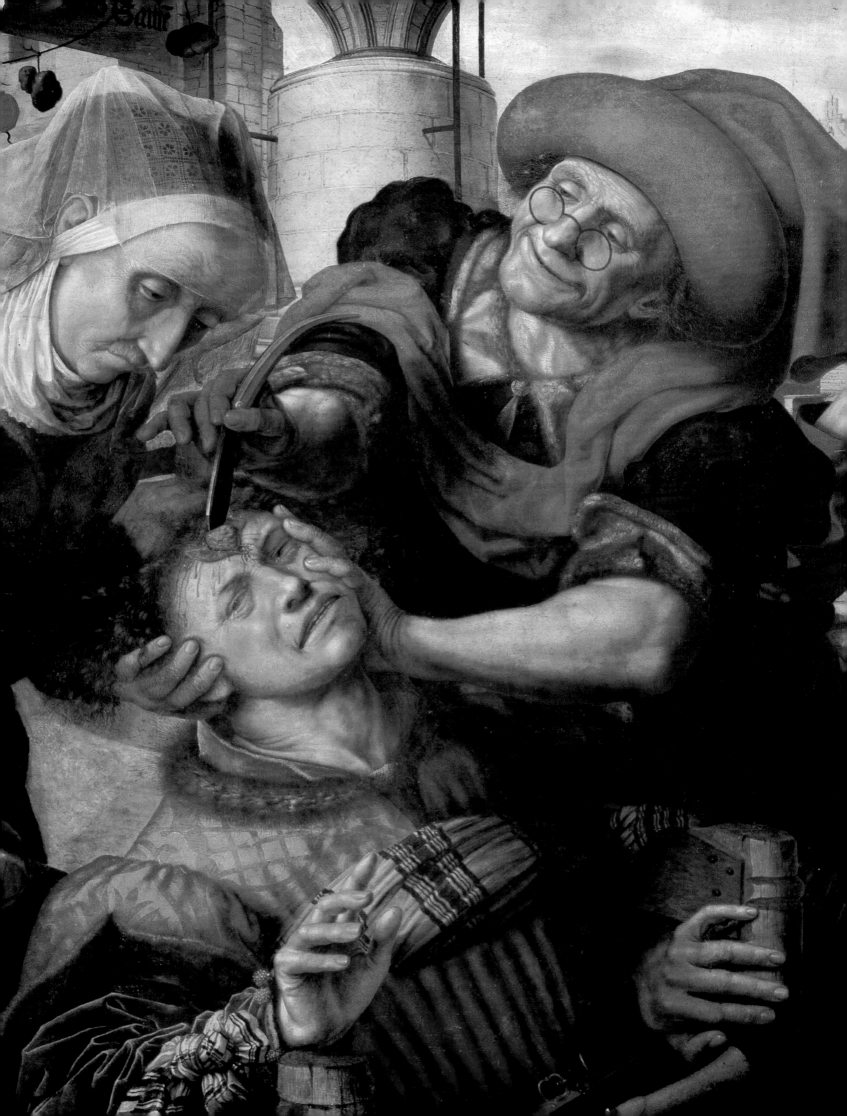

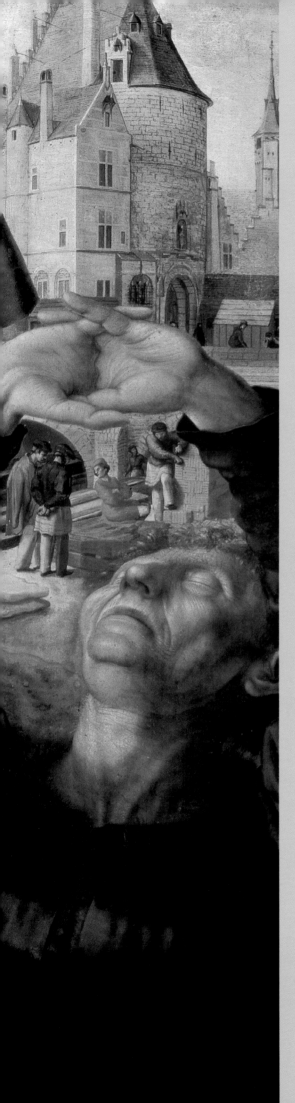

TRAUMA SURGERY

Vertigo, vomiting, stupidity, haemorrhage, loss of sense, either partial or total, are the symptoms of this kind of mischief…

PERCIVAL POTT
The Chirurgical Works of Percival Pott (1778)

Detail. *Extraction of the Fool's Stone,* oil on wood by Jan Sanders van Hemessen (1500-1557)

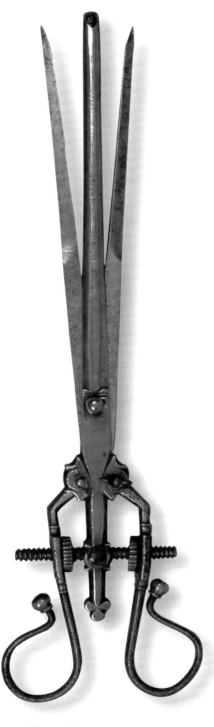

arring nations have always given physicians both the obligation and the opportunity to find new ways in which to treat trauma (figures 150, 151). Despite the fact that invasive surgery was not possible prior to the nineteenth century discovery of anesthesia, many important innovations resulted from desperate efforts made by military surgeons whose wards were suddenly overrun with battered troops.

NEUROSURGERY

Head trauma resulting in the development of a subdural hematoma, or blood clot around the brain, was not an uncommon medical condition faced by physicians after military confrontations. These clots needed to be removed and made trepanning (the excision of a section of skull) a fairly routine practice throughout early medical history. This was also the first documented operation performed in prehistoric times as early "healers" hoped to allow the departure of evil spirits whose presence was suggested by such symptoms as seizures, headaches, depression, or any bizarre behavior. Healed wounds found in ancient skulls, including a trepanned skull found in the village of Ensisheim on the boarder of France and Germany (7000 B.C.), attest to the fact that many patients seem to have survived these early operations (figures 152, 153). Some skulls have shown evidence of trepanning at different periods of the patient's life, and there is evidence that several procedures were performed at the same time. In ancient Greece, a drill-bore called a trypanon was used to create small holes in the cranium that were united to form a larger hole with a chisel. Trepanning was accepted as an important neurosurgical procedure well into the nineteenth century (figures 154–157).

Since a specific diagnosis could only be made on the basis of a neurological examination, physicians often managed patients in a conservative way, as demonstrated in this excerpt from the ancient Egyptian Smith papyrus:

CASE 6
Instructions concerning a gaping wound in his head, penetrating to the bone, smashing the skull, rending open the brain of his skull.

If thou examinest a man having a gaping wound in his head, penetrating to the bone, smashing his skull, rending open the brain of his skull, thou shouldst palpate his wound. Shouldst thou find that smash which is in his skull those corrugations which form in molten copper, something therein throbbing

150. Above. Arrow remover (ca. 1540)
151. Multiple trauma in *Feldtbüch der Wundartzney* (1517) by Hans von Gersdorff

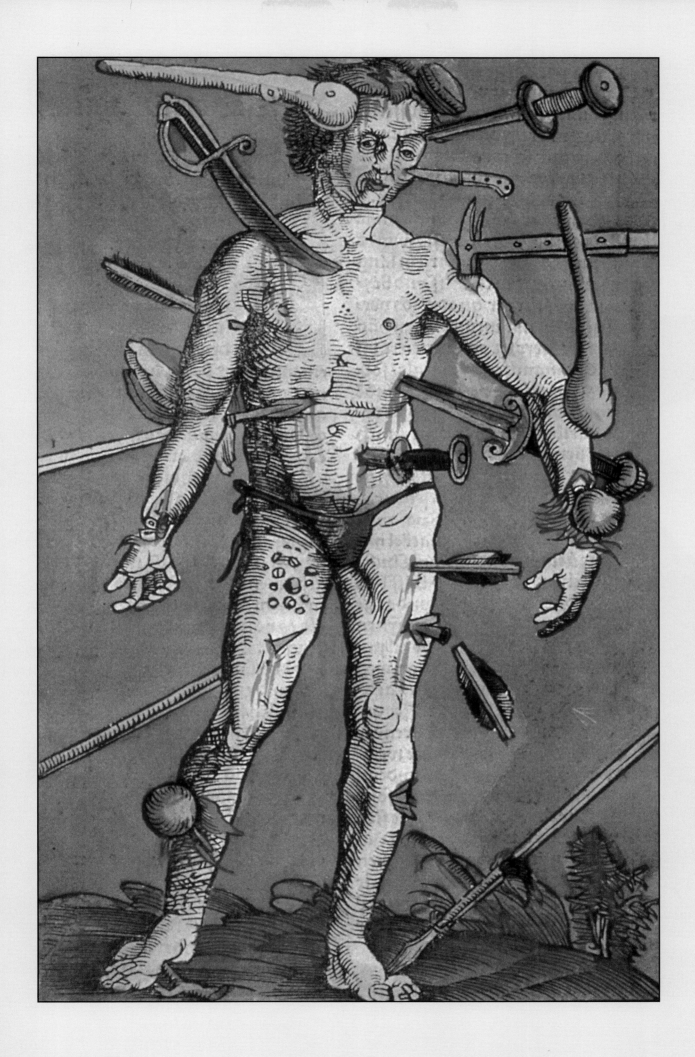

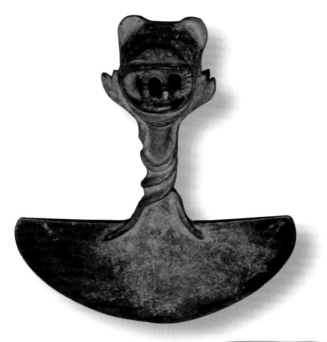

(and) fluttering under the fingers, like the weak place of an infant's crown before it becomes whole—when it has happened there is no throbbing (and) fluttering under thy fingers until the brain of his skull is rent open—he discharges blood from both nostrils, he suffers with stiffness in his neck.

Thou shouldst say: 'An ailment not to be treated.'

Thou shouldst anoint that wound with grease. Thou shalt not bind it; thou shalt not apply two strips upon it: until thou knowest that he has reached a decisive point.

The following description addressed an infrequent complication of head trauma:

Instruction concerning a dislocation of a vertebra of his neck:

If you examine a man having a dislocation of a vertebra of his neck, should you find him unconscious of his arms and legs on account of it, while his phallus is erected on account of it and sperm drops from his member without his knowing; his flesh has received wind; his eyes are blood-shot—then you should say concerning him: 'He has a dislocation of a vertebra of his neck, since he is unconscious of his legs and arms, and his sperm dribbles. An ailment which cannot be treated.'

A more common result of head trauma is the development of a seizure disorder, and medical thera-py was always considered before resorting to surgery. Following is the etiology, diagnosis, and treatment of epilepsy according to Philip Woodman in *The Modern Physician* (1712):

An Epilepsy or Falling Sickness is a sudden Abolition of sense, accompanied with alternate convulsive Motions of the limbs, and Prostration on the Ground.

The Epilepsy is produced either from internal or external Causes; the internal Causes are a disorderly motion of the Animal Spirits . . . Acrimony of the Humours is produced sever-al ways as from a depraved Digestion of the Stomach, a stoppage of the Menses, a too long retention of the Semen in Hot, Youthful Constitutions, and from the stoppage of any wonted Evacuation. . . .

The external Cause is from a Puncture of the Nerve or Tendon . . . Or from hearing of some sudden disagreeable News . . . also Wounds of the Head.

152. Inca tumi knife with puma and intertwining snakes (ca. 1500–1700?)

153. Peruvian skull (elongated by early banding) with partially healed trephine surgery (age unknown)

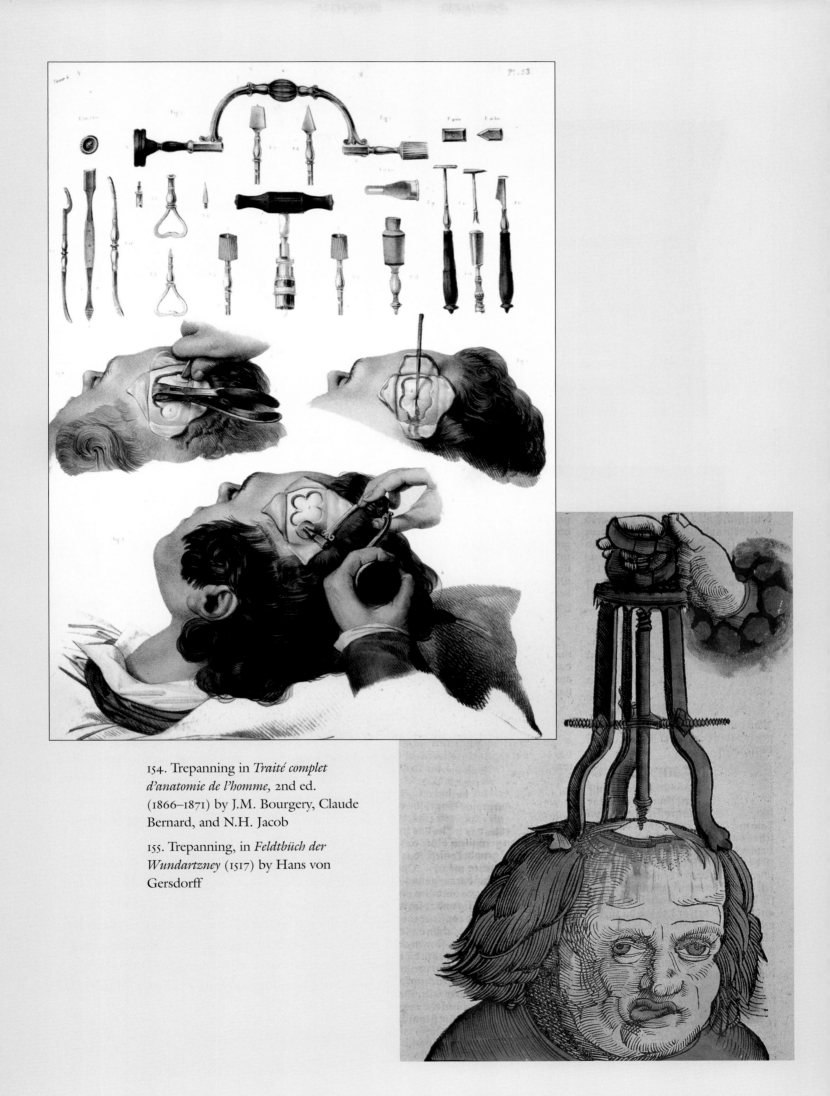

154. Trepanning in *Traité complet d'anatomie de l'homme,* 2nd ed. (1866–1871) by J.M. Bourgery, Claude Bernard, and N.H. Jacob

155. Trepanning, in *Feldtbüch der Wundartzney* (1517) by Hans von Gersdorff

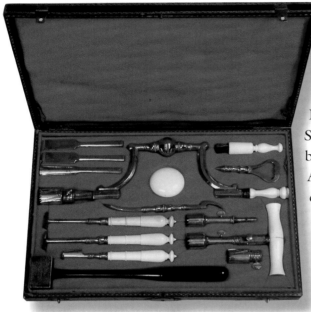

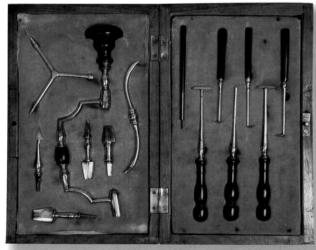

156. Trepanning set (ca. 1780) by Grangeret

157. Trepanning set with trephine brace and Galt's trephine, raspatories, lenticulars, and elevator (ca. 1760)

The following medicated Ale hath done Wonders, in totally curing this Disease; as, take Oak, Fern, and male Penny Roots Fresh, of each Four Ounces, Mistletoe of the Oak cut small, and Sassafras Word of each two Ounces, the Dung of a Peacock, and of Pidgeons, of each one Ounce and half, Raisins of the Sun Stoned ten Ounces, all being cut small, put into a bag, and hang it in three Gallons of New Small Ale. After it has done Working; let this continue eight or ten days, then let the Party drink a quarter of a Pint, every Morning Fasting, and about eleven a Clock, and at Night going to bed.

The following Powder taken Morning and Evening has cured many. Take of the Ashes of a Mole burnt, two ounces, Earth worms cleansed, dryed and powdered, Humane and Cinnabar of Antimony, of each half an Ounce: mix them well, and give it from sixteen to twenty four Grains, twice a day, three days before and after every New and Full Moon.

Percival Pott pointed out the appropriate time for neurosurgical intervention in *The Chirurgical Works of Percival Pott* (1778): "Vertigo, vomiting, stupidity, haemorrhage, loss of sense, either partial or total, are the symptoms of this kind of mischief. . . ." Benjamin Bell added in *Lectures on the Principles and Practice of Surgery, with Additional Notes and Cases* (1824–1827): "Giddiness; dimness of sight; stupefaction; loss of voluntary motion; vomiting; an apoplectic stertor in the breathing; convulsive tremors in different muscles; a dilated state of the pupils, even when the eyes are exposed to a clear light; paralysis of different parts, especially of the side of the body opposite to the injured part of the head; involuntary evacuation of the urine and faeces; and oppressed, and in many cases an irregular pulse; and when the violence done to the head has been considerable, it is commonly attended with a discharge of blood from the nose, eyes, and ears."

Hermann Boerhaave described the natural progression of untreated head trauma in *Boerhaave's Aphorisms: Concerning the Knowledge and Cure of Diseases* (1715): "When the Scull is depress'd in Children, or in grown People after a Fracture the Brain is squeezed; and according to the different places of it thus press'd, the different bigness, depth, sharpness, and pricking of the pressing Body; are produced, a Dumness, Drowsiness, Vertigo, Tinkling, Cloudiness, Delirium, vomiting of Choler, Head-ache,

Convulsions, Palsie, involuntary Stools and Urine, Apoplexies, Fevers, and Death."

Laurence Heister's acceptance of Galen's advice regarding the importance of balanced humors is evident in *A General System of Surgery, in Three Parts* (1743):

> 1. Open a Vein, and draw away as much Blood as the strength of your Patient will admit; this will take off the Impetus of the vessels, and Prevent the Extravasion of more Blood. 2. Prescribe a pretty brisk Purge, to lesen the quantity of Fluids, for which purpose you may also give sharp Clysters. 3. Foment the Head with medicated Bags, and apply a melilot Plaster to it. 4. Endeavor to rouse the Patient by volatile applications to his Nostrils. . . .
>
> This method does not immediately procure the desired effect, therefore it must be continued for some time, and the Prescriptions frequently repeated; and more particularly when the Symptoms seem by degrees to abate. The repetition of bleeding in this case may seem strange to some, but it must be to those who are ignorant of the good effects it produces by lessening the quantity of Fluids, and by restoring the course of the stagnating Blood. If the Patient finds a little relief from the first bleeding, it will be proper to repeat the Operation a second and a third time, especially if he is young and athletic, and to apply remedies which we have recommended above in the Intervals, till the Disorder is entirely removed.
>
> But when you find, notwithstanding these applications, that the Symptoms rather encrease than abate, you will be abliged to make Perforation in the *Cranium* with the *Trepan*, that there may be a Passage for the discharge of the confined grumous Blood. When you cannot discover the Part of the Head which is principally affected, you must perforate the Skull in several places, till you hit upon the right.

The following case described by Percival Pott in his *Chirurgical Works* exemplifies medical care and trepanning in the eighteenth century:

> CASE XVIII
>
> A young man playing at cudgels in Moorfields received a stroke on his forehead; it did not seam either to himself or the spectators to have been a severe one, but as it produced blood it was deemed by the laws of the game a broken head, and he was obliged to yield to his antagonist.
>
> As it gave him no trouble, he took no notice of it; was for several nights afterwards engaged in the same diversion, and fol-

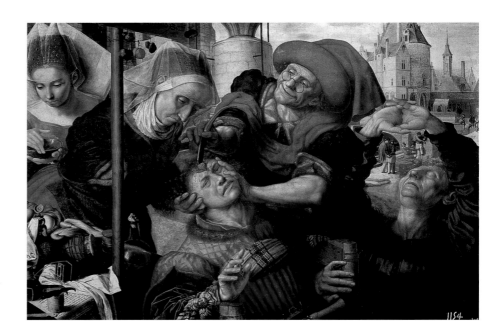

158. *Extraction of the fool's stone*, oil on wood by Jan Sanders van Hemessen (1500–1557)

lowed his daily labour. On the ninth day from that on which he received the blow he thought that his forehead was somewhat swollen, and felt tender to the touch, on the eleventh it was more tumefied and more painful, and on the twelfth he found himself so much out of order, that he applied to be received into St. Bartholomew's hospital.

An incision was made into the tumor; a thin brown ichor was discharged, and a bare bone being discovered, a circular piece of the scalp was removed, which discovered a fracture. The trephine was applied twice along the track of the fracture, by which means it was almost totally removed. The dura matter was found discoloured, and beginning to have matter on its surface. The patient was let blood, and ordered to take the sal absinth. mixture with a few grains of rhubarb in it every six hours. The succeeding night was passed ill; the patient complained much of pain, and got little or no sleep. On the fourteenth his fever was high, his skin hot, and his pulse full and hard; fourteen ounces of blood were taken from one of the jugulars; and as he still continued costive, a lenitive purge was given a few hours afterwards. On the seventeenth every thing bore a bad aspect, both as to his wound and his general state: he got no rest, his fever was high, and the wound very ill-conditioned. His head was again very carefully examined, in order if possible to discover some other injured part. No such injury was found; and it being impossible that he should remain in his present state, evacuation seemed to be his only chance, and therefore fourteen ounces more of blood were drawn from one of the temporal arteries, by which he fainted, and after which he seemed to be somewhat easier.

For three days from this time he seemed to be considerably better; but on the twenty-first he was again in as much pain as ever, and the sore again begun to put on a bad aspect.

The benefit which he had once already received from phlebotomy had been manifest; and as his pulse was well able to bear it again, the temporal arteries were again opened, and he was bled till his pulse failed so much and so suddenly that I was not a little alarmed. By proper care he was brought to himself, and I had no other trouble during his cure than what proceeded from the extreme weakness, which the bark soon removed.

Although this man may very justly be said to have been saved by the frequent repetition of phlebotomy, yet as matter was beginning to be formed on the surface of the dura matter, and as such matter could have no outlet whereby to escape, it is very clear, that unless the cranium had been perforated he must have perished.

Of course, early quack physicians found an opportunity here and roamed the countryside curing the insane or possessed by removing the "stone of insanity." The healer made an incision in the forehead of those afflicted, and, while palming a stone, he appeared to remove it for a cure. The present day expression describing one who exhibits unusual behavior as having "rocks in the head" is probably derived from that practice (figure 158).

ORTHOPEDIC SURGERY

Prehistoric skeletons have commonly demonstrated evidence of healed fractures, and certainly physicians have always been faced with the need to address broken bones and displaced joints. Some of the finest early illustrations were those of the skeletal system, and orthopedic repair was a subject of some of the earliest medical texts (figures 159–164). Percival Pott provides an insight into the repair of fractures in his *Chirurgical Works* (1778) with the following recommendations:

In order to accomplish this, we are directed, if the fracture be of the thigh or leg, to place the patient in a supine posture, and the broken limb in a straight one; then having the upper part of it held firm and steady, by proper assistants, we are ordered, by means of hands, ligatures, lacs, or even in some cases by pieces of machinery, to make such an extension or stretching of the limb lengthways, as shall enable the surgeon to place the ends of the broken bone in as apt, that is, in as even a position, with regard

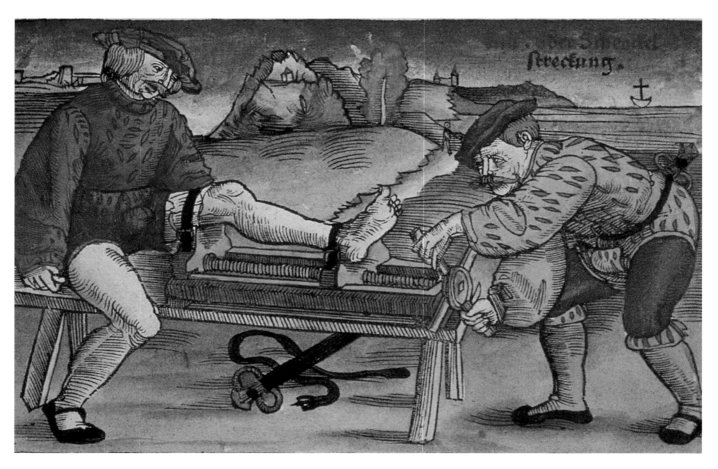

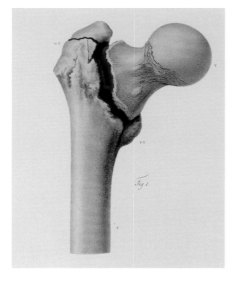 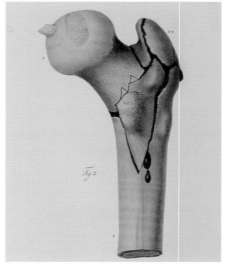 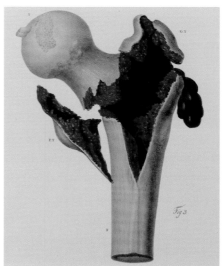

159. Top. Repair of a fractured leg in
Feldtbüch der Wundartzney (1517) by
Hans von Gersdorff

160. Fractured femurs from *Anatomia
Pathologique du corps Humain*, book 2
(1835–1842) by J. Cruveilhier

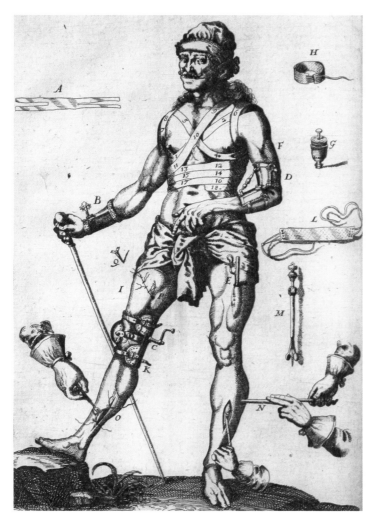

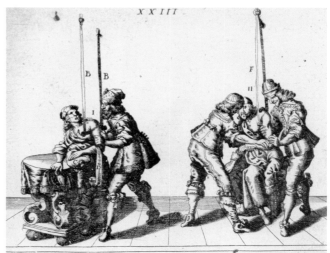

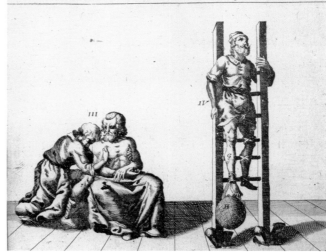

to each other, as the nature of the fracture will admit. —This is a short description of what in the vulgar phrase, is called setting a broken bone; and is most commonly a painful operation to the patient, a fatiguing one to the operator and his assistants; and what is worse, is in many instances found to be inefficacious; at least, not fully to answer the intention of the bone, or the expectation of the other.

Pott then went on to describe the consequences of a compound fracture (in which bone pierces the skin):

Gangrene and mortification are sometimes the inevitable consequences of the mischief done to the limb at the time that the bone is broken; or they are the consequences of the laceration of parts made by the mere protrusion of the said bone.

    They are also sometimes the effect of improper or negligent treatment; of great violence used in making extension; of irritation of the wounded parts, by poking after, or in removing fragments or splinters of bone; of painful dressings; of improper disposition of the limb, and of the neglect of phlebotomy, anodynes, evacuation, &c. Any or all these, are capable either of inducing such a state of inflammation as shall end in a gangrene,

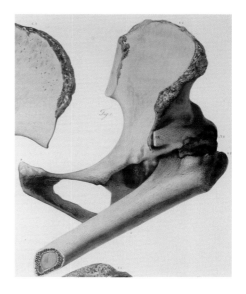

161. Multiple trauma in *Armamentarium Chiruigicum* (1655) by Joannis Scultetus

162. Repair of a fracture and dislocation in *Armamentarium Chiruigicum*

163. Dislocated femur from *Anatomia Pathologique du corps Humain*, book 2 (1835–1842) by J. Cruveilhier

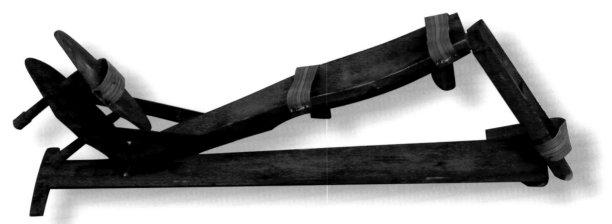

164. Wooden leg splint (ca. 1850) by
A.M. Day of Bennington, Vermont

or of permitting the inflammation, necessarily attendant upon such accident, to terminate in the same event.

When such accident or such disease is the mere consequence of the injury done to the limb, either at the time of or by the fracture, it generally makes its appearance very early; in which case also, its progress is generally too rapid for art to check. For these reasons, when the mischief seems to be of such as that gangrene and mortification are most likely to ensue, no time can be spared, and the impending mischief must either be submitted to or prevented by early amputation. I have already said, that a very few hours make all the difference between probable safety and destruction. If we wait till the disease has taken possession of the limb, even in the smallest degree, the operation will serve no purpose, but that of accelerating the patient's death.

The death rate from compound fractures was well over fifty percent until Joseph Lister incorporated the use of aseptic procedures in surgery. Following is a jubilant letter written by Lister to his father on May 27, 1866, on the benefits of his aseptic technique: "One of my cases at the hospital would, I think, interest thee. It was a compound fracture with a rather large wound, and with great loss of skin and bleeding in the tissues, which caused much swelling. Though I hardly expected any success, I tried carbolic acid on the wound, to prevent blood decomposition and thus avoid the awful result of pus formation in the leg. Well, it is now eight days since the accident, and the patient has reacted just as if there had been no open wound—as though the fracture had been a simple one. Appetite, sleep, etc. have been good and the leg has gradually decreased in girth without any sign of pus formation. A truly dangerous injury seems to have been robbed of its most perilous element."

ALTERNATIVES TO AMPUTATION

Certainly the most reasonable repair for the loss of an extremity is reimplantation, and the earliest reported application of that technique was outlined in the Indian *Susruta-samhita*. This document was written in Sanskrit between 800 and 600 B.C. by the famous Hindu physician and author Susruta, and it is the foundation of surgical care in India. In India, the practice of amputating a nose was a common punishment for adultery, treason, and other egregious crimes for thousands of years and is still practiced in some parts of the country today. As a result, reconstructive rhinoplasty, or *nacta* in the Hindu language, has been a fairly common procedure and one uniquely attributed to Indian medicine. Because the upper castes, or Brahmins, avoided personal contact, surgery was left to lower-caste physicians, including the Kshatriyas and Vaishyas. The following is a description by Susruta of repair for an amputated nose: "First the leaf of a creeper, long and broad enough to fully cover the whole of the severed or clipped off part, should be gathered; and a patch of living flesh, equal in dimension to the preceding leaf, should be sliced off (from down upward) from the region of the cheek (or forehead) and, after scarifying it with a knife, swiftly adhered to the severed nose. Then the cool-headed physician should steadily tie it up with a bandage decent to look at and perfectly suited to the end for which it has been employed. The physician should make sure that the adhesion of the severed parts has been fully effected and then insert two small pipes into the nostrils to facilitate respiration, and to prevent the adhesioned flesh from hanging down." After a period of healing, the attachment between the forehead and the nose was divided. This was called the "Indian method," and, in about 1550, surgeon Gasparo Tagliacozzi modified the procedure by connecting a flap from the patient's arm to his nose. This alternate technique is known as the "Italian method" (figure 165).

Successful reattachment was the exception, however, and amputation has always been the norm for diseased or traumatized limbs. Rarely were functional prostheses available, though Pietro De Marchetti (1589–1673) reported this excellent result in *Observuatiomum Medico-Chirurgicarum Raiorum Sylloge* (1664):

> Nerves and tendons must never be sutured, for this practice is often followed by fatal tetanus. The ingenious surgeon should rather remedy deformities by appropriate splints, as I did in the case of a distinguished Marshal of France, of the family of Montmorency. He received a sword cut on the right wrist, dividing the extensor tendons of the thumb. When the wound healed the thumb was drawn across the palm of the hand, so that he could not hold sword, dagger or lance, and was entirely incapacitated for the profession of arms, apart from which he declared life was not worth living. So he consulted me about amputating his hand, to which I could in no wise consent, but devised an

165. Rhinoplasty: (top) the Indian method; and (bottom) the Italian method in *Traité complet d'anatomie de l'homme,* 2nd ed. (1866–1871) by J.M. Bourgery, Claude Bernard, and N.H. Jacob

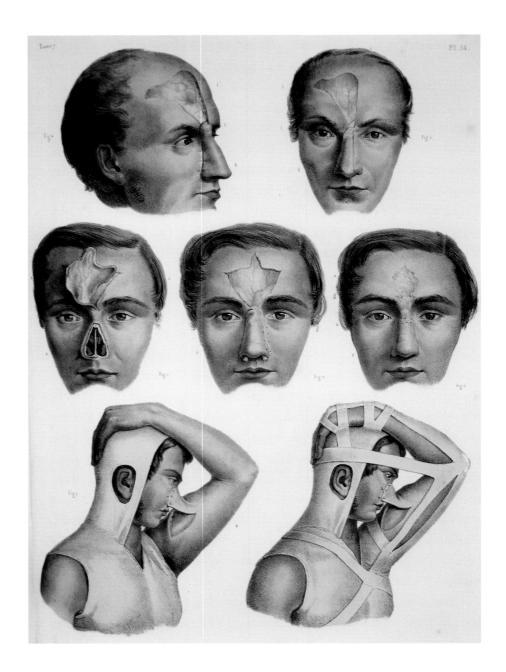

iron case to hold the thumb out, fixed by two cords to bracelets round the wrist, and so he was able to hold and use all kinds of weapons.

In the nineteenth century, surgical sets became specialized for the care of orthopedic injury (figures 166, 167).

GUNSHOT WOUNDS: BELL AND THE BULLET

Though gunpowder had been in use for thousands of years, the invention of firearms in the fifteenth century presented physicians with new challenges regarding the removal of foreign bodies. The surgical problems were indeed formidable, and Laurence Heister described one drastic method of treating gunshot wounds in the eighteenth century: "When a large Piece of Bone is driven away by a Pistol or Musquet Ball, it is better to cut off the lower Part of the Limb, since the two Ends of the Bone are never likely to unite, than to deceive the Patient with the fruitless Hopes of a Cure, and weaken him to the last Degree, with the Attempt. But when only a small Piece of the Bone is carried off in this Manner, you may safely enough attempt the Union of the Parts, but the Limb will be ever shorter than other; and if the Injury is in the Foot, he will be always lame."

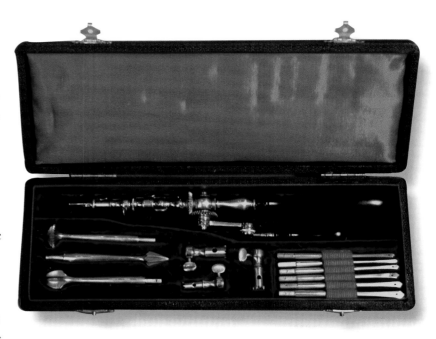

It was not until the use of X-rays and aseptic technique in the twentieth century that surgeons were able to effectively intervene in the removal of foreign bodies (figures 168–170). The assassination of President James Garfield in 1881 graphically illustrates the difficulties that physicians faced when treating gunshot wounds and the peril that patients faced. James Abram Garfield was born in Cuyahoga County, Ohio, on November 19, 1831, and was the last president to be born in a log cabin. He was quite well-read and attended Williams College, graduating with the highest honors in 1856. Garfield was a professor of Greek and Latin and had assumed the college presidency at the age of only twenty-six. Soon after the beginning of the Civil War, he entered the Union Army as a lieutenant colonel and quickly rose to the rank of major general as a reward for leading his troops to a number of victories in the South. Following the war, Garfield served in the House of Representatives, and represented Ohio for seventeen years before assuming the presidency on March 4, 1881. After only two hundred days in office and while on his way to a Williams College reunion, Garfield was shot by a disgruntled lawyer, Charles Julius Guiteau. He died after eighty days of illness on September 19, 1881.

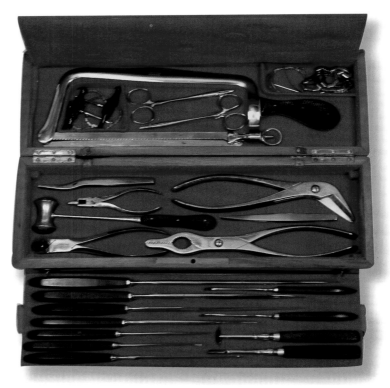

166. Bone-drilling set (ca. 1880)

167. Cased orthopedic set (1877) by Lindenmaier

President Garfield was passing the waiting room of the Baltimore and Potomac railroad depot when he was shot twice by Charles Guiteau with an English bulldog .44-caliber pistol, the first bullet harmlessly grazing his arm, but the second entering his right posterior thorax.

168. Right. Bullet forceps in *Armamentarium Chiruigicum* (1655) by Joannis Scultetus

169. Sheathed bullet screw (ca. 1540)

170. Nineteenth-century bullets and bullet removers: (top to bottom) 2 canister shot, unfired .58-caliber Minie ball, deformed Minie ball after impact, porcelain tipped Nelaton bullet probe by Tiemann, bullet forceps with .69-caliber musket ball, Coexter bullet remover with Colt's army pistol bullet, bullet screw with sheath (ca. 1860)

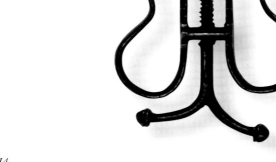

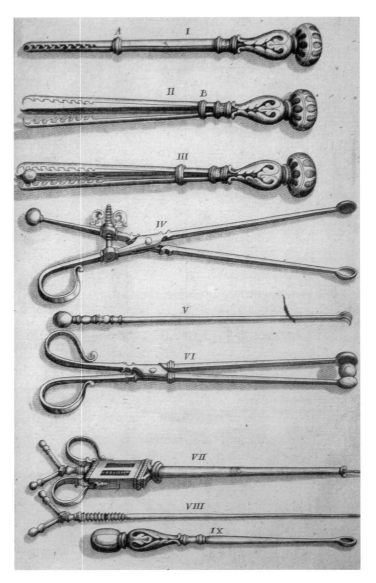

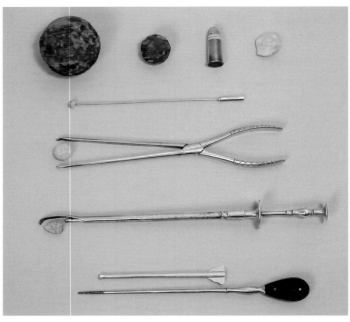

Physicians at the time felt that any projectile entering an organ was automatically fatal, so without a way to determine the bullet's location, every effort was made to remove it. The first surgeon on the scene was Dr. Willard Bliss. His decision was to try to remove the fragment by first using his (unwashed) finger and then an unsterilized silver probe. Bliss was the first of sixteen doctors to probe the wound with unwashed fingers, including the army surgeon general who reached the president's ribs, and the navy surgeon general who, in fact, punctured his liver. The initial wound of three-and-a-half inches eventually enlarged to an area of draining pus twenty inches in length, stretching from Garfield's ribs to his groin.

In the hot Washington, DC, summer, doctors treated Garfield with quinine, morphine, and calomel. He was fed brandy and milk while doctors argued over the location of the bullet and debated therapeutic options. The president's medical condition was discussed nationally in newspapers, and the frustration that physicians had in finding the bullet was regularly highlighted. At about that time, Simon Newcomb of Baltimore reported the production of a "hum" when metal was placed near electrified coils in an article in the *Washington National Intelligencer*. He suggested that his discovery might be helpful in finding the missing bullet, though the sound needed to be amplified. Alexander Graham Bell had read the article while he was in Boston and contacted Newcomb with the thought that perhaps his newly discovered telephone could provide the necessary amplification. Bell went to Baltimore, where the two came up with a metal detector that consisted of two coils, a battery, and Bell's telephone, the so-called "Induction Balance." A hum could be heard when a piece of metal was placed near the circuit breaker, and the device was tested by the two inventors with bullets hidden in various places, including in bags of grain and at different parts of the body. Finally, the two tested Civil War veterans at their residence in the Old Soldier's Home in Washington, DC, for old lodged bullets. The device worked well, and on July 26, Newcomb, Bell, and his assistant, Charles Sumner Tainter, went to the White House where they passed a wand over the president, who was fearful of being electrocuted by the new invention. In front of five White House doctors, the procedure failed since there was a faint hum no matter where they placed the wand. Bell was accused in the newspapers of being a "publicity seeker," and the inventor left wondering what had gone wrong.

The trio remained resolved, and they returned to their laboratory in Baltimore. Once again, all experiments were successful there and at the Old Soldier's Home, so they convinced the White House doctors to give them another chance. Unfortunately, the same generalized hum resulted no matter where they moved the wand over the president's body. The three were incredulous, and Bell returned to Boston having given up trials on his new invention. Several weeks later, on September 19, 1881, President Garfield died, probably of a myocardial infarction related to his long bout with infection.

After Garfield's death, several interesting facts came to light, including the reason for the failure of the Bell and Newcomb electromagnetic induction balance metal detector. The metal coil spring mattress had just been invented and, unknown to Bell, Garfield was one of the first to have one. Had Bell moved the president to another bed, the bullet might have been found, and his invention would have been a success, perhaps saving Garfield's life. The postmortem examination showed that the bullet had passed through the L1 vertebral body and had lodged in a safe area near the spine. The president might have survived had his physicians not been so aggressive in trying to remove the bullet; ironically, the first doctor to introduce his finger (with foreign organisms) in search of the bullet, Willard Bliss, later died of an infection with probably the same organisms that he had received from dressing Garfield's wound. Bliss was forced to publicly admit his error, and many newspapers, including the *Washington Post,* accused the White House physicians of malpractice. In fact the assassin, Charles Guiteau, used that argument in his defense, shouting, "Your honor, I admit to the shooting of the president, but not the killing."

Though Guiteau's defense was medical malpractice, he did not convince the jury, and he was convicted after only five minutes of deliberation. Guiteau was hung for the murder of President Garfield about one year after the shooting despite his great fear of that form of execution. Prior to the assassination, he had hired a cab to wait for him at the depot to take him to jail so that he might avoid being lynched by an angry mob. Additionally, Guiteau's sister had unsuccessfully attempted to spare him of a hanging by smuggling in a bouquet of roses that concealed a vial of arsenic. Against the wishes of his family, the body was fully dissected, and the bones were to be put on public display, though that never took place. Fortunately, the number of physicians who continued to discount the importance of asepsis declined after this national disaster and the debate that followed.

CIVIL WAR MEDICINE

The Civil War was a seminal event in American history as combatants decided whether or not the United States would ultimately become a great nation. Physicians were also faced with important choices and options after having been presented with two of the greatest discoveries in the history of medicine: anesthesia and surgical asepsis. The signifi-

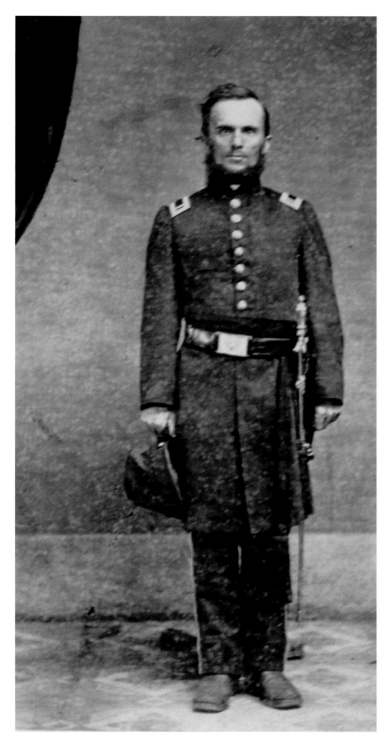

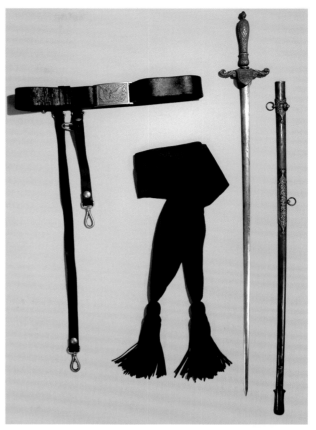

171. Typical Civil War medical officers uniform with belt, medical green sash, and dress sword by the Ames Manufacturing Company of Chicopee, Massachusetts

172. Carte-de-visite (CDV) of a Union medical officer in formal dress (ca. 1865)

cance of both were known by the beginning of the war, though many Civil War surgeons refused to avail themselves of either discovery during the conflict . . . or for many years that followed.

A large part of the problem with the provision of medical care during the Civil War was the fact that very few physicians had surgical training when the war broke out, and none had any forewarning of the flood of injured and maimed that they were about to encounter (figures 171, 172). There were only a few medical schools in the United States at the time, and the Union had just 30 surgeons and 83 assistant surgeons; 3 of those surgeons and 21 assistants resigned to join the South at the beginning of the war. Most of the military training for surgeons on both sides of the conflict had come from earlier medical experience during the Crimean War, where Turkey had opposed Russia over the control of Constantinople and its outlet to the Mediterranean Sea. The British and French aided the Turks, and it was the documentation of their surgical care that provided a basis for military training in the United States. On July 21, 1861, Confederate Medical Steward E.A. Craighill commented on the level of medical training in the United States at the time: "Of course, there are surgeons in our army older than I was, who had more experience, but none of us up to that time had seen much of gunshot wounds, and we had to unlearn what we had been taught in college in books as almost worthless, and only experience was useful in treatment and forming a correct or even an appropriate opinion of results from wounds particularly and sometimes from disease." Conscripted physicians barely out of school were suddenly faced with treating thousands of shattered and mutilated soldiers, many in shock, with equipment that was not much more than a knife, a saw, and a tourniquet.

Early medical care was made more chaotic by the lack of adequate logistical support, and an organized system of patient transport was not available until later in the war. There were few hospitals to handle the large number of casualties, and the nursing care was haphazard at best. The carnage was often truly overwhelming, as recounted by Union nurse Emma Edmonds during the initial shock at the Battle of Bull Run: "Still the battle continues without cessation; the grape and canister fill the air as they go screaming on their fearful errand; the sight of the field is perfectly appalling; men tossing their arms wildly calling for help; they be bleeding, torn and mangled; legs, arms, and bodies are crushed as if smitten by thunderbolts; the ground is crimson with blood; it is terrible to witness."

As is the case in all conflict, the Civil War provided physicians with an invaluable learning experience, and by the end of the war, surgery had become a respected branch of medicine, no longer considered to be a trade practiced by barber-surgeons. Significant medical progress was made during the war, but the cost in lives was almost unimaginable, and was by far higher than in any other war in US history. The toll to the Union Army was estimated at about 110,000 who died directly in battle, while the mortality from peri-operative infection and diseases such as typhus, pneumonia, infectious diarrhea, typhoid, and tetanus, was a staggering 250,000. The number of Confederate soldiers losing their lives directly from wounds was approximately 95,000 and from other causes 165,000, a loss even higher when considered as a percentage of the southern population. Surgeons themselves were not immune to the onslaught, and according to Surgeon General Joseph Barnes (1817-1883), the losses to the medical department were "proportionately larger than that of any other staff corps." By the end of the war, 39 Union medical officers had died either directly or indirectly as a result of the war.

Surgery was performed under oil lamps in an assembly line fashion, and only those who had any chance of survival were given the privilege of being operated on. Surgeons did not wear gloves and had no time or concern for cleanliness. They often wore the same gown for all procedures throughout the day and wiped off instruments on their aprons between cases. Conditions were often appalling by any medical standard. Gen. Carl Schurz, commander of the 11th Union Corps, described the operating theater at Gettysburg: "Most of the operating tables were placed in the open where the light was best, some of them partially protected against the rain. There stood the surgeons, their sleeves rolled up to their elbows, their bare arms as well as their linen aprons smeared with blood, their knives not seldom held between their teeth while they were helping the patient on and off the table or had their hands otherwise occupied. Around them were pools of blood and amputated arms or legs in heaps sometimes more than a man high" (figures 173, 174). The wounds were frequently dressed with an adhesive plaster containing benzene and turpentine, a formula similar to one in use as far back as the fifteenth century.

Postoperative care was no better. In August 1861, Asst. Surgeon S.H. Melcher of the 5th Missouri Volunteers said, "The flies were exceedingly troublesome after the battle, maggots forming in the wounds in less than an hour after dressing them, and also upon any clothing or bedding soiled by blood or pus. The wounded left on the field in the enemy's hands were swarming with maggots when brought in. After several ineffectual attempts to extirpate these pests, I succeeded perfectly by sprinkling calomel freely over the wounded surface." Some surgeons, however, discovered that the use of maggots improved the survival of their patients because of their ability to debride wounds. Following his service in Danville, Virginia, Confederate physician John Forney Zacharias wrote, "I first used maggots to remove the decayed tissue in hospital gangrene and with eminent satisfaction. In a single day they would clean a wound much better than any agents we had at our command. I used them afterwards at various places. I am sure I saved many lives by their use, escaped septicaemia, and had rapid recoveries."

Sickrooms contained "fumigators" filled with herbs, and sometimes even formaldehyde, to clean the air that some felt contained the material

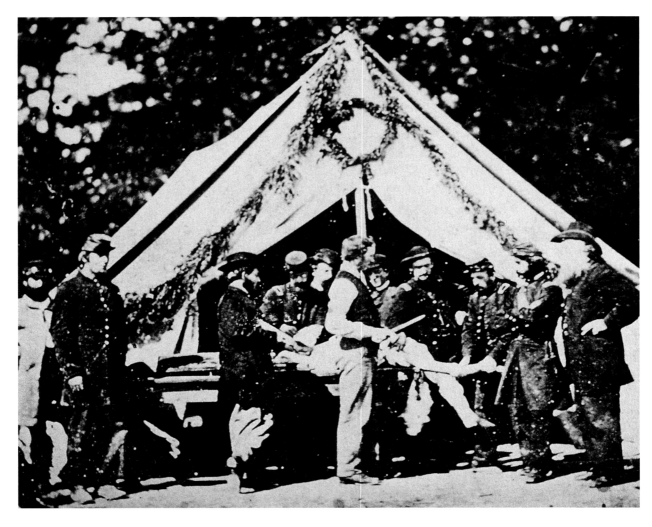

173. Amputation purportedly performed by Dr. James T. Calhoon on Maj. Gen. Daniel Sickles in Camp Letterman at the battle of Gettysburg on July 2, 1863. General Sickles presented his amputated leg to the newly established Army Medical Museum in Washington, DC, where he later visited it and where it now resides. (Earlier on February 27, 1859, Sickles had shot and killed the son of Francis Scott Key, Philip Barton Key, because Key had been having an affair with his wife. Sickles pleaded temporary insanity. He was the first person to successfully use that defense for murder in a US court.)

174. *A Morning's Work*, Civil War albumin print (CDV) named by Reed Brockway Bontecou, MD, surgeon in charge of the Harewood United States Army General Hospital in Washington, DC

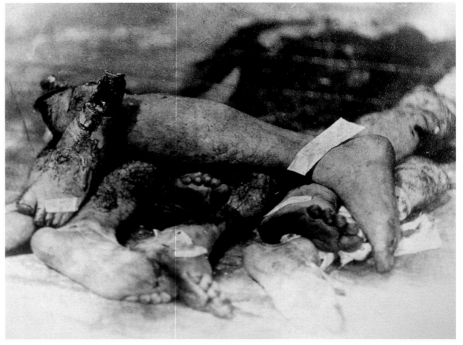

that was causing the dreaded "hospital gangrene" (figure 175). In some ways, medicine had not changed from the ancient time of Galen since the formation of pus two to three days after surgery was still thought to be a sign of recovery and an indication that body "humors" were being released to allow a more balanced internal environment. Surgeons used the terms "laudable pus" or "favorable pus" to describe this encouraging finding.

A Life-Saving Amputation

Battles were often fast and furious, and the casualties were unusually high because of the confrontational battle strategy fought throughout most of the war. The effective weaponry also resulted in high mortality and morbidity figures. The rifle with Minie ball, invented by French army Capt. Claude Etienne Minié, became a deadly weapon during the war because of the devastating damage that resulted from the accuracy of this soft lead projectile that flattened on impact. Surgeons were left to face the challenge of treating overwhelming infections without antibiotics and wounds without the availability of adequate anesthesia for surgery (figures 176, 177). There was never a lack of patients, and one surgeon wrote to his wife after operating for four straight days, ". . . yet there are a hundred cases of amputation waiting for me. Poor fellows come and beg almost on their knees for the first chance to have an arm taken off. It is a scene of horror such as I never saw." Seventy-five percent of all operations in the Civil War were amputations as surgeons soon discovered that the quick removal of a traumatized limb was the most effective way to save lives. Civil War survivors with limb prostheses became a common sight throughout the latter part of the nineteenth century (figures 178, 179).

The US Sanitary Commission was a civilian volunteer corps created in 1861. Early recommendations favored a liberal approach regarding amputation in most battlefield conditions:

> In army practice, on the field, amputation, when necessary ought to be primary. Patients, in most cases, cannot bear removal from the field without increased danger, neither can they have afterwards the hygienic attentions which secondary amputations most necessarily require, therefore:

1. Amputate with as little delay as possible after the receipt of the injury in those cases where there is intensive suffering from the presence in the wound of bone spicule or other foreign bodies, which the fingers or forceps cannot reach.

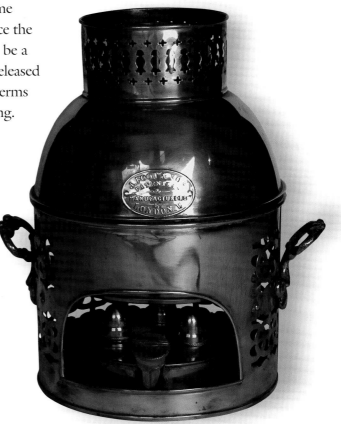

175. Sick room herb fumigator (ca. 1870) by J. Foot and Sons

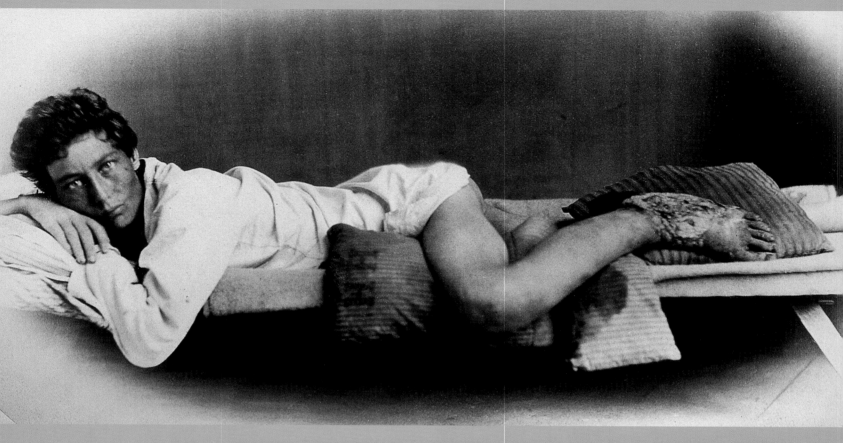

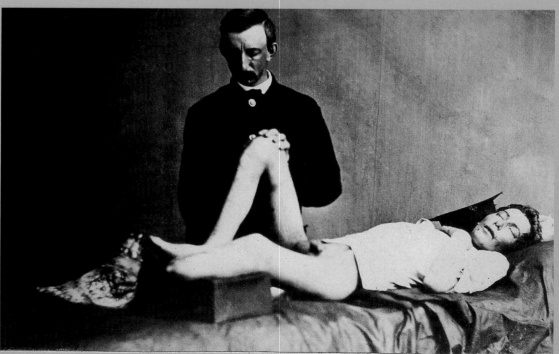

176. CDV of Private John D.
Parmenter, 67th Pennsylvania
Volunteers prior to an amputation of
his gangrenous left foot on June 21,
1865

177. CDV of Private Parmenter on the
operating table just after the amputation

2. In those cases where a limb is nearly torn off, and a dangerous hemorrhage is occurring which cannot be arrested.

3. In army practice, attempts to save a limb which might be perfectly successful in civil life, cannot be made. Especially in this case in compound gunshot fractures of the thigh, bullet wounds of the knee joint and similar injuries to the leg, in which, at first sight, amputation may not seem necessary. Under such circumstances attempts to preserve the limb will be followed by extreme local and constitutional disturbance. Conservative surgery is here in error; in order to save life, the limb must be sacrificed.

In 1871, Stephen Smith issued a final report to the Sanitary Commission regarding amputation:

1. Immediate amputations, or those performed *before the shock*, give good results in military surgery.

2. Amputations performed between the first and sixth hour after injury, or *during the shock* are more successful than when performed at a later period, but are not probably more successful than when performed immediately.

3. Amputations performed between the sixth and forty-eighth hour, or in the period of reaction, are more successful than at any subsequent period, but are not nearly as successful as amputations performed previously to the sixth hour.

4. Amputations performed between the forty-eighth hour and seventh day, or in the intermediary period, are more fatal than at any time prior to or subsequent to that period.

5. Amputations performed after the seventh day, or in the secondary period, are more fatal than amputations performed at any time prior to the forty-eighth hour after the receipt of the injury.

Ninety-four percent of the wounds suffered in the Civil War resulted from gunshots, and the survival was astonishingly low, no matter where the injury occurred. The mortality was fifty percent in patients whose limb was amputated, while two-thirds of those with a compound

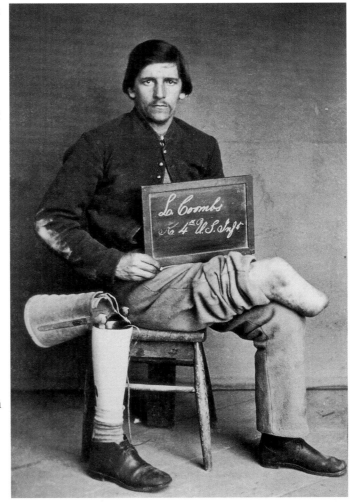

178. CDV of Private L. Coombs, 4th US Infantry seated with his prosthesis (ca. 1865)

179. Lady's prosthesis (ca. 1880)

fracture expired. Since intra-abdominal surgery was not an option on the battlefield, the death rate of those having gunshot wounds of the abdomen was over ninety percent.

The Medical and Surgical History of the War of the Rebellion

In 1862, William Alexander Hammond held the post of army surgeon general. Hammond's medical career was an interesting one, beginning with his graduation from medical school at the University of New York in 1848. He served in the army for eleven years where he took part in campaigns against the Sioux Indians in the southwest. In 1860, Hammond assumed the chair of physiology and anatomy at the University of Maryland, though at the outbreak of the war, he returned to the army and was appointed by President Lincoln at the age of thirty-four to the post of surgeon general. Hammond's personality and that of the secretary of war, Edwin Stanton, clashed, resulting in his dismissal from the army after a court-martial encouraged by Stanton in which Hammond was found guilty of irregularities related to the purchase of medical supplies. He left penniless and in disgrace, though with a keen intellect and an adventurous spirit, Dr. Hammond set up a neurology practice in New York where his fortunes significantly improved. He was appointed professor of psychiatry and nervous diseases in the College of Physicians and at University of the City of New York, and, following an impartial review of the charges, he was exonerated of his earlier conviction by an act of Congress. William Hammond was one of the seven founding members of the American Neurological Association, and he established the Army Medical Museum.

Early in the war, Dr. Hammond had ordered that measures be taken "to secure more detailed and exact reports of sick and wounded." It was under his authority that a massive six-volume account of the war was compiled that included the names, ranks, and the nature of injury relating to over 200,000 casualties. It was the first large-scale epidemiological study produced in the United States, and it took over eighteen years of research and analysis before it was ready for publication. *The Medical and Surgical History of the War of the Rebellion* (1870–1888) was written by J.H. Brinton, J.J. Woodward, G.A. Otis, and Charles Smart under the direction of Hammond's successor, Joseph Barnes, and published by the surgeon general's office. According to the army medical director, Surgeon H.S. Hewit, this was "the complete medical and surgical history . . . the most valuable contribution that could be made to the literature of military medicine. . . ." Following are several examples from that work:

PRIVATE JESSIE M. JONES (figure 180)
Private Jones was injured in 1862 in Baton Rouge, Lousiana.

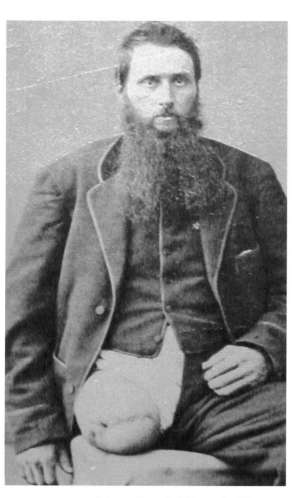

180. Private Jesse M. Jones in *The Medical and Surgical History of the War of the Rebellion* (1870–1888)

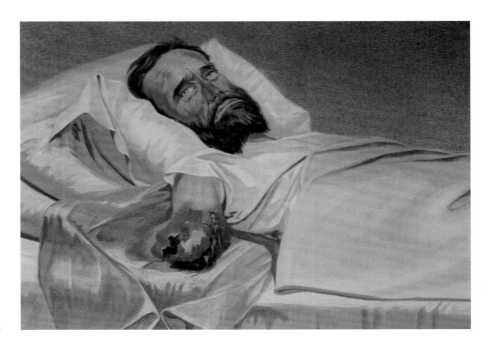

181. Private Milton E. Wallen

The wound remained unhealed for seven years until his leg required amputation, as pictured in a CDV that was taken at the Medical Museum in Washington, DC upon his visit there following the war.

PVT MILTON E. WALLEN (figure 181)

Private Wallen, age 41, of the 1st Kentucky Cavalry was hospitalized Aug. 3, 1863 and while a prisoner in Richmond, was shot by guards. He developed "hospital gangrene," and required an amputation on Aug. 24.

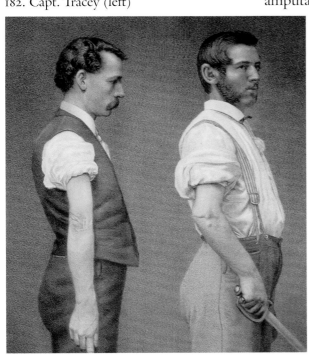

182. Capt. Tracey (left)

"For a few days afterward the stump was dressed with charcoal and yeast poultices, and a generous diet and an ample allowance of ale and other stimulants was allowed. By Aug. 30, 1863, the sloughing process was entirely arrested, and from this date the patient steadily improved. In October he was furloughed from the hospital, and was reported as having deserted on furlough April 5, 1864." In 1873, Pvt Wallen made applications for a pension, stating that "he was captured at Rowena, on the Cumberland River, May 26, 1863, and carried to Atlanta, Georgia, then from there to Richmond, and placed in Castle Thunder, and while there was shot by the guards, July 4, 1863."

CAPT TRACEY (figure 182)

Capt Tracey was wounded at Chancellorsville, May 2, 1863 by musket-ball to the right humerus. Surgeon HE

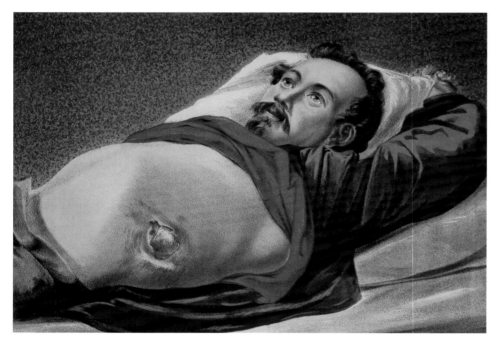

183. Capt. Robt S.

Goodman excised the joint, removing 4¹/₂ inches:

"I returned to the Army August 15th, the wound being perfectly healed, the bones remaining disunited, and I continued to serve on the staff of General Slocum until the close of the war. My arm has become about three inches shorter. The muscles have never withered away, and sensation is perfect in the limb. I can write as well as ever (with great elegance, it may be remarked, in passing), but experience some difficulty in raising my arm."

CPT. ROBERT S. (figure 183)
Cpt. "S" of the 29th New York volunteers was wounded by a musket ball on May 2, 1863 at Chancellors-ville. With his lung collapsed, he walked 1¹/₂ miles to a field hospital where physicians unsuccessfully attempted to reduce the hernea, which contained lung and "some portion of the alimentary canal." The following day, hostilities forced Cpt S to be evacuated and he subsequently had to walk another 1¹/₂ miles. The musket ball passed in his stool on May 7th, and the wound, which contained lung and stomach, eventually granulated in. He was one of a small minority of wounded who survived such major trauma in this pre-antibiotic era.

PVT. CHARLES BETTS (figure 184)
Pvt. Betts of the 26th New Jersey Volunteers was wounded by a three ounce grapeshot in 1863 as he charged Fredericksburg. At one point, his aortic arch was outwardly visible, though Betts eventually recovered.

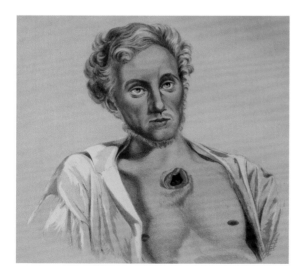

184. Private Charles Betts

PVT. EDSON D. BEMIS (figure 185)
"Private Edson D. Bemis, Co. K, 12th Massachusetts Volunteers, was wounded at Antietam by a musket ball which fractured the shaft of his left humerus. The fracture united kindly, with very slight angular displacement and quarter of an inch shortening. Promoted to be corporal, Bemis received May 6th, 1864, at the battle of the Wilderness a wound from a musket ball in the right iliac fossa. He was treated in the Chester Hospital, near Philadelphia. There was extensive sloughing about the wound,

but it ultimately healed entirely. . . . On February 5th, 1865, Corporal Bemis was again severely wounded at the engagement at Hatcher's Run, near Petersburg, Virginia . . . the ball entered a little outside of the left frontal protuberance, and passing backward and upward, removed a piece of the squamous portion of the temporal bone, with brain substance and membranes. When the patient entered the hospital of the 1st division of the Second Corps, brain matter was oozing from the wound. There was considerable hemorrhage, but not from any important vessel. Respiration was slow; the pulse 40; the right side was paralyzed and there was total insensibility. On February 8th, the missile was removed from the substance of the left hemisphere. . . . The patient's condition at once improved. He told the surgeon his name, and seemed conscious of all that was going on about him. . . . On February 28th he was able to walk about the ward. . . . He recovered perfectly, and in May was furloughed . . . suffering only slight dizziness in going out in the hot sun. In July he went to Washington to apply for a pension, and entered Campbell Hospital. He was discharged on July 13th, 1865, on surgeon's certificate of disability. At this date he was photographed at the Army Medical Museum. The wound in the head was then nearly healed. There was a slight discharge of healthy pus from one point. The pulsations of the brain could be felt through the integument. The mental and sensory faculties were unimpaired. . . . Mr. Bemis was pensioned at eight dollars per month. On October 30th, 1870, he wrote to the editor of the surgical history from his home in Suffield, Connecticut, as follows: 'I am still in the land of the living. My health is very good considering what I have passed through at Hatcher's Run. My head aches some of the time. I am married and have one child, a little girl born last Christmas. My memory is affected, and I cannot hear as well as I could before I was wounded.'"

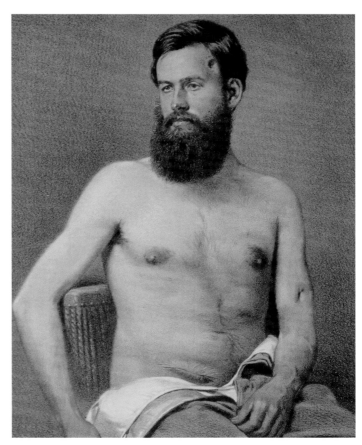

185. Private Edson Bemis

Sepsis among the Troops

Despite the extraordinarily high death rate from infection, proper sanitation became a part of routine medical care only at the end of the war. Ironically, surgeons unknowingly transmitted bacterial infections, and the largely iatrogenic problem of "hospital gangrene" was almost always fatal without amputation. Florence Nightingale, a nurse in the Crimean conflict, demanded that her wards be clean and well ventilated, and that all dressings be changed regularly. Her aseptic techniques reduced the death rate in the Crimean conflict from forty-two percent to two percent, and eventually lessons regarding sanitation translated into improved survival rates in many hospitals during the Civil War. The prognosis improved for many of the injured because of an increase in the use of Middleton Goldsmith's bromine, and, by the end of the war, substantial inroads had been made into the devastating problem of sepsis.

Pain Control

Medical staff physicians were well aware of recent discoveries regarding anesthesia, though they could not always provide these agents to front line troops. Surgeons used chloroform only at the beginning of surgery because most of the procedures lasted only a few minutes, leaving patients to depend on alcohol and opiates postoperatively. The expression to "bite the bullet" may have come from the custom of patients having been given a shot to chew during a painful procedure when no other anesthesia was available. Bullets from the war are noted to have tooth marks, though some would debate the authenticity of this practice since there is no written documentation. Despite the obvious benefit of using anesthesia with chloroform, a number of surgeons argued against its use. Some felt that anesthetics increased the incidence of postoperative shock, while others suggested that they retarded wound healing and increased the chances of sepsis and hemorrhage.

THE BATTLE OF COLD HARBOR

There were many confrontations during the Civil War, and looking in detail at one battle sometimes can be useful in understanding all others. In early June 1864, the Union Army, under the direction of General Ulysses Grant, was advancing toward the capital of the Confederacy in Richmond, Virginia, with the intent of ending the war by its capture (figure 186). Union troops numbered about 110,000 and were pitted against a Confederate force of 60,000. Unfortunately, some of Grant's forces got lost on the way, allowing the Confederates twenty-four hours to build trenches along a six-mile front. During a misty rain at 4:30 on the morning of June 3, 1864, 31,000 Union troops assaulted those of Gen. Robert E. Lee just outside Richmond at Cold Harbor, a decision leading to one of the bloodiest days of the Civil War. Grant lost about 7,000 men that day, most reportedly dying in the first hour as he ordered a frontal attack

186. Gen. Ulysses S. Grant at Cold Harbor, Virginia, June 1864

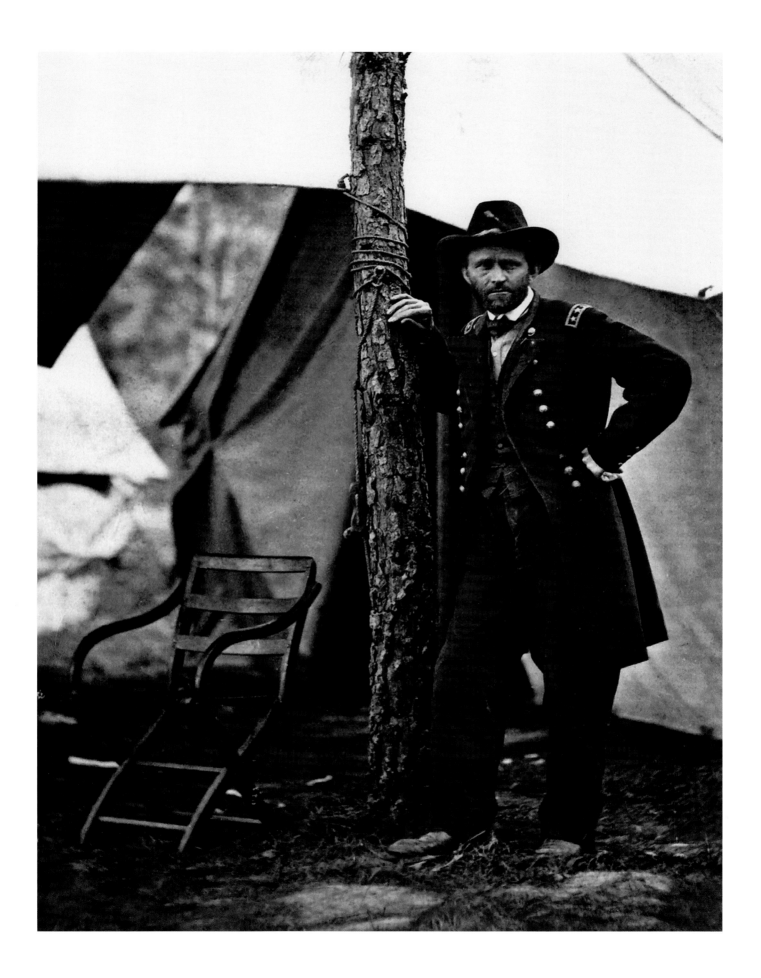

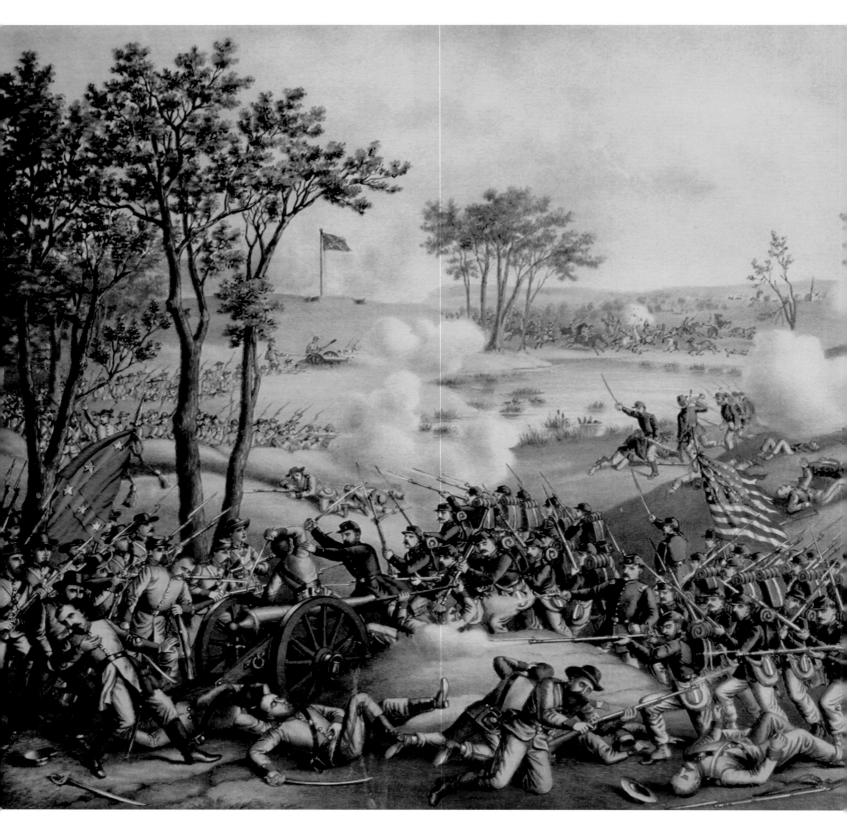

187. Kurz and Allison's (Chicago) spin
control color print (1888) showing
Grant "triumphantly" advancing on
Lee at Cold Harbor, Virginia

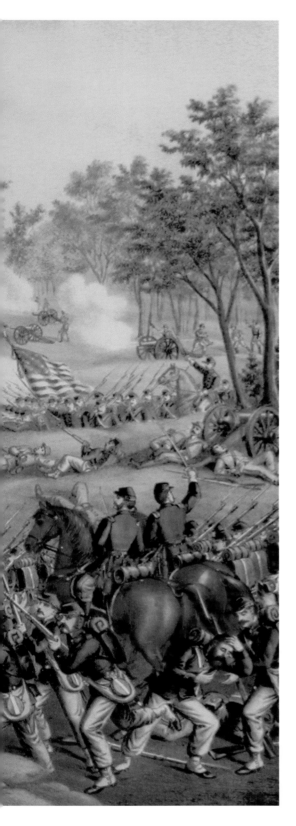

against well-entrenched Confederate forces. In no previous battle of the war had troops been killed so rapidly, and many described the encounter not unlike a field of wheat being cut down (figure 187).

Statements later made by Union soldiers reflected the ferocity of the battle: ". . . volleys of hurting death poured from the rebel lines," "dreadful storm of lead and iron . . . seemed more like a volcanic blast than a battle," and "the ground was swept with canister and rifle-bullets until it was literally covered with the slain." From the Confederate viewpoint, "the lines seemed to wave like wheat in a breeze, then dissolve, with men gathering in bunches and being shot down," and Confederate Gen. Evander M. Law later stated, "It was not war, it was murder." In fact, Grant had planned a second assault, though was refused when a Union officer said, "I will not lead my men in another such charge if Jesus Christ himself comes down and orders it." Prior to the assault, Union soldiers had written their names on pieces of paper and pinned them to their uniforms so that their bodies could be identified later for return to their families.

The Battle of Cold Harbor could have been a significant political turning point in American history since it occurred just prior to the Republican convention that was to be held on June 7, 1864. Some Republicans wanted to replace Lincoln as president, and Grant was looking for a victory before the convention to bolster Lincoln's chances of renomination, though the Battle of Cold Harbor was a Union disaster. Normally a truce would be called immediately after a major battle so that the wounded and dead could be attended to; this was not the case at Cold Harbor. Most of the injured were not cared for, (presumably because of a disagreement regarding the terms of the cease fire between Grant and Lee), and the true consequences of the battle were not reported until after the June seventh convention and nomination of Lincoln. Grant minimized the report of a death toll that had been significantly increased because of the injured thousands who had been left unattended for several days. General Grant issued the following dispatch, which was reported on June 6 in the *New York Times*: "We assaulted at 4:30 A.M., driving the enemy within his entrenchments at all points, but without gaining any advantage. Our troops now occupy a position close to the enemy, some places within fifty yards, and are remaining. Our loss was not severe, nor do I suppose the enemy to have lost heavily. We captured over three hundred prisoners, mostly from Breckinridge." Had this huge defeat been publicized, Lincoln might not have been nominated, and the course of the war might have been significantly different.

The Battle of Cold Harbor was to have marked the implementation of a newly established ambulance system to transport the wounded to field hospitals. Two years earlier, the son of prominent Harvard professor of medicine Henry Ingersoll Bowditch had died a horrible death after having been unattended for two days following an abdominal gunshot wound. Through the efforts of his father, the Ambulance Corps Act of 1864 was passed, and the first four-wheeled horse-drawn wagons appeared at the Battle of Cold Harbor, though too late for professor Bowditch's son or for the great majority of combatants at Cold Harbor because of the large number of casualties. The suffering must have been unimaginable, not only to the injured, but to those troops unable to give assistance.

LETTERS:
"IF WE COULD ONLY LIVE IN PEACE. . ."

Combatants on both sides of the conflict were quite literate, and letters written by troops have left us with personal insights into the lives of those who fought. Following is a letter written by Thomas Fanning Wood, MD (1841–1892), Confederate assistant surgeon in the 18th North Carolina Infantry, to his sister concerning the June 3 Battle of Cold Harbor. Wood was with Lee at Appomattox and graduated from the University of Maryland School of Medicine in 1868. His comments regarding the treatment of the wounded, the design of his hospital camp, the deaths of friends, and the reasons for Grant's success ("In his stubbornness consists his greatness. . .") leave us with a unique view of the battle:

> Rodes Division Hospital
> Old Battle Field of Cold Harbor
> June 10th, 1864
>
> Dear Lydia,
>
>   I received your letter of the 5th, mailed the 7th in Wilmington, with a great deal of pleasure. It had a comfortable ring of the Home about it, that almost made me feel that I was very near about the "frog-pond". The thoughts of home for the past week or so have not been few. I am writing now upon the farm where McClellan, the little Yankee Napoleon had his Head Quarters when the battle of Cold Harbor was fought; and in the rear of the field the Yankees camped. The House is now occupied by Gen. Lee as Head Quarters. Our Hospital camp is in an apple orchard. Let me give you a description of a Hospital Camp taking an old Brigade as a model. Each Brigade has a Hospital wagon, and each Division I for transporting Hospital Stores, cooking utensils, tents, etc. Each tent is marked the name of the Brigade, and laid out in regular order. One large tent fly is located centrally as a tent for operations. This constitutes a Hospital Camp. The wounded are placed in the tents, and are

operated upon in such order that suits the case of a patient. When we have wounded, we of course have shelter for ourselves. But as long as it doesn't rain, I like to sleep out of doors.

There has been some change lately in our lines. The Yankees seem determined to make a desperate effort in the neighborhood, as they take it to be the key to Richmond. Such an attempt would be exactly what we want. We are massed very strongly at this point, which affords us time to rest and recruit. Men are constantly coming in from the camps instruction and the hospitals, swelling out ranks no little. As for my regiment though, we number about 30 for duty. Col. Thurston has resumed command, and has in addition to his own the 1st N.C. which numbers about 40—making a command of about 70 men. I have no regular duties to perform now, being sometimes on the field, sometimes in the Hospital. During the last week or so we have had two men very badly wounded in our small company. I have never seen more frightful lacerations then these men had.

No one can now complain of Confederate rations. We get *plenty* of everything. Bacon of all sorts, coffee and sugar, molasses, vegetables and alternately wheat, meal, and sometimes a ration of baker's bread. So you see we are doing very well. In fact, there has been no time since the war that the men have been better fed than now. There is no one that can grumble now about the fair, if grumbling would do any good we might say something about the duration of this continual fight. For several days there has been but little fighting. One day a Flag of Truce was out for the purpose of burying the dead. It was said to be a strange sight (it occurred in front of Gen. Hokes' division) when the signal gun announced the commencement of the truce. Previously nothing but sharp shooters had been showing themselves, as everyone who exposed himself was shot at by a hundred muskets. But as soon as the signal was given, three solid lines of blue draped Yankees rose as if by magic and *four* lines of well dressed confederates (it was once a fact that the Yankees were better dressed than our men, but it is no longer so). The two contending parties were soon mixing up with each other as though they had been a few minutes before engaged in deadly strife. The number of Yankee slain was great—I have forgotten the figures.

The enemy is now visibly engaged digging parallels or zig zags, in order to dig us out and we find fighting only weakens them to no purpose. The insane idea of accomplishing anything in this way would occur to anyone but Grant. In his stubbornness consists his greatness. . . .

Affectionately your brother,

Thomas F. W.

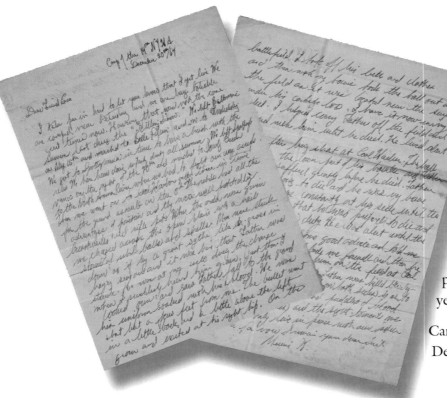

188. Letter from Merari Bunajah
Stevens to his friend Ezra on
December 20, 1864

Written from the other side of the battlefield, the
following is a touching letter sent home by
eighteen-year-old farmer Merari Bunajah
Stevens (figure 188). This document reflects
the lack of medical care available to combatants at the time as Stevens described the loss
of his father. He recognized his honor and
duty as a soldier, though his ambivalent feelings about the war were shared by many. Of
interest is the fact that probably because of his
wartime experiences, Stevens went to medical
school at the University of Michigan and then
practiced surgery in Defiance, Ohio, for many
years.

Camp of the 14th N.Y.H.A.
December 20/64

Dear Friend Ezra,
I take pen in hand to let you know that I yet live.
We are camped near Petersburg and we are having tolerable
good times now. However, that was not the case last Summer
during the "Killing Season". We left Baltimore on May 15th and
marched to Belle Plain and on to Fredericksburg. We got to
Spottsylvania on the night of the 20th and marched to Bowling
Green and to the North Anna River where we had to fight our
way across. Then we went on to Coal Harbor getting there in
time for the grand assault on the 3rd. The rebs had all the advantages of position and they were well protected by breastworks
and rifle pits. When the order was given we charged across the
open plain into a hail storm of rebel balls and shells. Men were
struck down as if by a great sythe like grass in haying time, and it
was here that Father was struck. He was at my side during the
charge when I suddenly heard him groan. Just then I looked
over and saw Father fall to the ground his uniform soaked with
blood. He was shot but a few feet from me. The bullet went in a
little back and a little above the left groin and exited near the
right hip. On the battlefield I took off his belts and clothes and
then with my bowie took the ball out on the field as it was located near the surface under his cartridge box. I have it now in my
pocket. Then I helped carry Father off the field and I stayed with
him until he died. He lived about a day after being shot at Coal
Harbor. The bullet went through the lower part of his bowels
and Father must have suffered greatly before he died. Father

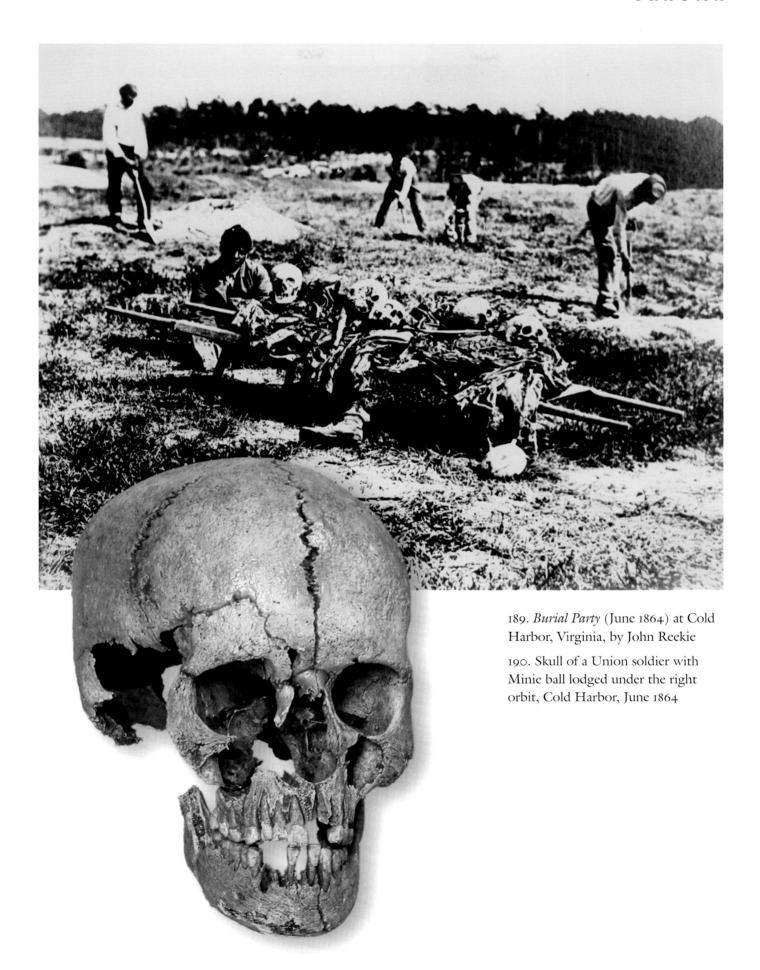

189. *Burial Party* (June 1864) at Cold Harbor, Virginia, by John Reekie

190. Skull of a Union soldier with Minie ball lodged under the right orbit, Cold Harbor, June 1864

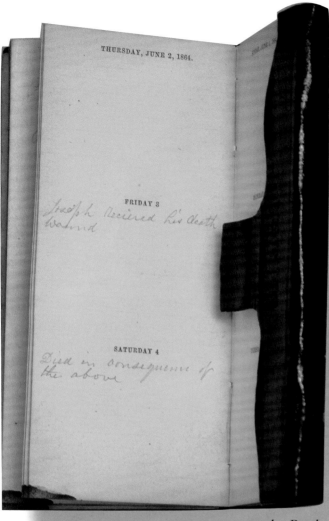

THURSDAY, JUNE 2, 1864.

FRIDAY 3

Joseph Recieved his death wound

SATURDAY 4

Died in consequence of the above

191. Diary kept by Sgt. Joseph Hume of Massachusetts, expired June 3, 1964

knew that he was going to die and he was very brave and calm. I was constantly at his side until the end. Father said that he was prepared to die and that he had done his duty. He was alert until the last and gave me some good advice and told me to be a good soldier. He bade me farewell and then he died in my arms. I buried him on the field at Coal Harbor. I am grief stricken yet as Uncle Luther was killed the day before Father. So much blood shed on both sides so as to be beyond description. The ground had puddles of blood from the mangled bodies and the sight torments me still. If we could only live in piece with our Southern brothers. No more for now. I remain your dear friend,

Merari

Many soldiers kept personal diaries of their experiences, and a number have survived. One soldier wrote, "June 3. Cold Harbor. I was killed," and, unfortunately, he was correct (figures 189, 190). Another artifact from that battle includes a diary kept by Sgt. Joseph Hume of Massachusetts, killed on the bloodiest day of the battle on June 3, 1864 (figure 191). He was a twenty-year-old mill hand who was born in Ashburnham, Massachusetts, and entered the "A Company"—MA 36th infantry—as a private on July 28, 1862. Hume was promoted to sergeant major as he traveled south to fight at the Battle of Cold Harbor. A compatriot completed his diary on June 3 with the words, "Joseph received his death wound," and the following day "Died in consequence of the above." The diary was apparently on Hume's person at the time of his death in light of the bloody stain in the corner.

The city of Cold Harbor had been named after a local hotel that provided shelter (a harbor), though not hot meals. Ultimately, the city became a "cold harbor" to Grant who had hoped to use it as a gateway to the defeat of the capital of the South in Richmond. This was the first battle in the Civil War in which Gen. Ulysses Grant was pitted directly against Gen. Robert E. Lee and was the most decisive in terms of casualties inflicted on the North. The Union lost 13,000, and the South 2,600, though this was also Lee's last victory of the war in a general engagement. Grant later admitted that his command at Cold Harbor was flawed and that this was "the one attack I always regretted ordering." The dramatic Northern defeat there ended forever the tactic of frontal attacks on well-prepared positions and marked the beginning of the type of trench warfare that was seen later in World War I.

MEDICAL ADVANCES FROM THE WAR

Many important advances in medical care resulted from the American Civil War. Physicians recognized the importance of rapid evacuation to field hospitals and the vital role played by good sanitation in saving lives. The significance of asepsis was beginning to be appreciated though, unfortunately, resistance to simple rules of cleanliness in the operating room and in follow-up wound care continued for many years after the war. The large number of causalities led to a dramatic increase in the number of physicians experienced in the use of anesthesia and, since pain control was improved, more innovative surgical procedures could be developed. Newer techniques led to innovations in the design of surgical equipment resulting in a rapid growth in the number of manufacturers in the United States, and the next forty years saw the production of some of the finest medical instruments ever made. Clara Barton founded the Red Cross, and nursing was established as a profession. Surgery finally became recognized as an important branch of medicine, no longer to be considered a craft practiced by tradesmen.

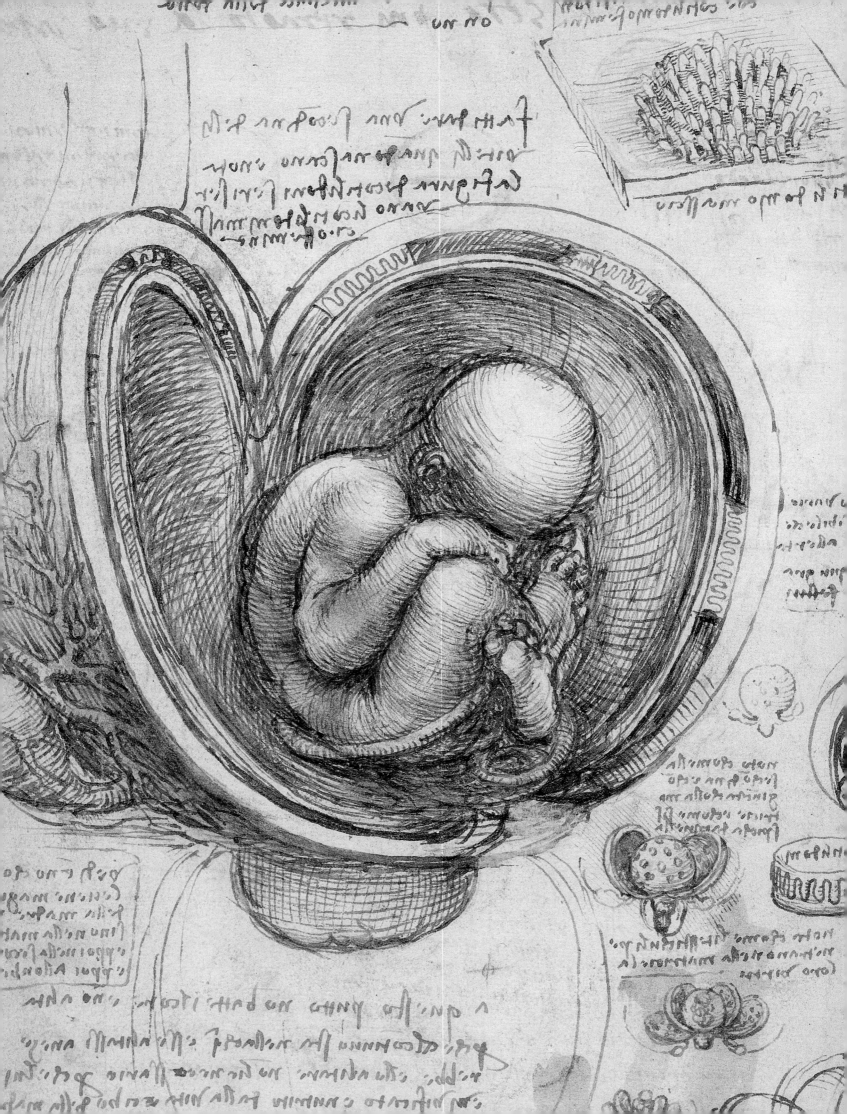

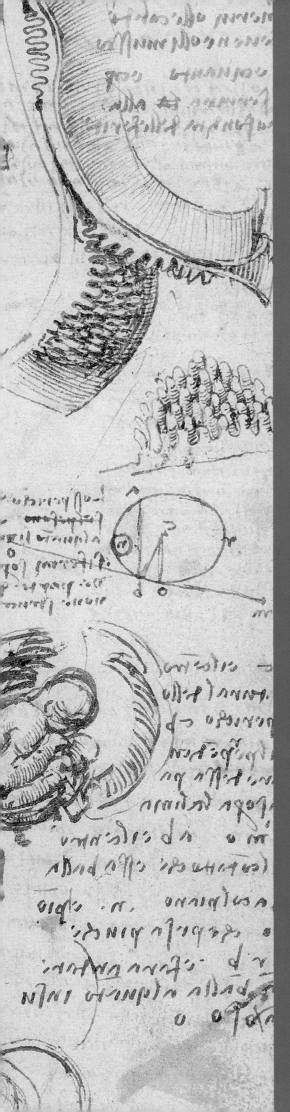

OBSTETRICS AND GYNECOLOGY

Where they save one, they murder many.

Dr. William Hunter (1718–1783)

Detail, sketch of gravid uterus
(ca. 1500) by Leonardo da Vinci.

It was only within the last several hundred years that the study and treatment of conditions affecting women were considered appropriate for review by the established medical community. Even into the nineteenth century, Victorian prohibitions and gender bias prevented an accurate and thorough evaluation of women's diseases. This attitude is illustrated in the famous image by J.P. Maygrier in *Nouvelles Démonstrations D'Accouchements* (1822) (figure 192).

OBSTETRICS

Egyptian papyri contain some of the first printed materials related to the diseases of women. The earliest was the Kahun papyrus, which dates back to 1825 B.C. and was discovered by Flanders Petrie in 1889. A number of matters related to female reproduction were addressed including the use of contraceptive pessaries containing honey and crocodile dung mixed in sour milk. When recently tested, this mixture has actually been shown to be effective after exposure to vaginal lactic acid. In another part of the papyrus, there is a test of fertility that required the expectant mother to place an onion in her vagina for one night. The result was positive (and the woman fertile) if she reported noticing an odor or taste the next morning, a demonstration that all passages were open. Also, according to the Kahun papyrus, the sex of the child could easily be determined since a pregnant woman's urine germinated wheat if the fetus were male and barley if female.

From the earliest medical records, the mother's role in reproduction was felt to be a passive one. Leonardo da Vinci, the first great medical artist, perpetuated that view in the sixteenth century when he sketched a direct anatomic relationship between the male reproductive organs and his brain and heart (figure 193). In reality, there is no such connection, and da Vinci's drawing reflects a pervasive view that the child was made up only of elements from the male's heart and soul. This anatomic representation was consistent with the animalculist theory introduced later in the seventeenth century, which suggested that a totally preformed individual, called a homunculus, was produced in the male seminal fluid and then transmitted to the female, the woman acting only as an incubator. This passive view of the female's role in reproduction was a reflection of the way in which the sexes have interacted on a social level for centuries.

In Ayurveda, or ancient Indian medicine, both parents participated in determining the sex of the child. Physicians believed that a child was formed by the union of semen and blood discharged from the uterus, and that it was the relative amount of each that decided the sex of the child. Because blood from the first menstrual cycle supposedly resulted

192. Examination of the expectant female in *Nouvelles Démonstrations D'Accouchemens* (1822) by J.P. Maygrier

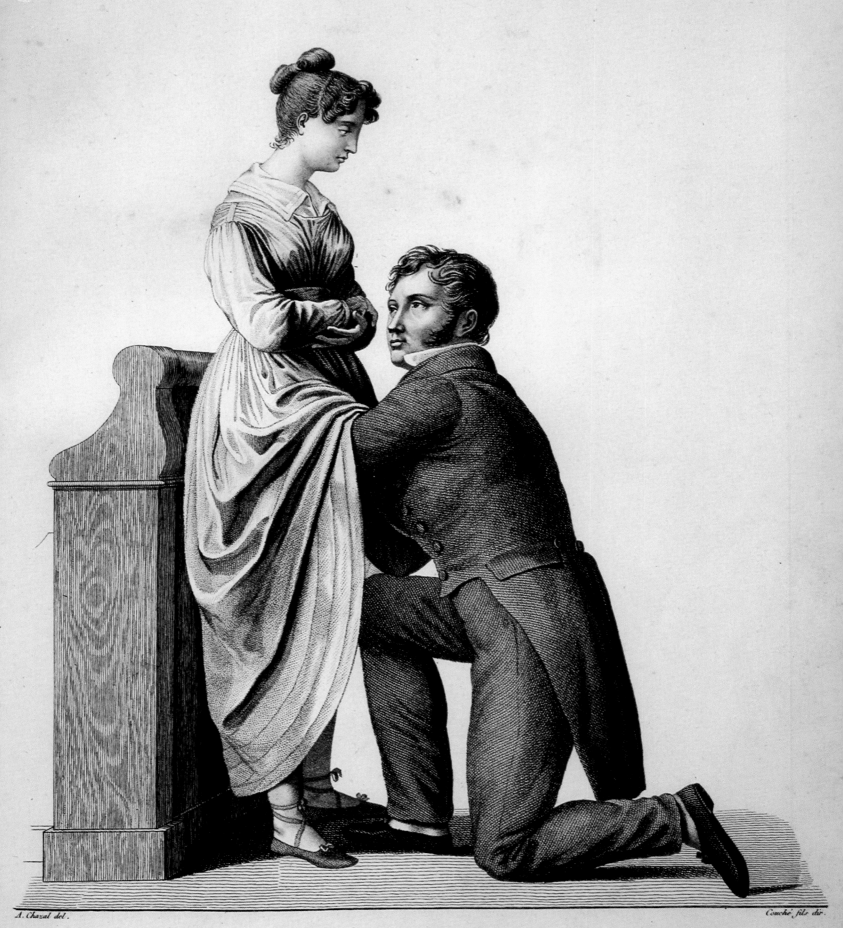

A. Chazal del.

Couché fils dir.

Toucher, la femme debout

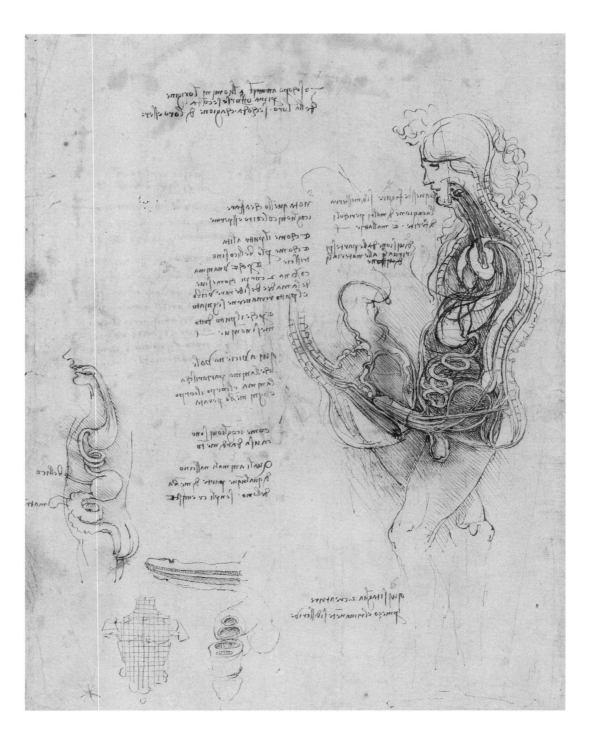

193. Sketch of procreation (ca. 1500)
by Leonardo da Vinci

in a particularly healthy offspring, early marriage for girls was, and remains, a long-held Indian custom.

Though her role in carrying the fetus was considered merely an inactive one in many European communities, the mother's behavior during gestation, however, was thought by some to be important. Nicolas Andry made the following suggestions in his work *Othopaedia: or, the Art of Correcting and Preventing Deformities In Children* (1743):

Women with Child, who, during their Pregnancy, drink a good

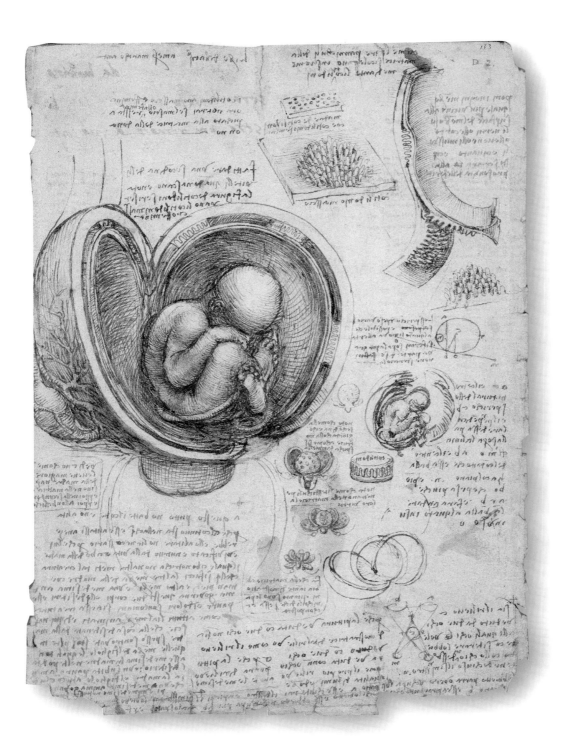

194. Sketch of a gravid uterus (ca. 1500) by Leonardo da Vinci

deal of Wine, and live upon too hot a Diet, render the Blood of their Children at this time too active . . . may make the Head too large; and they who drink nothing but Water, and live upon Food of a cold Quality, render the Blood of their Children too slow, which, by the contrary Reason, may make the heads too little. Thus, in this respect, it may be said in some measure, that Women with Child are as it were the Mistresses for forming the Heads of their Children. They ought therefore to shun all kinds

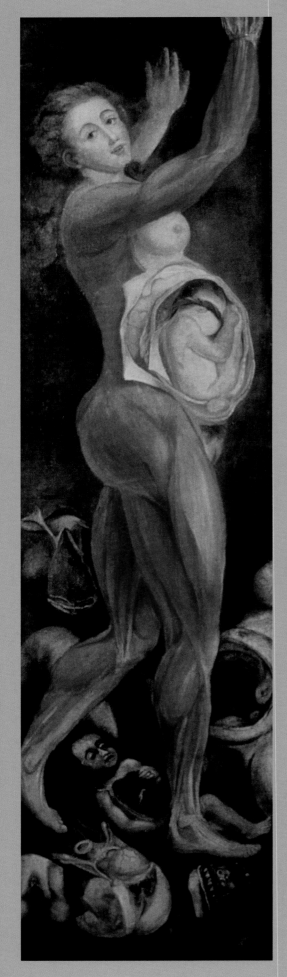

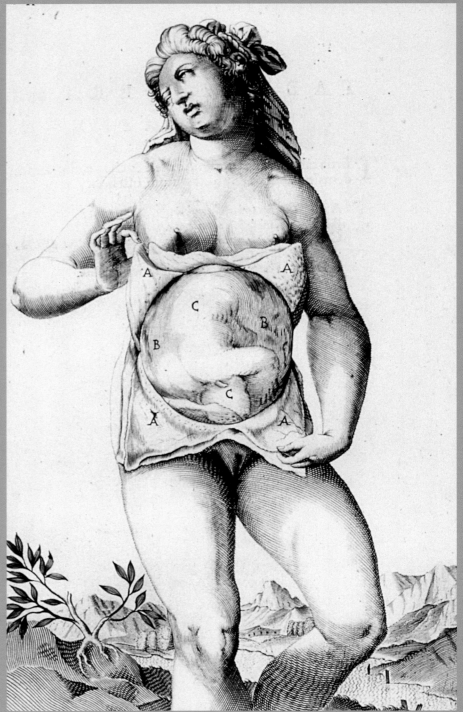

195. Female with child in *Anatomie des parties de la génération de l'homme et de la femme* (1773) by Jacques Fabien Gautier D'Agoty

196. A women showing her fetus in *De formato foetu liber singularis geneis figures exornatus in Opera quae extant omna* (1645) by Adrianus Spigelius

244

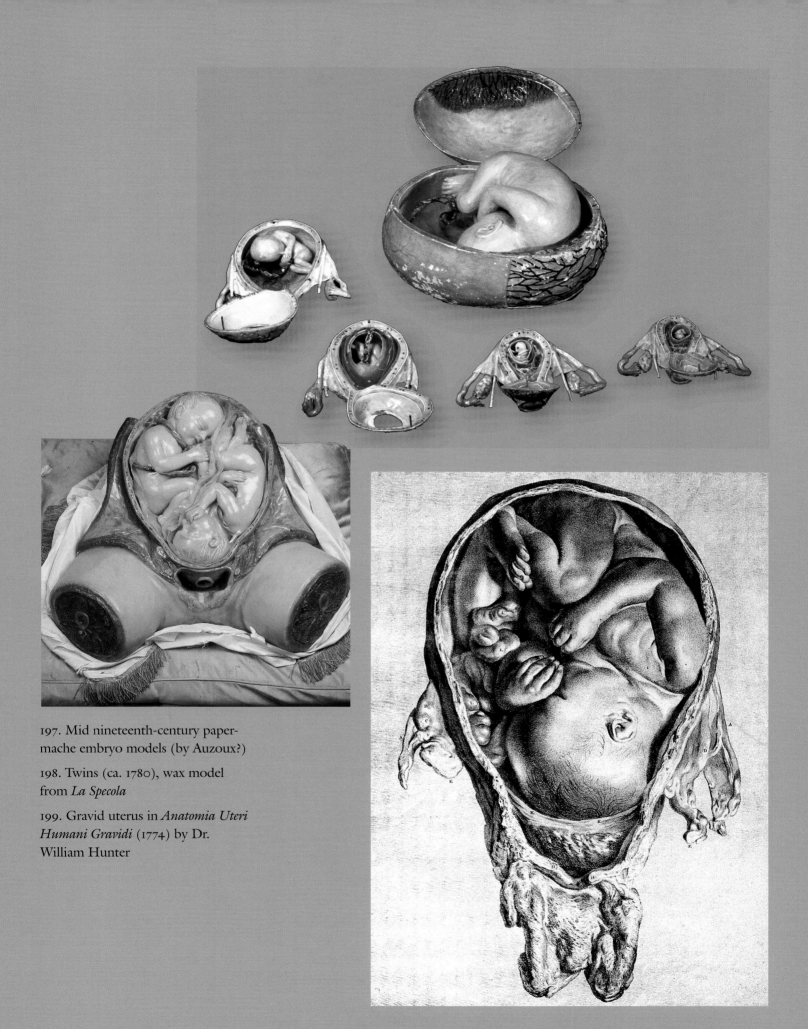

197. Mid nineteenth-century paper-mache embryo models (by Auzoux?)

198. Twins (ca. 1780), wax model from *La Specola*

199. Gravid uterus in *Anatomia Uteri Humani Gravidi* (1774) by Dr. William Hunter

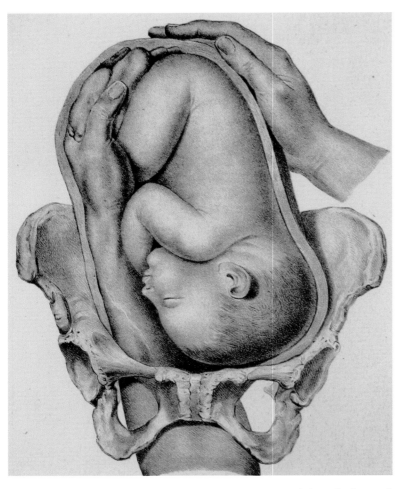

200. Turning the foot in *A Practical Treatise on Midwifery: Exhibiting the Present Advanced State of the Science* (1844) by F.J. Moreau

201. *A Rose Garden for Expectant Women and Midwives* (1513) by Eucharius Rösslin

of Food that are either too hot, or too cold, and guard themselves in the mean time against all the Passions which agitate the Blood too much, as likewise from a Life too indolent and inactive, by which Conduct their Children will neither have the Head too large or too little; at least, if no hereditary accidental Causes prevail to occasion it; and even in that case, the Regimen which we have advised, may help very much to diminish the Force of these Causes.

The most famous image of a gravid uterus was the sketch drawn by Leonardo da Vinci (figure 194), though a number of fine artisans turned their attention to this subject with wonderful results (figures 195–199).

THE ROLE OF THE MIDWIFE

Prior to the seventeenth century, obstetrics was primitive by today's standards, and without adequate anesthesia or surgical intervention, only the most uncomplicated deliveries were successful. The mother was usually left to her own devices, and both the mother and child remained at high risk should the delivery be at all delayed. Sometimes, however, help came from a female assistant, or "midwife," and physicians, who were always male, remained reluctant to become involved. They were, in fact, prohibited from viewing the birthing process until the sixteenth century. In 1522, Dr. Wertt had to dress as a woman in Hamburg, Germany, in order to witness several deliveries, and when found out, he was burned at the stake.

Over the centuries, the role of the midwife changed from simply that of an assistant to a more active one in which she actually aided in the delivery. Soranus of Ephesus (A.D. 78–117) introduced the technique of "turning the foot," or the podalic version, to aid in the delivery of a malpositioned fetus by allowing the midwife to place her hand in the uterus and pull down one of the legs (figure 200). Podalic version was described by Eucharius Rösslin, in his book *Der Schwangern Frauwen und Hebammen Roszgarten* (*A Rose Garden for Expectant Women and Midwives*) (1513) (figure 201). This first book for midwives was extraordinarily popular, and Thomas Raynalde reprinted it in many English editions as *The Byrth of Mankynde* (ca.1540).

Jacob Rueff (1500–1558) described a typical sixteenth-century preparation for delivery that required four female aids:

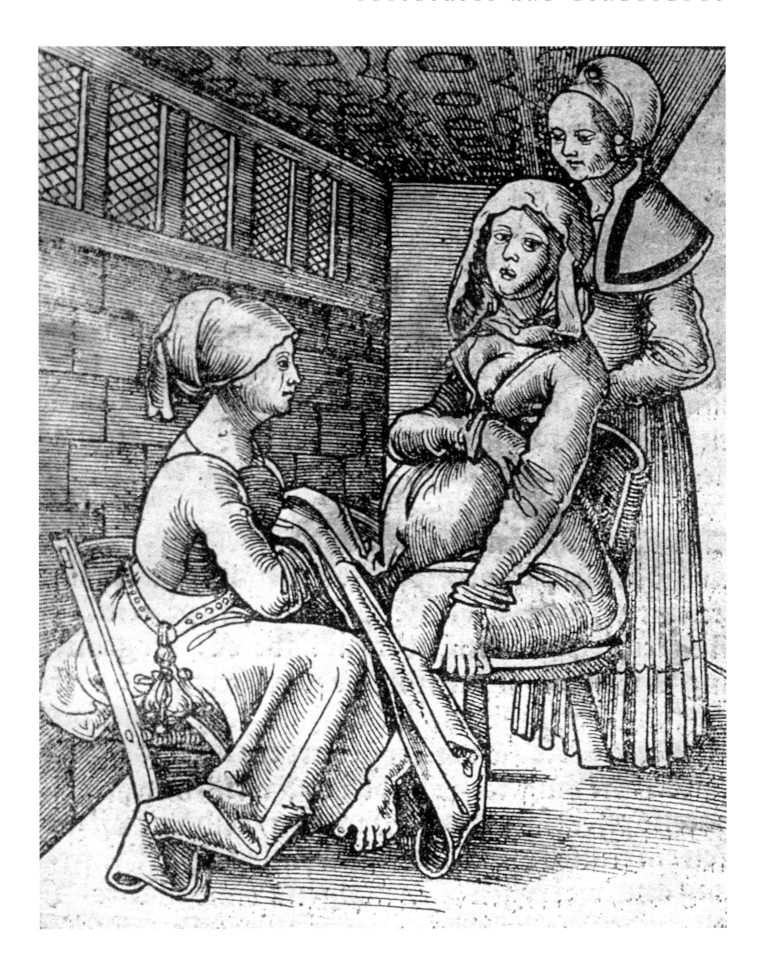

Let the stoole be made compassewise, under-propped with foure feet, the stay of it behind bending backward, hollow in the midst, covered with a blacke cloth underneath, hanging down to the ground, by that means the labouring woman may be covered, and other women sometimes apply their hands in any place, if necessity require. Let the stoole be furnished and covered with many cloths and clouts at the back and other parts, that the labouring woman be placed in her chaire about to be delivered, the midwife shall place one woman behind her back which may gently hold the labouring woman, taking her by both the arms, and if need be, the pains waxing grievous may stroke and presse downe the wombe, and may somewhat drive and depress the infant downward. But let her place other two by her sides which may both, with good words, encourage and comfort the labouring woman, and also may be ready to helpe and put to their hand at any time. This being done, let the midwife herself sit stooping forward before the labouring woman, and let her annoint her own hands and the womb of the labouring woman with oils and lillies, of sweet almonds and the grease of a hen, mingled and tempered together. For to do this doth profit and help them very much which are gross and fat and them whose secret parts are strict and narrow, and likewise them which have the mouth of the matrix dry, and such women as are in labour with their first child.

Ambrose Paré (1510–1590) finally legitimized the practice of obstetrics when he established the first school for midwifes at the Hôtel Dieu in Paris. He was responsible for interesting physicians in the practice of obstetrics and brought back Soranus' innovation of podalic version. Malposition of the fetus presented the most serious danger to the lives of both the fetus and the mother. Prior to the use of this technique, there was nothing that could be done to aid in delivery, and the adoption of podalic version by male physicians marked the birth of the specialty of obstetrics. In 1649, Thomas Johnson published *The Workes of that Famous Chirurgion, Ambrose Parey,* which contained his account "of the chirurgical extractions of the childe from the womb either dead or alive":

Therefore first of all the air of the chamber must bee made temperate, and reduced unto a certain mediocritie, so that it may neither bee too hot nor too cold. Then shee must bee aptly placed, that is to say, overthwart the bed-side, with her buttocks somewhat high, haveing a hard stuffed pillow or boulster under them, so that shee may bee in a mean figure of situation, neither fitting altogether upright, nor altogether lying along on her back; for so shee may rest quietly, and draw her breath with eas, neither shall the ligaments of the womb bee extended so as they would if shee lay upright on her back, her heels must be drawn up close to her buttocks, and there bound with broad and soft linen rowlers. The rowler must first com about her neck, and then cros-wise over her shoulders, and so to the feet, and there it must cross again, and so bee rowled about the legs thighs, and then it must bee brought up to the neck again, and there made fast, so that shee may not bee able to moov her self, even as one should be tied when he is to bee cut of the stone. But that shee may not bee wearied, or lest that her bodie should yeeld or sink down as the Chirurgian draweth the bodie of the infant from her, and so hinder the work, let him caus her feet to bee set against the side of the bed, and then let som of the standers by hold her fast by the legs and shoulders. Then that the air may not enter into the womb, and that the work may bee don with the more decencie, her privie parts and thighs must be covered with a warm double linen cloth. Then must the Chirurgian, haveing his nails closely pared, and his rings (if hee wear anie) drawn off his fingers, and his arms naked, bare, and well anointed with oil, gently draw the flaps of the neck of the womb asunder, and then let him put his hand gently into the mouth of the womb, haveing first made it gentle and slipperie with much oil; and when his hand is in, let him finde out the form and situation of the childe, whether it bee one or two, or whether it bee a Mole or not. And when hee findeth that hee commeth naturally, with his head toward the mouth or orifice of the womb, hee must life him up gently, and so turn him that his feet may come forwards, and when hee hath brought his feet for-wards, he must draw one of them gently out at the neck of the womb, and then hee must binde it with som broad and soft or silken band a little above the heel with an indifferent slick knot, and when hee hath so bound it, hee must put it up again into the womb, then he must put his hand in again, and finde out the other foot, and draw it also out of the womb, and when it is out of the womb, let him draw out the other again whereunto hee had before tied the one end of the band, and when hee hath them both out, let him join them both close together, and so by little and little let him draw all the whole bodie from the womb. Also other women or Midwives may help the endeavor of the Chirurgian, by pressing the patient's bellie with their hands downwards as the infant goeth out: and the woman herself by holding her breath, and closeing her mouth and nostrils, and by driveing her breath downwards with great violence, may verie much help the expulsion.

Dr. William Smellie (1697–1763) is thought of as the "Father of English Obstetrics." His *A Treatise on the Theory and Practice of Midwifery* (1752) was the finest obstetrical text published to that time, and he was the first to accurately describe the mechanism of birth. There was a continuing controversy regarding the specific responsibilities of the physician and the midwife during delivery, and, prior to Smellie, men were not asked to attend deliveries except as a last resort. Dr. Smellie was at the vanguard of the new specialty of obstetrics as early male practitioners struggled with their identity, calling themselves "man-midwives" or "accoucheurs." He described the prerequisites for a midwife in his classic text:

A Midwife, though she can hardly be supposed mistress of all these qualifications, ought to be a decent, sensible woman, of a middle age, able to bear fatigue; she ought to be perfectly well instructed with regard to the bones of the *Pelvis*, with all the contained parts, comprehending those that are subservient to generation; she ought to be well skill'd in the method of touching pregnant women, and know in what manner the womb stretches, together with the situation of all the abdominal *Viscera*; she ought to be perfectly mistress of the art of examination in time of labour, together with all the different kinds of labour, whether natural or praeternatural, and the methods of delivering the *Placenta*; she ought to live in friendship with other women of the same profession, contending with them in nothing but in knowledge, sobriety, diligence, and patience; she ought to avoid all reflections upon men practitioners, and when she finds herself difficulted, candidly have recourse to their assistance: on the other hand, this confidence ought to be encouraged by the man, who called, instead of openly condemning her method of practice, (even though it should be erroneous) ought to make allowance for the weakness of the sex, and rectify what is amiss, without exposing her mistakes. This conduct will as effectually conduce to the welfare of the patient, and operate as a silent rebuke upon the conviction of the midwife; who finding herself treated so tenderly, will be more apt to call for necessary assistance on future occasions, and to consider the accoucheur as a man of honour and a real friend. These gentle methods will prevent that mutual calumny and abuse which too often prevail among the male and female practitioners, and redound to the advantage of both: for, no accoucheur is so perfect, but that he may err sometimes; and on such occasions, he must expect to meet with retaliation from those midwives whom he may have roughly used.

Smellie provided an example of the friction that sometimes existed between midwives and physicians in his *Smellie's Treatise on the Theory and Practice of Midwifery*:

1724. Winston. A midwife, who never had any education, and who had formerly vaunted that she always did her own work, and would never call in a man to her assistance, was called to a case, in which the child presented wrong. After she had, with great difficulty, brought down the body, she could not deliver the head, from the woman's being of a small size and the child large. During the time of her making these trials, the husband sent in a great haste for me. In the meantime, when the midwife found that her endeavors were in vain, she rested, to recover from her fatigue, and told those who were present, that she would not wait for the assistance of the woman's pains. One of the servants seeing me at a distance, went in a hurry, and told her I was come. She, not knowing that I was called, fell to work immediately, and pulled at the child with great force and violence. Finding, as she imagined, the child coming along, she called out, 'that now she had got the better of him!' The neck at that instant separating, the body was pulled from the head, and she fell down on the floor. As she attempted to rise, one of the assistants told her that it wanted a head; a circumstance that shocked her so much (being a woman of violent disposition) that she was immediately seized with faintings and convulsions, and obliged to be put to bed in another room. I just then arrived, and was surprised to find the house in such confusion.

After being informed of what had happened, I found that the woman's pulse was pretty good, and that there had been no discharge of blood from the uterus, but what came now was only from the child's head; which, to my great joy, I found lying in the vagina and pelvis. I let her lie a little, to recover of the former fatigue; then examining more particularly, I found part of the skin of the neck without the os externum. After I had put her in a supine position, I introduced the fingers of my left hand, and found the mouth at the right side and lower part of the sacrum. Introducing two of my fingers into it, I tried with that hold to bring along the head; but finding that this would not be sufficient, and being afraid that the underjaw would separate if I used greater force, I pushed up, my fingers farther, and along the face, and with my right hand introduced the crochet to the upper part of the forehead. Here I fixed it; and again taking the former hold in the mouth with my fingers, by pulling with them and the crochet, I delivered the head much easier than I expected. After having extracted the placenta, and put the woman into an easier position in bed, I went and recovered the midwife, by giving her some volatile spirits in water. The child appeared to have been dead several days; and I was persuaded, that if the neck had not give way, but had stood another pull, the head had been delivered. This accident was lucky for me, and rendered the midwife more tractable for the future.

A (SECRET) LANDMARK DISCOVERY

One of the most important discoveries in the history of medicine was that of the obstetric forceps. Some have called the forceps "the most valuable of all surgical instruments" (figures 202, 203). A variant of the type used today was available to physicians in the Middle East in A.D. 1000, though the knowledge of that discovery was lost for centuries until rediscovered by Peter Chamberlen in the seventeenth century. The story of the discovery of this most important instrument began when the lance of a reluctant captain of the Scottish Guard, Gabriel de Montgomery, fatally pierced the eye of French King Henry II during a jousting tournament. The king died despite the valiant efforts of the most illustrious physicians of the day, including Dr. Andreas Vesalius and Dr. Abroise Paré. Henry II's successor was François II who marked his reign by a campaign against the Protestants (Huguenots) that resulted in three French wars between 1562 and 1570. Francois II died suddenly, and Catherine de Medici assumed control of the country, though attacks on the Protestants did not abate. On the Feast of St. Bartholomew, August 24, 1572, over 18,000 Huguenots were massacred throughout France. Many had left the country prior to the massacre, including surgeon and accoucheur William Chamberlen, who had fled France on July 3, 1569 to open a medical practice in Southampton, England.

Chamberlen was a barber-surgeon and had two sons named Peter (the elder and the younger), both of whom were barber-surgeons practicing obstetrics. The elder was inducted into the guild of barber-surgeons in 1598 and probably was the inventor of the modern obstetric forceps. He was the barber-surgeon to Queen Anne, wife of King James I, though with fame came resentment from the Royal College of Physicians that resulted in his confinement at the Newgate Prison for practicing medicine without a license; he was subsequently released

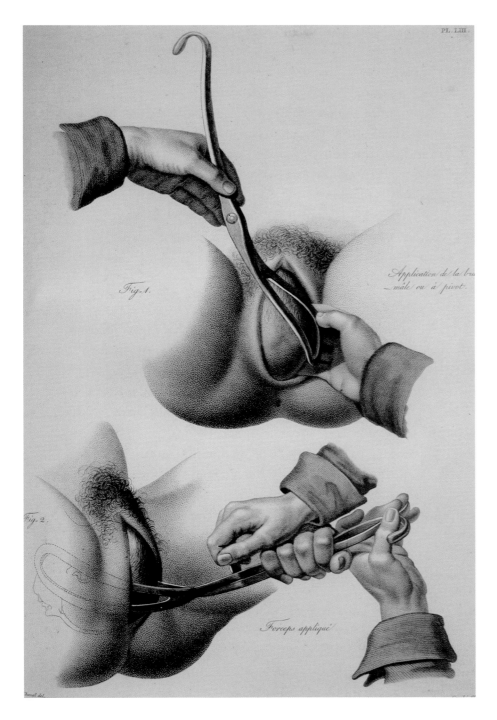

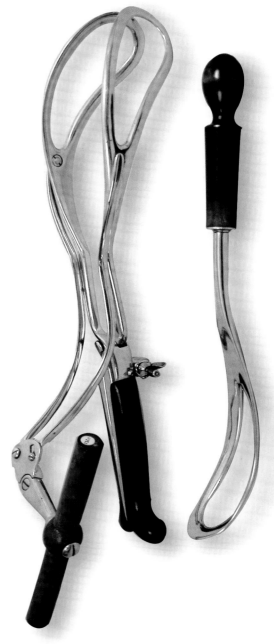

under the good auspices of the queen and the archbishop of Canterbury.

The good doctor, however, elected to keep his life-saving discovery a family secret, thus transforming this into a story of power, fame, and greed. When delivering a child, Peter (the elder) Chamberlen mysteriously brought a large ornate box into the operating room that was carried by two assistants and covered with a black cloth. He performed his deliveries under a sheet, ringing a bell when the procedure was complete, and kept his discovery within his family where it stayed for generations. On his tombstone is the following inscription:

202. Traction forceps by J. Ellis and Son; vectis (both ca. 1870)

203. Application of the forceps in *Nouvelles Démonstrations D'Accouchemens* (1822) by J.P. Maygrier

The said Peter Chamberlen toock ye degree of Doctor in Physick, in fever all Universities born att home and abroad and lived such above three score years being physician in ordinary to three Kings and Queens of England. viz.

King James and Queen Anne; King Charles ye first & Queen Mary; King Charles ye second & Queen Katherine; & also tosome forraine Princes; having travelled most of partes of Europe and speaking most of the languages.

As for his religion he was Christian keeping ye Commandments of God & faith of Jesus, being baptized about ye year 1648, & keeping ye 7th day for ye saboth above 32 years.

To tell his learning and his life to Men: Enough is said by here lyes Chamberlen.

The secret of the forceps was passed to the next generation in the hands of another Peter Chamberlen, the son of Peter Chamberlen the younger. This member of the family was the first to actually earn a medical degree, having attended Cambridge, Oxford, and the prestigious medical university in Padua. He became a member of the Royal College of Physicians in 1628 and participated in the birth of Charles II, though it was rumored that he had "used instruments of iron." The doctor moved to Mortimer Hall in Essex, where he died in 1683, and, at his death, Dr. Peter Chamberlen's widow buried the secret instruments under a trapdoor in his attic. A wine merchant bought the Essex estate and, while restoring it in 1813, Mrs. Kembell found three pair of the original forceps, which are now housed at the Royal College of Obstetricians and Gynecologists. The discovery of the forceps was recounted by H.H. Carwardine in *Medico-Chirurgical Transactions* (1862):

Two or three years ago, a lady with whom I am intimately acquainted (and from whom I had the particulars) discovered in the floor of the upper closet a hinge, and tracing the line she saw another, which led to the obvious conclusion of a door; this door she soon found means to open. There was a considerable space between the floor and the ceiling below, and this vacancy contained divers empty boxes, etc. Among these was a curious chest or cabinet, in which was deposited a collection of old coins, trinkets, gloves, fans, spectacles, etc., with many letters from Dr. Chamberlen to different members of his family, and also the obstetric instruments. Being on terms of intimacy with the family resident at Woodham Mortimer Hall, these instruments have been presented to me, and I have now the gratification of depositing them with your society for the gratification of

public curiosity, and to secure to Chamberlen the need of
posthumous fame due to him for his most useful discovery.

Dr. Peter Chamberlen had three sons, Hugh (senior), Paul, and John,
and all assumed the use of this magic instrument though they all kept
their discovery within the family. Hugh amazed physicians and patients
alike with his surgical prowess and was the accoucheur to Queen
Catherine, wife of Charles II. He drifted into debt and offered the secret
of his obstetric forceps to Jules Clement, the personal physician to King
Louis XIV of France. Clement refused to pay the 10,000-crown price
requested by Hugh when he visited Paris in 1670. The next offer went to
François Mauriceau, a well-known physician and head of the faculty of
the famous Collegium of Paris surgeons at St. Côme . Mauriceau was
opposed to the concept of delivery by forceps, but was willing to give
Chamberlen a trial by challenging him to deliver the child of a dwarf.
Chamberlen failed after three hours of excruciating labor on the part of
both the mother and the doctor, and he admitted defeat. The fetus had
expired during the ordeal, and after attempts to deliver it by Caesarean
section, the mother also died. Mauriceau refused to pay Chamerlen for
his discovery. They remained friends, however, and it was Hugh
Chamberlen who translated Mauriceau's 1668 text on obstetrics, *Traité
des maladies des femmes grosses et accouchées*, which was a significant book
in the history of medicine in that it established obstetrics as a science.
Chamberlen included the following commercial preface in the translation: "My father, my brothers and myself (but no one else in Europe)
have by the grace of God and our own industry developed an instrument which we have been using for a long time to deliver women in
childbirth, in cases of head presentation, without any risk to them or the
infants; whereas others must place in jeopardy, if not destroy with
hooks, one or the other life, or both."

Hugh Chamberlen lost his position as the royal accoucheur when he
was late in arriving at court following the Queen's delivery of James III,
and he fled the country for Amsterdam in 1699. There he finally found a
willing customer, though what followed was one of the great swindles in
the history of medicine, leading to this description by one critic: "To
give you his character truly complete, he's doctor, projector, man-mid-
wife, and cheat." Hugh sold the use of his forceps to Dutch obstetrician
Dr. Eric van Roonhuyze. Rather than completely give away the family
secret, Chamberlen sold him only one rather ineffective blade. About
fifty years later, van Roonhuyze then sold the "secret" to Drs. de
Vusscher and van de Poll, beginning a black market that included the
son of the original buyer, Rogier van Roonhuyze. Hugh finally sold the

licensing authority of the "Chamberlen technique" to the Amsterdam College of Physicians and Pharmacists, the members quite indignant by that time regarding trafficking in the use of this important instrument. They were responsible for a 1746 decree that only those who could demonstrate proficiency in the Chamberlen technique would be allowed to deliver children in Amsterdam. At the same time, the examiners themselves were not too indignant to require 2,500 guilders for instruction in the use of the forceps.

Amsterdam became the center for obstetrical care in Europe—until Hugh's son and friend of the Duke of Buckingham, Hugh (junior), finally gave the "secret" to the public. Hugh's statue was placed in the Westminster Abbey, where it remains today. The medical community then, as now, was averse to anyone profiting from the development of a surgical technique at the expense of the public. Dr. Gillaume Manquest de la Motte (1655–1737) was a contemporary of Hugh Chamberlen (senior) and addressed the Paris Academy of Medicine regarding his behavior, "He deserved to be tied to a barren rock and have his vitals plucked out by vultures."

Dr. William Smellie was familiar with the use of obstetric forceps and delivered babies with a sheet that extended from the mother's shoulders to his neck. He kept one blade in each pocket and covered each blade with leather so that there would be no telltale clink of metal that might frighten his patient. He described their use in his *Treatise on the Theory and Practice of Midwifery* (1752):

> The woman being laid in a right position for the application of the forceps, the blades ought to be privately conveyed between the feather-bed and the cloaths, at a small distance from one another, or on each side of the patient: that this conveyance may be the more easily affected, the legs of the instrument ought to be kept in the operator's side-pockets. Thus provided, when he sits down to deliver, let him spread the sheet that hangs over the bed, upon his lap, and under the cover, take out and dispose the blades on each side of the patient; by which means he will often be able to deliver with the forceps, without their being perceived by the woman herself, or any other of the assistants. Some people pin a sheet to each shoulder, and throw the other end over the bed, that they may be the more effectually concealed from the view of those who are present: but this method is apt to confine and embarrass the operator. At any rate, as women are commonly frightened at the very name of an instrument, it is adviseable to conceal them as much as possible, until the character of the operator is fully established.

Despite the great success many had with the use of obstetric forceps, there remained a number of opponents, one of the most prominent being Dr. William Hunter (1718–1783), older brother of the great surgeon Dr. John Hunter. He attended patients with a pair of aged forceps covered in rust, stating, "where they save one, they murder many." His argument took a blow in 1819 when Princess Charlotte, daughter of the Prince Regent, died with her child after fifty-two hours of labor when her physician, Sir Richard Crofts, refused to use forceps, thus allowing Queen Victoria to come to the throne. The accoucheur subsequently shot himself, and the use of forceps in delivery was instantly more acceptable to the medical community.

By the end of the eighteenth century, the traditional female midwife began to be displaced by the accoucheur, who was armed with a degree from a medical school and his obstetric forceps. The obstetric forceps continued to be used with a mystique never before associated with any other medical instrument.

THE DANGERS OF DELIVERY

Carrying a pregnancy to term has always been a risky undertaking, both to the lives of the child and the mother. Many did not survive because of inadequate prenatal care, but a significant mortality accompanied anatomic incompatibilities that did not allow the fetus to pass easily. The cesarean section was an operation performed prior to the nineteenth century, but only to save the life of the fetus when the mother was either dead or dying. In legend, the Greek god Apollo performed the first cesarean section when he delivered his son, Asklepios, the eventual god of medicine. Images of this procdure appeared in many ancient cultures, including those of the Egyptians, Chinese, and Greeks (figure 204). The term has been attributed to the birth of Julius Caesar, though this origin is likely erroneous since Caesar's mother, Aurelia, was apparently alive during her son's invasion of Great Britain years later. The term may have originated from the Latin term *caedare,* which means "to cut," or perhaps it's related to the laws enacted under Roman emperors called "Caesarean Laws." At the time, the removal of a child from a dead mother was a "Caesarean operation."

This type of surgery remained crude for centuries, as did the understanding of the relevant anatomy and physiology. For example, in 1280, the Council of Cologne passed a decree that on the death of the mother while in labor, her mouth was to be kept open so that the baby would not suffocate prior to being removed by cesarean section. It was not until 1500 that the first documented procedure took place on a living

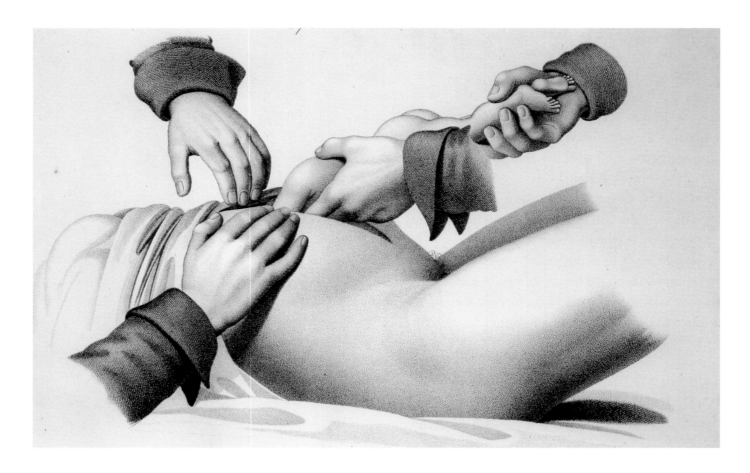

204. Cesarean section in *Nouvelles Démonstrations D'Accouchemens* (1822) by J.P. Maygrier

woman when a sow-gelder from Switzerland, Jacob Nufer, delivered his own child. Thirteen midwives had assisted the mother for days without success and, with permission from the authorities, Nufer successfully performed the operation. The baby lived to the age of seventy-seven, and his wife went on to have five more children.

Even when the delivery was "normal," there were potentially devastating consequences to the mother. A vesicovaginal fistula was first described in the final section of the Kahun papyrus and was a connection between the bladder and vagina resulting from difficult labor that could last several days. Prolonged pressure of the fetal head on the delicate walls of the vagina, bladder, and rectum caused tissue necrosis, and sometimes a connection developed between the three that led to incontinence of urine and stool. This dreadful condition was vividly described by Johann Dieffenbach (1792–1847) in *Med. Zeitung* (1836):

> A sadder situation can hardly exist than that of a woman afflicted with a vesicovaginal fistula. A source of disgust, even to herself, the woman beloved by her husband becomes, in this condition, the object of bodily revulsion to him; and filled with repugnance, everyone else likewise turns his back, repulsed by the intolerable, foul, uriniferous odor. As a result of the seepage from the open-

ing, whether large or small, the usual retention of the urine in the vaginal folds makes it even sharper and more pungent. The labia, perineum, lower part of the buttocks, and inner aspect of the thighs and calves are continually wet, to the very feet. The skin assumes a fiery red color and is covered in places with a pustular eruption. Intolerable burning and itching torment the patients, who are driven to frequent scratching to the point of bleeding, as a result of which their suffering increases still more. In desperation many tear the hair, which is coated at times with a calcareous urinary precipitate, from the mons pubis. The refreshment of a change of clothing provides no relief, because the clean undergarment, after being quickly saturated, slaps against the patients, flopping against their wet thighs as they walk, sloshing in their wet shoes as though they were wading through a swamp. The bed does not soothe them, because a good resting place, a bed or a horsehair mattress, is quickly impregnated with urine and gives off the most unbearable stench. Even the richest are usually condemned for life to a straw sack, whose straw must be renewed daily. One's breath is taken away by the bedroom air of these women, and wherever they go they pollute the atmosphere. Washing and anointing do not help; perfumes actually increase the repugnance of the odor, just as foul-tasting things become even worse when coated with sugar. This horrendous evil tears asunder every family bond. The tender mother is rejected from the circle of her children. Confined to her lonely little room, she sits there in the cold, at the open window, on her wooden chair with a hole cut in its seat, and may not cover the floor with a carpet even if she could. Indifference overtakes some of these unfortunates; others give themselves over to quiet resignation and pious devotion. Otherwise they would fall victim to despair and would attempt suicide.

American surgeon James Marion Sims (1813–1883) finally found a surgical remedy, which he described in his 1852 paper "On the Treatment of Vesico-Vaginal Fistula." Sims' discovery came after placing his patient in a knee-chest position as he attempted to restore a retroverted uterus. He was then able to directly visualize the fistula with a specially developed instrument—made out of a bent pewter soup spoon (figure 205). Though others had used the "Sims position" for the repair of vesico-vaginal fistulae, his new technique resulted in a worldwide change in the treatment of this devastating condition. Sims described his epiphany in *Silver Sutures in Surgery, the Anniversary Discourse, before the New York Academy of Medicine* on November 18, 1857:

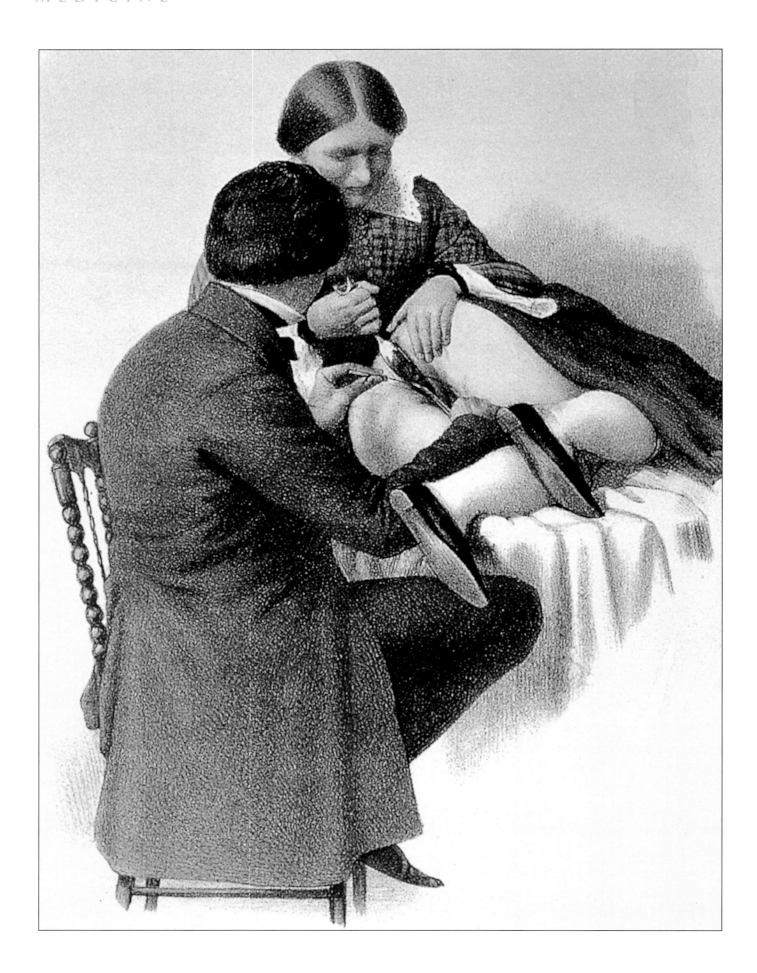

I cannot, nor is it needful to describe my emotions, when the air rushed in and dilated the vagina to its greatest capacity, whereby its whole surface was seen at one view, for the first time by any mortal man. With this sudden flash of light, with the fistulous opening seen in its proper relations, seemingly without any appreciable process of ratiocination, all the principles of the operation were presented to my mind. . . . And thus in a moment, in the twinkling of an eye, new hopes and new aspirations filled my soul, for a flood of dazzling light had suddenly burst upon my enraptured vision, and I saw in the distance the great and glorious triumph that awaited determined and persevering effort. . . . I thought only of relieving the loveliest of all God's creation of one of the most loathsome maladies that can possibly befall poor human nature. . . . Full of sympathy and enthusiasm, thus all at once I found myself running headlong after every class of sufferers that I had all of my professional life most studiously avoided.

205. Lithograph of the repair of a vesicovaginal fistula in *The surgery, surgical pathology, and surgical anatomy of the female pelvis organs,* 5th ed. (1882) by Henry Savage

Sims also discovered that the use of silver sutures significantly improved the success of his repair. His work was not without controversy, however, since his first experimentation was on his African-American slaves Anarcha, Betsy, and Lucy. In his 1884 autobiography, Sims commented, with delight, "This was the thirteenth operation performed on Anarcha. She was put to bed . . . and the next day the urine came from the bladder as clear and as limpid as spring water. . . ."

MEDICAL ABORTION

Since the life of the mother was always in question, debate over the ethics of abortion in difficult deliveries remained largely moot prior to the twentieth century. In 1809, Xavier Bichat presented a popular argument in his classic text *Physiological Researches upon Life and Death*, providing moral justification for some of the destructive obstetric procedures performed at that time. The topic remains controversial today:

. . . we may, I think, confidently conclude, that in the foetus animal life is null, and that all the acts attached to this age, are in a dependance on organic life. The foetus has nothing in its phenomena which can particularly characterize the animal; its existence is the same as that of the vegetable; its destruction cannot be considered that of an animated being, but of a living being only. In the cruel alternative, therefore, of being compelled to sacrifice it, or to expose the mother to an almost certain death, the choice should not be for a moment doubtful.

The crime of destroying its life is more relative to animal than to organic life. It is the being who feels, who reflects, who wills, who performs voluntary actions, and not the being who respires, digests, is nourished, and has circulation, secretions, &c. whom we regret, and whose violent death is accompanied with all those horrible images under which homicide is painted to our minds. In the series of animals, in proportion as the intellectual functions decrease, the painful feeling which the sight of their destruction causes us, is gradually weakened; it becomes extinct when we come to vegetables, which possess organic life only.

At about the same time, the British drew the line for legal abortion to before the moment of quickening, or the first fetal movement that occurs between the fourth and fifth month. After then, Lord Ellenborough's act of 1803 made abortion illegal:

> . . . be it therefore further enacted, That if any Person or Persons . . . shall wilfully and maliciously administer to, or cause to be administered to, or taken by any Woman, any Medicines, Drug, or other Substance or Thing whatsoever, or shall use or employ, or cause or procure to be used or employed, any Instrument or other Means whatsoever, with Intent thereby to cause or procure the Miscarriage of any Woman not being, or not being proved to be, quick with Child at the Time of administering such Things or using such Means, that then and in every such Case the Person or Persons so offending, their Counsellors, Aiders, and Abettors, knowing of and privy to such Offence, shall be and are hereby declared to be guilty of Felony, and shall be liable to be fined, imprisoned, set in and upon the Pillory, publickly or privately whipped, or to suffer one or more of the said Punishments, or to be transported beyond the Seas for any Term not exceeding fourteen Years, at the Discretion of the Court before which such Offender shall be tried and convicted.

In the case of the dead or undeliverable fetus, rapid evacuation was called for because of the inherent risk to the mother. This raised the difficult question of determining the viability of the fetus, though several guidelines could be found in *Boerhaave's Aphorisms: Concerning the Knowledge and Cure of Diseases* (1715): "'Tis known to be dead, if it is unmoveable, if the Umbilical Arteries are felt to rest up-on the Navel-string, and chiefly near the Body of the Child; If there comes from the Womb faetid Matters; If the Mother feels a greater dead weight than a little while before; If she has sudden and continual Motions to go to Stool; If she Faints away often; her Hairs stand on end; her Breath stinks much; and of a dead Corps; Looks of a livid Colour; If she is not deliver'd long after the Waters are all come away; If the Skin of the Child feels loose, and comes off easily; and his Bones are moveable and soft."

Once a decision had been made that the fetus was not viable, medical abortion was always preferable to surgical intervention. Trotula of Salerno (ca. 1097) described noninterventional techniques later printed in a fifteenth-century text, *A Medieval Woman's Guide to Health*:

> In order to deliver a woman of a child and to kill it if it cannot be brought out: take rue, savin, southern wood, and iris, and let her drink them. Also take 2 drachms each of the juice of hyssop and of dittany, and 2 scruples of quicksilver, and this medicine is proved to be effective. Also take 4 drachms each of the juice of iris and bull's gall, 2 drachms of suitable oil, mix all these together, put it in a pessary, give it to the woman, and this medicine will bring out all the decomposed matter of the womb. And it will deliver a woman of a dead child, and of her secundines, and it brings on menstruation. Again, give to the pregnant woman 2 drachms of asafetida 3 times daily, and let the stomach and back be anointed with oil and gall, and afterward let oil, ox gall, and asafetida be placed in the vulva with a feather.

This is Boerhaave's recommendation for a simple extraction if medications failed: "As soon as the Foetus is known to be dead, it ought to be drawn out for fear of communicating a Gangrene to the Mother, throwing her into fainting Fits, Convulsions and Death; and that ought to be done by the feet if possible, because there is the best hold, which is material, when the Child doth not help it self."

INSTRUMENTS OF DESTRUCTION

After the determination had been made that an abortion was indicated, the procedure was done with some immediacy since only the life of the mother was of concern and was in great danger. The instruments were often gruesome. They were constructed without regard to aseptic considerations, leading to a significant level of mortality in the mother, though a mortality lower than the almost universal death rate faced by those with an undeliverable fetus (figures 206–212).

William Smellie discussed some of the details of this dramatic effort to save the mother's life by either a rapid delivery or by abortion in his classic text, *A Treatise on the Theory and Practice of Midwifery* (1752). Note some of the ethical dilemmas that continue to be of concern today:

> . . . when all the common methods have been used without success, the woman being exhausted, and all her efforts vain; and when the child cannot be delivered without such force as will

206. Right. Smellie's perforator in *Nouvelles Démonstrations D'Accouchemens* (1822) by J.P. Maygrier

207. Below. Ramsbotham cranioclast in *The Principles and Practice of Obstetric Medicine* (1836) by A. Davis

208. Opposite page, top left. Mid nineteenth-century instruments of destruction: (left) Thomas' perforator; (top center) Holmes' Cranioclast by S. Maw, Davis perforator, Jacquemier's embryotome caché by Mathieu ; (right) plain crochet

209. Opposite page, top right. Late eighteenth-century abortion instruments: (top) Tarnier's basiotribe by Collin, Cephalotribe du Dr. Bailly by Klein Glitsehka Gand, Trepan de Leisurg et Diwisch by Thuerrigl

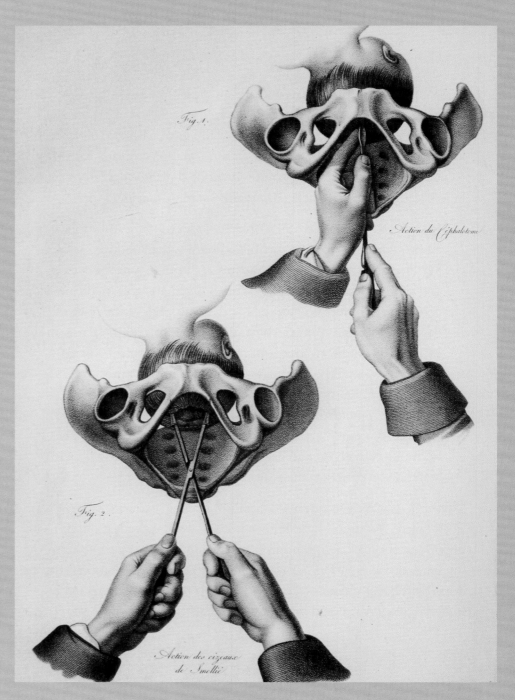

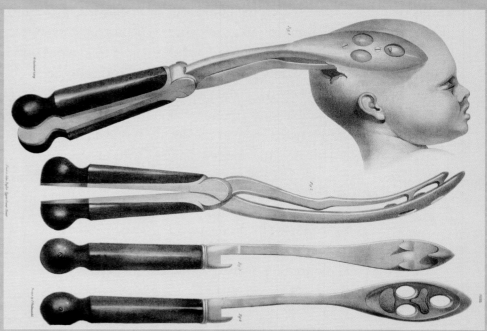

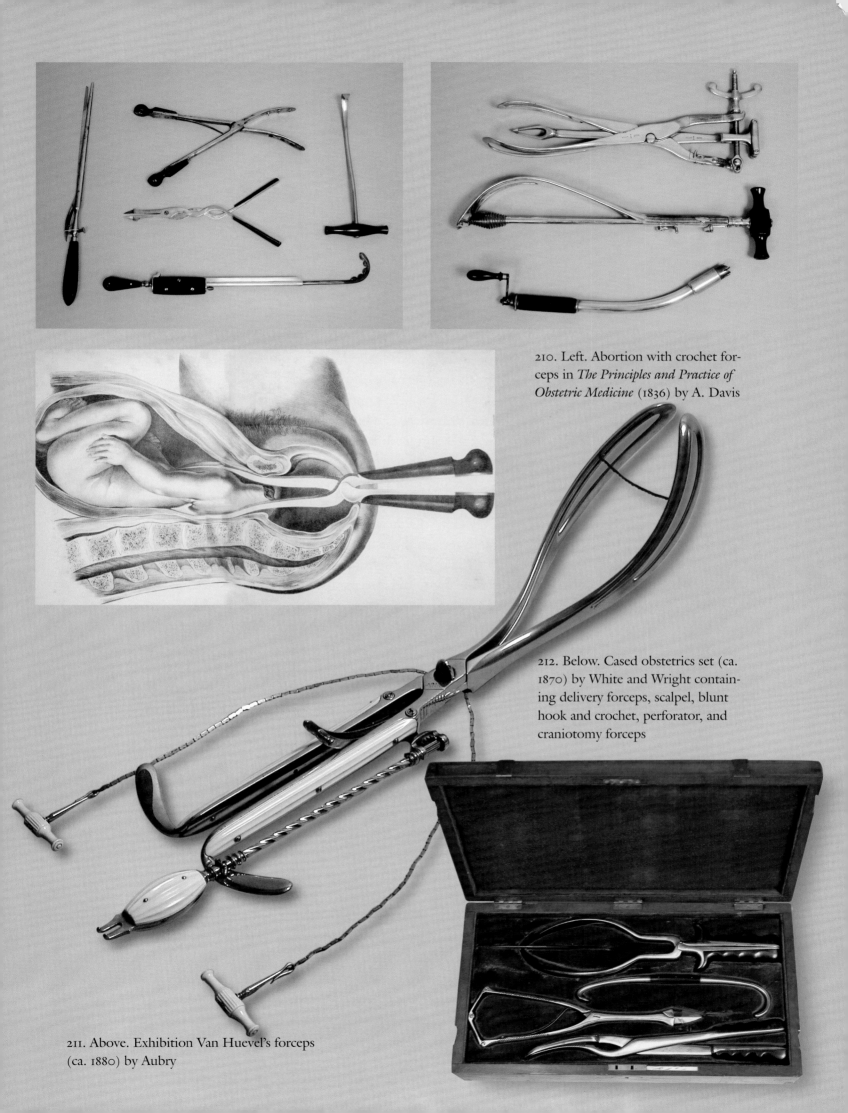

210. Left. Abortion with crochet forceps in *The Principles and Practice of Obstetric Medicine* (1836) by A. Davis

212. Below. Cased obstetrics set (ca. 1870) by White and Wright containing delivery forceps, scalpel, blunt hook and crochet, perforator, and craniotomy forceps

211. Above. Exhibition Van Huevel's forceps (ca. 1880) by Aubry

endanger the life of the mother, because the head is too large or the *Pelvis* too narrow; it then becomes absolutely necessary to open the head, and extract with the hand, forceps, or crochet. Indeed, this last method formerly was the common practice when the child could not be easily turned, and is still in use with those who do not know how to save the child by delivering with the forceps: for this reason, their chief care and study was to distinguish, whether the *Foetus* was dead or alive; and as the signs were uncertain, the operation was often delayed until the woman was in a most imminent danger; or when it was performed sooner, the operator was frequently accused of rashness, on the supposition, that the child might in time have been delivered alive by the labour-pains. . . .

When the head presents, and such is the case, that the child can neither be delivered by turning, nor extracted with the forceps, and it is absolutely necessary to deliver the woman to save her life, this operation must then be performed in the following manner.

The operator must be provided with a pair of curved crochets, made according to the improvements upon those proposed by *Mefnard*, together with a pair of scissars about nine inches long, with rests near the middle of the blades, and the blunt hook.

The patient ought to be laid on her back in the same position in the use of the forceps; the operator must be seated on a low chair, and the instruments concealed and disposed in the same manner, and for the same reason, mentioned in treating for the forceps. . . .

The head is commonly kept down pretty firm by the strong contraction of the *Uterus* round the child; but should it yield to one side, let it be kept steady by the hand of an assistant, pressing upon the belly of the woman: let him introduce his hand, and press two fingers against one of the sutures of the *Cranium*; then take out his scissars from the place in which they were deposited, and guiding them by the hand and fingers till they reach the hairy scalp, then push them gradually into it until their progress is stopped by the rests. . . .

The scissars being thus forced into the brain, as far as the rests at the middle of the blades, let them be kept firm in that situation; and the hand that was in the *Vagina* being withdrawn, the operator must take hold of the handles with each hand and pull them asunder, that the blades may dilate and make a large opening in the skull; then they must be shut, turned, and again pulled asunder, so as to make the incision crucial; by which means, the opening will be enlarged, and sufficient room made for the introduction of the fingers: let them be afterwards closed, and introduced even beyond the rests, when they must again be opened, and turned half round from side to side, until the structure of the brain is so effectually destroyed, that it can be evacuated with ease. This operation being performed, let the scissars be shut and withdrawn; but if this instrument will not answer the last purpose, the business may be done by introducing the crochet within the opening of the skull. The brain being thus destroyed, and the instrument withdrawn, let him introduce his right hand into the *Vagina,* and two fingers into the opening which hath been made, that if any sharp splinters of the bones remain, they may be broken off and taken out, lest they should injure the woman's *Vagina,* or the operator's own fingers. . . .

Although many people have exclaimed against the crochets as dangerous instruments, from ignorance, want of experience, or a worse principle, as formerly observed; yet I can assure the reader, that I never either tore or hurt the parts of a woman with that instrument. I have indeed several times hurt the inside of my hand, by their giving way . . . and before we had the curve crochet, I have been so fatigued from the streight kind slipping their small hold so often, that I have scarcely been able to move my fingers or arms, for many hours after; and if this force had not been used, the mother must have been lost as well as the child.

AFTER THE BLESSED EVENT

In the event of a successful delivery, a number of devices were manufactured to aid the new mother with her nursing since breast-feeding was popular and an inexpensive way to provide nutrition for the newborn. It was not uncommon for children to nurse well until the time they had teeth, so that many mothers sought the help of breast pumps and nipple shields. Some shields were made of lead, which was absorbed with the breast milk, causing potentially toxic consequences (figure 213).

INSTRUMENTS DESIGNED FOR WOMEN

Aside from cesarian section and mastectomy, there was little invasive surgery available to women prior to the discovery of anesthesia in the mid nineteenth century. Male physicians had been quite reluctant to examine and treat women, a concern illustrated by this quote from *Hints to Husbands* (1857): "We allude to the speculum. The adoption of this instrument as we are informed, is now becoming general; and its employment plunges its wretched victim, woman, into the lowest depths of infamy and degradation. We will not pollute these pages by describing its methods of action; suffice it to say, that, to the sense of touch,

213. (Top) cased breast pumps by Elam, and Maw, Son, and Thompson; (bottom) Wansbrough's Metallic Nipple Shields, and glass nipple shields, nipple shell (all mid nineteenth century)

214. Roman trivalve vaginal speculum with replica screw (ca. 99 B.C.–A.D. 400) found in Lebanon

common to all midwifery practices, is added, in its application, that of sight; exposure the most complete of all which modesty in the most abject of races, invariably conceals." Despite this admonition, vaginal specula had been in use from the time of the ancient Roman Empire (figure 214) and evolved in a number of ways into the nineteenth century.

The growing female market in the early twentieth century was reflected by a great diversity in devices manufactured for the treatment of women's diseases. Instruments were made for feminine hygiene and for minor surgery, including ecrasures to remove uterine polyps (and later hemorrhoids) by crushing them with a chain (figures 215, 216). Male physicians often attributed various women's disorders such as pain, dysmenorrhea, and mood swings to an abnormally placed, or "dropped" uterus, and the obvious therapy was to reposition this organ with an instrument called a repositor.

Despite the fact that gynecology is now a recognized branch of medicine, female gender bias continued to play a significant role in the practice of medicine until the latter part of the twentieth century when attention to diseases specifically affecting women became comparable to that spent on other disorders. Many clinical trials are now gender sensitive and, with some irony, now recognize the increasing risk to women of classically male medical problems, including lung cancer and cardiovascular disease.

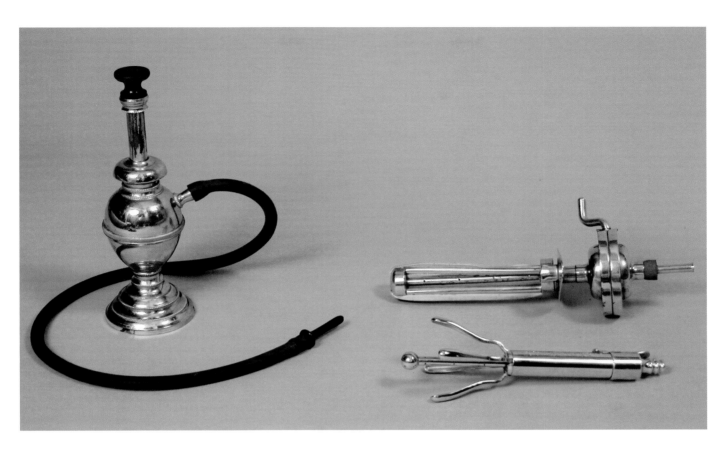

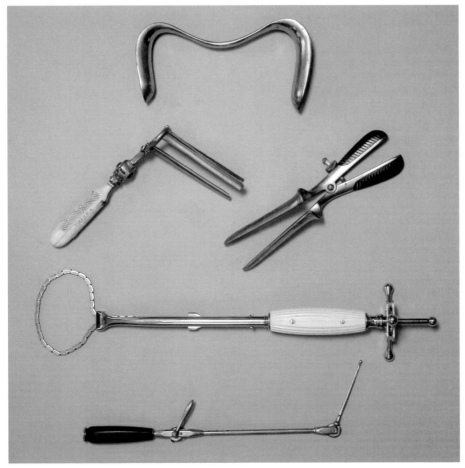

215. Instruments designed for female hygiene (ca. 1900): (left) Hygieno-phile by G. Huclin and Co.; (top right) Lawson's vaginal washer; (bottom) Vagex by American Vagex Corp.

216. Sims vaginal speculum by Tiemann, trivalve speculum Weiss, bivalve speculum by Tiemann, Edward's ivory ecraseur, repositor by Sharp and Smith

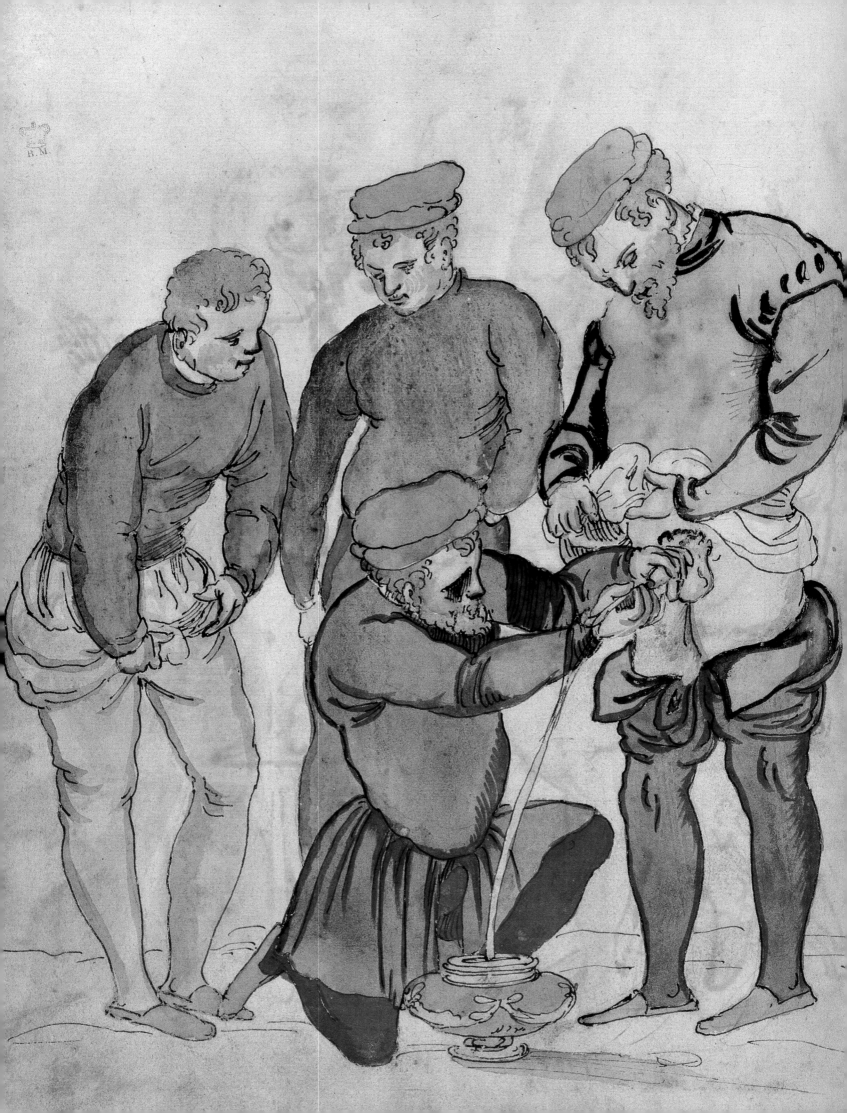

"The cure itself is something horrible, grave, and perilous. The mind recoiled at the thought of so frightful a remedy, but what remedy seems frightful when it carries hope to people in peril of death?"

Anon, 16th century

Short-robed Surgeon Catheterizes a Patient (ca 1510) by Heinrich Kullmaurer and Albrecht Meher

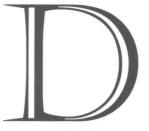

isorders of the urinary tract have played a prominent role in the history of medicine because venereal disease and kidney stones have always been common, painful, and often fatal conditions, quickly demanding the attention of patients and physicians alike. Artists were interested in the anatomy of the kidneys well before physicians understood the pathophysiology of any of these conditions (figures 217, 218).

EARLY MEDICAL THERAPY

Venereal disease was widespread prior to the discovery of antibiotics. Nicholas Culpeper discussed early medical options in his *Culpeper's School of Physick* (1659):

> *Of Ulcers in the Yard*
> The causes are clearly sharp and gnawing humors.

- Make a decoction of Sage in white Wine, and inject it often into the Yard.
- If the Yard be swelled, anoint it with warm Oyl of Roses.
- If much sharp humors resort to the place, as usually there doth in such cases; take of those Cakes called *Trochifi albi Rhazis* with *Opium* one dram, Plante-water four ounces, beat the Troches with powder, and mix them with the Plante-water, and inject it into the Yard with a syringe, a little at a time, not all at once.

Of course, mercury remained popular for the treatment of venereal disease well into the nineteenth century, though its use was accompanied by a number of toxic side effects, one of which ironically was kidney failure.

Obstructive uropathy, or the blockage of urine, was an unexpected and very painful consequence not only from syphilis and gonorrhea, but from kidney stones as well. Culpeper outlined some of the early therapeutic regimens used by physicians to increase the flow of urine when this serious and urgent problem developed:

> *Of the Strangury.*
> In the Strangury, the Urine comes away by drops with much pain; with a great desire to piss.

- Ox dung mixed with honey, and applied warm to the neck of the Bladder, is very good.
- The neck of the Bladder anointed with the Grease of a Hedge-hog, is exceeding good to open the stoppage of Urine.
- Raddish-roots scraped clean, and sliced thin, and infused all night in

217. Renal system (abdomen) in *Traité complet d'anatomie de l'homme,* 2nd ed. (1866–1871), by J.M. Bourgery, Claude Bernard, and N.H. Jacob

218. Kidneys, ureters, and bladder (ca. 1780), wax model from *La Specola*

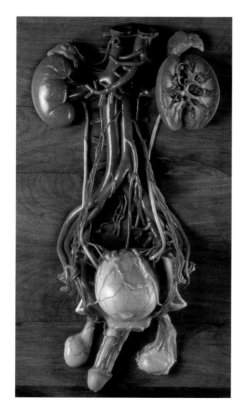

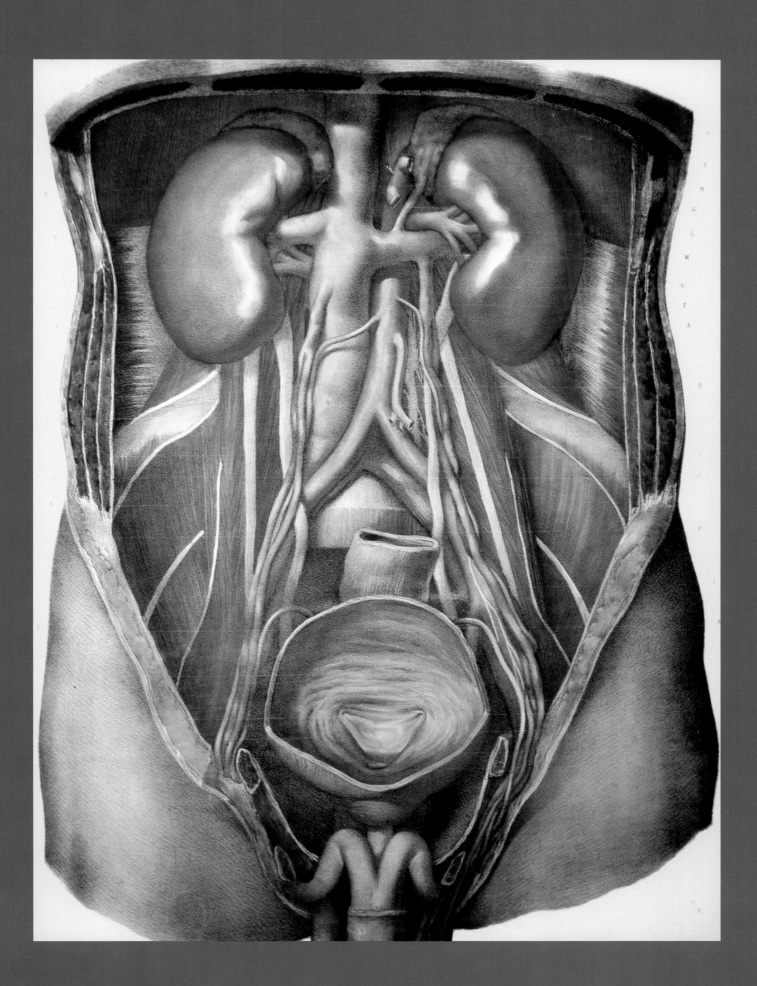

White Wine, and stopped close, and a quarter of a pinte taken the next morning, is a mighty great provoker of Urine, but it hath no very pleasing taste.

- Warm Eggs applied to the neck of the Bladder, wonderfully provoke Urine.
- The best remedy in the world against the Strangury, is this; to save all the water the diseased party maketh, and let the diseased party drink it down back again, and that in very few dayes will cure him.

Physicians injected caustics like silver nitrate for strictures (figure 219), though urinary catheterization was a less traumatic option, if it could be accomplished. John of Gaddesden (1280–1361), physician to Edward II, reportedly passed the first urinary catheter, and that procudure was illustrated in some of the earliest texts (figures 220, 221). Laurence Heister discussed the proper use of a urinary catheter in *A General System of Surgery, in Three Parts* (1743):

> Though the passing of a Catheter into the Bladder may appear a slight and trivial Operation in the Eye of an inconsiderate Person; yet so arduous is sometimes the Task, that it even baffles the Skill of the most expert Surgeon, and is through various Impediments impracticable, even in the dextrous Hand, which is frequently versed in the Operation. There are usually two principal Causes, for which this Instrument is applied in both Sexes. The first is, to be satisfied with regard to the Existance of a Stone in the Bladder, in as much as the other Symptoms of the Stone, such as Pain in the Bladder, Suppression of the Urine, a Strangury or *Ischuria*, &c. are often found to be fallacious, and not to be confided in; because the same Symptoms may arise from an Inflammation, Abscess, or Ulcer in the Bladder, from a Tumor or Excrescence in the Neck of the Bladder, &c. The second Case, in which the Use of the Catheter is necessary, is to discharge the Urine in an *Ischuria*, or when the Patient cannot make any Water at all, or but very little, and with difficulty, from some Defect in the Bladder, so that the Urine is thereby retained, until the Bladder is extremely distended, with violent Pain, and other bad Symptoms. For if the Patient be not relieved in such a Case, by a timely Application of this Instrument; the Neglect will certainly be attendede with an Inflammation, Mortification, or Rupture of the Bladder, or Death will be the End, in the Extremities of Pain, Anguish, and Convulsions.

When a tube could not be passed into the bladder to relieve the obstruction, other procedures were devised, some quite novel, though

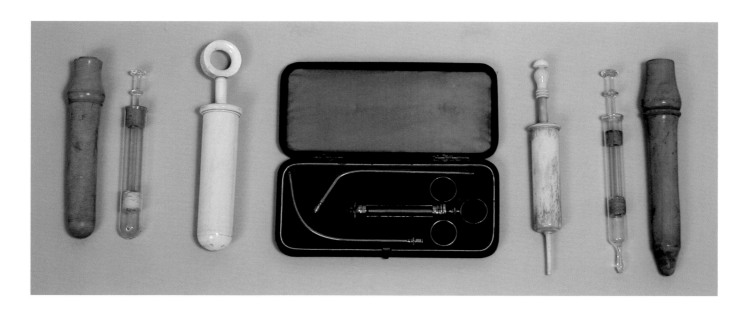

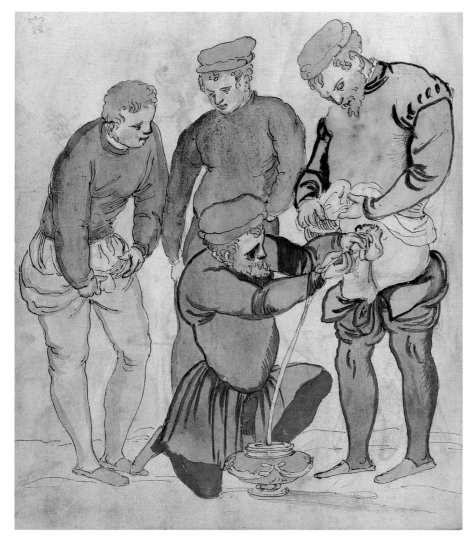

219. Nineteenth-century devices for infusion and irrigation: (left to right) female glass treen cased and ivory syringes, cased urethral syringe, male ivory and glass treen cased syringes

220. *Short-robed surgeon catheterizes a patient* (ca. 1510) by Heinrich Kullmaurer and Albrecht Meher

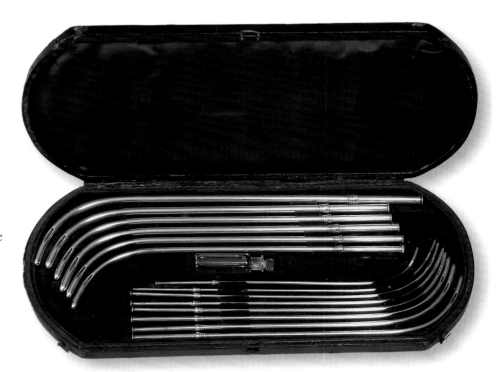

221. Silver urinary catheters with oil (ca. 1860)

222. Dupuytren's double bistoury caché in *Traité complet d'anatomie de l'homme comprenant l'anatomie chirurgical et la médicine opératoire*, 2nd ed. (1866–1871) by J.M. Bourgery, Claude Bernard, and N.H. Jacob

223. Dupuytren's double bistoury caché by J.J. Teufel

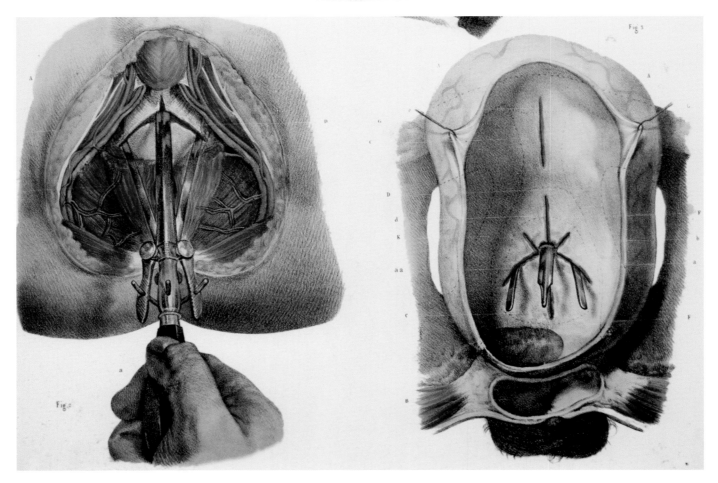

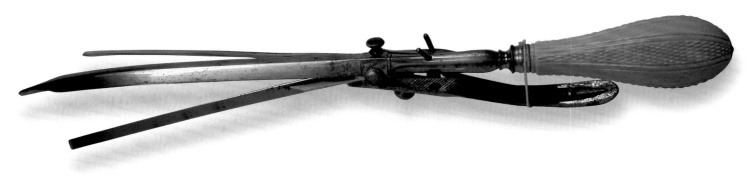

all probably as painful and dangerous as the condition itself. Remember that these instruments were all used prior to the discovery of anesthesia and aseptic techniques (figures 222–224).

Urinary retention is not always mechanical, and one of the earliest urinals became popular in early French churches. A Jesuit priest named Louis Bordeloue (1632–1704) gave a most beautiful and lengthy sermon, so lengthy in fact that young ladies passed around a female urinal, now called a "bordeloue" in his honor, so that they might not miss his oratory (figure 225).

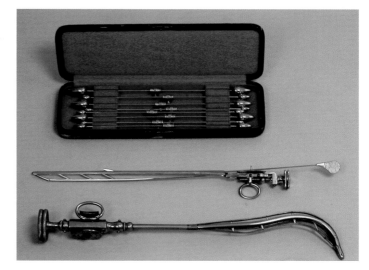

KIDNEY STONES—THE CAUSE

Bladder stones were much more common prior to the nineteenth century than they are now, perhaps because of increased food and water impurities. A number of famous personalities suffered from this condition, including Leopold I, Napoleon III, Francis Bacon, Isaac Newton, Peter the Great of Russia, Louis XIV of France, Oliver Cromwell, George IV of England, and Dr. Thomas Sydenham, the latter one of the greatest physicians of all time. Sydenham commented, "The patient suffers until he is finally consumed by both age and illness, and the poor man is happy to die."

In *A Complete Treatise of the Stone and Gravel* (1710), Dr. John Greenfield attributed the development of kidney stones to several causes, including eating unfermented bread, smoked goat's flesh, scaleless fish, or unripe fruits, drinking yeast in beer, or having a birthday in the eighth house under Saturn and Mercury. Further, "the immoderate and more than brutish Salaciousness, which some indulge themselves in, most certainly promotes the rise and growth of the Stone, heating and obstructing the Urinary Parts."

Hermann Boerhaave discussed the etiology and diagnosis of kidney stones in *Boerhaave's Aphorisms: Concerning the Knowledge and Cure of Diaseases* (1715):

- Whenever in a Humane Body another certain Body altogether insoluble stops, there soon gathers upon it and about it a Crust more or less stony.
- If this happens in the Kidneys from the earthy part of the Blood dried up, there follows and grows a Stone in the Kidneys, taking its Birth chiefly at the end of the smallest arteries there in the shape of a Sand.
- Which increasing there gradually doth stop up the Kidney and

224. Above. Mid nineteenth-century urethral instruments: (top) cased set of Bougie á boule, Otis Dilating urethrotome with dissecting blade, internal dilating urethrotome

225. Below. Mid eighteenth-century urinals: (top) Bordeloue for females; and (bottom) floral ceramic for males

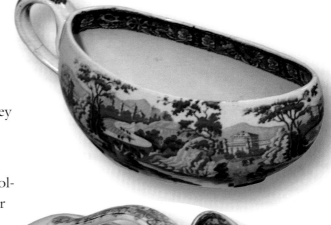

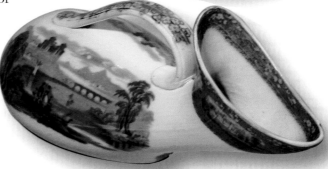

277

choakes its flesh, consuming the same and drives out the same in the form of clotts of Blood, Pus, Caruncles and Skins, and corrupts the whole at last, exciting bloody Urine, pissing of Pus and foetid black and ulcerous Matters; and doth even occasion an Ulceration and Inflammation of the neighbouring Parts.

- The Stone in the Kidneys is known from an obtuse Pain there, from a pissing of Blood after riding in a Coach, or other great motion upon the Stones and rough Roads, upon any other violent motion or straining of the Body, from having often voided some Stones, Skins, Pus, or Strings.

- That there is a Stone in the Bladder is known, from the pain in making Water, before and after it; from the Water being made only by drops, white with a mucous, thick, heavy Sediment to a great Quantity, from an itching at the Gland or Head of the Yard; by putting the Fingers up the Fundament and pressing towards the Neck of the Bladder, and by probing with the Catheter, and by observing the Symptoms.

The Medical Treatment of Stones

After recognizing the certain fatality of untreated obstructing bladder stones and the high risk of surgical intervention, physicians were anxious to provide a medical alternative. Since no treatment was clearly effective, approaches to medical therapy were quite numerous and often bizarre. Phil Woodman, in *The Modern Physician* (1712), suggested the use of enemas: "The Belly must be Kept Loose either with Laxatives or Specifick Emollient Clysters; these latter must not be injected in a large Quantity, especially in Big-belly'd Women, for fear of encreasing the Pain, from too much distending the Parts. After the Bowels are very well emptied, inject now and then one of the following Lubricating Diuretic Clysters; Take Urine of a young found Lad eight Ounces, Oils of Rue, Chamomil, Linseed of each six Drams, Turpentine (opened with the Telk of an Egg) one Ounce, Syrup of Marsh-mallows one Ounce and a half: mix and inject it warm." According to Richard Lower (1631–1691), "To alleviate a stone-attack and the usually consequent retention of urine, take snail-shells and bees in equal quantities, dry them in a moderately hot oven, and grind them to a very fine powder. Take as much to this as a six pence holds, dissolve it in a quarter-mug of bone meal powder, and give it on an empty stomach, followed by two hours of fasting, every day for three days in a row. It has often been found to break down the stone and drive the urine forth."

Nicholas Culpepper discussed the medical treatment of kidney stones in his *School of Physick* (1659):

- A Hedge-sparrow is of a notable vertue, for the guts detracted, and the feathers taken off, and so either kept in Salt, or converted into Mummy and eaten, (the Birds I mean, not the guts or feathers) it will break the stone, either in the Reins or Bladder, and bring it forth.

- Also it is an excellent remedy to break the Stone, to drink the blood of a Fox either alone by it self, or mixed with white Wine. And to make the truth of this appear clearly, take a Pebble-stone, and put it into the blood of a Fox, and it will dissolve it; yet in my opinion, and my opinion is grounded upon reason, if the Stone lie in the Reins, it is best to drink the blood of a Fox; but for the Stone in the Bladder, it is best to inject it with a Syringe.

- And here take notice by the way, that many times people in avoiding gravel have some great Stone stick by the way in the passage of the Yard, which is many times forced to be taken out by cutting; in such a case, if the party did but hold his Yard in the warm Blood of a Fox, it would be in a short time be made small enough to come out of it self, without any such troublesome or painful remedy.

- Take all the blood and the whole skin of a Hare, put them into a new pot that hath a cover, lute it up close, and burn it in the fire to ashes; the Hares skin, and blood I mean, and not the pot: Give the Patient a small spoonful of these ashes in White Wine; it mightily breaks and drives out the Stone.

- The Stone that hath been taken out of a man, or the Gravel which men void, being taken back again inwardly, a drachm at a time, doth wonderfully break and bring away the Stone, and is indeed the most exquisite remedy that I know.

- Take of Goats Blood, the Liver, Lungs, Reins, Yard, and Stones of the Goat; make puddings thereof in the great Gut of the said Goat; order them well and boyl them as you do Hogs puddings; and let him that is troubled with the Stone eat them as meat, not as Medicine; their wonderful effects in breaking the Stone will be admirable in your eyes.

- Goats piss drunk, breaketh and expelleth the Stone.

Hermann Boerhaave took a pragmatic approach to the medical treatment of obstructive uropathy. According to him, the stone may be removed "by loosening the Vessels with Baths, Glysters, and relaxing oily Liniments; By making the passages slippery with moistening Emollients, soft and gentle oily Medicines; Opening them with Opiates and Anodynes; Driving them on with gentle Motion, such as that of a Boat or a very easy going Horse."

The Surgical Treatment of Stones

The surgical treatment of bladder stones originated in India several thousand years ago and was limited to physicians of the lower castes who did not object to "hands on" care. As described in about 800 B.C. in the *Susruta-samhita*, the procedure began by the surgeon placing two fingers that had been lubricated with fat into the patient's rectum in order to palpate the stone in the bladder and move it downward as far as possible. A knife was then inserted into the perineum between the scrotum and the anus, through the prostate, and the stone was then removed. The incision was left to heal, though occasionally fistulae resulted from the surgery.

For centuries, the practice of removing stones, or lithotomy, was looked down on by the medical profession in Europe as a trade best left to traveling barber-surgeons, who included in their resume other minor surgical procedures such as dental extractions, bloodletting, abscess drainage, and fracture repair. The procedure was often quite crude, and the first simple removal of a kidney stone using forceps was attributed to John of Gaddesden in the fourteenth century (figure 226). Death was certain unless the obstruction was relieved, and patients who consented to this gruesome operation experienced over a fifty percent mortality rate, succumbing from bowel perforation, uncontrolled bleeding, and infection. The fortunate who survived often had to suffer from a chronic draining fistula-in-ano with constant leakage of urine and stool. Hippocrates was well aware of the high surgical mortality when he included as part of his famous oath to be taken by physicians: "I will not cut, even for the stone, but I will leave such procedures to the practitioners of that craft."

In his *Apologie Et Voyages* (1585), Ambrose Paré described the preparation of the patient in his chapter titled "Of Cutting for the Stone" (figure 227), and one gets an idea of the horror and uncertainty faced by these patients:

> Seeing wee cannot otherwise helpe such men as have stones in their bladders, we must come to the extreme remedy, to wit, cutting. But the patient must first be purged, and if the case require, draw some blood; yet must you not immediately after this, or the day following hasten to the work, for the patient cannot but be weakened by purging & bleeding. Also it is expedient for some daies before to foment the privities with such things as relaxe and soften, that by their yielding, the stone may the more easily be extracted. Now the cure is thus to be performed; The patient shall be placed upon a firm table or bench with a cloth many times doubled under his buttocks, and a pillow under his loynes & back, so that he may lie halfe upright with his thighs lifted up, and his legs and heels drawn back to his buttocks. Then

shall his feet be bound with a ligature of three fingers breadth cast about his ankles and with the heads thereof being drawn upwards to his neck, and cast about it, and so brought downewards, both his hands shall bee bound to his knees, as the following figure sheweth.

The patient thus bound, it is fit you have foure strong men at hand; that is, two to hold his armes, and other two who may so firmely and straightly hold the knee with one hand, and the foot with the other, that he may neither move his limmes, nor stirre his buttocks, but be forced to keep in the same posture with his whole body. Then the Surgeon shall thrust into the urinary passage even to the bladder, a silver or iron and hollow probe, annoynted with oyle, and opened or slit on the out side that the point of the knife may enter thereinto, and that it may guide the hand of the workman, and keep the knife from piercing any farther into the bodies lying thereunder.

Because of the nature of the cure and the associated high mortality, many developed a rather strong antagonism toward "stone cutters," as well as toward all members of the medical profession. Prolific sixteenth-century essayist Michel de Montaigne (1533–1592) graphically expressed this disdain in his autobiography, *Gravel and the Doctors*:

I am at grips with one of the worst diseases—painful, dreadful, and incurable. Yet even the pain itself, I find, is not so intolerable as to plunge a man of understanding into frenzy or despair. At least I have one advantage over the stone. It will gradually reconcile me to what I have always been loathe to accept—the inevitable end. The more it presses and importunes me, the less I will fear to die. . . .

It may be that I inherited my hatred of doctoring, but in any case I have strengthened it by arguments and reasons. In the first place, the experience of others makes me fearful of it. No one, I see, falls sick so often and takes so long to recover as those who are enthralled by the rules of medicine. Their very health is weakened and injured by their diets and precautions. Doctors are not satisfied to deal with the sick; but they are forever meddling with the well, in order that no one shall escape from under their thumbs. I have been sick often enough to learn that I can endure any disease (and I have had a taste of all sorts) and get rid of it as nicely as anyone else, and without adding to it the vileness of their prescriptions. . . .

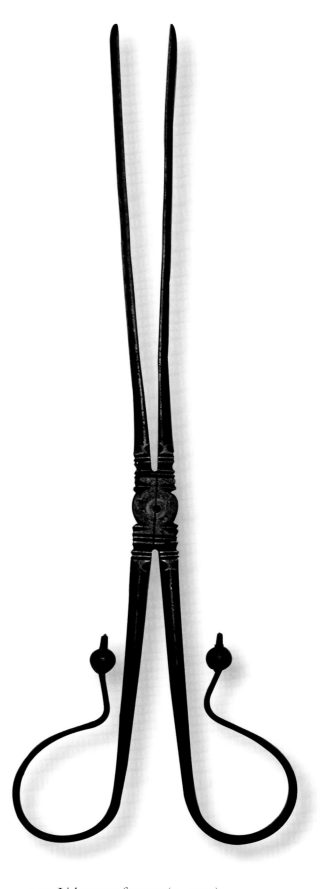

226. Lithotomy forceps (ca. 1540)

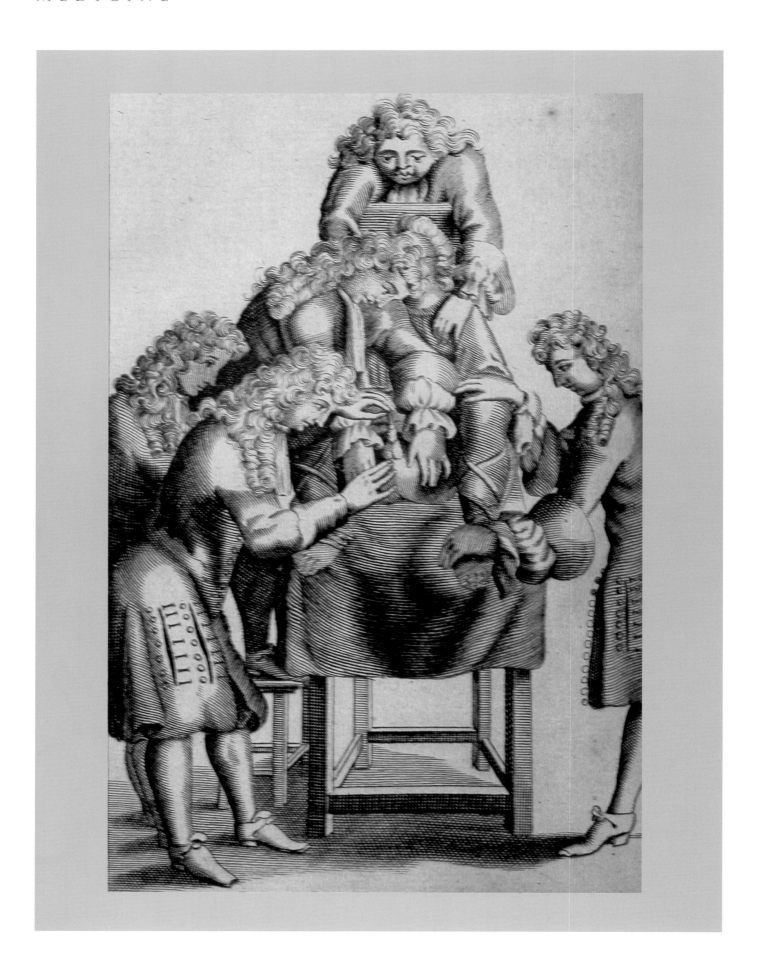

Doctors have a clever way of turning everything to their advantage. Whenever nature, luck, or anything else benefits our health, they lay it to their medicine. When things go badly they disown all responsibility and throw the blame on their patient. . . .

How often we see one physician impute the death of a patient to the medicine of another physician! Yet how, God knows, shall a doctor discover the true symptoms of a disease when each is capable of an endless variety? How many controversies have raged between them on the significance of the urine? For my part, I would prefer to trust a physician who has himself suffered the malady he would treat. The others describe diseases as their town-criers do a dog or horse—such color, height, and ears. But bring the beast to him, and he can't recognize it.

In my own sickness I have never found three doctors of the same opinion. Aperients, I am advised, are proper for a man afflicted with the stone—by dilating the vessels they help discharge the viscous matter out of which the gravel is formed. Again, aperients are dangerous, because, by dilating the vessels, they help the formative matter to reach the kidneys which naturally seize and retain it.

It is good, they say, to urinate frequently, for this prevents the gravel from settling in the bladder and coagulating into a stone. But frequent urinations are bad, because the deposits cannot be voided without grave violence to the tissues. It is good to have frequent intercourse with women, for that opens the passages; and it is bad, because it inflames, tires, and weakens the kidneys. Hot baths are good because they relax the parts, and they are bad because they help bake and harden the gravel. Because the doctors were afraid of stopping a dysentery lest they put the patient in a fever, they killed me a friend who was worth more than the whole of them together.

Thus they juggle and prate at our expense. They can't furnish me one argument than I'll not find a contrary of equal force. . . .

In short, I honor physicians not for their services, but for themselves. I have known many a good man among them, and most worthy of affection. I do not attack them, but their art. Nor do I blame them for taking advantage of our folly, for most men do as much. Many professions, both of greater and lesser dignity, live on gulling the public.

When I am sick, I send for them if they are near at hand, merely to have their company; and I pay them as others do. I give them leave to order me to keep myself warm, for I like to do it anyway. I let them recommend leeks or lettuce for my soup,

227. Opposite. Surgical treatment of kidney stones in *A Compleat Treatise of the Stone and Gravel* (1710) by John Greenfield, MD

put me on white wine or claret, or anything else that is indifferent to my taste and habits.

I know right well that I am not coddling them in this, for to them bitterness and strangeness is the very essence of a remedy. A neighbor of mine takes wine as an effective medicine for fever. Why? Because he abominates it.

Yet how many doctors do we see who, like myself, despise taking medicine, who live on a liberal diet and quite contrary to the rules they prescribe to their patients? What is this but sheer abuse of our simplicity!

It is the fear of pain and death, impatience at being ill, and reckless search for cures, which blind us. It is pure cowardice that makes us so gullible. Yet most men do not so much believe in doctors as submit and consent to them.

De Montaigne joined what was a legion of authors disenchanted with the medical profession. In the seventeenth century, Francis Quaries wrote the following in *Hieroglyphics of the Life of Man*:

Physicians, of all men, are most happy:
Whatever good success soever they have, the world proclaimeth
And what faults they commit, the earth covereth.

Of Bladder Stones and Nursery Rhymes

The recommended technique for the removal of stones remained controversial for hundreds of years. A midline perineal incision was popular, though the mortality was high, the pain almost unbearable, and the postoperative complications, especially fistula-in-ano, were common. William Cheselden (1688–1752), one of the leading surgeons of the eighteenth century, popularized the "high," or suprapubic approach that allowed him to remove a stone within sixty seconds. Unfortunately, bleeding remained a significant complication until a vagabond physician dramatically changed the prognosis for this condition with his clever innovation.

Jacques De Beaulieu (1651–1714) was the apprentice of an Italian stonecutter, and called himself "Frère Jacques" in order to provide himself with some safety during his travels about the countryside. The popular nursery rhyme was actually based on the life of this traveling surgeon: "Frère Jacques, Frère Jacques, dormez vous? dormez vous? . . ." or

Are you sleeping, are you sleeping,
Brother John, Brother John?

Ring the bell for matins,
Ring the bell for matins,
Ding, dang, dong,
Ding, dang, dong.

Frère Jacques took his examination for a license to operate at the Hôtel Dieu Hospital, though failed because he had not preoperatively bled and purged his patient. Many criticized the manner in which Jacques performed his lithotomies, including the famous Benjamin Bell in *A System of Surgery* (1746):

> The original invention of the lateral operation is due to a French Ecclesiastic, commonly known by the name of Frère Jacques. This operator first appeared at Paris in the year 1697, when, by the successful event of a few cases, he was desired to operate upon a great number. But it soon appeared to practitioners of discernment, that the fame he has acquired would not probably be of long duration. For with a very imperfect knowledge of the anatomy of the parts concerned in the operation, a bad assortment of instruments, and a total neglect of his patients after the operation, it was scarcely possible that much success could result from his method.
>
> In consequence of this unpardonable neglect, and by frequently cutting parts in the course of the operation which he ought to have avoided, a great proportion of those on whom he operated died; no less, we are informed, than twenty-five of sixty. Hence Jacques soon fell into disrepute; and although he afterwards made many improvements in his method of operating, particularly in using a grooved staff instead of a solid one, and in being more attentive to the subsequent management of his patients, yet his reputation in Paris never again gained ground; nor do we find that his method was ever attended with much success, either in Holland, or in the various parts of Germany where he afterwards practised.

Jacques was temporarily restricted from operating, though he was later reinstated after further modifying his lithotomy procedure. He developed a new technique called a lateral cystotomy, entering the bladder by way of a lateral perineal incision. In 1703, it so happened that the wealthy Marechal de Lorges became the victim of a painful stone and solicited Jacques' help because of the success of his new technique. In order to be certain that the new operative procedure was safe, de Lorges invited twenty-two patients with a similar problem to his mansion for the removal of their stones. Following Jacques' successful surgery on all, de Lorges consented to have the procedure done on himself. It did not go well, and the aristocrat died. Jacques de Beaulieu spent the rest of his life traveling all over Europe removing kidney stones, while the famous surgeon Dr. William Cheselden adopted his technique and reduced the operative mortality for lithotomy to an astounding ten percent.

Surgical sets specifically manufactured for lithotomy became quite ornate and expansive by the end of the nineteenth century when the safety and comfort of this procedure became bearable (figures 228–231).

EARLY UROLOGIC SURGERY

Urologic surgery prior to the nineteenth century was fairly brutal, and anecdotal evidence was relied upon since there were no controlled studies to determine the true efficacy of any of the procedures performed. Modern surgery for hydrocele is relatively safe and painless, though that was not always the case, as seen in *The Chirurgical Works of Percival Pott* (1778):

A poor man was brought from the neighbourhood of Rosemary-lane, to St. Bartholomew's Hospital.

228. Use of the bow Civiale lithotriptor in *Traité complet d'anatomie de l'homme,* 2nd ed. (1866–1871) by J.M. Bourgery, Claude Bernard, and N.H. Jacob

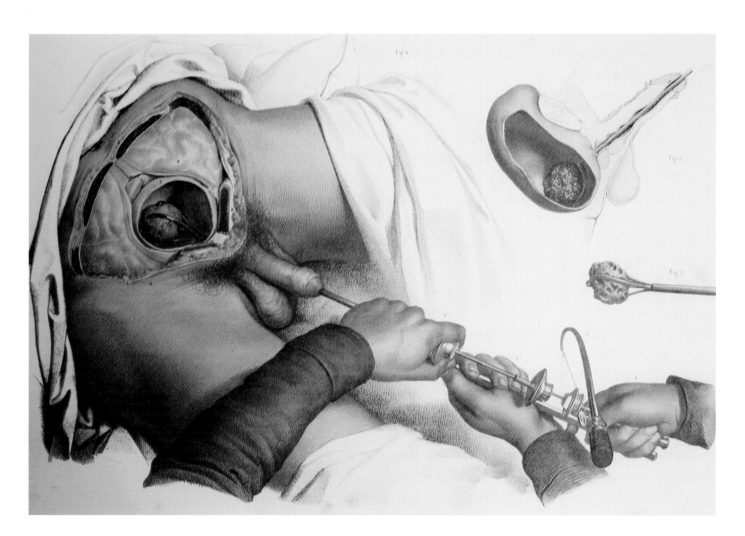

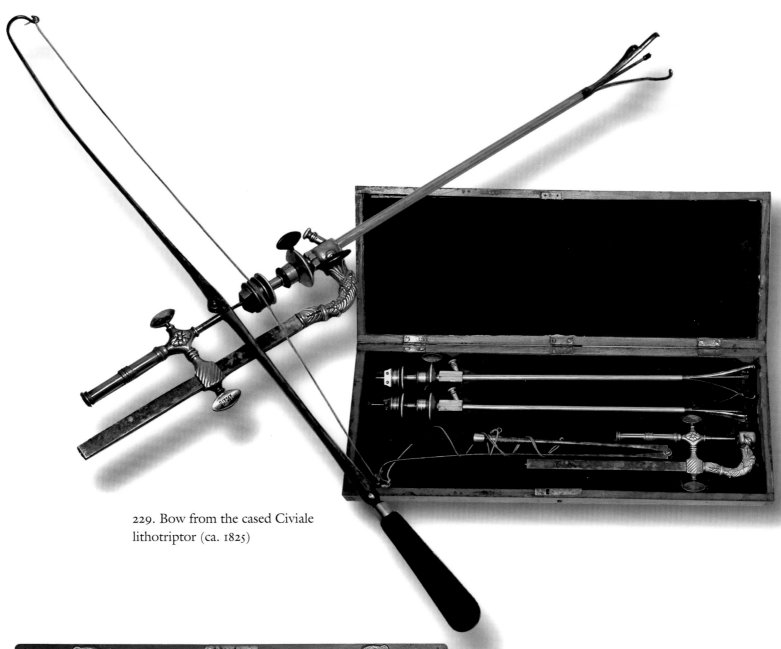

229. Bow from the cased Civiale
lithotriptor (ca. 1825)

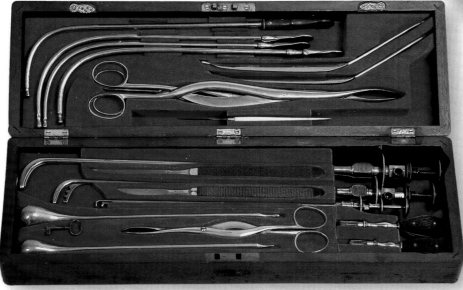

230. Above. Cased bow Civiale
lithotriptor (ca. 1825) by Samson

231. Left. Cased lithotomy set (ca.
1840) by George Tiemann containing
urinary catheters, gorgets, stone forceps, and Ferguson's lithotrites for
crushing stones

His scrotum was of prodigious size; very hard excessively inflamed quite up to his groin; it was of a dusky red colour; extremely painful to the touch; and in one part seemed inclined to sphacelate; the spermatic process also was considerably thickened. He had a hard, full, rapid pulse; a hot skin, a flushed countenance, great thirst; and complained of a most excruciating pain in his back.

The account he gave was, that he had for some years, been troubled with a swelling on the right side of his scrotum, which some of the surgeons of St. Thomas's Hospital had told him was a water-rupture, and would have tapped: that he had also applied to several rupture-doctors, each of whom had sold him a bandage, and some of them had pretended to cure him by medicines and applications: that finding no relief from any of these, he had a few days before given an itinerant stage-quack three guineas to cure him. That this operator laid him on his back, on a couch, and lifting up the tumor, thrust an instrument into it. That no discharge followed but blood. That it bled for near a quarter of an hour, and then stopped upon his fainting away. That from the time of this operation (which was two days) he had been in extreme pain; and, that his operator, not coming to take any care of him, his friends had brought him to the hospital. He was immediately bled, had a glyster injected, and the scrotum was enveloped in a soft, warm, poultice, and tied up in a bag truss. When he had passed a stool, I ordered him a grain of extract. thebaic. to be taken immediately and repeated again at the distance of six or eight hours. Next day he was much the same in every respect; his pain was excessive, particularly in his back, and he had not closed his eyes. I bled him again freely, (he had two stools in the night) and gave him two grains of opium, and direction to repeat one grain every six hours until he got ease and sleep. His scrotum was well fomented, and the cataplasm continued. Two days more were spent in this manner, before we obtained any remission of the symptoms; when that was done, I pierced the anterior part of the tumor, and drew off more than a pint of bloody serum. The testicle now appeared very much inlarged, and hardened; but, by persisting in the antiphlogistic method, he at length got well.

Here Pott presents an example of surgery for venereal disease:

A poor labouring man in Essex, got venereal hernia humoralis. As his daily work would not permit him to take proper care of himself, it was a considerable while before he had got rid of his inflammation symptoms; and when he had so done, a part of the testicle and the whole epididymis were left hard, and rather too large. In getting over a high style he missed his footstep, and struck his scrotum with violence against the upper rail: the blow gave him excessive pain for some minutes; but that soon ceased, and he went on with his day's work. Next day his testicle appeared swelled, and was painful, to the touch; but as the man had no subsistence but from is labour, he was obliged to follow it. At the end of a week, he was so much worse that he could go out no longer; and making his case known to some gentlemen, who used to employ him, a neighbouring practitioner was desired to visit him. A fluctuation being felt, it was supposed to be matter; and a warm adhesive plaster was applied to forward it. In a few days an opening was made for discharge of the supposed *pus*, but nothing followed except a very small quantity of bloody serum. The smallness of the quantity, and the nature of the fluid, joined to the very small subsidence of the tumor, induced the surgeon to think he had not gone deep enough: and to thrust a lancet farther in: this was attended with acute pain, and followed by a copious haemor-rhage, which was not easily restrained; or, to speak more properly, did not soon cease. Inflammation, pain, tumefaction, &c. followed this method of proceeding; and at the end of the week, the man was brought to St. Bartholomew's Hospital.

Upon mere sight of the part, I should have supposed the case to have been a schirrhus of the malignant kind: the testicle, or scrotum, was large, hard, unequal, of a deep red dusky colour, with distended veins, and so painful that it could not bear the slightest touch; and the spermatic process was far from being in a natural or a healthy state. The man complained of constant pain in his back, the wound discharged a bloody, offensive gleet and long pain, and want of rest, had given him a very diseased aspect.

Nothing but clear, and circumstantial account, which both the man, and the surgeon who had attended him (and who came with him to the hospital) gave, could have induced me to have thought the case to be any other than what I have just mentioned; but they were so positive, and so consistent, that I thought myself obliged to regard what they said, and to act accordingly.

By phlebotomy, evacuations, anodynes, rest, a low regimen, and the general antiphlogistic method pursued vigorously, and long, he got cure.

THE MOVEABLE KIDNEY

By the beginning of the nineteenth century, the understanding of human anatomy was fairly clear, though physicians still struggled at times to correlate anatomy with clinical disease. A malpositioned kidney was called *ren mobilis,* or moveable kidney, and, according to C.W. Suckling,

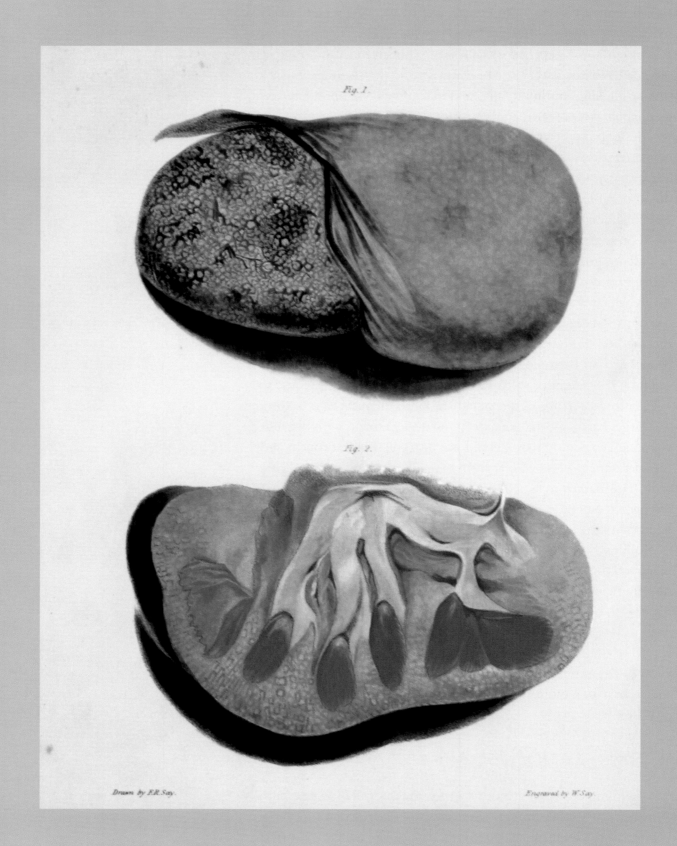

Fig. 1.

Fig. 2.

Drawn by F.R.Say.

Engraved by W.Say.

MD, MRCP, in 1905, it was felt to be "a cause of insanity, headache, neurasthenia, insomnia, mental failure, and other disorders of the nervous system, a cause also of debilitation of the stomach." The cure was surgical and involved nephropexy, or internal fixation.

Sir William Osler was one of the most prominent physicians of all time. He took issue with Suckling's conclusion in his landmark textbook of medicine regarding ren mobilis: "In a large majority of cases there are no symptoms, and if detected accidentally it is well not to let the patient know of its presence." Suckling responded acerbically in his text, "I am sure that had Professor Osler made a special study, or read the up-to-date literature on the subject, or even had some of the cases and results which I am willing to demonstrate to him at any time, he would never have published that paragraph." Controlled studies later that century vindicated Osler and made Suckling's position ludicrous.

BRIGHT'S DISEASE

Renal failure remained a uniformly fatal condition until the middle of the twentieth century when dialysis became an option. The first to recognize the association between "dropsy" (fluid retention), albuminuria, elevated urea, and pathologic changes in the kidney was a British physician at Guy's Hospital, Dr. Richard Bright (1789–1858), after whom "Bright's Disease" was named (figure 232). The chemical determination of albumin in urine as an aid in making the diagnosis of renal disease was, in fact, one of the first instances in which physicians were able to employ the basic sciences in their care of patients. Clinicians, however, resisted the use of chemical analysis and, according to the *Lancet* (1842), "the information of the medical profession, generally, on matters of natural science, is very little greater than that of the people at large. This is an extremely humiliating fact."

Bright's classic description of the symptoms and progression of kidney failure appeared in his *Guy's Hospital Reports, Cases and Observations* (1836):

The first indication of the tendency to this disease is often haematuria, of a more or less decided character: this may originate from various causes, and yet may give evidence of the same tendency: scarlatina has apparently laid the foundation for the future mischief: . . . Intemperance seems its most usual source; and exposure to cold the most common cause of its development and aggravation. . . .

The history of this disease, and its symptoms, is nearly as follows:

A child, or an adult, is affected with scarlatina, or some other

232. Hand-colored plate of the pathologic specimen of John King, first case in *Reports of Medical Cases* (1827) by Richard Bright, MD

acute disease; or has indulged in the intemperate use of ardent spirits for a series of months or years: he is exposed to some casual cause or habitual source of suppressed perspiration: he finds the secretion of his urine greatly increased, or he discovers that it is tinged with blood; or, without having made any such observation, he awakes in the morning with his face swollen, or his ankles puffy, or his hands oedematous. If he happen, in this condition, to fall under the care of a practitioner who suspects the nature of his disease, it is found, that already his urine contains a notable quantity of albumin: his pulse is full and hard, his skin dry, he has often headache, and sometimes a sense of weight or pains across the loins. . . . After a time, the healthy colour of the countenance fades, a sense of weakness or pain in the loins increases; headaches, often accompanied by vomiting, add greatly to the general want for comfort; and a sense of lassitude, of weariness, and of depression, gradually steal over the bodily and mental frame. Again, the assistance of medicine is sought. If the nature of the disease is suspected, the urine is carefully tested; and found, in almost every trial, to contain albumin, while the quantity of urea is gradually diminishing. . . . If, in the attempt to give relief to the oppression of the system, blood is drawn, it is often buffed, or the serum is milky and opaque; and nice analysis will frequently detect a great deficiency of albumin, and sometimes manifest indications of the presence of urea. The swelling increases and decreases; the mind grows cheerful, or is sad; the secretions of the kidney or the skin are augmented or diminished, sometimes in alternate ratio, sometimes without apparent relation . . . the swelling increases, the urine becomes scanty, the powers of life seem to yield, the lungs become oedematous, and, in a state of asphyxia or coma, he sinks into the grave; or a sudden effusion of serum into the glottis closes the passages of the air, and brings on a more sudden dissolution. Should he, however, have resumed the avocations of life, he is usually subject to constant recurrence of his symptoms; or again, almost dismissing the recollection of his ailment, he is suddenly seized with an acute attack of pericarditis, or with a still more acute attack of peritonitis, which, without any renewed warning, deprives him, in eight and forty hours, of his life. Should he escape this danger likewise, other perils await him; his headaches have been observed to become more frequent; his stomach more deranged; his vision indistinct; his hearing depraved: he is suddenly seized with a convulsive fit, and becomes blind. He struggles through the attack; but again and again it returns; and before a day or a week has elapsed, worn out by convulsions, or overwhelmed by coma, the painful history of this disease is closed.

Renal replacement therapy became a possibility in 1861 when Thomas Graham, a professor of chemistry at Anderson's University in Glasgow, extracted urea from urine, and first used the term *dialysis*. In 1913, John Abel utilized the anticoagulant hirudin produced by leeches obtained from Parisian barbers to perform the first dialysis on an animal. With great foresight, he wrote, "this apparatus might be applied to human beings suffering from certain toxic states, especially if due to kidney damage, in the hope of tiding a patient over a dangerous chemical emergency." Credit for the first human dialysis goes to German George Haas in 1924 when he performed a fifteen-minute dialysis on a patient with kidney failure "because this was a condition against which the doctor stands otherwise powerless." The rotating drum dialysis machine of Willem J. Kolff in 1943 was the first effective replacement for kidney failure, and his innovation has saved the lives of millions. It was only eleven years later on December 23, 1954 that Joseph E. Murray, MD performed the first successful kidney (and organ) transplant at the Peter Bent Brigham Hospital in Boston, Massachusetts.

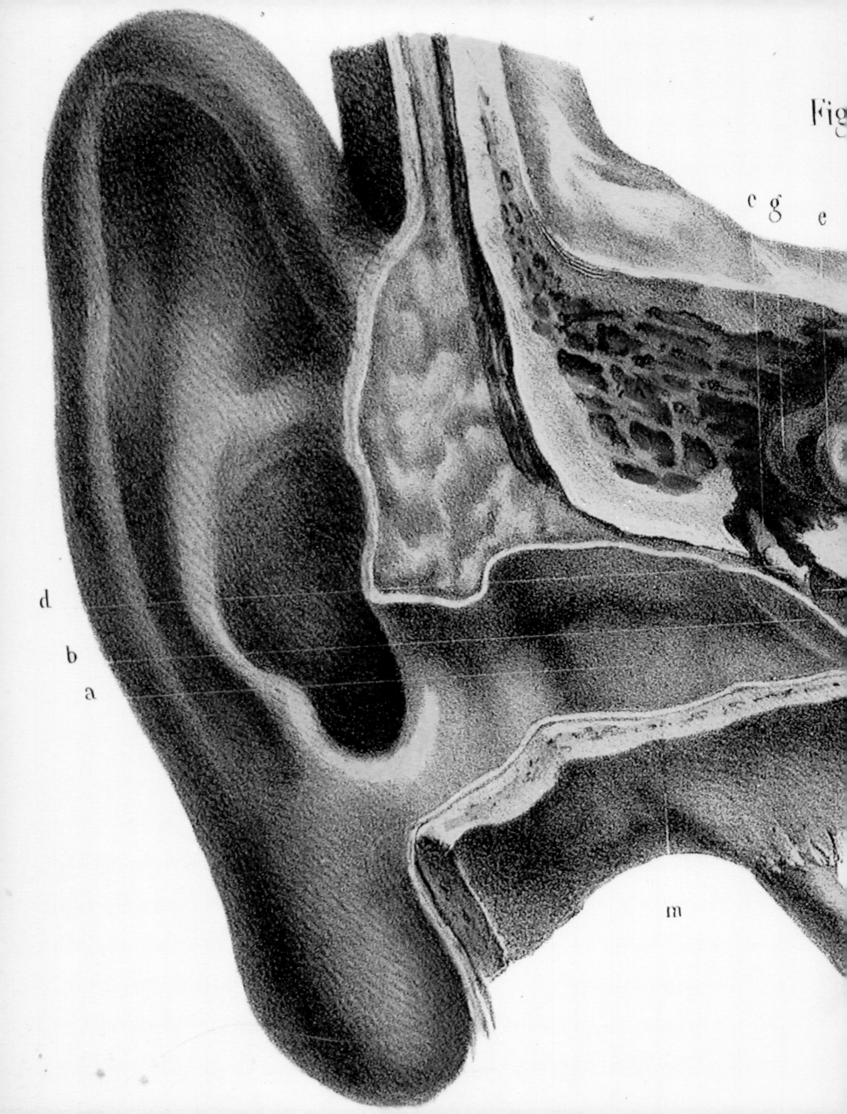

Fig.

c g   e

d

b

a

m

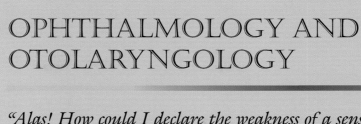

OPHTHALMOLOGY AND OTOLARYNGOLOGY

"Alas! How could I declare the weakness of a sense which in me ought to be more acute than in others..."

Ludwig van Beethoven (1802)

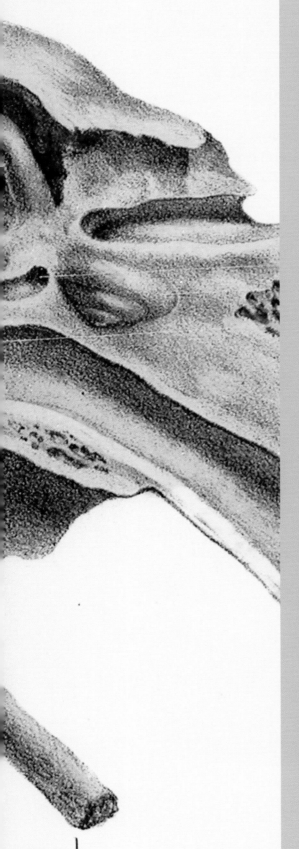

External and internal ear in *Traité complet d'anatomie de l'homme,* 2nd ed. (1866–1871) by J.M. Bourgery, Claude Bernard, and N.H. Jacob

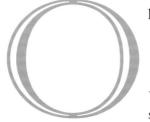

Ophthalmology and otolaryngology are fairly modern medical specialties, though physicians have always been faced with the challenge of treating patients with disorders of the head and neck. Early therapy for the loss of vision and hearing was largely ineffective, and barber-surgeons did their best to repair the consequences of trauma in battle. It was not until the middle of the nineteenth century and the discoveries of anesthesia and aseptic technique that physicians began to take a special interest in this area of the body since they could then finally offer their patients a reasonably painless experience with some hope of survival. Additionally, an exploding population in the United States offered manufacturers economic incentives that encouraged the development of highly specialized instruments, thus at last giving physicians an opportunity to perform new surgical procedures related to disorders of the eyes, ears, nose, and throat.

OPHTHALMOLOGY

Aside from very crude topical palliative therapy, there was little that could be done to treat diseases affecting the eyes until recently. A great

233. Facial anatomy in *Traité complet d'anatomie de l'homme,* 2nd ed. (1866–1871) by J.M. Bourgery, Claude Bernard, and N.H. Jacob

234. Opposite. Color mezzotint of the Circle of Willis in *Exposition anatomique des organs des sens . . .* (1775) by Jacques Fabien Gautier D'Agoty

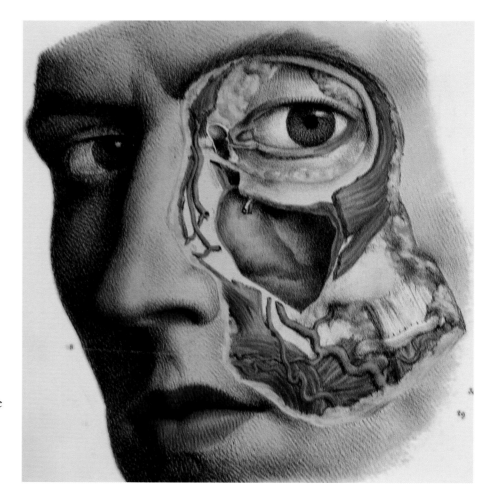

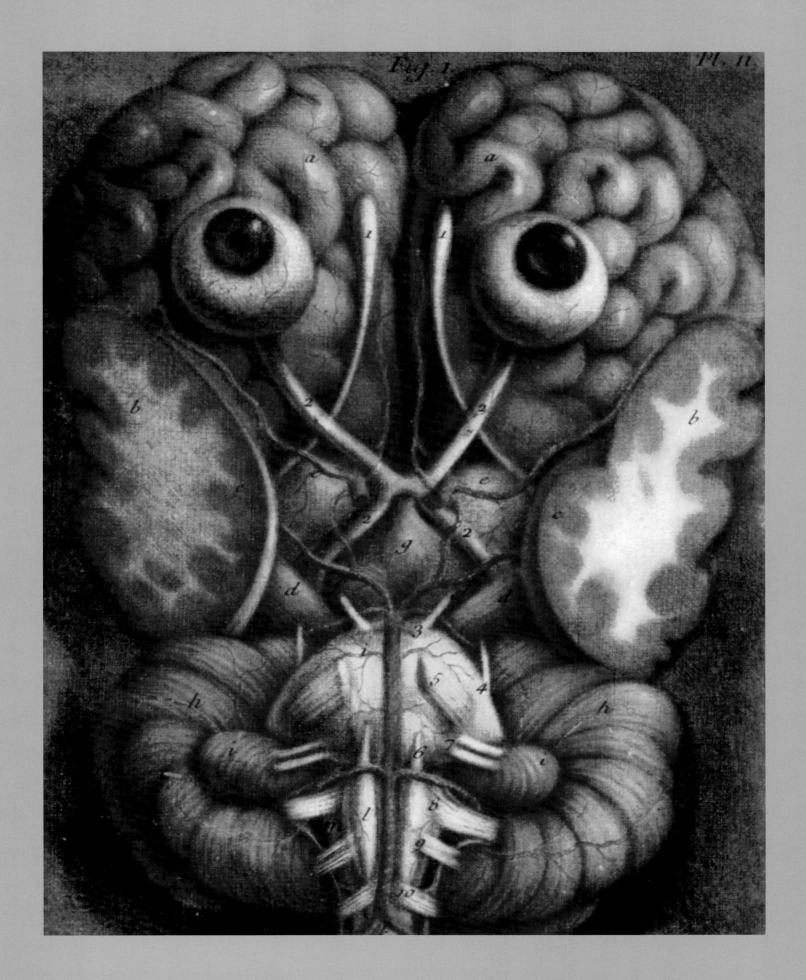

Fig. 1.

Pl. II.

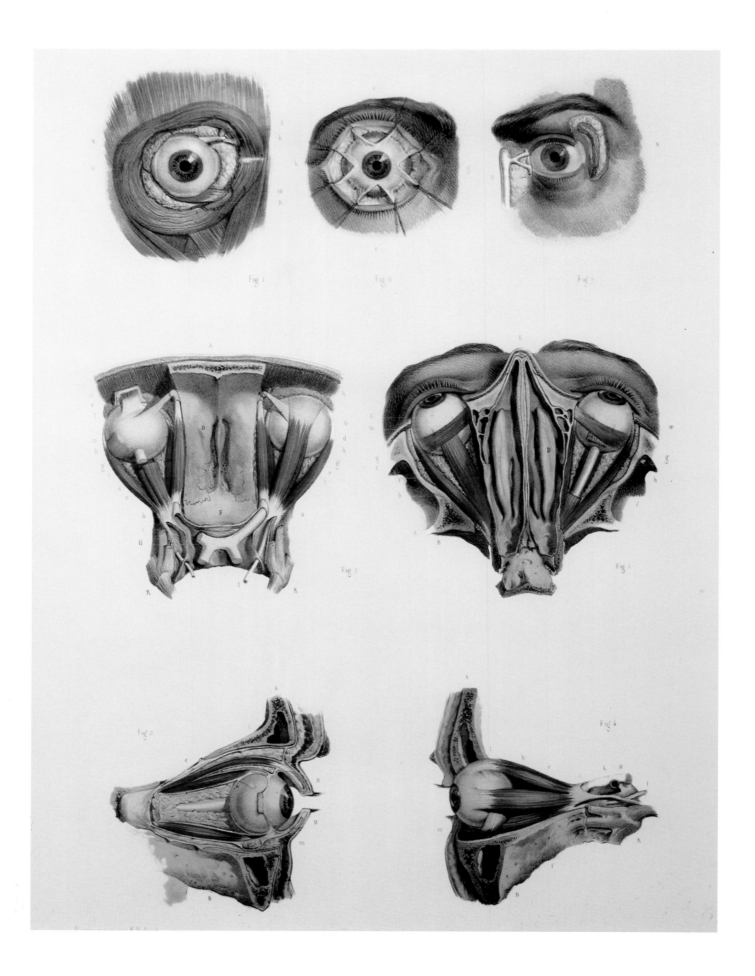

deal was left to home remedies and supernatural cures in early recorded history since malpractice penalties, as outlined in the Code of Hammurabi, provided a significant disincentive to those who considered new and innovative forms of therapy. For example, a physician could have both of his hands cut off if his surgery led to a loss of sight or worse the loss of life. The treatment of diseases affecting the eye remained crude for thousands of years since whatever advancements were made in the basic sciences of anatomy (figures 233–235) and physiology were of little consequence without an understanding or application of the scientific method. Acceptance finally came in the latter part of the nineteenth century, and, with the discovery of anesthesia and aseptic techniques, ophthalmology was quickly propelled into the "modern era."

Cataract Surgery

The only procedure routinely performed on the eye in early recorded history was the removal of cataracts, popular in sixth-century India and continued by barber-surgeons as they traveled throughout Europe. This minor surgery was widespread, though unfortunately many patients suffered at the hands of incompetent physicians, including composers George Frederic Handel who lost his eyesight and Johann Sebastian Bach who lost his life to British quack oculist John Taylor. Patients and physicians feared surgical intervention, so there was never a shortage of ideas for the medical treatment of cataracts. The following is an example by Nicholas Culpeper in his *School of Physick* (1659): "The head of a Cat that is all black burned in a new pot or crucible, and made into fine ashes, and a little of it blown with a quill into an eye that hath a web or pearl growing before it, three times a day, is a most sovereign remedy."

Medical therapy having failed, the next step was surgical intervention with the popular couching needle as described by Laurence Heister in his *A General System of Surgery* (1743) (figures 236–239):

> But first it may be proper for us to admonish Surgeons to make themselves better acquainted with the Operation for couching Cataracts, and to be more conversant in the Practice thereof, and not to leave the Business to Quacks and itinerant Pretenders, as we have seen it done but too much of late. If the Practice is, as we see often, well enough executed by these boasting Pretenders, what might we not expect from the Hands of the more prudent and regular Surgeon, were he to engage more in the Practice, which is, in reality, attended with less Danger or Hazard than the common Operation of Phlebotomy; for in couching a Cataract, you run no risque of wounding a Nerve, Tendon, or Artery, as you do in opening a Vein. But lest our Reader should

235. Opposite. Muscles of the eye in *Traité complet d'anatomie de l'homme,* 2nd ed. (1866–1871) by J.M. Bourgery, Claude Bernard, and N.H. Jacob

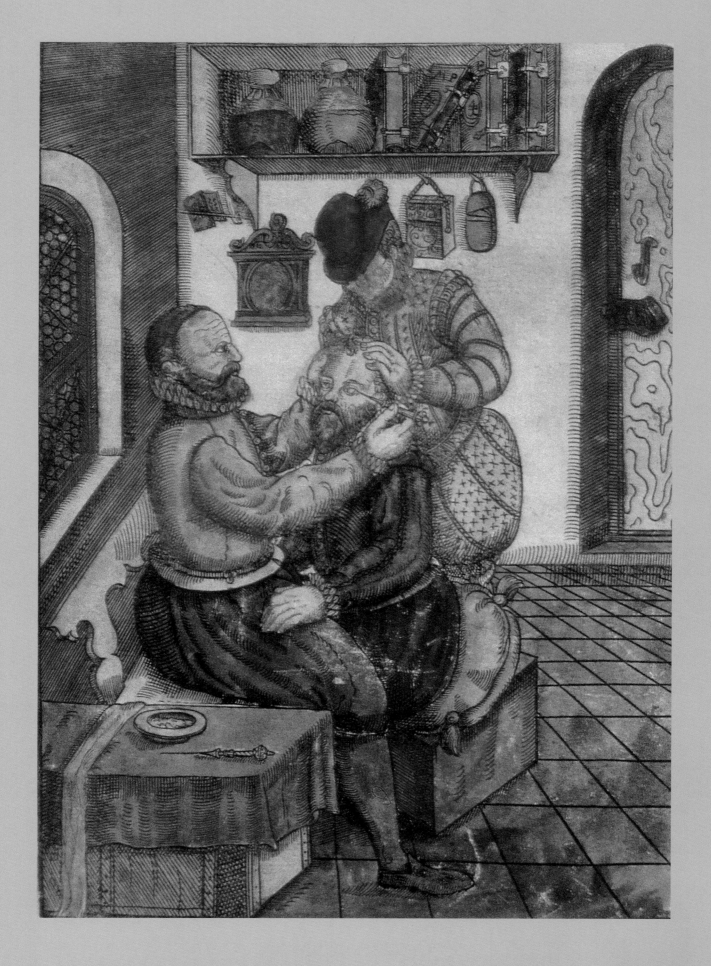

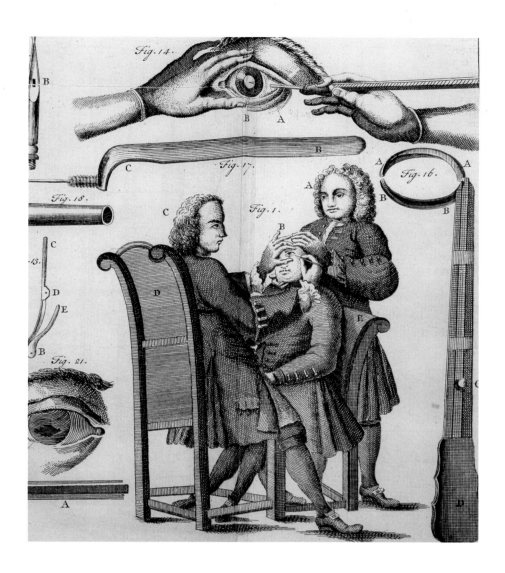

think we are recommending the Operation, for its Easiness, to the Practice of every one, though ever so unskillful, we shall here enumerate the several necessary Qualifications for an Oculist, whom we may venture to trust in the Cure of this Disorder. I. He must be very well versed in the anatomical Structure, and in the Functions of the several constituent Parts of the Eye, that he may avoid injuring any of them ignorantly. 2. He must be well acquainted with the best Instruments and Methods of operating, to be learned from a frequent and close Attention to the Practice of some expert Master. 3. His Mind must be intrepid, his Hand steady, and his Eye sharp and quick-sighted. 4. He should be equally ready with his left as with his right Hand; that he may couch the left Eye with his right Hand, and the right Eye with his left Hand. 5. He must have made himself previously expert in the Practice, by repeated Trials upon the Eyes of Brutes, and of dead Men, before he ventures to couch the Eyes of the Living.

But, in order to the more successful and easy Performance of

236. Opposite. Cataract surgery in *Das ist Augendienst* (1583) by Georg Bartisch

237. Above. Cataract surgery in *A General System of Surgery* (1743) by Laurence Heister

238. Opposite. Cataract surgery in *Traité complet d'anatomie de l'homme*, 2nd ed. (1866–1871) by J.M. Bourgery, Claude Bernard, and N.H. Jacob

this Operation, it will be previously necessary for the Surgeon to appoint the most convenient Time, and to prepare his Patient in the best manner, by a proper Regimen and Medicines. With regard to the first, a Season should be chose, in which the Air is pretty temperature as to Heat and cold as in Spring and Autumn. The Day appointed for the Operation should especially be serene and clear, and the Hour generally in the Forenoon; not but the Afternoon will do very well, and may be in some Cases preferable for weak and timorous Patients, who are usually in better Spirits after a moderate Dinner. The Apartment for couching the Patient in will be fitter as it lighter, provided the Sun does not shine in upon you; for so strong a Light as the Sun's Rays will cause the Pupil to contract itself, so that you cannot have so large a View of the Parts and Instrument within the Eye. As for the Preparation of the Patient, he should not only observe a proper Regimen and Diet a few Days before the Operation, but he should also in that time take some alternative and evacuating Medicines, with the Use of Phlebotomy, to prevent the Eye from being molested by intense Pain, Inflammation, Suppuration, and perhaps a Loss of the whole, after the Operation has been performed. It may also be generally convenient to give the Patient a Clyster, if he has not eased himself lately: And, that his Courage may not fail him, the Operator should take care that he may have some Gravy-Soop, or other strengthening Suppings in the Morning, before he begins his Operation. Lastly, nothing can more conduce to the Patient's Recovery, and the Prevention of Accidents, after the Operation, than to procure him a sound Sleep afterwards by an Anodyne Draught of Emulsion, by which the Faculties both of his Body and Mind will be recruited, and the lately suppressed Cataract will not be apt to ascend again. . . .

There now remains but one more Prerequisite before the Surgeon enters on his Work, and that is, to fix and secure the Patient in the most convenient and advantageous Posture. . . . If the Patient can see either perfectly, or but in part with the Eye, which is not couched, it must be first covered or blindfolded with a Handkerchief, or Bandage, lest, by feeling the Instrument.

Approach, he should move his Eye, and disturb the Operation. Upon which account it may be also proper to admonish the Patient, that if his Eye should recover its Sight very suddenly in the Operation, as is not unfrequent he may not stir, or make any Exclamations of Joy till it is over, lest, by small

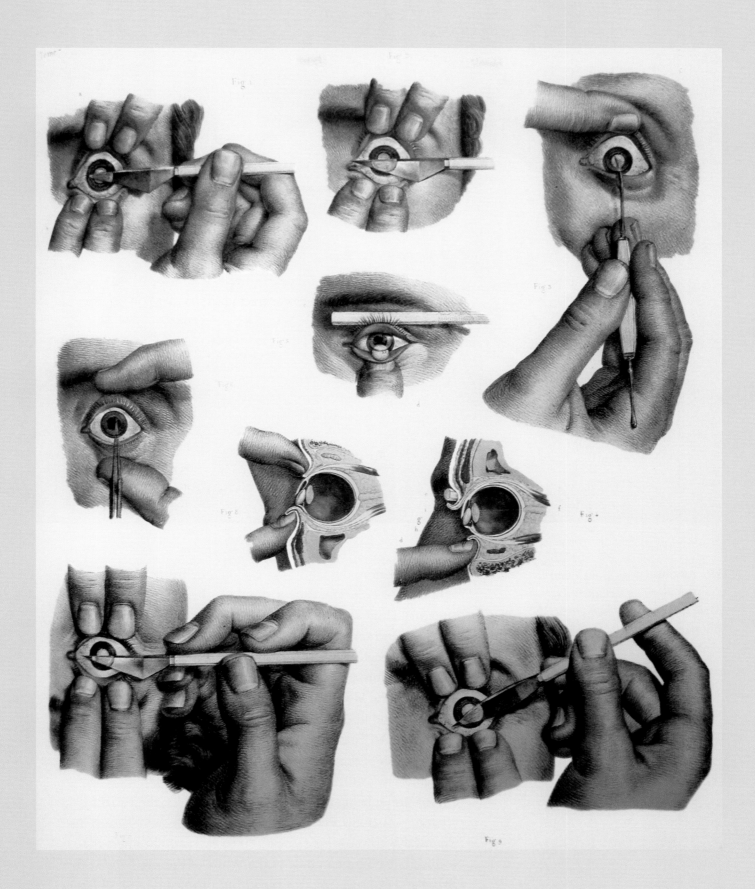

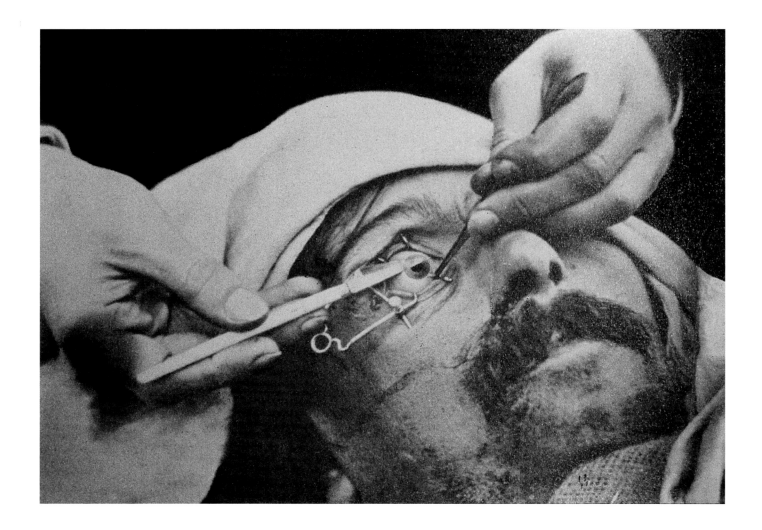

239. Albumin print from *Cataract Surgery: Teaching a Student How to Make a Superior Incision* (1870) by Edouard Meyer

irregular Motion, the whole Cure should be frustrated, and his Sight lost for ever. The Patient should fix his Hands on the Surgeon's Thighs, and his Legs also betwixt those of the Operator; and sometimes it may be proper for an Assistant to hold up his Feet, that he may not rise out of the Chair before the Operator is finished. Behind the Patient must stand the Assistant A, securing the Head with his left Hand on the Forehead, and his right Hand upon the Chin, which he must press close to his Breast, so as to hold the Head firm and steddy; because a very small Motion of the Head may cause perpetual Blindness, as we are assured by sad Experience. . . .

Every thing being thus prepared in Readiness, the Patient is ordered to open his Eye-lids as wide as possible, and to turn his Eye inwards towards his Nose . . . then he carefully enters the Needle almost in the middle of the White of the Eye betwixt the *Cornea* and external Angle of the Orbit, proceeding, not obliquely, but straight, through the Coates of the Eye over-against the Cataract, to avoid wounding the Blood-vessels. As soon as the

Needle is perceived to be through the Coats of the Eye, which may be known by your losing the Resistance, its Point is then inclined towards the Cataract which being entered by the End of your Instrument, you thereby endeavour to depress it gently below the Pupil to the Fundus of the Eye whether it be a Membrane or an Opacity in the crystaline Lens . . . if, upon elevating your Instrument again, the Cataract does not rise above the Pupil, your Operation is well performed; and therefore the Needle is now to be drawn out of the Eye in a straight Line as it entered. . . .

It is a common Practice with Mountebanks and Itinerant Oculasts, to hold up their two Fingers extended, or else a Glass of Wine, before the Patient's Eye, as soon as the couching Needle is extracted, calling out to know what the Object is, or of what Colour it appears, and if the Patient can distinguish, and answer rightly, they then conclude the Operation to have been well performed. But this is, by the more prudent Surgeons and Oculists, judged to be a pernicious Method, because by the Patient's straining his Eye too soon to view the Objects, the Cataract is often roused and elevated again. It is therefore much better to defend the Eye immediately after Couching with a Compress dipt in some Collyrium, and secured by a Handkerchief, that the *Retina* may not be injured by a too strong Action of the Light. It will be necessary to bind up both Eyes, though you couched but one, because if you leave the sound Eye uncovered, it will perhaps be looking at Objects, and will consequently draw or strain he diseased Eye in the same Direction, which may remove the Cataract, and cause it to ascend again, or else induce an Inflammation, or other bad Accidents. . . .

A few Hours after the Operation it will be convenient to bleed the Patient in proportion to his Strength and Fulness of Habit, to prevent an Inflammation in the wounded Eye, and to repeat the same, if necessary, with the Use of *Collyria* externally, and cooling Purges internally. 'Tis very remarkable, that the Patient is often troubled with a Vomiting an Hour or two after the Operation. . . . However, this Symptom of Vomiting is no good Presage, because the Patient's straining in this Action often causes the Cataract to ascend. In the Evening after the Operation you should order the Patient an anodyne Emulsion, to compose him to Rest, because Watchings and Restlessness very often occasion the Cataract to ascend again above the Pupil. The Diet and Regimen here must be ordered the same as we have directed in

Wounds and inflammatory Disorders. Lastly, if the Patient does not go to Stool freely without straining, it will be proper to help him with a Clyster; nor should he be permitted to disturb his Head by rising out of Bed for this Office, but, for the first few Days after the Operation, it will be more convenient to use a Bed-pan; all which Precautions are necessary, to prevent the lately depressed Cataract from being disturbed or raised again above the Pupil.

Always a Place for Bleeding

In the same text, Heister described the use of phlebotomy in order to "cleane the Eye, and abate its Inflammation." In the absence of adequate anesthesia, this was certainly a brutal procedure, greatly taxing the faith of any patient, as well as any physician practicing eye surgery at the time:

> To scarify the Patient's Eye, he must be first seated on his Chair or Bed in an advantageous Posture against the Light, with his Head secured from moving by an Assistant, after which the Operator presses his Thumb and Fore-finger on the Eye-lids, so as to elevate, or open, and turn them outward, that their interior red Surface may come into View, which may be done with most Ease in the lower Eye-lid. He now takes the scarifying

240. Above. Herman von Helmholtz's original ophthalmoscope (1850)

241. Below left. Late nineteenth-century Morton's Chain of Lenses ophthalmoscope by Maw, Son, and Thompson

242. Below right. Loring's ophthalmoscope by Luer (ca. 1880)

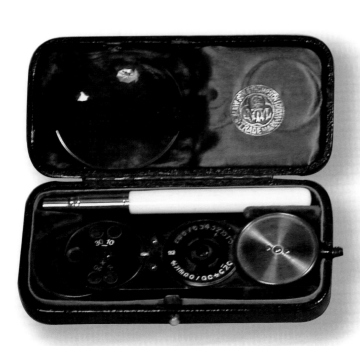

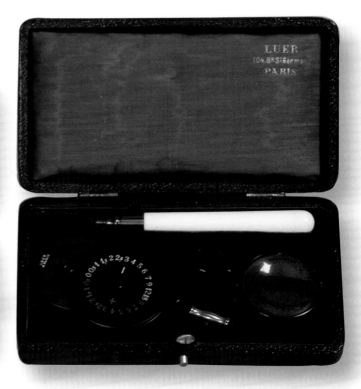

Instrument in the other Hand, and rubs it backward and forward with great Swiftness upon the internal Surface of the Lid, and upon the White of the Eye itself, if he thinks proper, and sometimes even upon the *Cornea*, moving from one Corner of the Eye to the other, so as to lacerate the small turgid Veins, and make them bleed plentifully. But this in general is an Operation much sooner learnt from Inspection, than a verbal Description.

An Explosion of Instrumentation

In 1850, Herman von Helmholtz (1821–1894) invented the ophthalmoscope, a device that enabled him to be the first to see the retina, and ophthalmology was on its way to becoming a specialized branch of medicine (figure 240). He described his landmark discovery in 1851:

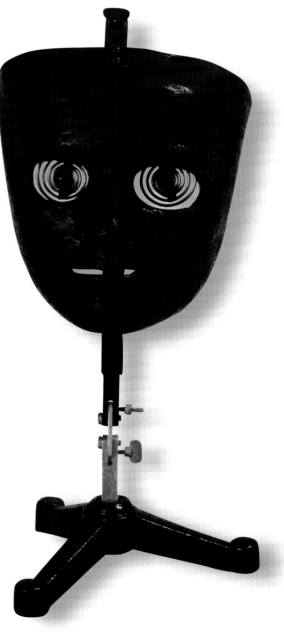

243. Ophthalmophantome by Luer (ca. 1870)

> I was endeavoring to explain to my pupils the emission of reflected light from the eye, a discovery made by Brücke, who would have invented the ophthalmoscope had he only asked himself how an optical image is formed by the light returning from the eye. In his research it was not necessary to ask it, but had he asked it, he was just the man to answer it as quickly as I did, and to invent the instrument. I turned the problem over and over to ascertain the simplest way in which to demonstrate the phenomenon to my students. It was also a reminiscence of my days of medical study, that ophthalmologists had great difficulty in dealing with certain cases of eye disease, then known as black cataract. The first model was constructed of pasteboard, eye lenses, and cover-glasses used in the microscopic work. It was at first so difficult to use that I doubt that I should have persevered unless I had felt that it must succeed; but in eight days I had the great joy of being the first who saw before him a living human retina.

This accomplishment was also a major breakthrough since by seeing the retina, von Helmholtz became the first ever to view the central nervous system of a living patient without surgical intervention. Over the next several decades, manufacturers further modified ophthalmoscopes for clinical use (figures 241, 242).

The complexity of surgery in treating diseases of the eye increased significantly throughout the nineteenth century, partly as a result of the discovery and use of the topical anesthetic properties of cocaine pioneered by ophthalmologist Carl Koller in 1884. Young physicians learned about surgery by practicing on pigs' eyes that were placed in surrealistic appearing ophthalmophantomes (figure 243), and surgical sets improved dramatically (figure 244). A great deal of morbidity resulted from the

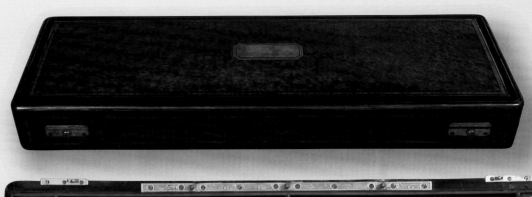

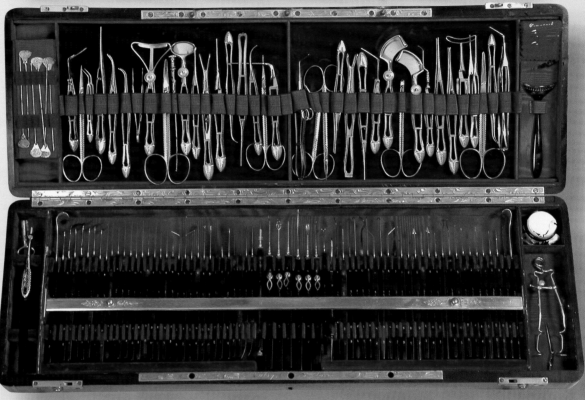

244. Exhibition ophthalmologic surgical set with polished steel, silver, gilt brass, and horn handled instruments in burl wood case by Aubry (ca. 1880)

245. Right. (Top) folding Chinese spectacles of brass and tortoiseshell with forehead rest (ribbons replaced) (ca. 1700), silver horn-rimmed Benjamin Martin type ("Martin's margins") with fish skin case (ca. 1770); (bottom) quizzer with case (ca. 1800) and silver folding lorgnette (ca. 1860)

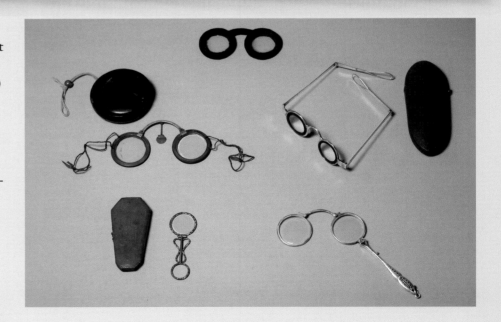

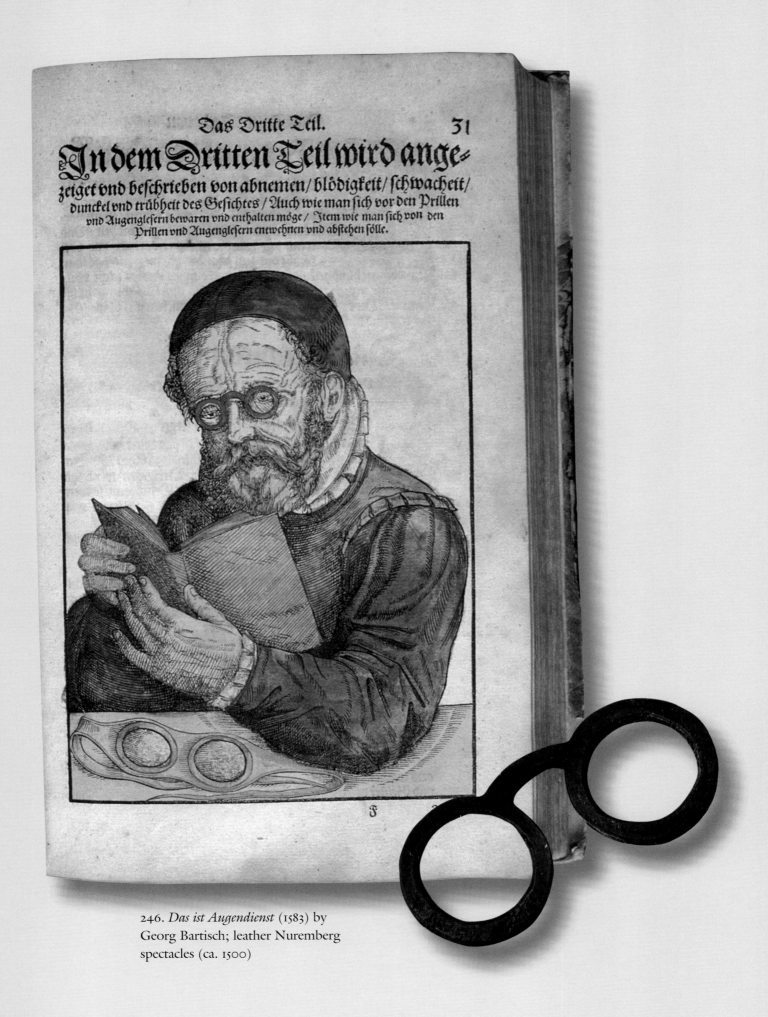

In dem Dritten Teil wird ange-
zeiget vnd beschrieben von abnemen/ blödigkeit/ schwacheit/
dunckel vnd trübheit des Gesichtes / Auch wie man sich vor den Prillen
vnd Augenglesern bewaren vnd enthalten möge / Item wie man sich von den
Prillen vnd Augenglesern entwehnen vnd abstehen sölle.

F

246. *Das ist Augendienst* (1583) by
Georg Bartisch; leather Nuremberg
spectacles (ca. 1500)

247. Cased set of trial lenses by Nachet and Fils (ca. 1880) distributed by James W. Queen and Co.

248. Mid to late nineteenth-century hand-painted glass artificial eyes: (bottom left) eye prosthesis resting on a French opalescent eye cup

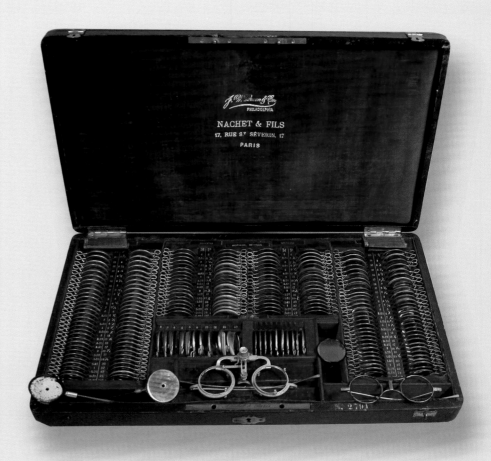

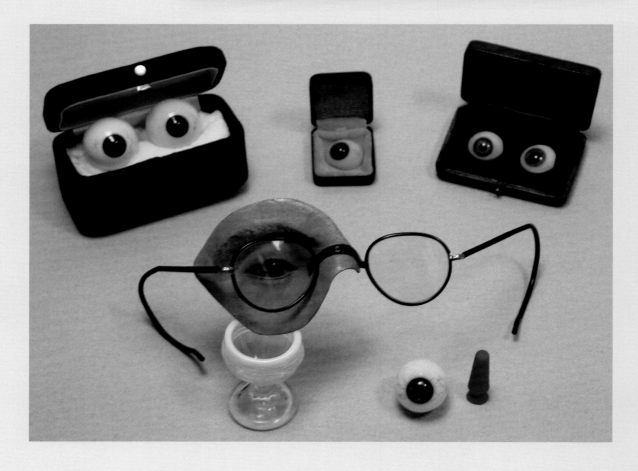

use of these instruments since they were made of materials that could not be adequately sterilized, and, in fact, the medical community had not yet unanimously accepted the principles of asepsis.

The specific origin of spectacles remains unclear, though the first reference to a device for the refraction of light was by the Roman philosopher and statesman Lucius Annaeus Seneca, the Younger (4 B.C.–A.D. 65), when he said that he had "read all the books in Rome" through a glass globe of water. The Chinese are generally given credit for the invention of eyeglasses, though they probably used the lenses to protect themselves from "evil forces" rather than for reading. The use of ground glass for reading probably was invented in Venice at the end of the seventeenth century, and, in 1768, Roger Bacon wrote in his *Opus Majus,* "If anyone examines letters or other minute objects through the medium of crystal or glass or other transparent substance, if it be shaped like the lesser segment of a sphere, with the convex side toward the eye, he will see the letters far better and they will seem larger to him. For this reason such an instrument is useful to all persons and those with weak eyes for they can see any letter, however small, if magnified enough." Early frames for eyeglasses were made of leather, iron, horn, and gold, and the demand for spectacles dramatically increased with the invention of moveable type and the printing press by Johannes Gutenberg (figures 245–247). He began work on his press in 1436 and was able to produce his famous Bible in 1455, which was, unfortunately, the same year that he went bankrupt. When a loss of vision resulted from injury, disease, or surgery, many types of prostheses were available by the end of the nineteenth century (figure 248).

OTOLARYNGOLOGY

Otolaryngology, or the study of diseases of the ear, nose, and throat, also became a recognized branch of medicine at the end of the nineteenth century with the discovery of anesthesia (figure 249). Battlefield medicine was heroic by any standard, and physicians have always been called upon to do their share of surgery on the head and neck. One example was recounted in the eleventh century by Arabic physician Albucasis in his *Altassif*: "For then, a man was wounded by an arrow at the angle of the eye and close to the root of the nose. I extracted it from the opposite side below the lobule of the ear. The man recovered without sustaining any complications on the part of the eye!" Further, "I extracted another from the throat of a Christian. It was an Arabian arrow with barbs. I incised over it, between the jugular veins: it had penetrated deeply into the throat; I operated with precaution and I succeeded in extracting it. The Christian was saved and recovered."

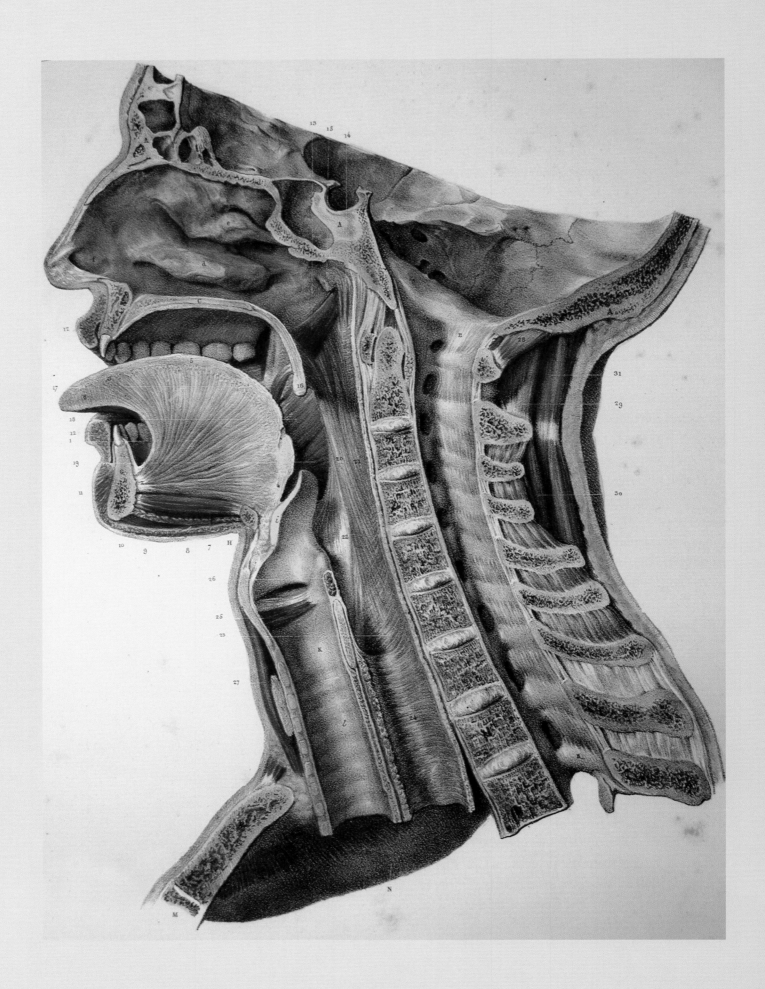

The Ear

Surgery on the ear in any meaningful way is only a recent phenomenon, and many remedies for disorders affecting that organ have been offered over the ages. For an earache, Nicholas Culpeper suggested the following in 1659: "If you fry Earth-worms in Goose-grease, and drop a drop or two of the Grease warm (being strained) in your ear, helps the pains thereof. I suppose you had best first slit them, and wash them in white wine."

Many rather bizarre therapeutic approaches regarding diseases of the inner ear were advanced during the nineteenth century, both patients and physicians suffering through medical conditions that might be easily treated today with either an antibiotic or a minor surgical procedure. The following case study is from *The Diseases of the Ear: Their Nature, Diagnosis, and Treatment* (1860) by Joseph Toynbee, FRS:

Case III. *Acute inflammation of the mucous membrane of the tympanum; ulceration of the membrana tympani; paralysis of the portio dura nerve; cure.*—EI, aged 23, was admitted under my care, at the St. George's and St. James's Dispensary. On February 28th, 1843.

History.—He stated that three months previously he was suddenly seized with a violent attack of pain in the right ear, which extended over the side of the head. After the pain had lasted for about twenty-four hours, he experienced a sensation of something bursting in the ear, followed by an abundant thick and offensive-smelling discharge. During the attack of pain he had much giddiness, lost the use of the right side of the face, and could not shut his right eye, while the mouth was drawn to the left side. On *examination*, an orifice was observed in the right membrana tympani; the mucous membrane of the tympanum was red and thick, and poured out a mucous discharge. He was ordered to apply a blister behind the ear, and became better, having no return of the pain till March 11th, when it suddenly reappeared in great violence, accompanied by a singing and by sensations of pumping and throbbing in the ear. These symptoms were much aggravated by coughing. The discharge was abundant, and the mucous membrane of the tympanum very red. Leeches were applied below the ear, which was often syringed with warm water; and after the pain was somewhat subdued, a blister was applied behind the ear. Calomel and opium were administered until the gums were rendered tender. The symptoms gradually subsided. . . .

249. Saggital section of the neck in *Traité complet d'anatomie de l'homme*, 2nd ed. (1866–1871) by J.M. Bourgery, Claude Bernard, and N.H. Jacob

Note that the recovery of the patient was likely secondary to the spontaneous drainage of the tympanic membrane with therapeutic measures offered by the treating physician coincidental. Sir Astley Cooper actually won the Copley Medal of the Royal Society in 1802 when he was the first to puncture a tympanic membrane and "cure" deafness.

Despite dramatic advances in the knowledge of anatomy and physiology (figure 250), patients remained at risk from well-meaning, though inexperienced caregivers. This report appeared in *The Cyclopedia of Practical Medicine* (1883) by Bennion: "In some cases considerable ingenuity is required to extract the foreign body from the ear. In one instance a small ivory ball had been detached from the top of a pen-holder in the case of a little boy. Syringing had done no good and the forceps failed to grasp it and only push it in further. At last it was extracted by bringing the point of a small brush, dipped in glue, in contact with its surface, allowing the glue to harden, and then removing brush and ball together. This is a hint that might be of service in difficult cases. The case is recorded of a nurse who, having failed to remove a button from a child's ear, actually tried to push it out the other side. We need hardly say that not only could such a thing be impossible but such treatment is highly dangerous."

Because surgery of the inner ear was not available until the twentieth century, instruments to amplify sound, beginning with a cow horn and progressing to devices made of silver and tortoise shell, were always in

250. External and internal ear in *Traité complet d'anatomie de l'homme,* 2nd ed. (1866–1871) by J.M. Bourgery, Claude Bernard, and N.H. Jacob

251. Opposite. Mid nineteenth-century hearing devices: (top) banjo-type ear trumpet, conversation tube with silk and ebony mounts, silver-plated dome by Rein and Son

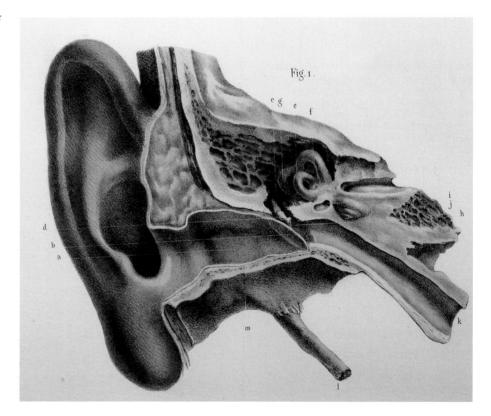

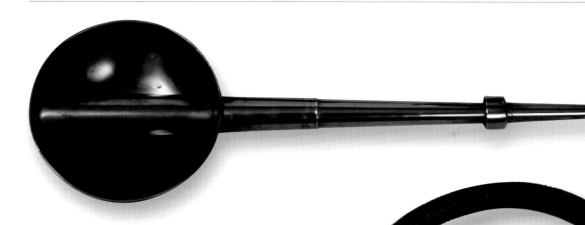

demand (figures 251, 252). Some individuals, however, lost their hearing entirely, and that loss certainly factored into their professional performance. Jonathan Swift suddenly became deaf, and the resultant cynicism likely played a significant role in the writing of *Gulliver's Travels*. The loss of Spanish artist Francisco Goya's hearing and subsequent despair both might well have been secondary to lead toxicity. According to Théophile Gautier, "He scooped his color out of tubs, applied it with sponges, mops, rags, anything he could lay his hands on. He trowelled and slapped his colours on like mortar, giving characteristic touches with a stroke of his thumb."

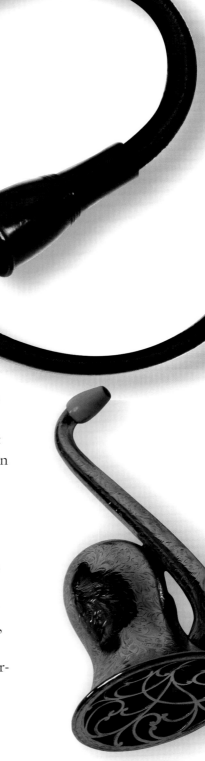

Probably the most famous and tragic of the hearing impaired was Ludwig van Beethoven (1770–1827). Frustration, embarrassment, and resignation were all reflected in the note he wrote to his brothers Carl and Johann in 1802: "Yet it was not possible for me to say to men; speak louder, shout for I am deaf. Alas! How could I declare the weakness of a sense which in me ought to be more acute than in others—a sense which formerly I possessed in highest perfection, a perfection such as few in my profession enjoy or have ever enjoyed." Beethoven went on in the *Heiligen-Städter Testament*: ". . . I must live like an outcast; when I approach a gathering I become fearful of revealing my condition. . . . What a dejection when somebody next to me heard a flute and I did not hear anything, or when somebody heard the shepherd singing and I could not hear even that—such incidents made me desperate, I was not far from putting an end to my life. It was only Art, my art that restrained me—oh, I felt unable to leave this world before I had created what I felt had been assigned to me; and so I endured this miserable life—really miserable." Beethoven's final words were "I shall hear in Heaven."

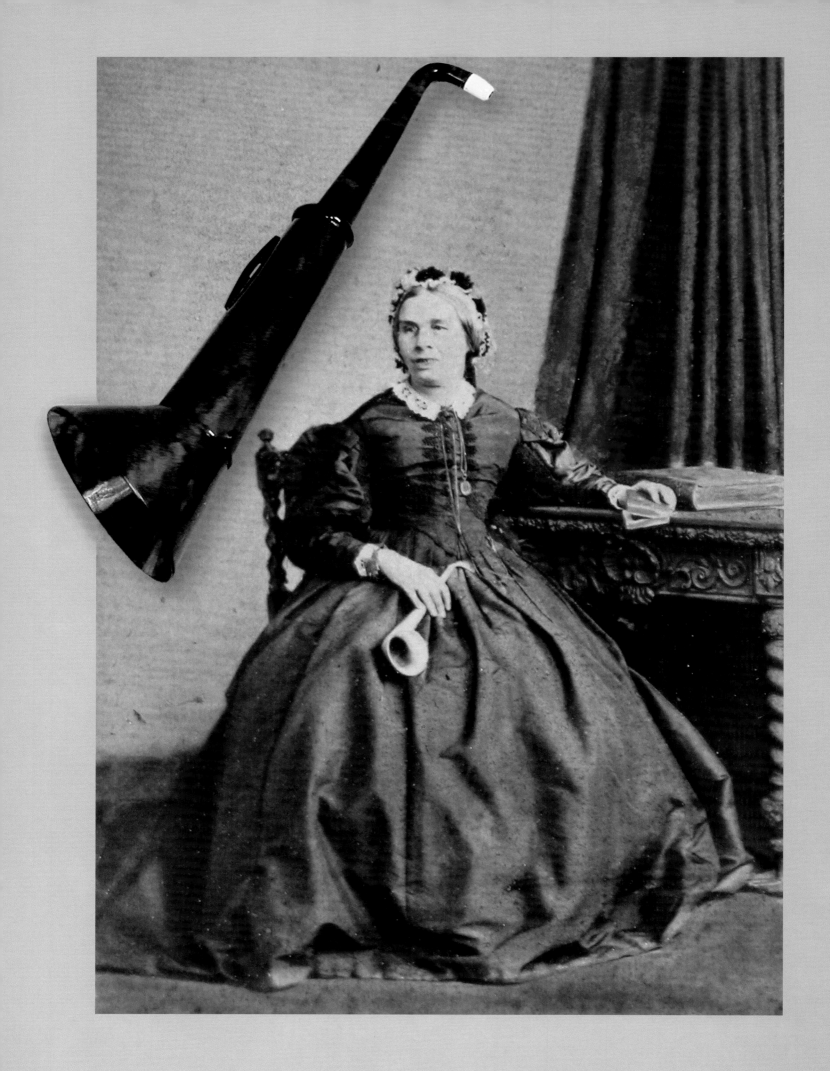

The Nose

One of the more common problems suffered by patients over the ages has been that of nosebleeds. Prior to the use of surgical intervention, physicians attempted medical therapy, though not always with success. In the seventeenth century, Culpeper recommended "Take nettles and stamp them and press out the juice, and let him that bleedeth at Nose take a spoonfool of the juice, and hold it in his mouth as long as he can, and spit that out and take another fresh spoonful, and hold that in the mouth likewise; also if you will you may moisten the Nettles after you have pressed the juyce out of them with a little Vinegar, and binde it on to the forehead."

Hippocrates related one of the earliest reports regarding surgery of the nose when he described the removal of nasal polyps (figure 253). He used three techniques, the first of which was to tie strings to a sponge that was inserted through the nose and into the pharynx. The sponge was dragged across the pharynx, bringing the polyps along with it. The physician inserted a snare in the second method, and cauterization with

252. Opposite. Albumin print of a woman holding a hearing horn (ca. 1860); (overprint) faux tortoiseshell Miss Martineau's Trumpet

253. Below. Nasal packing in *The Principles of Surgery* (1812) by John Bell

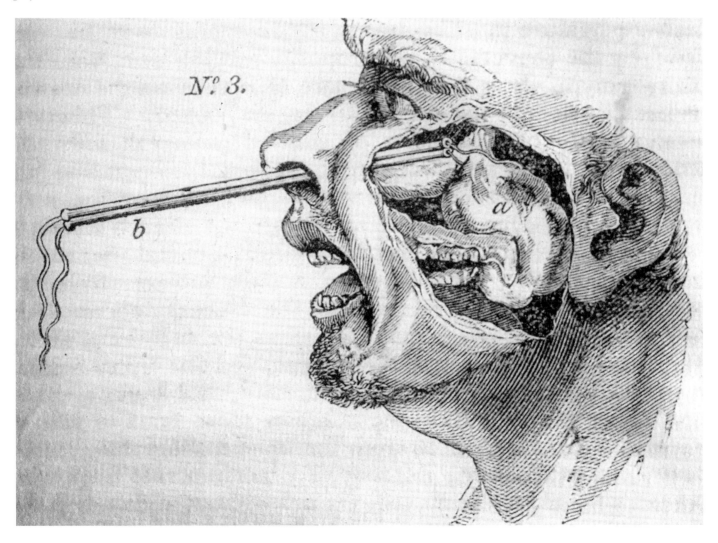

a hot iron was a last resort. This technique was used throughout the medieval period and was described by the seventh-century Greek surgeon Paulus Aegineta:

> Malignant polypi we burn with cauteries, knob-shaped; and, after the burning, we have recourse to the treatment for burnt parts. After the operation, having sponged the parts carefully, we inject oxycrate or wine into the nose, and, if the fluid descend by the roof of the mouth to the pharynx, the operation will have been rightly done; but if it does not descend, it is clear that about the ethmoid bones, or the upper parts of the nose, there are fleshy bodies which have not been reached with the polypus instruments. Taking, then, a thread moderately thick, like a cord, and having tied knots upon it at the distance of two or three fingers' breadths, we introduce it into the opening of a double-headed specillum upwards to the ethmoid openings, passing it by the palate and mouth, and then drawing it with both hands, we saw away, as it were, with the knots of the fleshy bodies.

The Throat

All diseases affecting children are tragic, though one of the most devastating is diphtheria because the treatment has been so dreadful and the suffering so heartbreaking. Greek physician Aretaeus of Cappadocia described diphtheria long ago in the first century (figure 254):

> Ulcers occur on the tonsils; some, indeed, of an ordinary nature, mild and innocuous; but others of an unusual kind, pestilential and fatal . . . but such as are broad, hollow, foul, and covered with a white, livid, or black concretion . . . and small pustules form, at first few in number, but others coming out, they coalesce, and a broad ulcer is produced. And if the disease spread outwardly to the mouth, and reach the columella (*uvula*) and divide it asunder, and if it extend to the tongue, the gums, and the alveoli, the teeth also become loosened and black; and the inflammation seizes the neck; and these die within a few days from the inflammation, fever, foetid smell, and want of food. But, if it spread to the thorax by the windpipe, it occasions death by suffocation within the space of a day. For the lungs and heart can neither endure such smells, nor ulcerations, nor ichorous discharges, but coughs and dyspnoea supervene. . . .
>
> The manner of death is most piteous; pain sharp and hot as from carbuncle; respiration bad, for their breath smells strongly of putrefaction, as they constantly inhale the same again into

254. Right. *Diphtheria Trying to Strangle a Small Child* (ca. 1910), watercolor by Richard Tennant Cooper

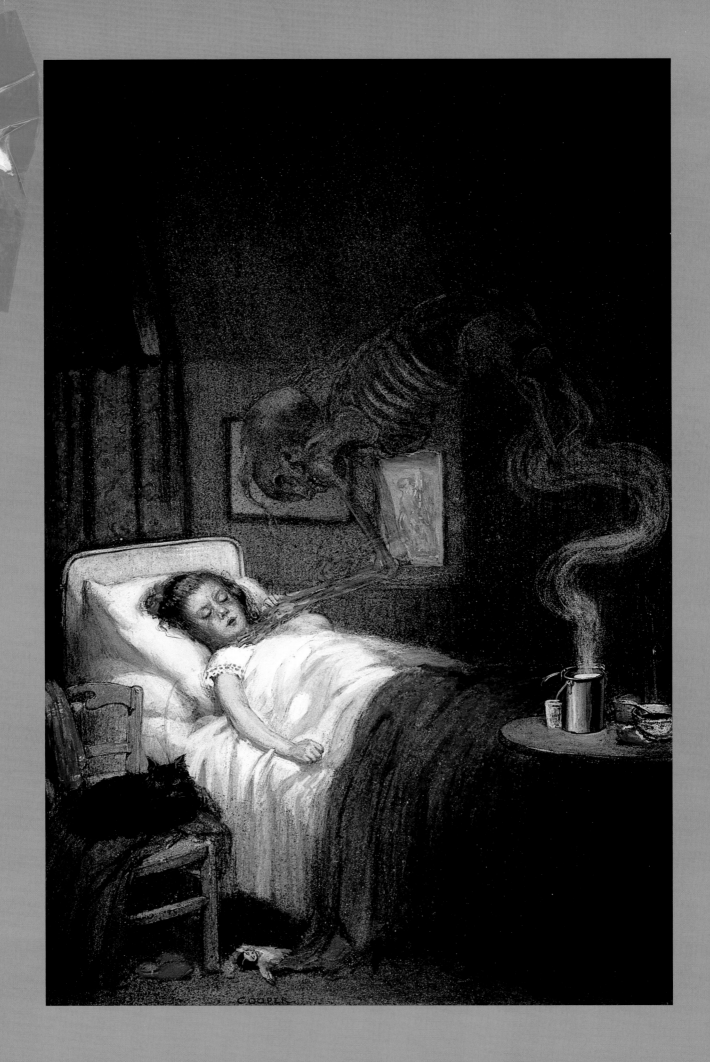

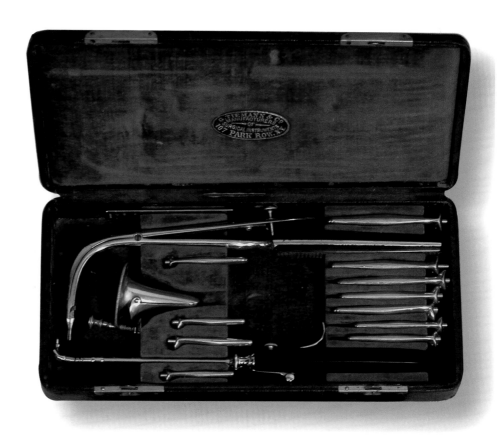

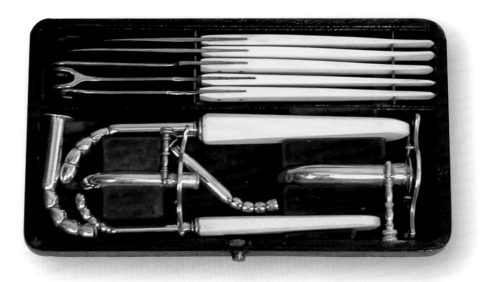

255. Late nineteenth-century tracheotomy sets: (top) O'Dwyer set with added nasal speculum by Tiemann; (below) Maw, Son, and Thompson

their chest; they are in so loathsome a state that they cannot endure the smell of themselves; countenance pale or livid; fever acute, thirst is if from fire, and yet they do not desire to drink for fear of the pains it would occasion; for they become sick if it compress the tonsils, or if it return by the nostrils; and if they lie down they rise up again as not being able to endure the recumbent position, and if they rise up, they are forced in their distress

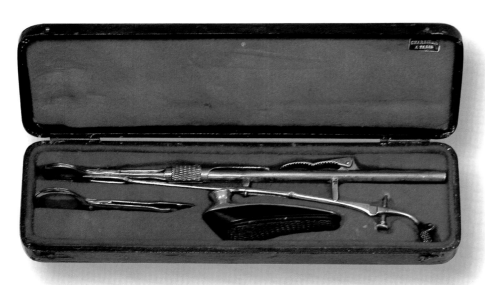

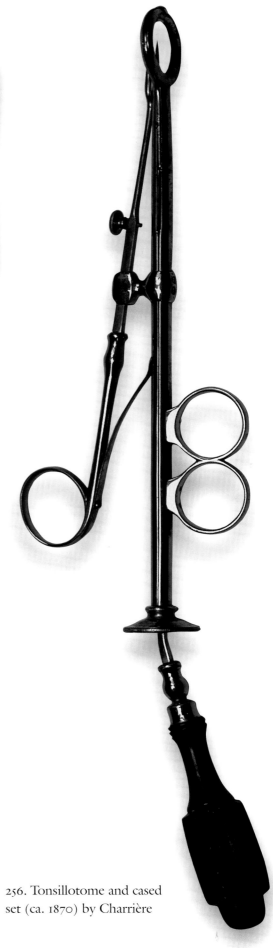

to lie down again; they mostly walk about erect, for in their inability to obtain relief they flee from rest, as if wishing to dispel one pain by another. Inspiration large, as desiring cold air for the purpose of refrigeration, but expiration small, for the ulceration, as if produced by burning, is inflamed by the heat of the respiration. Hoarseness, loss of speech supervene; and these symptoms hurry on from bad to worse, until suddenly falling to the ground they expire.

Tracheotomy, or surgical opening of the windpipe, was the only definitive way in which to treat acute obstruction of the upper respiratory tract secondary to diphtheria (figure 255), though in the pre-antibiotic era, other infections could also progress to the same life threatening condition from a peri-tonsillar abscess (known as quinsy). A tracheotomy was depicted on an Egyptian tablet as early as 3,600 B.C., and there was a recorded repair in the Hindu Rig Veda (ca. 2000 B.C.): "the bountiful one who, without a ligature, can cause the windpipe to re-unite when the cervical cartilages are cut across, provided they are not entirely severed." Greek ruler Alexander the Great was rumored to have carried out a tracheotomy in the fourth century B.C. when he used the tip of his sword to open the trachea of a choking soldier. The first to be given credit for having performed this procedure was Asclepiades of Bithynia (ca. 124-40 B.C.), and Antonio Musa Brasavola first documented a successful tracheotomy in 1546.

Aretaeus opposed this sort of intervention in his *Therapeutics of Acute Diseases*: "But those who, in order to guard against suffocation in quinsy, make an incision in the trachea for the breathing, do not appear to me to have proved the practicability of the thing by actual experiment; for the heat of the inflammation is increased by the wound, and thus con-

256. Tonsillotome and cased set (ca. 1870) by Charrière

tributes to the suffocation and cough. And, moreover, if by any means they should escape the danger, the lips of the wound do not coalesce; for they are both cartilaginous, and not of a nature to unite."

Tonsillitis sometimes progressed to quinsy, and a tonsillectomy was the medical recommendation frequently chosen. Though considered a simple procedure today, it carried a significant risk well into the nineteenth century (figure 256). Morell Mackenzie (1837–1892) recounted a procedure gone dramatically awry:

> The larger tonsil had been excised with the bistoury with comparatively little bleeding, so little that the excision of the other one was proceeded with immediately. As I cut into this, the hemorrhage was at once so profuse as to conceal the field of operation from view; but the excision was completed as rapidly as possible, and by the time the divided portion of the gland was withdrawn—less time than it has taken to narrate the circumstance—several ounces of blood had been lost. I immediately applied the dry persulphate of iron, slapping it upon the bleeding surface with my fingers, which held it there with some difficulty on account of the struggles of the patient to eject the blood streaming into her mouth. Shortly after the hemorrhage was controlled the patient fainted. She was placed prone on the floor and soon recovered. Upon examination, a few minutes after the administration of some alcoholic stimulant, I found that I had not removed the lower portion of the tumor, having cut the knife out just above it. With some persuasion the patient permitted me to remove this portion, but no bleeding followed it. I was subsequently informed by the physician who had brought the patient to me, that secondary hemorrhage took place a few days after, which necessitated a renewal of the application of the persulphate of iron. A few weeks afterwards the patient called upon me perfectly well, but she had not yet recovered the rosy complexion she had before she made my acquaintance.

When clinicians failed in their efforts to check tonsillar infections, they could only hope that a postmortem examination might provide them with information to help in the next case. Giovanni Battista Morgagni (1682–1771) made an early and important physical finding during the public autopsy of a forty-year-old woman who had died suddenly during an asthmatic attack. He noted that the viscera, chest, and cranium were normal, though on examining the larynx, he commented, "And when I laid it open by longitudinal incision behind what we were seeking was at once manifest. For a whitish mass of ash-looking pus, of a pultaceous character, like a cork, obstructed the cavity of the larynx far

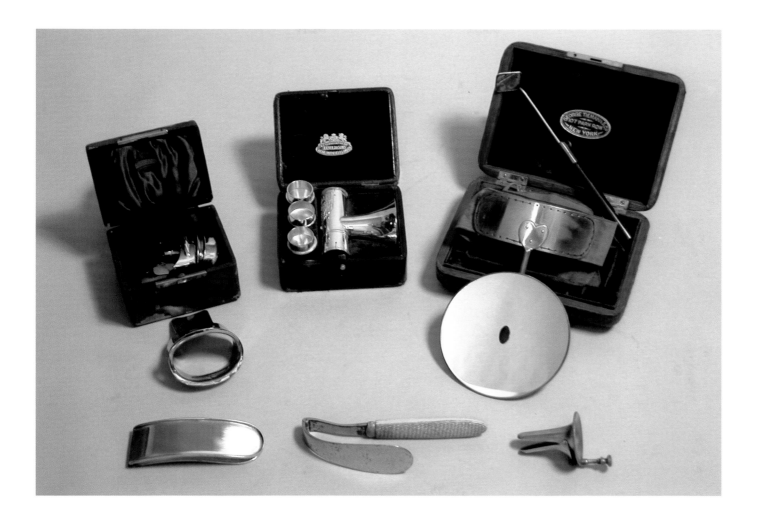

down below the glottis, and there the investing membrane of the larynx was ulcerated, as well as where it covered the nearest rings of the trachea, though to a less extent."

Surgeons began to perform more invasive and intricate procedures in the nineteenth century, and craftsmen responded by manufacturing instruments of ebony, ivory, brass, and silver for diagnosis and treatment (figure 257). Some would mark the beginning of the specialty of oto-laryngology with the discovery of the laryngoscope by Dr. Manuel Garcia, a scientist and professor of singing. This was Garcia's excited description of his first look through the instrument he had just invented:

> . . . suddenly I saw the two mirrors of a laryngoscope in their respective positions as if actually present before my eyes. I went straight to the surgical instrument maker and asked if he had a small mirror with a long handle and was informed that he had a dentist's mirror which had been one of the failures of the London Exhibition of 1851. Having obtained also a hand mirror, I returned home, impatient to begin my experiments. I placed against the uvula the little mirror, which I had heated in warm

257. Late nineteenth-century ENT devices: (top) cased set of mouth gags by Mellier Drug Co., silver cased oto-scope set by Arnold and Sons, head mirror by Tiemann; (bottom) folding silver tongue blade, ivory folding tongue blade by Tiemann, nasal speculum by Klein, Gund

water and carefully dried. And then flashing on its surface with the hand mirror a ray of sunshine, I saw at once, to my great joy, the glottis wide open and so fully exposed that I could perceive a portion of the trachea. When any excitement had somewhat abated, I began to examine what was passing before my eyes. The way in which the glottis silently opened and moved in the act of phonation filled me with wonder.

William Shakespeare (1564–1616) frequently referred to the practice of medicine in his plays. In 1602, he moved to a residence in London on Silver Street close to the annual public anatomy demonstrations at the Barber-Surgeons' Hall, and the St. Paul's churchyard bookstalls with their many medical texts. Shakespeare's eldest daughter married a prominent physician in 1607, Dr. John Hall (1575–1636), who wrote *Select Observations On English Bodies or Cures Both Empirical and Historical performed upon very Eminent Persons in Desperate Diseases*. In one of the most famous passages of *As You Like It* (act 2, scene 7), Shakespeare referred to the ultimate fate of the organ systems reviewed in this chapter, as Jacques says:

All the world's a stage
And all the men and women merely players
They have their exits and entrances,
And one man in his prime plays many parts,
His act being seven ages. At first the infant,
mewling and puking in the nurse's arms.
Then the whining school-boy, with his satchel
and shining morning face, creeping like snail
unwilling to school. And then the lover,
sighing like furnace, with a woeful ballad
made to his mistress's eyebrow. Then a soldier
full of strange oaths, and bearded like the pard,
jealous in honor, sudden and quick in quarrel,
seeking the bubble reputation even in the
cannon's mouth.
And then the justice in fair round belly with good
capon lin'd,
with eyes severe and beard of formal cut,
full of wise saws and modern instances; and so he
plays his part.
The sixth age shifts into the lean and slipper'd
pantaloon,
with spectacles on nose and pouch on side,

his youthful hose, well shav'd a world too wide for
his shrunken shank;
and his big manly voice, turning again toward
childish treble,
pipes and whistles in his sound.
Last scene of all, that ends this strange eventful
history,
is second childishness and mere oblivion,
sans teeth, sans eyes, sans taste, sans everything.

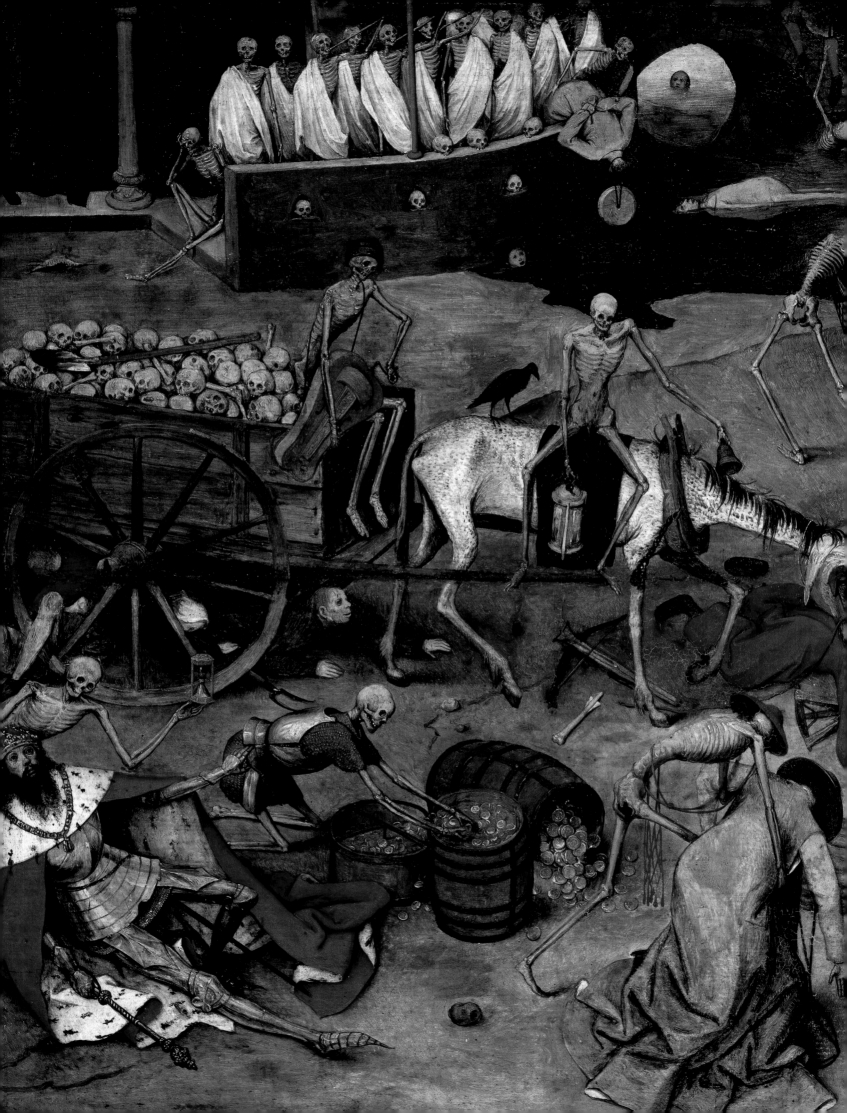

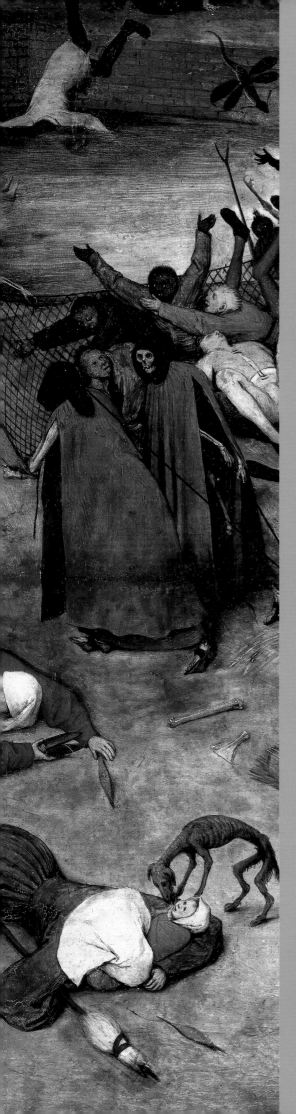

MEDICINE

The practice of medicine is an art, not a trade, a calling, not a business, a calling in which your heart will be exercised equally with your head.

William Osler, MD
The Master-word in Medicine, 1903

Detail, *The Triumph of Death* (1562-1563), oil on wood by Pieter Brueghel the Elder

327

hysicians were unable to enter the head, chest, and abdomen in a meaningful way for millions of years, so they resorted to an almost endless variety of medications to treat often fatal conditions. This chapter deals with the types of noninterventional therapy available to patients prior to the discovery of anesthesia in the middle of the nineteenth century.

ANCIENT CHINESE MEDICAL CARE

Traditional Chinese medicine dates back thousands of years. The Yellow Emperor, Huang Ti (2698–2599 B.C.) produced the greatest medical work in Chinese history, the *Nei Ching* (*Canon of Medicine*) written on strips of bamboo in about 200 B.C. In that work, the universe was based on two cosmic laws, the *yin* and the *yang,* which were both part of the underlying principle of the universe called the Tao (figure 258). As noted by the Yellow Emperor in his *Nei Ching*, "Those who rebel against the rules of the universe sever their own roots and ruin their true selves. Yin and Yang, the two principles in nature, and the four seasons are the beginning and the end of everything and they are also the cause of life and death. Those who disobey the laws of the universe will give rise to calamities and visitations, while those who follow the laws of the universe remain free from dangerous illness, for they are the ones who have obtained Tao, the Right Way." The familiar symbol that represents both the yin and yang shows that they are both part of a whole, they flow into each other, and though they are separate, each contains a seed of the other.

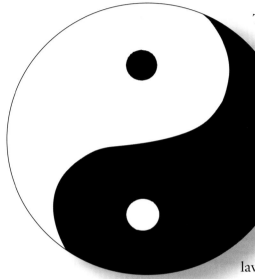

258. Yin and Yang

The yin was felt to be feminine and symbolized darkness, coolness, and passivity. The yang was masculine and represented what was light, active, and hot, though both were omnipresent in varying degrees. Each complimented the other in the same way that hot and cold, and wet and dry are related in a continuum, neither able to exist alone. For example, the relationship between yin and yang explained why severe and repeated heat (fever) resulted in chills and why those who had chills soon became febrile. During a dialogue in the *Nei Ching*, Qi Bo stated, "When Yang is the stronger, the body is hot, the pores are closed, and people begin to pant; they become boisterous and coarse and do not perspire. They become feverish, their mouths are dry and sore, their stomachs feel tight, and they die of constipation. . . . When the Yin is stronger, the body is cold and covered with perspiration. People realize they are ill; they tremble and feel chilly. When they feel chilled, their spirits become rebellious. Their stomachs can no longer digest food and they die."

According to the *Nei Ching,* five organs managed all functions of the body and influenced individual behavior as well. The heart was the most important and controlled the pulse and spirit, while other organs included the liver (blood and soul), spleen (nutrition and thought), lungs (breath and energy), and the kidneys (reproduction and will). These organ systems interacted on a daily basis and sometimes were in conflict, with the adversary relationship between the heart and the kidneys a good example. In fact, the cardiovascular and renal systems function more effectively in opposite states of hydration, so that cardiologists and nephrologists battle each other on a daily basis regarding proper fluid management for their hospitalized patients.

Similar to a number of principles characteristic of Western medical thought, the ancient Chinese felt that good health was only achieved when both the yin and yang were in balance, and that disease occurred as a result of a disruption in the relationship between these two forces. A disturbance could be diagnosed after an evaluation of the patient's appearance, temperature, pulse, tongue, urine, and stool. One suspected yang signs if the face were flushed, the tongue red, and the pulse rapid and full, while the yin was most active if the face were cool, the tongue pale, and the pulse slow and weak.

The body was felt to be an energetic system composed of twelve meridians with about 365 energy channels surrounding the various organs, each nourishing a part of the body with the life force, or *qi.* (figure 259) Disease (and a pathologic qi) resulted from an interruption in those channels because of a number of factors: 1) external sources such as a change in the weather—heat, cold, moisture, or dryness; 2) internal sources including anger, grief, or fear; and 3) other causes such as gluttony, malnutrition, and trauma. It was the task of early Chinese physicians to recreate a balance between the yin and yang by increasing the flow of qi through the stimulation energy points in one of the meridians that channeled energy to a diseased organ. This was accomplished in a number of ways, and one of the earliest was the still popular acupuncture first described by Shen Nung in about 2800 B.C., though acupuncture did not become routinely practiced until the Tsin dynasty (A.D. 263–420). Once a particular problem was identified, physicians placed needles at the relevant channel to stimulate the flow of qi to correct the imbalance between the yin and yang, and thus an internal disorder could be treated without surgical intervention.

Other methods employed to stimulate the flow of qi by those practicing traditional Chinese medicine included *Tui Na* (massage) and bone manipulation. Counterirritation by dry cupping and moxibustion were also popular, the latter technique probably having been imported from ancient Egypt. Moxibustion involved the placement of small com-

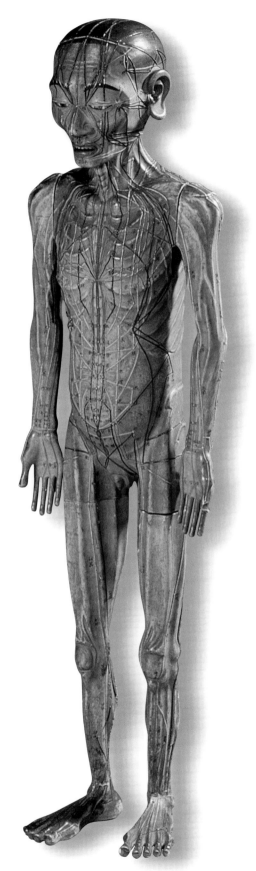

259. Wooden Chinese acupuncture figure from the Ming Dynasty (late seventeenth century)

bustible cones made of powdered mugwart, called moxas, at one of the meridian points of the skin. They were then ignited, and the resulting blisters caused an increase in the flow of qi. Bloodletting was forbidden, and the only surgical procedure condoned by Chinese religious leaders was castration.

ANCIENT INDIAN MEDICAL CARE

The history of India dates back to civilizations in west India and Pakistan that were conquered by Aryans during their invasion in about 1600 B.C. It was after an amalgamation of many cultures that the Sanskrit language became popular in an emerging Hindu civilization. The earliest and most holy of Hindu books are collectively called the *Veda,* and the earliest of those concerned with medical care is the *Atharva Veda* (ca. 1000 B.C.), though it is quite primitive and primarily contains sorcery and spells that were intended to remove the evil spirits responsible for disease. Over the centuries, medical care became more sophisticated, and Hindu physicians incorporated all their medical literature in the *Ayurveda* ("knowledge of life").

Ayurvedic medicine was a compilation of information from a number of early medical authors, many influential in India between 300–200 B.C. There is debate regarding the time frame of their lives, but certainly the most important Ayurvedic physicians were Charaka (ca. A.D. 100) and Susruta (ca. A.D. 400). The *Susruta-samhita* ("collection of the Susruta") was the foundation of Hindu medical care for centuries. It dealt primarily with surgery, and contained early descriptions of lithotomy, cataract removal, amputation, fracture repair, and rhynoplasty. A number of common medical conditions were also described, including leprosy, diabetes mellitus, and tuberculosis. Susruta's influence through the ages has been immense, and much of his philosophy remains relevant today: "A physician, well versed in the principles of the science of medicine but unskillful in his art through want of practice, loses his wit at the bedside of his patient, just as a coward. . . . On the other hand, a physician, experienced in his art but deficient in knowledge . . . is condemned by all good men as a quack, and deserves capital punishment at the hands of the king. Both these classes of physicians are not to be trusted, because they are inexpert and half educated. Such men are incapable of discharging the duties of their vocation, just as a one-winged bird is incapable of taking flight in the air."

The Buddhist religion based many if its beliefs on a world comprised of five primordial elements—earth, water, fire, air, and space. Out of these came the body *doshas* ("humors"), and disease resulted from disturbances in relationships between these three systems: the *kapha* or

260. Bhaisajyaguru, the medicine Buddha Thangka holding in his left palm an alms bowl filled with healing nectar and the medicinal plant myrobalan. Gouache painting by an unknown Tibetan artist (date unknown).

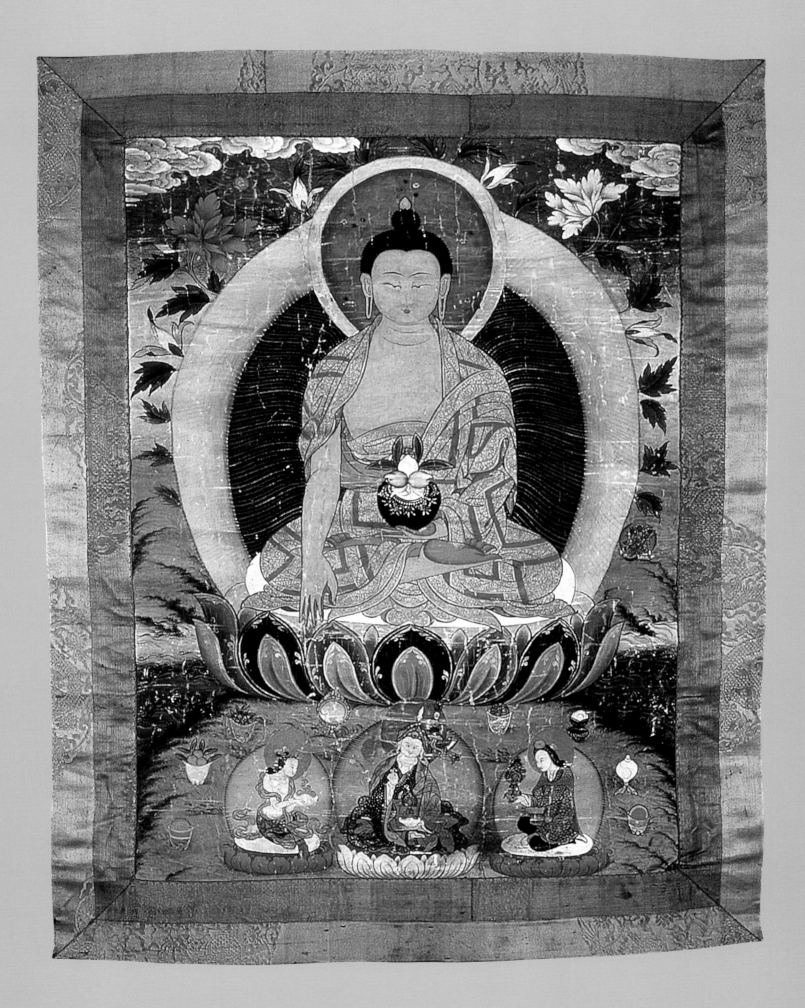

phlegm (water and earth—physical form and hereditary traits), *vata* (space and air—circulation of blood, thoughts, breathing, and the senses), and *pitta* or bile (fire and water—control of metabolism and digestion). After collecting a detailed history, the physician would determine how these doshas had fallen out of balance by examining the urine, pulse, and tongue. The recommended treatment plan usually included dietary changes, herbal remedies, massage, exercise, cleanliness, and spiritual guidance, along with the occasional use of venesection, cathartics, and emetics.

The influence of Hindu medicine was widespread, and over the centuries extended by way of trade routes and invading armies throughout Indo-China, Central Asia, and Japan. In Tibet in the fourth century, Ayurveda, as described by Hindu physician Charaka in the *Charaka-samhita*, was influential in the medical care provided by Buddhist monks. Disease was felt to be the result of ignorance, hatred, or passion, and therapy was practiced from a multidisciplined approach incorporating the mind, the body, and the natural world. As a result of Indian influences, Tibetan physicians added an extensive pharmacopoeia based on the use of butter, oil, honey, and molasses. Several centuries later, Tibet's foremost physician, Yutok Yonten K. Gongpo (A.D. 708–833), incorporated Chinese and Persian methods in the *Rg yud-bzi* (*Four-Part Medical Tantras*), and later in the eleventh century, Tibetans adopted Buddhist based systems. Early Tibetan therapy included behavioral modification in the form of meditation, spiritual advice, exercise, and diet. Herbal medications and contemplation were also employed in an attempt to understand the nature of life (figure 260).

RELIGION AND THE ROOTS OF WESTERN MEDICINE

The principles of Indian medicine spread throughout Asia analogous to the way in which Greek medicine influenced physicians in Europe. The two disciplines interacted with each other in many ways, and the Greeks of Alexander were well aware of Indian medicine in the fourth century B.C. The *Samhita* was translated into Persian and Arabic in about A.D. 800, and, since Arabic medicine continued to be the chief authority for European physicians until the Renaissance, the West was continually exposed to Asian medical philosophies. Both disciplines adhered to a holistic approach regarding diagnosis and treatment, and health was only achieved when the humors, or doshas, were in balance. Greek physician Hippocrates might have agreed with Susruta when the latter said in his *Susruta-samhita*, "an intelligent physician should preserve the state of health in the healthy individual, while he should increase or decrease the quantity of bodily humours, vital fluids, or excrements in a sick patient according to the exigencies of the case until his health is perfectly restored."

A great deal of early medical care involving the use of herbs and potions was ineffective in both the East and West, driving patients into the arms of religious leaders in search of an explanation for the causes, treatment, and prevention of their devastating conditions. This was especially true in India from 800 B.C. to A.D. 1000 when the practice of medicine was primarily in the hands of Brahman priests. They were often unable to chase out the demons responsible for disease, and it was not uncommon for religious leaders to accuse those afflicted of having sinned; punishment was proper, and so the illnesses were thereby justified.

Many Greek temples were built specifically for the Greek god of medicine, Asklepios, and that is where a great deal of early treatment took place in the West (figure 261). Asklepios is first mentioned in Greek literature in Homer's *Iliad* as the father of two physicians, Machaon and Podalirius, both of whom served in the siege of Troy in about 1180 B.C. As the stories of his great medical prowess grew, Asklepios' legend took on religious connotations. He was eventually thought of as a half-god since his father was the Greek god Apollo and his mother was Coronis, princess of Thessaly. Coronis had been betrothed to her cousin Ischus during Asklepios' conception, and, in order to save Asklepios embarrassment, his twin sister Artemis had Coronis killed while Apollo slew Ischus. (Apollo had been informed of the marriage by his spy, a white raven, which he turned black, that color to forever become a sign of morning.) Before Coronis was burned at the stake, Apollo removed Asklepios from her body and delivered the future Greek god to a goat to be nursed and to the centaur Chiron to be given instruction in the art of medicine.

For nearly one thousand years (500 B.C.–A.D. 500), those seeking medical treatment traveled to one of about two hundred Greek Temples of Asklepios to take part in a healing ritual called incubation. The temples, or Asclepieia, were sprawling complexes comprised of a central structure devoted to worship and healing surrounded by baths, gymnasiums, and perhaps a theater. Women who were near delivery and those close to death were not permitted inside the temple, but all others were welcome to the Asclepieia with the only requirement being that "pure must be he who enters

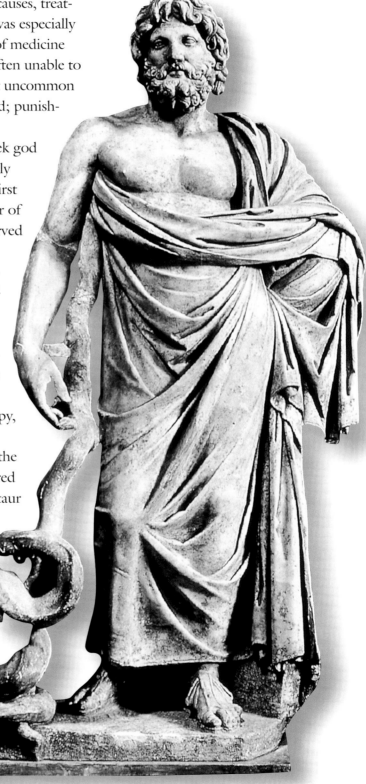

261. Second-century marble statue of Aesculapius

the fragrant temple; purity means to think nothing but holy thoughts." While those requesting therapy were asleep in the temple, Asklepios appeared with his daughter, Hygiae (goddess of health care and origin of the word "hygiene"), and the snake that Asklepios carried licked the wounds of the diseased to cure them.

In addition to Hygiae, Asklepios had several other children who entered the medical field, including Telesphorus (convalescent care), Panaceion (protectress of healing plants from whom the term *panacea*, or "treatment that cures all diseases," is derived), Podalirius (psychiatry), and Machaon (surgery). With time, Asklepios became so proficient in his art that he was even able to bring back the dead, a talent that angered Hades, the lord of the underworld. With his population dwindling, Hades complained to Zeus, who then vanquished Asklepios with a thunderbolt.

The medical staff of Asklepios with a snake wrapped around it likely has its origin from the legends surrounding Greek mythology, and is probably the first recognized medical symbol. One of the first references to the cypress staff can be found in the Bible in Numbers 21:8: "And the Lord said unto Moses, Make thee a fiery serpent, and set it upon a pole: and it shall come to pass, that every one that is bitten when he looketh upon it shall live." The filarial worm (*Dracunculus medinensis*) was a rather common parasite in ancient times that crawled around under the skin, and may, in fact, have been the origin of this medical symbol. The treating physician made an incision just ahead of the worm's path for it to exit, and then wrapped the worm around a stick to fully remove it. It became customary for physicians to use an image of this successful cure in their advertising.

In about the seventh century, another image, the caduceus, became linked to healing, and it is the symbol most associated with medicine today. This familiar emblem is a staff with wings at the top and entwined snakes below. It was initially the magic wand given to Hermes (the Roman god Mercury) by Apollo in order to help guide the souls of the dead to the lower world. Hermes was an ambassador of peace and threw his magical rod between two fighting snakes, which then stopped their battle and wrapped themselves around the rod. The wings were added as a result of the image of Hermes as a swift messenger. This symbol developed a closer relationship to medical care with the association of Hermes to alchemy in the Middle Ages, and practitioners were then referred to as "Hermeticists." Beginning in the early sixteenth century, printers used both the staff of Asklepios and the caduceus of Hermes to symbolize medical texts, though the caduceus became more prominent when the Medical Department of the United States Army adopted it as their official insignia in 1902.

The early provision of medical care continued to take place in religious centers for centuries since the etiology and transmission of devastating diseases remained poorly understood, and the afflicted could only pray for relief and protection. Amulets have been worn as a safeguard against disease and evil spirits for centuries. The term is derived from the Arabic "hamalet" and the variety of protective charms has been extraordinary, including Egyptian scarabs, bits of crania from ancient trephined skulls, teeth from the mouths of corpses, and widows' wedding rings, among many others. A rabbit's foot has been a sign of fertility since 600 B.C., though it was also carried as a guard against rheumatism. Those wishing to protect themselves from epilepsy wore a ring made out of a coffin nail, and many have considered bezoars (concretions from animals) an excellent way to prevent poisoning, bezoar meaning "to expel poison" in Persian. The present custom of crossing one's fingers for luck dates back to sixteenth-century England when the fear of harm by the supernatural led people to make the sign of the cross after feeling threatened.

The prognosis of serious conditions could only be guessed at, and since sinful behavior and disease have always been bound together, it is not surprising that the progress of an ailment was often forecast in a religious setting. Following the release of birds from the temple, a prognosis was good if they flew to the right and bad if they flew to the left. For that reason, the word *sinister,* which means "left," developed the negative connotation that it still carries today.

Without a scientific basis, predictions were frequently inaccurate, so a variety of Roman Catholic saints were charged with the protection and care of those who were afflicted with serious illnesses and had nowhere else to turn. A short list includes: St. Agatha (breast disease), St. Anthony (inflammation), St. Benedict (stones), St. Bonosa (smallpox), St. Cadoc (deafness), St. Cosmas (blindness), St. Erasmus (cholic), St. Eutrope (dropsy), St. Fiage (syphilis), St. Jude Thaddeus (desperate causes), St. Margaret of Antioch (difficult childbirth), St. Marus (convulsions), Sts. Rochus and Sebastian (plague), St. Sigismund (fever), and St. Valentine (epilepsy).

Religious leaders began to break away from their traditional duties of treating the sick in 1123 when Pope Callistus II demanded that priests and monks confine their activities to only those of a religious nature. Shortly thereafter in 1163 at the Council of Tours, Pope Alexander III specifically prohibited priests from studying medicine with the threat of excommunication should his decree be ignored. However, his ultimatum remained largely disregarded, and, in 1215, Pope Innocent II stated that no priest should perform operations that employed instruments of steel or fire, his justification being that the church abhorred cruel practices.

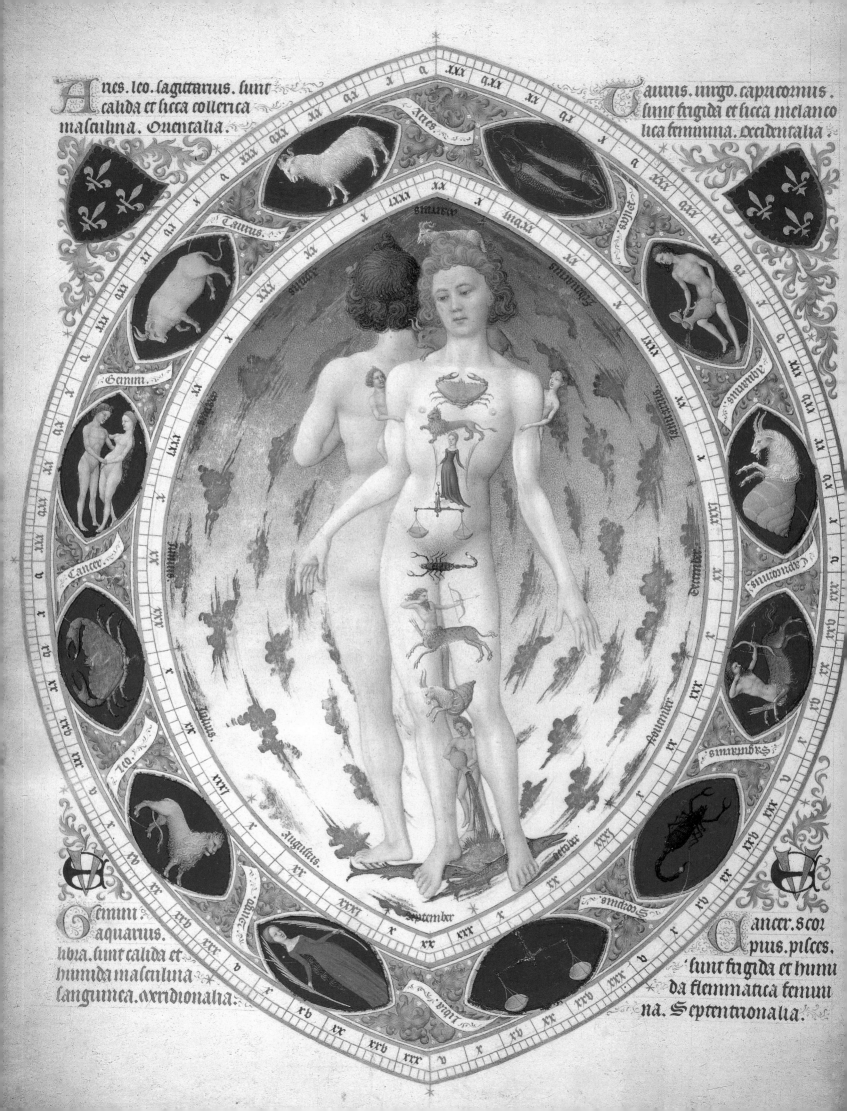

Aries. leo. sagittarius. sunt calida et sicca collerica masculina. Oriencalia.

Taurus. virgo. capricornus. sunt frigida et sicca melancolica feminina. occidentalia.

Aries.
Taurus.
Gemini.
Cancer.
Leo.

gemini.
aquarius.
libra. sunt calida et humida masculina sanguinea. oxridionalia.

September.

Cancer. scorpius. pisces. sunt frigida et humida flemmatica feminina. Septentrionalia.

Only after the Pope issued a special bull allowing physicians to marry did theology finally separate from medicine.

In addition to religion, astrology played an important role in the early provision of medical care, and astrological signs were assigned to various parts of the anatomy. Each of the seven known heavenly bodies had special influence over various human organs: the sun (heart), Jupiter (liver), Saturn (spleen), Mercury (lungs), Mars (bile), Venus (kidneys), and the Moon (brain). Those born under each sign of the zodiac were felt to be more susceptible to a certain disease or medical condition. An individual born under the sign of Gemini, for example, tended to be phlegmatic since Gemini was related to water, while plague and smallpox were the result of deadly emanations from the alignment of Mars and Saturn, according to the Jesuit Athanasius Kirchner. Aristotle believed that various phases of the Moon influenced disorders of women, and others were of the opinion that the Moon's rays affected all behavior, thus the genesis of the term "lunatic" from the word *lunar*.

Physicians literally looked to the heavens for advice, following the relationships of the stars and phases of the Moon carefully for guidance in their selection of the proper medication and appropriate timing for surgery, bleeding, and purging (figure 262). Medical advice based on the zodiac was included in the first printed document to discuss therapy, the German *Aderlasskalender* ("Calendar for Bloodletting") (1457), which guided physicians for centuries on the best times of the month for bloodletting. According to a quote from *The Husbandman's Practice, or Prognostication for ever* (1664), it was "good to purge with electuaries, the moon in Cancer; with pills, the moon is Pisces; with potions the moon in Virgo; good to take vomits, the moon being in Taurus, Virgo, or the latter part of Sagittarius; to purge the head by sneezing, the moon being in Cancer, Leo, or Virgo; to stop fluxes and rheumes, the moon being in Taurus, Virgo, or Capricorn; to bathe when the moon is in Cancer, Libra, Aquarius, or Pisces; to cut the hair off the head or beard when the moon is in Libra, Sagittarius, Aquarius, or Pisces."

The influence of astrology in the history of medicine continues to be reflected by some of the medical terms we use today. For example, the sign of the zodiac for cancer is the crab, and according to Galen "when the tumor extends its feet from all sides of its body into the veins, the sickness produces the picture of a crab." Geoffrey Chaucer (ca. 1343–1400) recognized the importance of an understanding of astrology in his *Picture of a good Physician*:

> With us there was a doctour of phisike;
> In al the world, was thar non hym lyk
> To speke of physic and of surgerye,
> For he was groundit in astronomie.

262. *The Anatomical Man and Woman*, zodiac representation in the calendar miniature from the *Trés Riches Heures du Duc de Berry* (1416) by the Limbourg brothers

EARLY HOSPITALS

Priests provided prayers and medications in their houses of worship for those still suffering after physicians had exhausted whatever resources they had available. In A.D. 390 in Rome, Christian convert Fabiola raised the necessary funds to establish the first hospital by selling all of her property. From *The Principal Works of Jerome*: "She was the first person to found a hospital, into which she might gather sufferers out of the streets, and where she might nurse the unfortunate victims of sickness and want. Need I now recount the various ailments of human beings? Need I speak of noses slit, eyes put out, feet half burnt, hands covered with sores? Or of limbs dropsical and atrophied? Or of diseased flesh alive with worms? Often did she carry on her own shoulders persons infected with jaundice or with filth. Often too did she wash away the matter discharged from wounds which others, even though men, could not bear to look at. She gave food to her patients with her own hand, and moistened the scarce breathing lips of the dying with sips of liquid." Over the next several hundred years, Christian hospitals were established throughout Europe only to provide "hospitality" to the aged and infirmed.

Between A.D. 641–649, Saint Landry founded the Hôtel Dieu in Paris where the sick were cared for in large halls that sometimes held eight hundred at a time. The conditions were appalling, as described by Max Nordau:

> In one bed of moderate width lay four, five, or six sick persons beside each other, the feet of one to the head of another; children beside gray-haired old men; indeed, incredible but true, men and women intermingled together. In the same bed lay individuals affected with infectious diseases beside others only slightly unwell; on the same couch, body against body, a woman groaned in the pangs of labor, a nursing infant writhed in convulsions, a typhus patient burned in the delirium of fever, a consumptive coughed his hollow cough, and a victim of some disease of the skin tore with furious nails his infernally itching integument. . . . The whole building fairly swarmed with the most horrible vermin, and the air of a morning was so vile in the sick wards that the attendants did not venture to enter them without a sponge saturated with vinegar held before their faces. The bodies of the dead ordinarily lay twenty-four hours, and often longer, upon the deathbed before they were removed, and the sick during this time were compelled to share the bed with the rigid corpse, which in this infernal atmosphere soon began to stink, and over which the green carrion-flies swarmed. . . .

It was not until 1181 that the Order of St. John set the standard for medical care in these institutions with the formation of its hospital in Jerusalem. During that same century, hundreds of cities throughout Europe established "lazarettos" (named after St. Lazarus) outside their city walls to house victims of the plague. The first hospital in England was built in York in A.D. 937, and six hundred years later, the Hospital of the Immaculate Conception in Mexico City became the first hospital in the New World. The Pennsylvania Hospital in Philadelphia was established in 1751 with the help of Drs. Thomas Bond and Benjamin Franklin, and is recognized as the first hospital in the United States. With a strong Quaker influence, that hospital's charter allocated services to "lunaticks or Persons distemper'd in Mind," and four of the first six patients were admitted for insanity.

INFECTIOUS DISEASE

The development of such signs and symptoms as fever, chills, and gangrenous changes leading to death must have been mysterious indeed, and it was not until fairly recently that physicians clearly understood the role that microorganisms play in most medical conditions. It took the discovery of the microscope before anyone believed that tiny creatures could live inside us, and even when microorganisms were first seen, not many believed that the little structures they saw were alive or could be the cause of illness. Most believed that diseases were transmitted through the air and used the term *miasma* well into the nineteenth century to describe the cause of disorders passed from one to another. Physicians visited patients wearing protective clothing and carried walking sticks that had strong fragrances to keep the bearer from inhaling "poisonous vapors." Numerous devices remained popular over the years to protect all from contamination (figure 263). In 1518, the mayor of Oxford attempted to control the spread of disease by confining the ill to their houses for forty days, and the word *quarantine* is derived from the Italian *quaranta giorni,* meaning forty days. This period of time may have been derived from the Bible since it was forty days that both Moses and Christ were isolated in the desert.

Shakespeare seemed to have had a fairly good understanding of the concept of communicable disease when, in *Cariolanus* (act 3, scene 1), Brutus said:

> Pursue him to his house, and pluck him thence:
> Lest his infection, being of catching nature,
> Spread further.

In the mid eighteenth century, Dr. William Cullen and John Brown of Edinburgh formally proposed a theory to explain the origin of inflam-

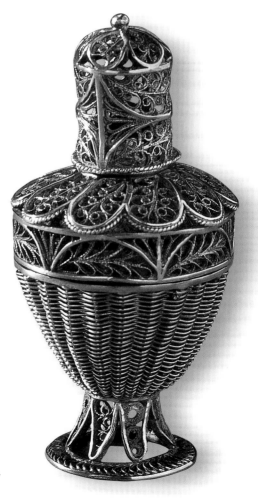

263. Silver pomander (ca. 1904), possibly Tunisian

mation. They believed that the etiology of infectious disease was "nervous irritability," or an over excitement and over stimulation of blood vessels and organs that led to the observed increase in pulse, temperature, chills, and ultimately seizures proceeding death. Many were of the opinion that the signs themselves were actually the pathologic processes rather than indicators of an underlying causative agent, so that is where physicians directed their therapy.

Dutch physician Hermann Boerhaave was more specific in his description regarding the etiology of these "nervous irritations" in his *Aphorisms: Concerning the Knowledge and Cure of Diseases* (1715):

> The nearer Singular Causes may be reduced under some Heads. α. The things received or conveyed into the Body being sharp and pricking, whether called Meat, Drink, Medicines, Preservatives or Poison, when endow'd with that propriety that they cannot be digested, moved, nor evacuated; or when taken to such a Quantity as to irritate the Stomach, to choak up, to obstruct, and to putrify with the Body. β. The things retain'd in the Body, which used to be evacuated each their proper Way, and that because of some Cold, Unctions, Vapours, some thick and fat Meat, Drink, medicines, Poisons, or Air; too long continued Rest, some usual Exercise omitted, Obstructions and Compressions from either the contain'd or surrounding Bodies. γ. The Gestures; as the too great disturbances of the Mind of Body, occasioning heat and tossings. δ. External Applications that are of sharp, pungent, gnawing, tearing, burning, or inflaming. ε. Those that change the Humors and their Motions much, which abundance of Externals as well as Internals will do; Hunger, great Evacuations; Collections of Pus, Water and watry blood in Dropsies and Empyemas, or sharp Serum; Choler being inflamed and burnt; Suppurations, Gangrenes, Cancers, too much Waking, too intense Studies of any Kind, and Excess of Venery.

Laurence Heister went into a bit more detail regarding the etiology and treatment of infectious diseases in his text *A General System of Surgery* (1743):

> If the Cause of the Inflammation is found to be external and obvious to the Senses, as Thorns, Splinters, the End of a Sword, Bullets, or any other foreign body stuck in the Part; nothing can be more serviceable than to speedily and carefully remove whatever is lodged there, if it can be done with Safety. So also when the Inflammation proceeds from a too strict Bandage in

Wounds, &c. or from a Luxation or Fracture; the first and principal business is to speedily relax the Bandage, or else to set the Fracture or reduce the Luxation.

When the external Causes are once removed, and when the Inflammation is great and proceeds from internal causes, it is in both Cases very useful to open a Vein either in the Arm or Foot, and to draw off a large Quantity of Blood, proportional to the Strength and Habit of the Patient; giving afterwards a brisk Purge; not one that heats the Body, but judiciously accommodated to the Age and Constitution of the Patient. Both these are very necessary here, and if the Symptoms do not remit and grow milder, they must be repeated at Discretion: But I would advise the Surgeon in this Case, where he can, to call in the Advice of some prudent Physician. . . .

The Plague

In the sixth century, more than one hundred million people died as a result of an infection caused by *Pasteurella pestis,* a bacterium transmitted to humans from fleas by way of infected rats. What came to be called The Black Death took the lives of up to sixty percent of those exposed as dark hemorrhages under the skin led to sepsis, gangrene, and ultimately death (figure 264). Initially, black pustules developed at the site of a fleabite, and buboes, or swollen and tender lymph nodes primarily in the inguinal and auxiliary areas, soon followed from which Bubonic Plague got its name. These lymph glands grew quite large and eventually became "plague sores," which discharged purulent, fowl smelling material. This was the usual pathology, though a less common "pneumonic" form spread from person to person by way of the respiratory tract. One of the earliest descriptions of the plague came from Rufus of Ephesus, a leading first-century Greek physician. According to him, "In the plague there is everything which is dreadful, and nothing of this kind is wanting as in other diseases. For there are delirium, vomitings of bile, distention of the hypochondrium, pains, much sweatings, cold of the extremities, bilious diarrhoeas, which are thin and flatulent; the urine watery, thin, bilious, black, having bad sediments, and the substances floating on it most unfavorable; trickling of blood from the nose, heat in the chest, tongue parched, thirst, restlessness, insomnolency, strong convulsions, and many other things which are unfavorable." Twenty-seven million died from this disease in the fourteenth century, and if subsequent epidemics are counted, Bubonic Plague claimed nearly half the lives of all Europeans by the late Middle Ages.

The first recorded outbreak of the plague took place in October 1347

264. Following pages. *The Triumph of Death* (1562–1563), oil on wood by Pieter Brueghel the Elder

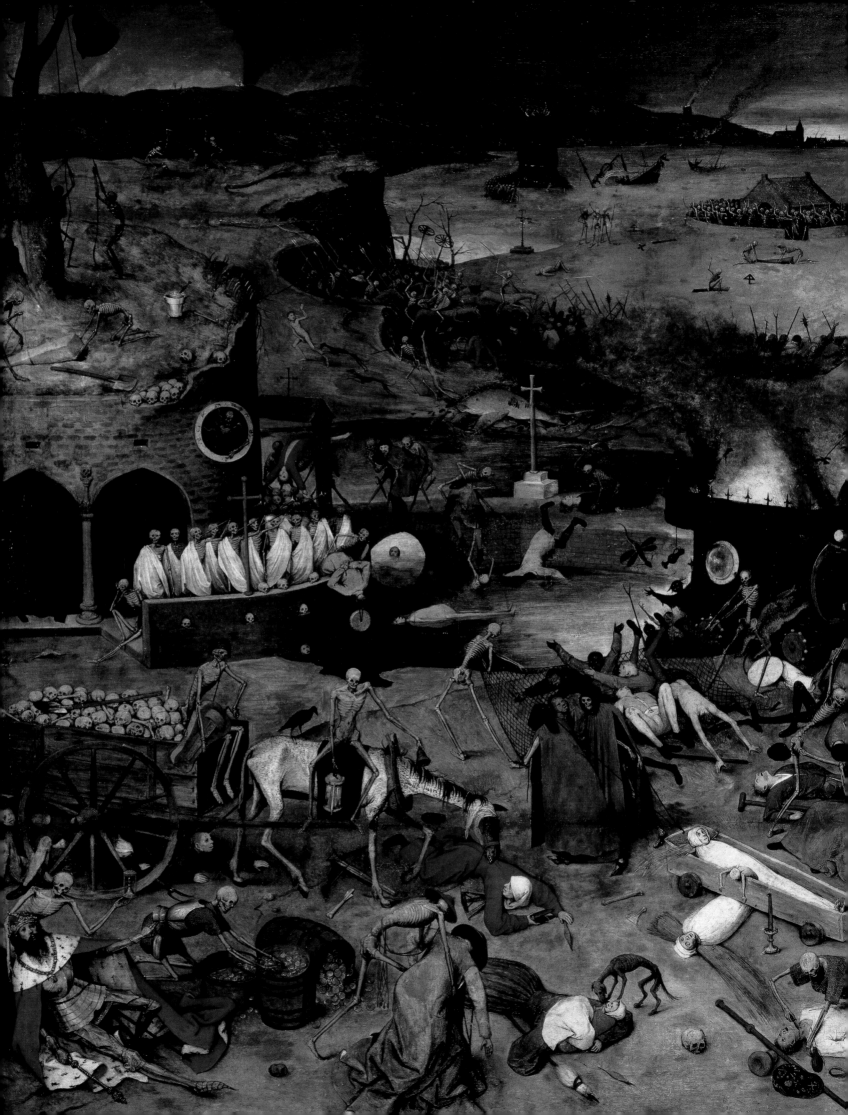

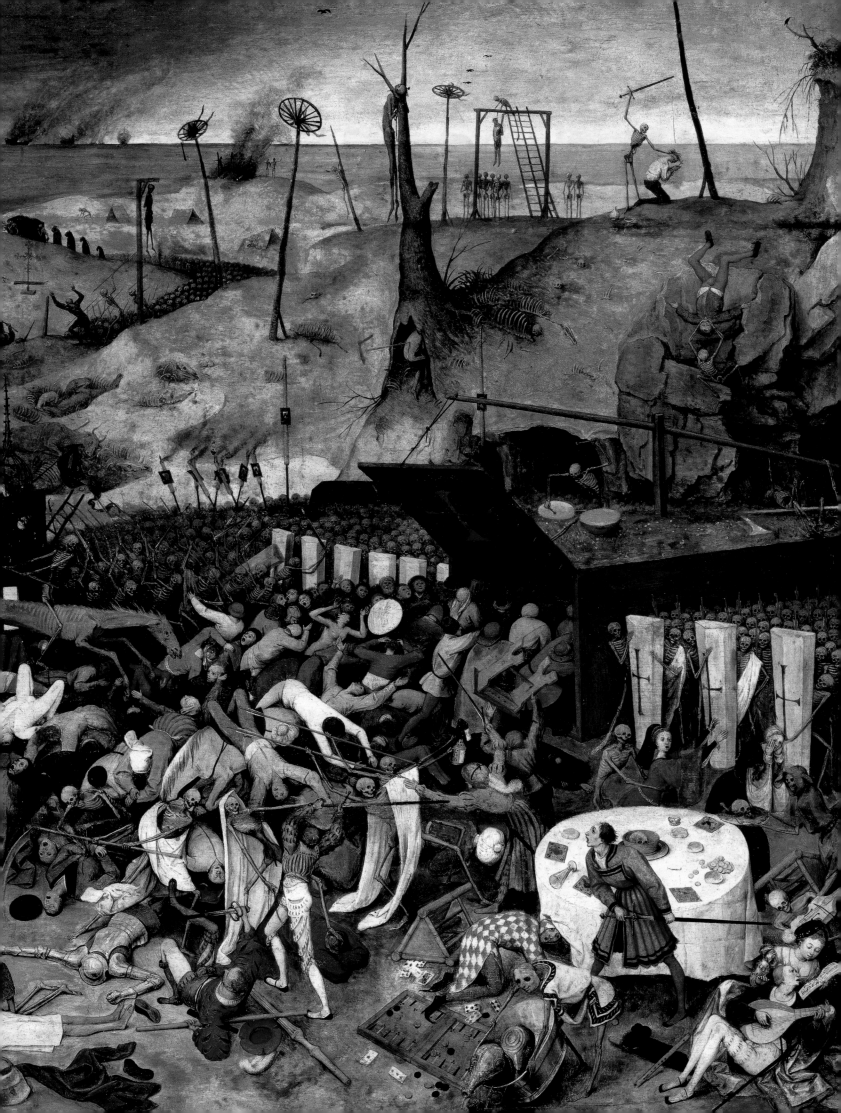

when infected sailors traveled to Sicily from China aboard Italian merchant ships returning from the Black Sea. The disease spread rapidly, and before the year was out, the plague had reached England with disastrous consequences. According to Italian novelist Giovanni Boccaccio (1313–1375) in his *Decameron,* those unfortunate enough to get The Black Death "ate lunch with their friends and dinner with their ancestors in paradise." The Venetians fought the epidemic by keeping out ships carrying the plague, the English lit coal fires and killed all the dogs, and the French and Italians fumigated the air with perfume, but no one paid attention to the rats with their infected fleas.

Boccacco commented on the European epidemic:

I say, then, that the years of the beatific incarnation of the Son of God had reached the tale of one thousand three hundred and forty eight, when in the illustrious city of Florence, the fairest of all the cities of Italy, here made its appearance that deadly pestilence, which, whether disseminated by the influence of the celestial bodies, or sent upon us mortals by God in His just wrath by way of retribution for our iniquities, had had its origin some years before in the East, whence, after destroying an innumerable multitude of living beings, it had propagated itself without respite from place to place, and so calamitously, had spread into the West. . . .

. . . in men and women alike it first betrayed itself by the emergence of certain tumors in the groin or the armpits, some of which grew as large as a common apple, others as an egg, some more, some less, which the common folk called gavoccioli. From the two said parts of the body this deadly gavocciolo soon began to propagate and spread itself in all directions indifferently; after which the form of the malady began to change, black spots or livid making their appearance in many cases on the arm or thigh or elsewhere, now few and large, then minute and numerous. And as the gavocciolo had been and still were an infallible token of approaching death, such also were these spots on whomsoever they shewed themselves. . . .

Those not infected changed their behavior in many ways in order to avoid a threat they could not recognize and did not understand: They therefore walked abroad, carrying in the hands flowers or fragrant herbs or divers sorts of spices, which they frequently raised to their noses, deeming it an excellent thing thus to comfort the brain with such perfumes, because the air seemed to be everywhere laden and reeking with the stench emitted by the dead and the dying, and the odours of drugs. . . . Tedious were it to recount, how citizen avoided citizen, how among neighbors was scarce found any that shewed fellow-feeling for another, how kinsfolk held aloof, and never met, or but rarely; enough that this sore affliction entered so deep into the minds of men and women, that in the horror thereof brother was forsaken by brother, nephew by uncle, brother by sister, and oftentimes husband by wife: nay, what is more, and scarcely to be believed, fathers and mothers were found to abandon their own children, unattended, unvisited, to their fate, as if they had been strangers. . . . Many died daily or nightly in the public streets; of many others, who died at home, the departure was hardly observed by their neighbors, until the stench of their putrefying bodies carried the tidings. . . .

In his 1961 publication *The Plague and the Fire,* James Leasor ignited an ongoing debate among those interested in folklore history when he suggested that the familiar nursery rhyme *Ring around the Rosie* referred to the 1347 epidemic. He further suggested that those verses may have been sung during the next great outbreak that occurred in England in 1665, an epidemic controlled only after the rats died in the great fire of London the following year. Though purportedly sung for five centuries, it was first published in Kate Greenway's *Mother Goose or The Old Nursery Rhymes* in 1881:

> Ring-a-ring o' roses,
> A pocket full of posies,
> Hush! hush! hush! hush!
> We're all tumbled down.

Many versions of this nursery rhyme remain popular today. The most familiar is probably the following, sung by children while holding hands and dancing in a circle:

> Ring around the rosie
> A pocket full of posies
> Ashes, ashes
> We all fall down.

Ring around the rosie: A maculopapular reddened area developed at the site of the fleabite, and later a rose-colored circular rash presented on the arms and legs.

A pocket full of posies: Physicians believed that the disease spread by air, so they carried flowers (posies) in their pockets when they treated their patients. Many dissolved these flowers in vinegar along with the powder

265. Seventeenth-century watercolor representation of a costume worn by physicians during an outbreak of the plague

of cloves, cinnamon, incense, and perfumed oils. This mixture was then placed in the long noses of masks they wore to protect themselves from contagion, and to hide the offensive odor of death (figure 265).

Ashes, ashes: This might have represented either the remains of corpses burned in mass graves or the darkened skin of those infected. The phrase "A-tishoo! A-tishoo!" is used in the British version and may have referred to the sneezing that attends early flu-like symptoms of the pneumonic form of the disease. Sneezing carried a bad prognosis, and during the sixth-century outbreak of plague, Pope Gregory the Great began the custom of saying "God bless you" to those who sneezed so that they might ultimately go to heaven. Those who were alone when they sneezed would say to themselves "God help me!"

We all fall down: The Black Death was very contagious, the course was short, and the death rate for the untreated was extraordinarily high.

According to Rufus of Ephesus, therapy for the plague included the following: "Care also must be had of the belly, and when there is phlegm in the stomach it must be evacuated by emetics. And when a fulness of blood prevails, a vein should be opened. Purgings also by urine, and otherwise by the whole body, are proper. . . . The following propoma may be used; of aloes, two parts; of ammoniac perfume, two parts; of myrrh, one part; pound these in fragrant wine, and give every day . . . but Galen says, concerning pestilential putrefactions, that to drink Armenian bole, and, in like manner, the theriac from vipers, is of great service. . . ." This therapy, however, was totally ineffective, and patients were driven away from classical medicine as taught by Hippocrates and Galen into the arms of religious leaders who continued to maintain that the disease was a punishment for those who had sinned by straying from church doctrine.

Physicians provided little relief to those suffering from the medical horrors that ravaged much of Europe. Pope Clement VI (1291–1352) was in power during the first great plague of 1347 when he received the following warning from Italian poet Francesco Petrarch:

I know that your bedside is beleaguered by doctors, and naturally this fills me with fear. Their opinions are always conflicting, and he who has nothing new to say suffers the shame of limping behind the others. As Pliny said, in order to make a name for themselves through some novelty, they traffic with our lives. With them—not as with other trades—it is sufficient to be called a physician to be believed to the last word, and yet a physician's lie harbours more danger than any other. Only sweet hope causes us not to think of the situation. They learn their art at our expense, and even our death brings them experience: the physician alone has the right to kill with impunity. Oh, Most Gentle Father, look upon their band as an army of enemies. Remember the warning epitaph which that unfortunate man had inscribed on his tombstone: 'I died of too many physicians.'

In 1348, Pope Clement VI granted absolution for all sins and a direct a path to heaven without first passing through purgatory to all those who traveled to Rome for the Holy Year. Over a million gathered in Rome, bringing with them not only an immense amount in offerings to the church, but the plague as well. Only about ten percent survived to return home, though the Pope remained safe by isolating himself in a room outside of the city at Avignon. The advice to remain there throughout the epidemic had been given to him by his personal physician, the famous Guy de Chauliac, who himself died of the plague.

Malaria

A tiny flea was responsible for the plague epidemics that were one of the greatest scourges of all time, though the true heavyweight in the history of medicine is the mosquito. Malaria derived its name from the words *mal aria* meaning "bad air," and is the oldest and most deadly disease in the history of mankind. There are about three hundred million now infected, and over two million continue to die yearly. Malaria is caused by one of several species of the protozoan *Plasmodium* that is transmitted to man by the female *Anopheles* mosquito. Symptoms include recurrent chills and fever, or "ague," along with anemia, chronic fatigue, and then death.

Malaria started in the warm climate of Africa, and widespread disease may have caused migrations out of that continent to cooler areas less hospitable to the mosquito. Some postulate that adaptations to those new varying conditions may have, in fact, led to the development of different racial features found throughout the world today. The disease might also have been responsible for significant social changes, first in ancient Italy where Roman citizens developed their now famous system of aqueducts as a way of protecting themselves from malaria in foul smelling nearby swamps, then called "Roman airs." The death toll from that disease was enormous, and may have contributed to a destabilized country that fell to outside invaders late in the fifth century. The small *Anopheles* mosquito later played a major role in history when malaria became a serious health problem in the New World, encouraging millions of settlers to migrate westward in order to avoid the characteristic shaking chills and fever of that disease.

Huan del Vego discovered the earliest successful therapy for malaria in 1640 when he used tincture of the cinchona bark, a substance that had been familiar to Peruvian Indians in the treatment of fever for centuries. It was not until the end of the nineteenth century, however, that Charles Laveran, a French army physician working in Algeria, first identified the causative agent and, in 1897, Sir Ronald Ross proved that the Anopheles mosquito was the vector for malaria. Current therapy is effective, though we now await an effective vaccine.

Leprosy

Throughout recorded history, the suffering from leprosy (*Mycobacterium leprae*) has been enormous. The disease was recognized in the Bible (Leviticus 13) where rules regarding the diagnosis and isolation of lepers was outlined in detail:

1. Then the Lord spoke to Moses and to Aaron, saying:
2. When a man has on the skin of his body a swelling or a scab or a bright spot, and it becomes an infection of leprosy on the skin of his body, then he shall be brought to Aaron the priest or to one of his sons the priests.

> 5. The priest shall look at him on the seventh day, and if in his eyes the infection has not changed and the infection has not spread on the skin, then the priest shall isolate him for seven more days.
>
> 6. The priest shall look at him again on the seventh day, and if the infection has faded and the mark has not spread on the

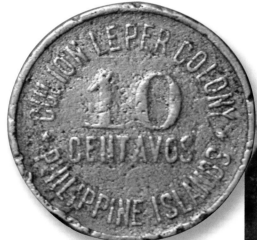

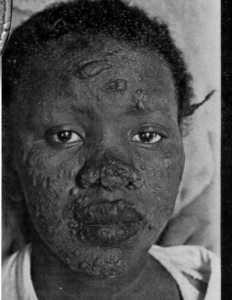
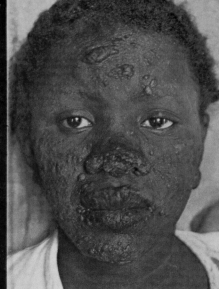

266. Sterioscopic views of leprosy (1910) by S.I. Rainforth, MD

267. Ten centavos coin from the Culion Leper Colony in the Philippine Islands (early twentieth century)

skin, then the priest shall pronounce him clean; it is only a scab. And he shall wash his clothes and be clean.

7. But if the scab spreads farther on the skin after he has shown himself to the priest for his cleansing, he shall appear again to the priest.

8. The priest shall look, and if the scab has spread on the skin, then the priest shall pronounce him unclean; it is leprosy.

45. As for the leper who has the infection, his clothes shall be torn, and the hair on his head shall be uncovered, and he shall cover his mustache and cry, 'Unclean! Unclean!'

46. He shall remain unclean all the days during which he has infection; he is unclean. He shall live alone; his dwelling shall be outside the camp.

Gilbertus Anglicus vividly described the grotesque appearance of a leper in the Middle Ages: "The eyebrows falling bare and getting knotted with uneven tuberosities, the nose and other features becoming thick, course, and lumpy, the face losing its mobility or play of expression, the raucous voice, the loss of sensibility in the hands, and the ultimate break-up of the leprous growths into foul running sores" (figure 266). Leper colonies were constructed to keep those inside isolated (figure 267), and the inhabitants were forced to give others a warning of their arrival by wearing colored clothes with bells, and by sounding leper rattles. In the thirteenth and fourteenth centuries, visitors breathed through cloth soaked in juniper to protect themselves. Lepers adhered to a number of strict regulations that suggested an early appreciation of the principles of communicable disease, though many in the church believed leprosy to be a punishment for immoral behavior:

I forbid you to ever enter Churches, or into a market, or a mill, or a bakehouse, or into any assemblies of people.

Also I forbid you ever to wash your hands or even any of your belongings in spring or stream of water of any kind; and if you are thirsty you must drink water from your cup or some other vessel.

Also I forbid you ever henceforth to go out without your leper's dress, that you may be recognized by others; and you must not go outside your house unshod.

Also I charge you if need require you to pass over some tollway through rough ground, or elsewhere, that you touch no posts or things whereby you cross, till you have first put on your gloves.

Also I forbid you to touch infants or young folks, whosoeve they may be, or to give to them or to others any of your possessions.

Also I forbid you henceforth to eat or drink in any company

except that of Lepers. And know that when you die you will be buried in your own house, unless it be, by favour obtained beforehand, in the Church.

The French Pox

Syphilis (*Treponema pallidua*) was always known to be a contagious disease, though its origin and transmission, like many maladies in the medieval era, were shrouded in mystery. Ulrich von Hutten (1488–1523) wrote the popular *De morbo Gallico* in 1519 and proposed a theory for the genesis of this widespread problem:

> The Physicians have not yet certainly discovered the secret Cause of this Disease, although they have long and diligently enquired after the same. In this all agree, which is very evident, that through some very unwholesome Blasts of the Air, which happened about that time, the Lakes, Fountains, and even the Waters of the Sea were corrupted, and the Earth for a large Tract, as it were poisoned thereby: The Pastures were infected, and venomous, Streams filled the whole Air, which living Creatures took in with their Breath; for this Distemper at first was found among the Cattle as well as among Men.
>
> The *Astrologers* deriving the Cause from the Stars, said, That it proceeded from the Conjunction of *Saturn* and *Mars*, which happened not long before, and of two Eclipses of the Sun; affirming, that hence they perceived were like to ensue many *cholerick* as well as *phlegmatick* Distempers, which would long continue, and slowly depart; such as *Elephantiasis*, *Lepra*, *Impetigo*, and all kinds of Scabs and Boils. . . .

The very name "venereal disease" meant a disease of Venus, giving the condition a divine origin with religious connotations.

Some feel that syphilis originated in the New World and was brought back with Columbus' crew, though the earliest recorded accounts of the disease date back to December 1494 when King Charles VIII sent his French army to Italy in order to conquer the Kingdom of Naples. That year marked the appearance of syphilis throughout all of Italy, and the French called it the Disease of Naples on their return home. The Neapolitans, on the other hand, gave it the name that lasted, the French Disease, because it had appeared for the first time with the French expedition. The name "syphilis" came from the 1530 poem by Girolamo Fracastoro (1478–1553) *Syphilis sive morbus Gallicus* in which Apollo punished the shepherd Syphilis with this disease for his pagan beliefs. Fracastoro, a philosopher, astronomer, and poet, may also be remembered as the first to clearly define infection as the spread of disease by living organisms rather than by their spontaneous generation in inanimate substances. Unfortunately, it took hundreds of years before his proposal was fully accepted by the medical community.

John Astruc was the physician to Louis XIV (1638–1715), and his objection to contemporary "theories" of contagion is now laughable:

> There are some, however, whom I forbear now to spend Time in imputing, such as Augustus Haupman and Christian Languis, who think that the Venereal Poison is nothing else but numerous School of little nimble, brisk invisible living things, of a very prolific Nature, which when once admitted, increase, and multiply in Abundance; which lead frequent Colonies to different Parts of the Body; and inflame, erode, and exulcerate the Parts they fix on; . . . in short, which without any Regard had to the particular Quality of any Humour, occasion all the Symptoms that occur in the Venereal Disease. But as these are mere visionary Imaginations, unsupported by any Authority, they do not require any Argument to invalidate them . . . if it was once admitted, that the Venereal Disease could be produc'd by invisible living things swimming in the Blood, one might with equal Reason alledge the same Thing, not only of the Plague, as Athanasius Kircher, the Jesuit, formerely, and John Saguens, a Minim, lately have done, but also in the small-pox, Hydrophobia, Itch, Tetters, and other contagious Diseases, and indeed of all Distempers whatsoever; and thus the whole Theory of Medicine would fall to the Ground, as nothing could be said to prove the Venereal Disease depending upon little things which might not be urged to prove that all other Diseases were derived from the like little living things though of a different Species, than which nothing can be more absurd.

Ulrich von Hutten accurately described the venereal nature of syphilis and warned: "In Women the Disease resteth in their secret Places, wherein are little pretty Sores, full of venomous Poison, being very dangerous for such as unknowingly meddle with them; the which Sickness, when contracted from these infected Women, is so much the more grievous, by how much they are much more inwardly corrupted and polluted therewith. . . . After this there will appear small Holes and Sores, turning *cankerous and fistulous*, which the more putrid they grow, the more they will eat into the Bones, and when they have been long corrupted the Sick grows lean, his Flesh wasting away, so that there remaineth only the Skin as a Cover for them: and by this many fall into Consumptions, having their inward Parts corrupted . . ." (figure 268).

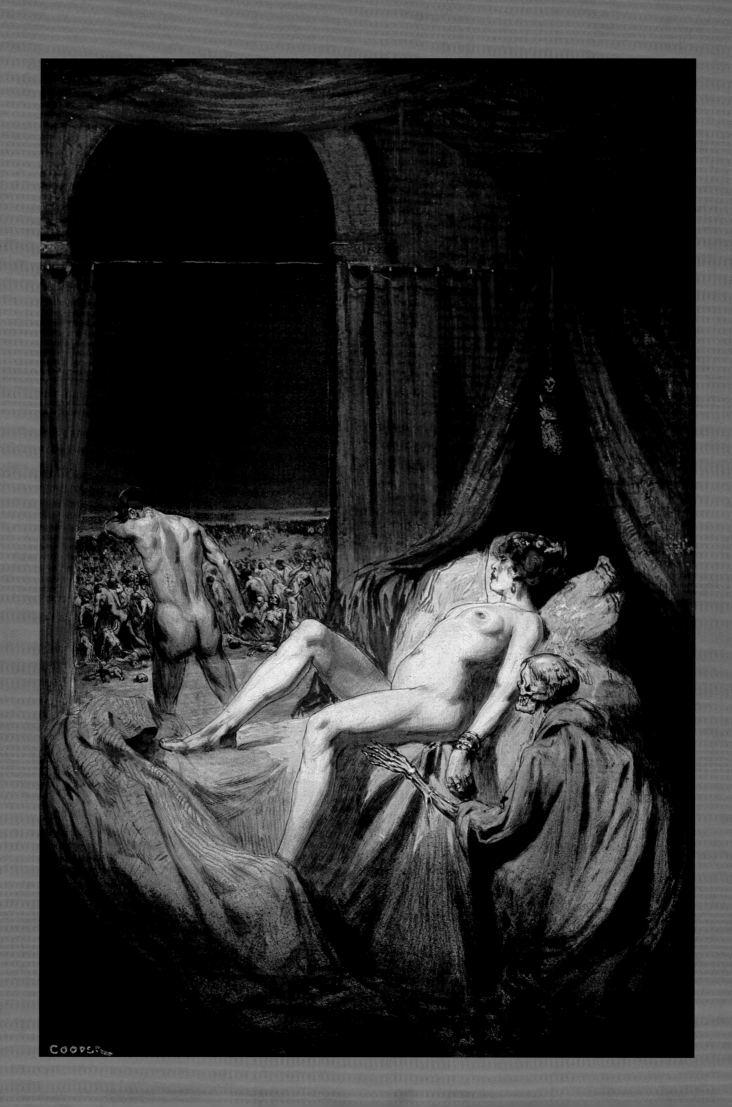

acastoro described syphilis and its consequences in *De contagione
ugiosis morbis* (1546):

> e affected were sad, weary, and cast-down; they were pale;
> f them had sores on the genital organs, ulcers similar to
those which are wont to develop themselves on those organs
after coition, and which are called caries, but of a very different
nature; they were obstinate. When they were cured in one place,
they appeared in another, and the treatment had to be recom-
menced. Afterwards, pustules arose on the skin, covered with a
crust; in some they appeared upon the head, which was the most
frequent place; in others they appeared elsewhere. At first they
were small; afterwards they increased to the size of an acorn,
which they resembled in shape, their appearance otherwise being
similar to the crusta lactea of children. In some cases these pustules were small and dry. In others they were large and moist; in
some livid; in others whitish and rather pale; in others hard and
reddish. They always broke in a few days, and constantly discharged an incredible quantity of stinking matter as soon as
open; they were so many true phagedaenic ulcers, which
destroyed not only the flesh, but even the bones. Those attacked
in the upper parts of the body suffered from malignant affec-
tions, which eat away sometimes the palate, sometimes the
fauces, sometimes the larynx, sometimes the tonsils; some lost
the lips, others the nose, others all the genital organs. Many had
gummy tumors of the limbs, which disfigured them, and were
often of the size of an egg, or of a small loaf; when they broke, a
kind of white mucilaginous fluid flowed from them. They
attacked chiefly the arms and legs; sometimes they remained cal-
lous until death.

But, as if all this were not sufficient, there ensued, moreover,
severe pains in the limbs, often at the same time with the pustules; sometimes before, sometimes after them. These pains,
which were persistent and unbearable, were chiefly felt in the
night, and were seated in the limbs themselves; and in the nerves
rather than in the joints; some, however, had pustules without
the pains, others pains without the pustules; most had both pustules and pains. However, all the limbs were in a languid condition; the patients were wan and emaciated, without appetite,
sleepless, always melancholy and ill-humored, and anxious to
remain in bed. Their faces and legs swelled, and a slow fever
sometimes supervened, but rarely. Some suffered pains in the
head, which were persistent, and did not yield to any remedy. If

268. Oposite. *The Tragedy of Syphilis*
(ca. 1910), watercolor by Richard
Tennant Cooper

269. Sterioscopic views of syphilis
(1910) by S.I. Rainforth, MD

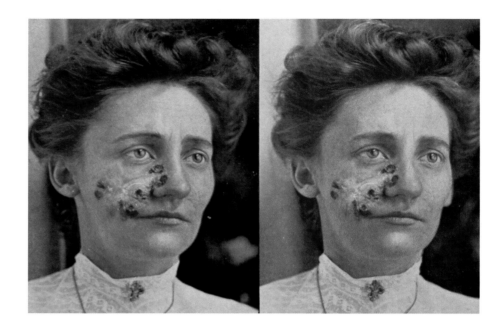

blood was drawn, it was found to be pure, and somewhat
mucous; the urine was thick and red; by this sign alone, super-
vening in the absence of fever, the disease might be recognized;
the stools were liquid and mucous. . . .

A circumstance which has astonished everybody is the falling
off of the hair of the head and other parts of the body, which
produces a ridiculous appearance; some have no beard, some no
eyebrows, some are bald. At first these results were attributed to
the remedies, especially to mercury. Now it is still worse: in
many the teeth become loose and in many they even fall out.
(figure 269).

270. Daguerreotype of a child with
congenital syphilis (ca. 1880)

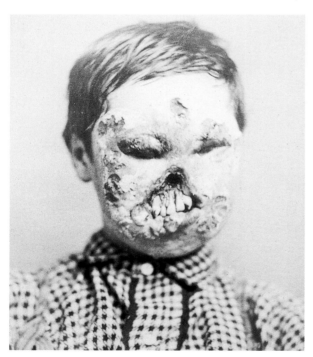

Prior to the antibiotic era, congenital syphilis was devastating to the young since it not only affected the skin and
teeth, but exposure resulted in the loss of vision and hearing. Ironically, these last two consequences of the disease
may have been fortunate to some patients because of their
tragic appearance (figure 270). Jonathan Hutchinson,
FRCS, who was one of the leading medical professors in
London at the time, wrote the following case report in *A
Clinical Memoir on Certain Diseases of the Eye and Ear, consequent on Inherited Syphilis* (1863). It is the typical description
of a child suffering from congenital syphilis:

Case XXXVIII—
Elizabeth H., aged 15, a patient at the City Hospital for
Diseases of the Chest in 1852. The eldest of three, the oth
ers reported healthy, but liable to eruptions. Father, a dis-

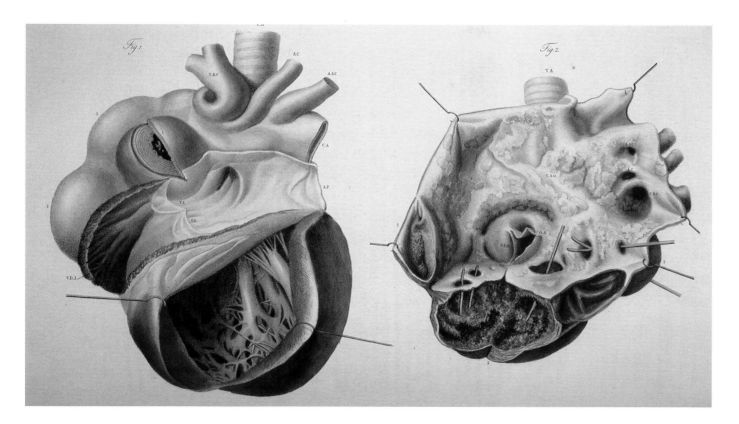

solute man, much subject to scaly eruption and sore throats. Although born healthy, the child, at the age of three weeks and from that to a year, suffered from severe snuffles; she also had the "thrush" badly. After that, however, until the age of five was a stout, healthy-looking child. The eyes then inflamed and soon afterwards the throat ulcerated, and subsequently she became deaf.

She was a puny girl of most marked syphilitic aspect. There was active ulceration of the posterior pharynx and pillars of the fauces, whilst the uvula and large part of the soft paate had already been destroyed. She was quite deaf, and suffered also from aphonia, with laryngeal whistling during cough.

Although the disease had commenced ten years ago the corneae were still so hazy that the irides could not be distinctly seen. The pupils, however, appeared to be partially adherent, and the iris structure thinned and slate-coloured.

The girl remained under Dr. Risdon Bennett's treatment for some months on account of her throat, and derived great benefits form mercurial fumigations and the administration of the iodides with tonics. No material change took place in the state of the eyes whilst she remained under my observation.

One of the manifestations of late, or tertiary, syphilis is the weakening of the thoracic aorta and the subsequent development of an aneurism (figure 271). This condition is rarely seen today because of easily available

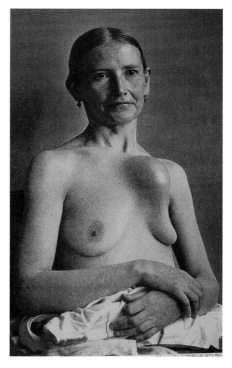

271. Aortic aneurism from *Anatomia Pathologique du corps Humain,* book 1 (1829–1835) by J. Cruveilhier

272. Heliotype of a syphilic aortic aneurism (1894) by Dr. H. Cruschmann

antibiotics that are effective against the spirochete, and this sort of aneurism is now surgically correctible. However, a syphilitic thoracic aortic aneurism was not a rare problem prior to the twentieth century, and the condition was not only frightening but always fatal. It would be difficult to imagine suffering from that disorder and feeling the pounding pulse almost every second, twenty-four hours a day, anticipating that inevitable final heart beat when a rupture would be fatal (figure 272).

Joannis Lancisii graphically described two cases of syphilitic aortic aneurysm in his *De Motu Cordis et Aneurysmatibus* (1745), the first illustrating the symptoms of untreated syphilis and the second an example of the debate that often took place regarding the need for surgical intervention. The differential diagnosis between an abscess and an aortic aneurysm was extremely important since surgery in the former was often curative, and was fatal in the latter.

> *Case 1.* A man over forty, corpulent, complexion swarthy, temperament melancholic and studious, disposed to gluttony, intemperate in the consumption of wine and acrid food of every kind . . . he was attacked by pricking pains in the chest, now here, now there, and palpitations over almost the whole body; then, in the following month he was afflicted with the most cruel pains in the right side of the thorax between the fourth and fifth ribs near the sternum, and although the torturing pains were not constantly present, yet they often distressed him seriously with the sensation of a sort of spasm. Next a buried pulsation became perceptible to the touch also; presently, difficulty of respiration supervened and finally the part affected became prominent as a tumor. Moreover, in the first stage of the disease the patient used to be able to lie on either side, though later it cost him considerable trouble to find the least painful position for lying down.
>
> But an indication that he would die soon was that, two days before, all the pains ceased; and the signs that he was dying were fainting fits, strangulation, asphyxia, and a noise that was heard even by those present, just as though a liquid was strained and pouring out within the thorax. . . .
>
> *Case 2.* His Eminence Cardinal Albani, now happily reigning as Pontifex Maximus, our most clement Pope, had as controller of his footmen a man named Plinio, healthy and strong, aged about 45, of square and stocky build. . . . Now since a rumor of this had been wafted to the ears of that Most Eminent Cardinal, he, with his usual innate and remarkable benevolence, urged me to examine the man. I therefore met in consultation two surgeons, one of whom gave the opinion that the disease was a deep-seated

abscess, the other that it was an aneurysm buried deep in the aorta. And since I myself had noted that the pulsation corresponded with the heartbeats and by its great pressure was driving the ribs outward, I did not hesitate to confirm at once the opinion of the surgeon who asserted that a genuine aneurysm of great size was concealed in the arch of the aorta. In fact, in the space of a few months (when the fluids also had been vitiated), his condition reached the point when no medicine gave any relief, but the ribs were eroded and pushed up till the spine was almost gibbous; moreover, a stretching and tearing pain extended as far as the shoulders. It was then that an extremely rash empirical quack, arguing from the fact that the violence of the pulsation had decreased and supposing that it was a buried abscess that lay concealed, without the knowledge of the wretched patient's friends and relatives, persuaded him to let himself be cut open at the spot, and promised for certain that the pus enclosed within would at once burst forth and the man would be snatched from the jaws of impending death. The time came for the terrible deed; but alas, to our grief, the stream of blood that was kept in bounds by the very weak wall of its thin covering, when that wall was cut through by that unskillful and cruel knife, at once burst out of its bed with such speed that it snatched away with it the soul from the body. So to the great terror of the empiric and as a warning to surgeons, the unhappy patient fell lifeless, the victim of a barbarous carelessness.

More than anyone, physicians appreciated the importance of properly differentiating an abscess from an aneurism. On March 10, 1858, Oliver Wendell Holmes, MD, delivered the valedictory address to the medical graduates of Harvard University. He said, "Sooner or later, everybody is tripped up in forming a diagnosis. I saw Velpeau tie one of the carotid arteries for a supposed aneurism, which was only a harmless tumor, and killed the patient. Mr. Dease of Dublin was more fortunate in a case which he boldly declared an abscess, while others thought it an aneurism. He thrust a lancet into it and proved himself in the right. Soon after, he made a similar diagnosis. He thrust in his lancet as before, and out gushed the patient's blood and his life with it. The next morning Mr. Dease was found dead and floating in his own blood. He had divided the femoral artery. . . . Be very careful; be very slow; be very modest in the presence of nature."

Syphilis spread rapidly, and in view of the devastating physical and social consequences, the search for an effective treatment proceeded with some urgency, though only by trial and error. Von Hutten listed a number of therapeutic options in the early sixteenth century: coral, burnt salt, rust of iron, turpentine, hogs-lard, goats and deer's suet, and red worms dried to powder. "With these, fewer or more, they anointed the sick Man's Joints, his Arms, Thighs, his Neck and Back, with other parts of his Body. . . ." An ancient remedy for scabes (an itchy skin disorder caused by mites) containing mercury was finally found to be effective against syphilis, and, in 1519, Ulrich Von Hutten recognized that fact: "Whilst the Physicians were thus confounded like Men amazed, the Surgeons as wretchedly lent a helping Hand to the same Error, and first began to burn the Sores with hot irons. But for as much, as there seemed no end to this Cruelty, they endeavoured now to avoid the same with their *Ointments*, but all in vain, unless they added *Quick-Silver* thereunto." Mercury was called "quicksilver" because of its appearance, and though somewhat helpful, a number of unpleasant side effects accompanied its use, including sweating, salivation, kidney failure, nerve damage, and behavioral changes. However, physicians continued to use mercury and mercury containing compounds for centuries; it was sometimes said that an hour with Venus led to a lifetime with mercury.

Heat was also a popular treatment, and patients were often exposed to mercury in the form of fumes containing powdered cinnabar. Von Hutten went on to describe this brutal therapy:

> The patient was shut up in a hot room which was steadily and most vigorously heated, some for twenty days, some for thirty, some for more; they anointed him and placed him on a bed laid in the hot room and with many covers over him forced him to sweat. The patient after being anointed barely the second time began to grow weak in remarkable fashion; such was the violent effect of the ointment that it forced the disease which had been on the surface of the body into the stomach; thence it rose to the brain and thence flowed through the throat and mouth to such an extent and with such violent injury that the teeth fell out in the case of those who had not cared well for their mouths; at the least in all cases the throat, tongue, and palate were ulcerated, the guts swelled, the teeth were loosened, sputum flowed without intermission through the lips with more stench than that of any foul matter and with such power of contagion that whatever it touched it immediately befouled and contaminated; whence the lips so touched contracted sores and the cheeks inside were infected. The whole house round about stunk and this type of treatment was so hard that many preferred to die of the disease rather than be cured in this way. . . . I have seen many perish in the midst of the treatment and I knew a certain man practicing

this method who wretchedly murdered three farmers whom he had shut up in an overheated hot room and who in their eagerness for the health which they had hoped they would get stood it more patiently than they should have until their hearts failed to such an extent through the violence of the heat that they did not know they were dying. I have seen others suffocate when their throats swelled so up to their jaws that there was no way out first for the poison which should have been thrown off in sputum and then even for the breath itself; some I have seen die because they could not urinate: altogether a few recovered, and these with such danger, such suffering, such misfortunes.

Syphilis was a fairly common disease, and those infected included the famous and influential from all walks of life: Christopher Columbus, Captain James Cook, Schubert, Beethoven, Gauguin, Goya, Keats, Goethe, Baudelaire, Dumas, Joyce, Wilde, Schopenhauer, Nietzsche, Peter the Great, Henry VIII, Mary Tudor, Napoleon, Pope Julius II, and Pope Alexander Borgia.

Consumption

Tuberculosis (*Mycobacterium tuberculosis*) was sometimes called "phthisis" though the more common name was "consumption" because the disease consumed its victims, leaving them weakened and pale before taking their lives. It is an ancient communicable disease of the respiratory tract that wreaked havoc on the lives of countless millions throughout history. Tuberculosis has been documented in the remains of a resident of Heidelberg ca. 5000 B.C., and evidence of the disease has been found in the bones of Egyptian mummies. The cause of consumption was unknown, though Greek and Roman physicians, including Hippocrates, suggested that individuals who were tall and fair had a special proclivity toward tuberculosis and its transmission, setting the stage for a bias against those from Scandinavian countries that lasted into the nineteenth century.

Dr. Thomas Sydenham (1624–1689) is sometimes referred to as the "English Hippocrates" and is considered by many to be the first great modern physician because of his attention to bedside manner and his detailed classification of diseases. Sydenham described tuberculosis in the following way: "The cough betrays itself, the phthisis comes in between the eighteenth and thirty-fifth years. The whole body becomes emaciated. There is a troublesome, hectic cough which is increased by taking food and which is distinguished by the quickness of the pulse, and the redness of the cheeks. The matter spit up by the cough is bloody or purulent. When burnt it smells fetid. When thrown into water it sinks. Night sweats supervene. At length the cheeks grow hard, the face pale, the nose sharp. The temples sink, the nails curve inward, the hair falls off, there is colloquitative diarrhoea, the forerunner of death."

Though primarily introduced by way of the respiratory tract, the disease sometimes spreads through the blood stream to the spinal column where it is referred to as Pott's Disease, first described in the eighteenth century by Percival Pott (1713–1788). The architecture of the vertebral bodies erodes, eventually leading to collapse and death from respiratory failure. Tuberculosis in the past was largely untreatable, and the consequences of Pott's Disease were devastating (figure 273).

On occasion, tuberculosis also presented as enlarged draining lymph nodes in the neck, that syndrome called scrofula after swine that were supposedly afflicted with the same disease. Another commonly used early term for this presentation was *morbus regius* ("the king's evil"), and those infected were purportedly cured by a king when he touched them with a newly minted gold coin bearing an image of an angel. That coin was then worn around the neck as a sign of healing and for future protection (figure 274). The first to perform the "king's touch" was Clovis in France in 494, though it was Edward the Confessor who established the tradition in 1045. A doctor refers to scrofula in Shakespeare's *Macbeth* (act 4, scene 3):

273. Daguerreotype of a patient with Pott's Disease (ca. 1879)

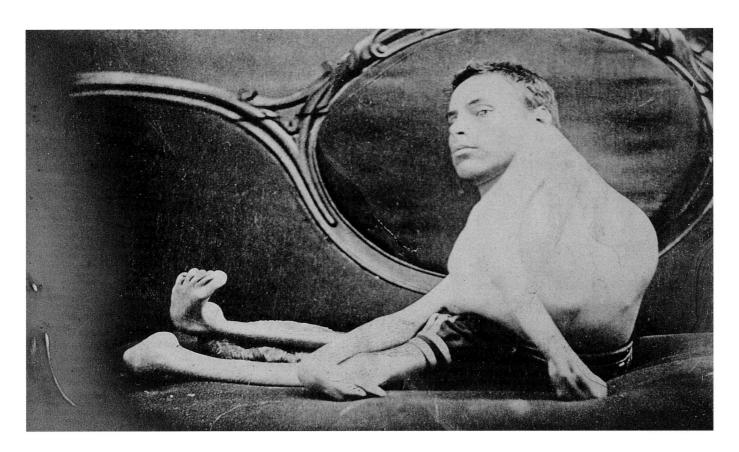

Malcolm Comes the King forth, I pray you?

Doctor Ay, sir. There are a crew of wretched souls
that stay his cure. Their malady convinces the
greatest essay of art, but at his touch, such
sanctity hath heaven given his hand.
They presently amend.

Malcolm Thank you, doctor.

Doctor exits.

Macduff What's the disease he means?

Malcolm 'Tis called the evil:
A most miraculous work in this good king,
which often since my here remain in England, I
have seen him do.
How he solicits heaven, himself best knows:
but strangely visited people, all swollen and
ulcerous, pitiful to the eye,
the mere despair of surgery, he cures,
hanging a golden stamp around their necks,
put on with holy prayers; and 'tis spoken,
to the succeeding royalty he leaves
the healing benediction.

Richard Wiseman (1620–1676), a famous seventeenth-century
English surgeon, said "I myself have been a frequent eye-witness
of many hundreds of cures performed by his majesty's touch
alone, without any assistance of chirurgery; and those, many of
them, such as had tired out the endeavors of able chirurgeons
before they came thither. . . . I must needs profess that what I
write will do little more than show the weakness of our ability
when compared with his majesty's, who cureth more in any one
year than all the chirurgeons of London have done in an age." The
tradition obviously had no merit, though Charles II touched 6,725 in
1660 and a total of 90,000 during his reign.

The following is a description from *Memoires of Evelyn*:

6 July, 1660. His majestie began first to touch for ye evil, according to costome, thus: his majestie sitting under his state in ye
banqueting house, the chirurgeons cause the sick to be brought
or led up to the throne, where they kneeling, ye king strokes
their faces or cheekes with both his hands at once, at which
instant a chaplaine in his formalities says, 'He put his hands
upon them and he healed them.' This is said to every one in particular. When they have ben all thouch'd they come up againe in
the same order, and the other chaplaine kneeling, and having

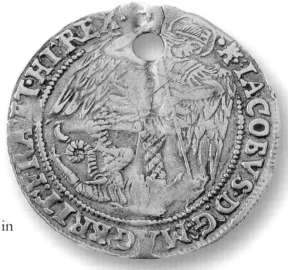

274. English Jacobean touch piece
issued by James I (1603–1625)

angel gold strung on a white ribbon on his arme, delivers them one by one to his majesty, who puts them about the necks of the touched as they passe whilst the first chaplaine repeats. 'That is ye true light who came into ye world.' Then follows an epistle (as at first a gospell) with the liturgy, prayers for the sick, with some alteration; lastly, ye blessing; and then the lo. chamberlaine and comptroller of the household bring a basin, ewer and towel, for his majesty to wash.

The demand for these cures was high, and Evelyn reported four years later, "There was so greate a concourse of people with their children to be touch'd for the evil, that six or seven were crush'd to death by pressing at the chirurgeon's doore for tickets."

Eighteenth-century monarch William III of Orange made the following statement as he touched a scrofula victim: "May God give you better health and more sense." French kings kept up the practice until 1776, and Charles X ended the tradition in 1824.

Physicians tried everything to cure tuberculosis, including incantations, prayer, and any number of bizarre therapies. Nicholas Culpepper said in his *School of Physick* (1659), "For a Cough or Consumption of the Lungs. Take a Cock, and when you have killed him, pull off the feathers while he is hot, then presently cut him through the back with a sharp knife, pull out all the bowels, and wipe him clean with a cloth, break all the bones, and put him into an Alimbeck, and distil him with a pottle of Sack, and as much red Cows Milk, so will you have an excellent Spirit for a Cough, or Consumption of the Lungs, if you take three or four spoonfuls of it in the morning fasting."

275. Mid nineteenth-century ceramic spittoon

With nineteenth-century industrialization came crowding in ever-enlarging cities, a circumstance that allowed tuberculosis to become a significant cause of death and disability (figure 275). Sufferers were treated as lepers since hospitals refused to admit tuberculosis patients, and those who could find lodgings at all were forced to pay exorbitant rents. Many writers in the eighteenth and nineteenth centuries had this disease, including Henry David Thoreau, Robert Louis Stevenson, D.H. Lawrence, Anton Chekhov, Rousseau, and Goethe. John Keats wrote to his finacée, "On the night I was taken ill—when so violent a rush of blood came to my lung that I felt nearly suffocated—I assure you I felt it possible I might not survive, and at that moment thought of nothing but you."

As might be expected, tuberculosis was portrayed in a great deal of literature at the time, including Charles Dickens' character Little Blossom in *David Copperfield*. Emily Brontë lost three sisters and a brother to tuberculosis, and alluded to consumption in her masterpiece *Wuthering Heights* before succumbing to that disease herself at the age of only thirty. She showed distain for her physicians in *The Valley of the Shadow of Death*: "One came, but that one was an oracle: he delivered a dark saying of which the future was to solve the mystery, wrote some prescriptions, gave some directions—the whole with an air of crushing authority—pocketed his fee, and went. Probably, he knew well enough he could do no good; but didn't like to say so."

The great composer Frédéric Chopin produced a number of memorable nocturnes after being banished to an abandoned island monastery. Unfortunately, his persistent coughing precluded anything more than a cargo ship of pigs for his long-anticipated passage back to Paris, where he died whispering, "The earth is suffocating. . . ." Tuberculosis also found its way into Puccini's *La Bohème* and Verdi's *La Traviata* as characters demonstrated the telltale bloody cough, followed by the ashen complexion, and a gradual deterioration characteristic of the "White Death."

Typhoid Mary

Infectious diseases of the gastrointestinal tract in the form of pain and diarrhea certainly tormented humankind long before recorded history, and one of the most significant organisms continues to be *Salmonella typhosa*, the culprit behind typhoid fever. This is one among many strains of the *Salmonella* bacterium, and is a cause of dysentery that has resulted in the death of millions who lived close together in unsanitary conditions or consumed contaminated food and water.

Large armies battling in close quarters frequently fought in miserable conditions, and typhoid was often the result of drinking and bathing downstream from communities that had used that water to carry away their waste material. During the Battle of Crécy in 1346, French bowmen laid in wait as thousands of British soldiers suffering from "the campaign

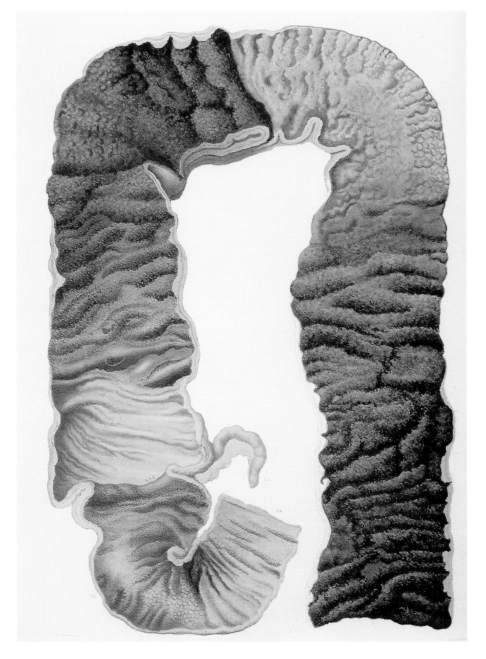

276. Dysentery from *Anatomia Pathologique du corps Humain*, book 2 (1835–1842) by J. Cruveilhier

disease" squatted down with their drawers around their ankles. More than 80,000 northern soldiers died in the American Civil War from typhoid fever and dysentery, almost the same number that died on the battlefield or later from their wounds (figure 276). The death toll was equally remarkable for the British during the Boer War of 1899–1901 when over 11,000 died from typhoid fever in South Africa, which was more than double the number of battle casualties.

Salmonella typhosa usually presents with gastroenteritis, though may also cause heart failure, pneumonia, or meningitis, and may involve almost any organ with a mortality rate of up to ten percent for those infected (figure 277). Unbeknownst to physicians in the early twentieth century, the organisms may reside in the gallbladder of a totally asymptomatic carrier, though may spread to others by way of stool. The most memorable example of this phenomenon in the history of medicine involved Mary Mallon, an Irish immigrant who had come to the United States in 1884 at the age of fifteen to work as a cook. Beginning in 1900, she left a deadly trail of typhoid fever throughout the eastern part of the country, never cooperating with authorities because she never accepted any responsibility for the epidemic she spread. Mallon was a cook for only a short time in Mamaroneck, New York, when the first outbreak was noted, soon followed by another in a Manhattan townhouse. Eight

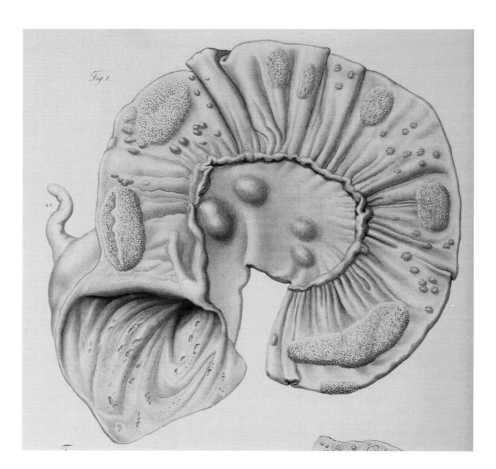

277. Follicular form of typhoid from *Anatomia Pathologique du corps Humain,* book 2 (1835–1842) by J. Cruveilhier

members of the next home became ill, then on to Sands Point, Long Island, in 1904 where several family members were hospitalized with the sweats and diarrhea of typhoid fever. The dutiful cook moved on after each outbreak to another unassuming family, only to witness a similar outbreak.

In the summer of 1906, New York banker Charles Henry Warren rented a home from George Thompson in Oyster Bay, Long Island. To their misfortune, they had hired Mary Mallon as their cook, and soon after on August 27, one of Warren's daughters contracted typhoid fever, followed by his wife, two maids, the gardener, and then another daughter (figure 278). The suspected etiology of the outbreak was either food or impure sources of water, and Thompson hired investigators to find the cause so that his property would be safe for future summer rentals. After an unsuccessful search, Thompson turned to George Soper, who was a civil engineer with experience investigating similar outbreaks.

Soper noted that all incidents seemed to be related to the employment history of a middle-aged, graying, heavy-set Irish cook who, in March 1907, had been working in the home of Walter Bowen. Typhoid fever was already active in the house, having taken the life of the family's daughter. Soper caught up with Mallon in the family's kitchen, and on his first encounter, "I was diplomatic as possible, but I had to say I suspected her of making people sick and that I wanted specimens of her urine, feces, and blood. It did not take Mary long to react to this suggestion. She seized a carving fork and advanced in my direction. I passed rapidly down the long narrow hall, through the tall iron gate . . . and so to the sidewalk. I felt rather lucky to escape." Soper followed Mallon to her home and again was angrily rebuffed, so he returned to the New York City Health Department to consider a different approach. Officials sent Dr. S. Josephine Baker to talk some sense into Mallon, though Baker met with the same fate as Soper. Determined to get her specimens, she returned with five police officers and an ambulance. Mallon was not at all intimidated, and after taking a swipe at

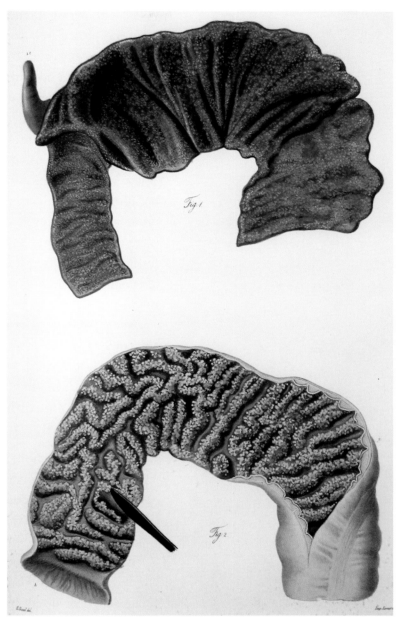

278. Typhoid enteritis from *Anatomia Pathologique du corps Humain*, book 2 (1835–1842) by J. Cruveilhier

Baker with a long kitchen fork, she disappeared for five hours, only to be found hiding in a closet. Baker gave the following description of Mary as she emerged: "She came out fighting and swearing, both of which she could do with appalling efficiency and vigor. I made another effort to talk to her sensibly and asked her again to let me have the specimens, but it was of no use. By that time she was convinced that the law was wantonly persecuting her, when she had done nothing wrong. She knew she had never had typhoid fever; she was maniacal in her integrity. There was nothing I could do but take her with us. The policemen lifted her into the ambulance and I literally sat on her all the way to the hospital; it was like being in a cage with an angry lion." The story was complete when all stool cultures came back positive for typhoid bacilli after testing at the Willard Parker Hospital in New York, and the cook admitted to her disregard for hand washing prior to beginning her work in the kitchen.

What followed was a medico-legal nightmare in that Mallon denied any responsibility for the epidemic and refused to stop her cooking. After much notoriety, "Typhoid Mary" was ultimately confined for three years to the Riverside Hospital on North Brother Island in the East River near the Bronx where she worked in the laundry. She, however, remained outraged:

> I never had typhoid in my life, and have always been healthy. Why should I be banished like a leper and compelled to live in a solitary confinement with only a dog for a companion?
>
> The contention that I am a perpetual menace in the spread of typhoid germs is not true. My own doctors say I have no typhoid germs. I am an innocent human being. I have committed no crime and I am treated like an outcast—a criminal. It is unjust, outrageous, uncivilized. It seems incredible that in a Christian community a defenseless woman can be treated in this manner.

While regularly collected samples were usually positive when tested by health officials, Mallon sent samples to a private lab where they all tested negative. On that basis, she sued the health department for her freedom, though lost and was sent back to her island sanctuary. In February 1910, however, Mallon promised never to cook again when interviewed by a new health commissioner, and she was given her freedom. She took several positions as a domestic, though she was not well paid. Enticed by higher wages in the kitchen and never really believing that she was a danger, Mary Mallon changed her name to Mary Brown and continued her career as a cook. With no great surprise, the deaths from typhoid fever again resumed in New York, and George Soper returned to the case. In 1915, he caught up with Mallon at the Sloan

Hospital for Women where typhoid fever had erupted from out of nowhere, resulting in the death of two of the twenty-five people infected. It was noted that an Irish cook had just departed, and she was arrested while working at a kitchen in Long Island. Having used up all the public goodwill from her first case in court, Mallon was returned to the North Brother Island, where she spent the rest of her life. She did various odd jobs in the hospital there until she suffered a debilitating stroke in 1932 and died six years later after having spent a total of twenty-six years on the island. At autopsy, Mallon's gallbladder was indeed found to be teeming with salmonella bacilli, though she remained incredulous of her role in the suffering and death that surrounded her for all those years.

Puerperal Fever

The development of puerperal, or childbed fever, following delivery was a major risk to the lives of new mothers until the end of the nineteenth century and the discovery of aseptic technique. This condition was probably secondary to a Group A Streptoccal infection, though physicians advanced many theories. For example, three hundred years earlier Hieronymous Mercurialis had suggested that puerperal fever was related to the common observation that some women failed to lactate after delivery. With some logic, though a poor understanding of physiology, he concluded that breast milk became purulent and then collected in the uterus rather than in the breasts.

This disease is as old as recorded medical history, and the following classic account was recorded by Hippocrates in *Greek Medicine* by A.J.Brock (1929):

> Epidemics, Book 1. Case iv.
> In Thasus, the wife of Philinus gave birth of a daughter; the lochial discharge was normal, and everything else was proceeding quietly, when, on the fourteenth day after delivery, she became feverish and had a rigor. There was pain at first in cardiac region of stomach and right abdomen. Pains in genital organs. Lochial discharge stopped. On the application of a pessary these symptoms were alleviated, but pains continued in the head, neck, and loins. No sleep; extremities cold; thirst. Bowels in overheated condition; scanty stools. Urine thin, and at first colourless.
>
> *Sixth Day*. At night she was very delirious; then came to once more.
>
> *Seventh Day*. Thirsty; stools scanty, bilious, high coloured.
>
> *Eighth Day*. Had a rigor; acute fever; many painful spasms; very delirious. On application of a suppository, she rose to stool, and had a copious motion, with bilious flux. No sleep.

Ninth Day. Convulsions.

Tenth Day. Mind slightly clearer again.

Eleventh Day. Slept; complete return of memory, but mind soon wandered again. She passed a large quantity of urine, accompanied by convulsions—her attendants seldom reminding her; this was thick and white, such as one sees when urine with sediment is shaken; but after standing for a long time it formed no sediment: in colour and consistence it resembled the urine of cattle. Such then was the urine which she passed, as I myself saw. On the fourteenth day there was twitching all over the body; much rambling talk; a short lucid interval, then quickly delirium again. On the seventeenth day she became speechless, and on the twentieth she died.

As can be seen in the following description by Alexander Gordon of Aberdeen , Scotland, in *Essays on the Puerperal Fever and Other Diseases Peculiar to Women* (1795), little changed over the next one thousand years:

A circumscribed crimson colour in the cheeks was a symptom which sometimes occurred towards the close of the disease, and was a mortal symptom.

A vomiting of bile, of a green colour, was a symptom which frequently occurred, especially when the patient was costive; and, when there were symptoms of mortification, what the patient vomited was black, and had a strong resemblance to the grounds of coffee.

A diarrhoea was a frequent symptom, and was a symptom rather to be desired than dreaded; for without a spontaneous or artificial diarrhoea, very few recovered. The stools were frothy, and of a yellow, greenish, or dark brown colour; and every discharge by stool seemed to give temporary relief; but, towards the end of the disease, they were frequently involuntary, and sometimes became black and very fetid, resembling moss-water, and were one of the symptoms of internal mortification.

The lochial discharge commonly continued to flow as usual, though in some the discharge was diminished; yet in few or none was it wholly suppressed. In those cases which terminated fatally, the secretion of the milk never took place; and in such as recovered, there was no secretion of it till after the crisis.

Dr. Alexander Gordon was the first to attribute the cause of puerperal fever to a transmissible agent in his book *A Treatise on the Epidemic Puerperal Fever in Aberdeen* (1795). He pointed out that "the cause of Puerperal Fever, of which I treat, was a specific contagion, or infection, altogether unconnected with a noxious constitution of the atmosphere." Gordon was also correct in his recommendations for prevention of the disease when he suggested that "the nurses and physicians, who have attended patients affected with the Puerperal Fever, ought carefully to wash themselves, and to get their apparel properly fumigated, before it be put on again." Gordon's treatment plan, however, missed the mark: "Bleeding and purging are the two great hinges, upon which the cure of the Puerperal Fever turns."

Despite Gordon's earlier work, most give credit to Oliver Wendell Holmes, MD, for his finding in 1843 that microorganisms could be the cause of infectious diseases. He described physicians as going "from bed to bed as rat-killers carrying their poison from one household to another," and he reported his theory in "The Contagiousness of Puerperal Fever" in *The New England Quarterly Journal of Medicine* (1843): "The disease known as Puerperal Fever is so far contagious as to be frequently carried from patient to patient by physicians and nurses. . . . In collecting, enforcing and adding to the evidence accumulated upon this most serious subject, I would not be understood to imply that there exists a doubt in the mind of any well-informed member of the medical profession as to the fact that puerperal fever is sometimes communicated from one person to another, both directly and indirectly." Oliver Wendell Holmes' report was largely overlooked, and, unfortunately, he did not act on his theory. He reminded physicians of their role in the spread of puerperal fever in this often quoted passage:

> It is a lesson rather than as a reproach that I call up the memory of these irreparable errors and wrongs. No tongue can tell the heart-breaking calamity they have caused; they have closed the eyes just opened upon a new world of love and happiness; they have bowed the strength of manhood into the dust; they have cast the helplessness of infancy into the stranger's arms, or bequeathed it with less cruelty the death of its dying parent. There is no tone deep enough for regret, and no voice loud enough for warning. The woman about to become a mother, or with her new-born infant upon her bosom, should be the object of trembling care and sympathy wherever she bears her tender burden, or stretches her aching limbs. The very outcast of the streets has pity upon her sister in degradation when the seal of promised maternity is impressed upon her. The remorseless vengeance of the law, brought down upon its victim by a machinery as sure as destiny, is arrested in its fall at a word which reveals her transient claim for mercy. The solemn prayer of the liturgy singles out her sorrows from the multiplied trials of

life to plead for her in the hour of peril. God forbid that any member of the profession to which she trusts her life, doubly precious at that eventful period, should hazard it negligently, unadvisedly or selfishly!

Ignaz Semmelweis: Medicine's Unsung Hero

Ignas Semmelweis (1818–1865), a Hungarian house officer on an obstetrics ward at the Allgemeines Krankenhaus in Vienna, also recognized the significant role that physicians played in the dissemination of postpartum infection. By clarifying the importance of asepsis, Semmelweis made one of the most important discoveries in the history of medicine.

The Vienna hospital had opened in 1794, though the maternal death rate significantly rose in 1821 when students began to perform their own postmortem examinations. That year, nearly one out of six of the 5,139 women who delivered there died. There were two wards in the obstetrics department at the University of Vienna, and in the First Clinic, students performed physical examinations on their patients immediately after having come from the dissecting room. Professors and students did not wash their hands, and the postpartum death rate was up to thirty

279. Puerperal fever from *Anatomia Pathologique du corps Humain*, book 1 (1829–1835) by J. Cruveilhier

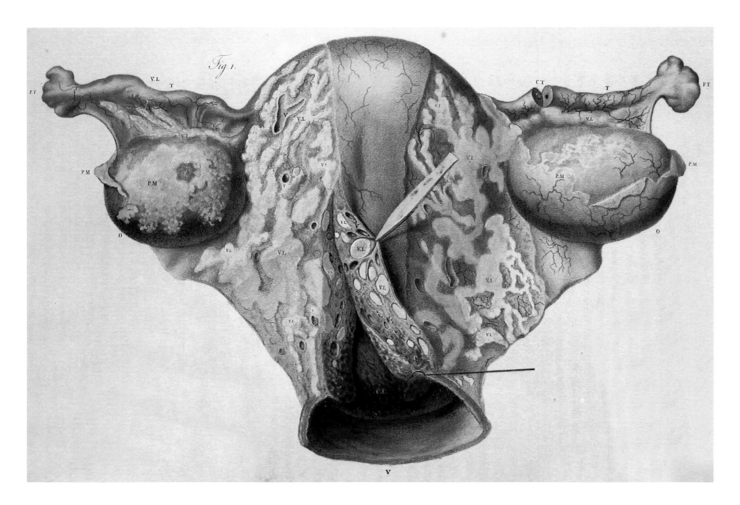

percent at times. This fatal disease was called childbed, or puerperal fever, and developed about four days after delivery, usually presenting with chills, fever, and almost certain death (figure 279). The Second Obstetrical Clinic, on the other hand, was attended by midwives, and the death rate was inexplicably much lower despite the fact that these were "street births" where conditions during delivery outside of the hospital suggested that the mortality rate should have been higher rather than lower.

Professor Jakob Kolletschka had been greatly admired by Semmelweis during his stay at the hospital but unexpectedly died while Semmelweis was away. In his autobiographical introduction to *Die Aetiologie, der Begriff und die Prophylaxis des Kindbettfiebers* (*The Etiology, the Concept, and the Prophylaxis of Childbed Fever*) (1861), Semmelweis presented the case history leading to his important discovery:

Kolletschka, Professor of Forensic Medicine, often conducted autopsies for legal purposes in the company of students. During one such exercise, his finger was pricked by a student with the same knife that was being used in the autopsy. I do not recall which finger was cut. Professor Kolletschka contracted lymphangitis and phlebitis in the upper extremity. Then, while I was still in Venice, he died of bilateral pleurisy, pericarditis, peritonitis, and meningitis. A few days before he died, a metastasis also formed in one eye. I was still animated by the art treasures of Venice, but the news of Kolletschka's death agitated me still more. In this excited condition I could clearly see that the disease from which Kolletschka died was identical to that from which so many maternity patients died.

Earlier, I pointed out that autopsies of the newborn disclosed results identical to those obtained in autopsies of patients dying from childbed fever. I concluded that the newborn died of childbed fever, or in other words, that they died from the same disease as the maternity patients. Since the identical results were found in Kolletschka's autopsy, the inference that Kolletschka died from the same disease was confirmed. The exciting cause of Professor Kolletschka's death was known; it was the wound by the autopsy knife that had been contaminated by cadaverous particles. Not the wound, but contamination of the wound by the cadaverous particles caused the death. Kolletschka was not the first to have died this way. I was forced to admit that if his disease was identical with the disease that killed so many maternity patients, then it must have originated from the same cause that brought it on in Kolletschka. In Kolletschka, the specific causal factor was the cadaverous particles that were introduced into his vascular system. I was compelled to ask whether cadaverous particles had been introduced into the vascular systems of those patients whom I had seen die of this identical disease. I was forced to answer affirmatively.

Because of the anatomical orientation of the Viennese medical school, professors, assistants, and students have frequent opportunity to contact cadavers. Ordinary washing with soap is not sufficient to remove all adhering cadaverous particles. This is proven by the cadaverous smell that the hands retain for a longer or shorter time. In the examination of pregnant or delivering maternity patients, the hands, contaminated with cadaverous particles, are brought into contact with the genitals of these individuals, creating the possibility of absorption. With resorption, the cadaverous particles are introduced into the vascular system of the patient. In this way, maternity patients contract the same disease that was found in Kolletschka.

Suppose cadaverous particles adhering to hands cause the same disease among maternity patients that cadaverous particles adhering to the knife caused in Kolletschka. Then if those particles are destroyed chemically, so that in examinations patients are touched by fingers but not by cadaverous particles, the disease must be reduced. This seemed all the more likely, since I knew that when decomposing material is brought into contact with living organisms it may bring on decomposition.

In May 1847, Semmelweis tested his theory by washing his hands with chloride of lime prior to all examinations and by requiring his students to do the same. The mortality rate from puerperal fever dropped precipitously from an average of eighteen to only one percent in the First Clinic. That year, a woman with an infected uterine carcinoma was placed on a ward with twelve others and, despite hand washing at the beginning of the examinations, eleven of twelve patients on that ward died of puerperal fever, leading Simmelweiss to the conclusion that the "poisonous material" could be transferred from both the living and the dead. He then required hand washing between patient examinations, and once again the death rate from puerperal fever plummeted.

Despite these landmark discoveries, the chief of obstetrics at the hospital, Professor Johan Klein, refused to accept the facts before him and denied Semmelweis reappointment to the medical staff in 1849. Semmelweis found himself in an atmosphere of professional jealousy and resentment, and was removed from direct patient care, having to teach obstetrics using only manikins. He had no choice but to leave Vienna, and took up a position at the University of Budapest, where he became a professor of obstetrics. He essentially eliminated puerperal sepsis in maternity wards at the old hospital of St. Roch in Budapest by requiring that the hands of treating doctors and nurses be disinfected prior to patient contact. Additionally, all bed linens and dressings were to be cleaned on a regular basis.

While in Budapest, Semmelweis published his landmark work, *Die Aetiologie, der Begriff und die Prophylaxis des Kindbettfiebers,* though it was poorly written and largely ignored. He made few friends because his personality was abrasive and accusatory. For example, Semmelweis wrote the following "open letter" on June 25, 1861: "Your teaching, Herr Hofrath, is based on dead bodies of lying-in women slaughtered through ignorance; and because I have formed the unshakable resolution to put an end to this murderous work as far as lies in my power so to do. . . . I denounce you before God and the world as a murderer, and the History of Puerperal Fever will not do you an injustice when, for the service of having been the first to oppose my life-saving *Lehre* it perpetuates your name as a medical Nero."

Semmwelweis was obviously not a good politician, and he never communicated well in Vienna since his native language was Hungarian. He faced constant battles with his peers and never got the credit he disserved while he was alive. In 1863, Semmelweis was declared insane (by three physicians who were not qualified as psychiatrists), and he was sent to a mental hospital in Vienna, taken there by his wife and a friend. Accounts vary, though some attribute Semmelweis' unusual behavior later in life to an early syphilitic infection that was exacerbated by the disappointment he felt for not having been given credit for his important discovery. While institutionalized, Semmelweis was reportedly beaten by attendants and, ironically, died from an infection that developed as a result of wounds that were inadequately treated.

Immunization: Smallpox, Rabies, and Tetanus

Immunization, or the prevention of a disease by previous exposure to the infecting agent, has been practiced for centuries, even before there was any real understanding of communicable disease. Smallpox, or variola virus, was the first infectious disease to be prevented by immunization, though for thousands of years, it was responsible for the death, disfigurement, and blindness of literally tens of millions in Europe and America (figure 280).

The first to describe smallpox was the great Persian physician Rhazes (Abu Becr Mohammed Ibn Zacariya Ar-Razi) (A.D. 864–930). Rhazes, along with Avicenna, are considered to have been the greatest of all Islamic physicians, and their influence continues to be important in the Muslim medical community today. Rhazes' *Kitab-al-hawi* (*Continens*) is the most extensive work ever written in Arabic, and while he relied on

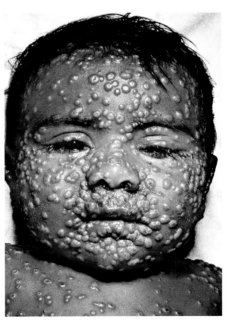

280. Child with smallpox (early twentieth century)

the precepts of Hippocrates and Galen, his diagnostic skills and practical approach to medicine resonated with physicians then the same way that Sir William Osler did a millennium later: "All that is written in books is worth much less than the experience of a wise doctor." Rhazes was the first to diagnose measles and smallpox, and his description of the latter remains a classic: "The eruption of the Small-Pox is preceded by a continued fever, pain in the back, itching in the nose, and terrors in sleep. These are the more peculiar symptoms of its approach, especially a pain in the back, with fever; then also a pricking which the patient feels all over his body; a fullness of the face, which at times goes and comes; an inflamed colour, and vehement redness in both the cheeks; a redness of both the eyes; a heaviness of the whole body; great uneasiness, the symptoms of which are stretching and yawning; a pain in the throat and chest, with a slight difficulty in breathing, and cough; a dryness of the mouth, thick spittle, and hoarseness of the voice; pain and heaviness of the head; inquietude, distress of mind, nausea, and anxiety. . . ."

The rapid conquest of the Aztecs in Mexico by Hernando Cortez in the early sixteenth century was in large part due to the smallpox that he and his men had imported. They exposed an unprotected population and caused the death of over eighteen million people. The religions indigenous to Peru and Mexico vanished quickly as natives converted to Christianity since Cortez' god had appeared to favor the (immunized) Spanish visitors. Members of the ruling classes across the sea, however, were certainly not immune since smallpox also affected Roman Emperor Marcus Aurelius, Charles IX, Louis XIV, Louis XV, William II of Orange, Emperor Joseph I of Germany, Peter II, Emperor of Russia, and Henry, Prince of Prussia.

In 1848, Thomas Macaulay described England in 1694 following the death of a young Queen Mary II from smallpox (*The History of England from the Accession of James II*): ". . . smallpox was always present, filling the churchyards with corpses, tormenting with constant fears all whom it had not yet stricken, leaving on those whose lives it spared the hideous traces of its power, turning the babe into a changeling at which the mother shuddered, and making the eyes and cheeks of the betrothed maiden objects of horror to the lover. Towards the end of 1694 this pestilence was more than usually severe. At length the infection spread to the palace and reached the young and blooming Queen. She received the intimation of her danger with true greatness of soul."

The Indians and Chinese immunized themselves by inhaling ground up smallpox scabs, and early Arabs scratched themselves with infected pustules, a process called "variolation," to ward off the disease. It was well known that milkmaids who had been exposed to the udders of cows infected with cowpox were protected from smallpox. Lady Mary Wortley

Montagu practiced the first Western inoculation in 1717 on her return from Turkey where she had witnessed this prophylactic procedure:

> Apropos of distempers, I am going to tell you a thing that will make you wish yourself here. The smallpox, so fatal, and so general amongst us, is here entirely harmless, by the invention of ingrafting, which is the term they give it. There is a set of old women who make it their business to perform the operation, every autumn, in the month of September, when the great heat is abated. People send to one another to know if any of their family has a mind to have the smallpox: they make parties for this purpose, and when they are met (commonly fifteen or sixteen together) the old woman comes with a nutshell full of the matter of the best sort of smallpox, and asks what veins you please to be opened. She immediately rips open that you offer to her, with a large needle (which gives you no more pain than a common scratch) and puts into the vein as much matter as can lie upon the head of her needle, and after that, binds up the little wound with a hollow bit of shell; and in this manner opens four or five veins. The children or young patients play together the rest of the day and are in perfect health until the eighth day, then fever seizes them and they keep their beds two days, very seldom three. They have rarely about twenty or thirty (pocks) on their faces, which never mark, and in eight days' time they are as well as before their illness.

Despite the long track record of vaccination, the practice was still met with skepticism by many. In 1720, a smallpox epidemic broke out, and the Prince and Princess of Wales were interested in having their two daughters protected, though they wanted to first convince themselves of the procedure's safety. With an offer of a pardon if the procedure went without complication, six prisoners allowed themselves to be variolated. The immunization was a success, though the prince and the princess were only satisfied after several children from an orphanage were similarly vaccinated.

In May 1796, Edward Jenner (1749–1823) took the next important step in making vaccination available to the masses when he removed infectious material from Sarah Nelms, a milkmaid who had been exposed to cowpox, and inoculated the arm of James Phipps (figures 281, 282). With great daring, Jenner vaccinated Phipps on July 1, 1796, and demonstrated that the boy had developed immunity. "On the seventh day, he complained of uneasiness in the axilla, and on the ninth he became a little chilly, lost his appetite, and had a slight headache. During the whole of this day, he was perceptibly indisposed, and spent the night with some degree of restlessness, but on the day following he was perfectly well."

Jenner named his procedure "vaccination" after *vacca* (the Latin word for *cow*). It was extremely controversial at the time since smallpox was a disease that carried a high mortality without a proven prevention or treatment. In 1797, Jenner submitted his findings to the Royal Society, but it was refused for publication with the admonition that Jenner "should be cautious . . . and ought not risk his reputation by presenting to the learned body anything which appeared so much at variance with established knowledge, and withal so incredible." Jenner understood the significance of his findings, though it took years before his discovery was recognized as one of the greatest in the history of medicine. "While the vaccine was progressive, the joy I felt at the prospect before me of being the instrument destined to take away from the world one of its great calamities, blended with the fond hope of enjoying independence and domestic peace and happiness, was often so excessive that, in pursuing my favorite subject in the meadows, I have sometimes found myself in a kind of reverie."

The importance of Jenner's monumental discovery became more apparent to others after his death. In 1847, Dr. James Simpson wrote, "During the long European wars connected with and following the French Revolution, it has been calculated that five or six millions of human lives were lost. In Europe, vaccination has already preserved from death a greater number of human beings than were sacrificed during the course of these wars. The lancet of Jenner has saved far more human lives than the sword of Napoleon destroyed. On these devastating European wars England lavished millions of money and freely bestowed honors, peerages, and heavy annual pensions upon the soldiers who were most successful in fighting their battles and destroying their

281. Cupping horn used by Edward Jenner to carry cowpox-infected material for vaccination

282. Cowpox and the hand of Sarah Nelmes in *An Inquiry into the Causes and Effects of the Variolae Vaccine* (1798) by Edward Jenner

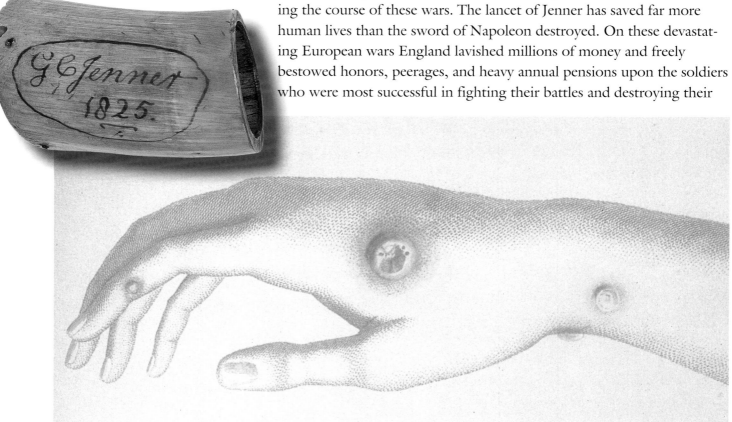

fellow-men. She grudgingly rewarded Jenner with 30,000 pounds for saving 30,000 of her subjects annually." During the Franco-Prussian War of 1870–1871, all members of the Prussian army were required to be immunized against smallpox, while there was no such requirement for French soldiers. It is no coincidence that the French lost the encounter after having suffered 23,400 casualties from smallpox while the death toll to the Prussians was only 297.

With the discovery of vaccination came protection from another previously untreatable disease, rabies. In *Richard III* (act1, scene 3), William Shakespeare wrote:

> Take heed of yonder dog!
> Look, when he fawns, he bites; and when he bites,
> His venom tooth will rankle to the death;
> Have not to do with him, beware of him;
> Sin, death, and hell have set their marks on him.

The following excerpts are from *The Extant Works of Aretaeus, the Cappadocian*, as translated by Francis Adams in 1856 regarding a third infectious disease now tamed by immunization, tetanus, or *Clostridium tetani* (figure 283). The disease was tragic, but Aretaeus (A.D. 120–180) does not fail to note the effects of this condition on the treating physician:

> Tetanus, in all its varieties, is a spasm of an exceedingly painful nature, very swift to prove fatal, but neither easy to be removed. They are affections of the muscles and tendons about the jaws; but the illness is communicated to the whole frame, for all parts are affected sympathetically with the primary organs. . . . Women are more disposed to tetanus than men, because they are of a cold temperament; but they more readily recover . . . whereas old men are most subject to the disease and most apt to die. . . . The face is ruddy and of mixed colours, the eyes almost immovable, or are rolled about with difficulty; strong feeling of suffocation; respiration bad, distension of the arms and legs; subsultus of the muscles; the countenance variously distorted; the cheeks and lips tremulous; the jaw quivering, and the teeth rattling. . . .
>
> Opisthotonos bends the patient backward, like a bow so that the reflected head is lodged between the shoulder-blades; the throat protrudes; the jaw sometimes gapes. . . . Should the mischief then seize the chest and the respiratory organs, it readily frees the patient from life; a blessing this, to himself, as being a deliverance from pains, distortion, and deformity . . . the patient is not only bent up into an arch but rolled together like a ball, so that the heads rests upon the knees, while the legs and back are bent forwards, so as to convey the impression of the articulation

of the knee being dislocated backwards.

An inhuman calamity! an unseemly sight! a spectacle painful to the beholder! an incurable malady! owing to the distortion not to be recognized by the dearest friends; and hence the prayer of the spectators, which formerly would have been reckoned not pious, now becomes good, that the patient may depart from life, as being a deliverance from the pains and unseemly evils attendant on it. But neither can the physician, though present and looking on, furnish any assistance, as regards life, relief from pain or from deformity. For if he should wish to straighten the limbs, he can only do so by cutting and breaking those of a living man. With them, then, who are overpowered by this disease, he can merely sympathise. This is the great misfortune of the physician.

Despite the ease and efficacy of vaccination (figure 284), many refused to accept this simple life-saving procedure, and joined the society of antivaccinationists that had been founded in England in 1812 (figure 285). Many refused to accept what is one of the most important discoveries in the history of medicine and joined the society of antivaccinationists that had been founded in England in 1812. In his youth, Benjamin Franklin had been a strong opponent to protection from smallpox, though his views changed when his son died of that disease in 1736. In his *Autobiography*, Franklin wrote, "A fine boy of four years old, by the smallpox taken in the common way. I long regretted bitterly, and still regret I had not given it to him by inoculation. This I mention for the sake of parents who omit that operation, on the supposition that they

283. *The Anatomy and Philosophy of Expression* (1847) by Charles Bell (tetanus)

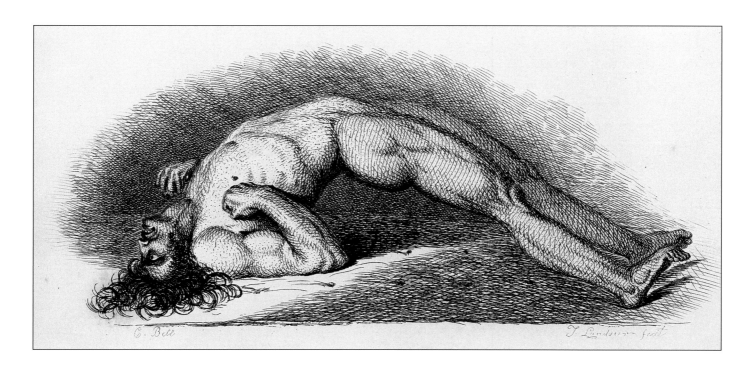

should never forgive themselves, if a child died under it, my example showing that the regret may be the same either way, and therefore that the safer should be chosen."

In opposition, Felix Oswald, MD, wrote the following as the preface to his book *Vaccination A Crime, With Comments on Other Sanitary Superstitions* (1901):

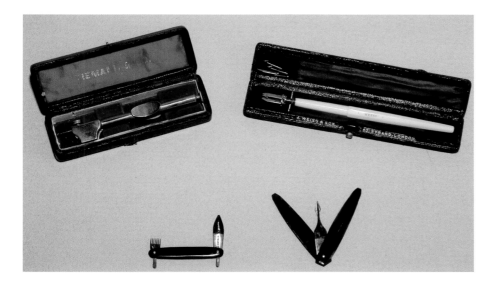

284. Nineteenth-century vaccination needles: (top) Tiemann and Co.'s vaccinating scarificator, vaccinating lancet by Weiss; (bottom) Wier's vaccinating lancet by Tiemann, vaccinating thumb lancet

285. Watercolor etching of Edward Jenner among patients in the Smallpox and Inoculation Hospital at St. Pancras (1802) by James Gillray

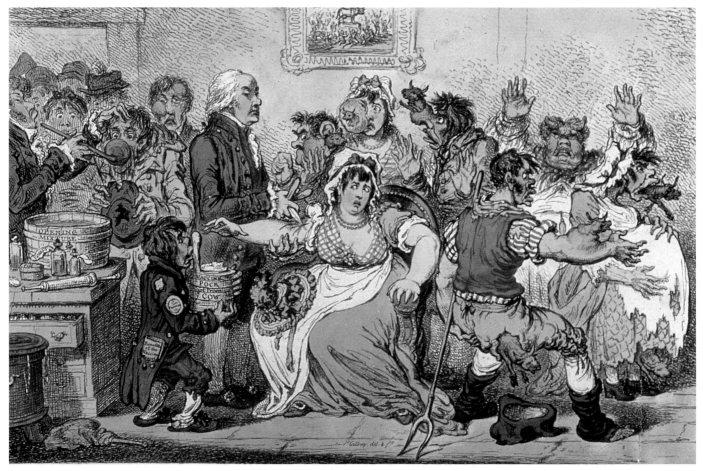

Compulsory vaccination ranks with slavery and religious persecutions as one of the most mischievous outrages upon the rights of the human race.

Vaccination yields fees to lymph-peddlers and baby-slashers. The sophisms of the Jenner doctrine have been so thoroughly exploded that the persistency of its defenders seems to imply a moral, rather than mental aberration; in other words, the collapse of all other supports justifies the suspicion of the hideous fact that the organization of the cowpox syndicate rests upon the deliberate sacrifice of truth to business considerations and corporation interests.

Vaccination has become a crime.

Growth of the Germ Theory

Advances in the understanding of the pathogenesis of infectious disease set the stage for the antibiotic era that followed several decades later. Louis Pasteur (1822-1895) was the first to prove the "theory" that infectious diseases were spread by microscopic organisms when he showed fermentation to be caused by "invisible" living creatures, and that heating those organisms for a few moments could act as a preservative (by "pasteurization"). He also demonstrated that previously immunized sheep could be protected from an exposure to anthrax, and, in 1885, Pasteur developed an attenuated form of the deadly rabies virus which he gave to a young boy who had been bitten by a rabid dog. Pasteur took an almost unimaginable risk in that circumstance since the rabies virus was too small to be seen even under the microscope: "The child's death appeared inevitable. I decided not without acute and harrowing anxiety, as may be imagined, to apply to Joseph Meister the method which I had found consistently successful with dogs." The boy's survival after a daily series of inoculations with rabbit spinal cord suspensions of progressively inactivated rabies virus was Pasteur's first important clinical discovery, and his contributions in the fields of bacteriology and immunology laid a foundation for future significant breakthroughs in many areas of clinical medicine. In 1854, Pasteur made the now famous statement that guided his landmark research: "In the field of observation, chance only favors prepared minds."

Robert Koch (1843-1910) went on to isolate the agents of many age-old deadly diseases, thereby proving the pathogenicity of previously unseen organisms. Some of the more important infections Koch studied were anthrax, tuberculosis, cholera, syphilis, diphtheria, and typhoid. Koch also provided prerequisites for the definition of communicable diseases in his famous four postulates: 1) The organism must be present in all cases of the disease; 2) The organism can be cultured; 3) Inoculation into animals of that cultured organism causes the disease; and 4) The organism can then be removed from the diseased animal and grown in culture. In 1905, Koch's groundbreaking discoveries earned him one of the first Nobel Prizes in medicine.

PULMONARY MEDICINE

The anatomy of the lungs and chest had been studied hundreds of years before there was an understanding of the underlying physiology and pathology (figure 286). Respiratory infections were described in texts as running a "natural course," and the mortality remained high despite the use of many different therapeutic regimens.

286. Anatomy of the respiratory system in *Traité complet d'anatomie de l'homme*, 2nd ed. (1866–1871) by J.M. Bourgery, Claude Bernard, and N.H. Jacob

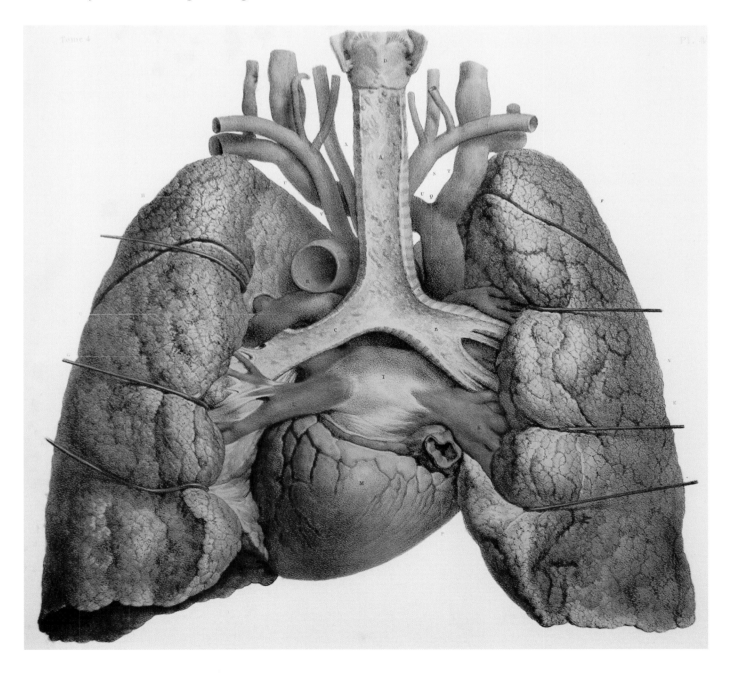

In his *Aphorisms: Concerning the Knowledge and Cure of Diseases* (1715), Dr. Hermann Boerhaave provides us with an early description of pneumonia in the preantibiotic era (figure 287):

If there be a great rattling in the Chest with a sad Countenance, the Eyes red and yellowish, with seeming dust in 'em, and dim; If the Spittle be in the beginning of divers colours; then do they often die on the third or the fifth Day. If the Patient Snoars much in his sleep, Spits nothing or with difficulty, the Pulse be languid, the Urine extremely high-colour'd: If there be a Looseness with watry, stinking, rotten Stools. . . . If the Blood coming out of the Vein appears very florid without the inflammatory Crust notwithstanding its discharge through a large Orifice, flowing briskly and received in a clean Porringer: If Spitting be suppressed leaving the difficulty of breathing behind, and that even increased with a pain and heaviness in the Chest, a hard, small, quick Pulse and a great heat; all which being grown much worse on the fifth Day do kill on the seventh: If the Urine is very red, dark, with a settling of mixed and various Colours, and not entirely separating at the Bottom or the Sides, that kills within fourteen Days: If the Sediment be black or broke into small particles like Bran, the Patient dies sooner: If the Pleuresie in gentle in the beginning, but grows worse on the fifth or sixth

287. Pneumonia from *Anatomia Pathologique du corps Humain*, book 1 (1829–1835) by J. Cruveilhier

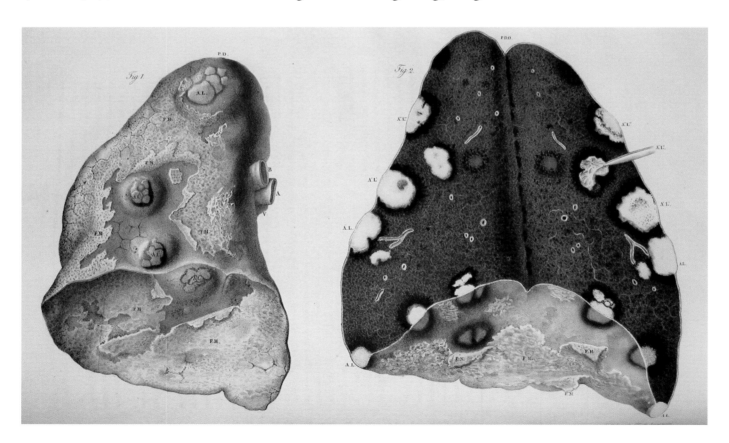

Day, the Danger is great on the seventh and twelfth Day, and they seldom do well unless they can overcome the struggles of the fourteenth Day. If the Back, Sides, Shoulders are heated with a Redness and a great Anguish, green loose Stools and very stinking. . . . If the Tongue is from the beginning dry, foul, livid, black, with a black Blyster or Pustule upon it; If any one of these Signs be present singly or more of them together, the Disease is most times Mortal of it self, not easie to be cured, but most times kills by a Gangrene. . . .

Boerhaave went on to graphically describe an advanced case of empyema, or fluid in the chest:

The Sharpness, Quantity, Putrifaction of the Pus increase daily; the Membranes, which do contain the same, are daily dilated, eaten and made thinner; The Blood and bronchial Vessels are converted into Pus; The whole Lungs or one of its Lobes is consumed into Pus also; a continual dry Cough, or one that continually rubs off Spittle with its shaking and forces it up, attends the Patient; all the Blood running upon the Ulcer is turn'd to Pus, the Vomica gains ground every Day into the substance of the Lungs, and that breaks at last into the Pipes of the Larynx; Sometimes the Patient is choak'd at once with the breaking and issuing forth of the Pus, or voids the same daily in great quantities with a Cough, and it generally stinks and runs together when spit out in a Bason with Water, it is sweet, fat, faetid, white, red, yellow, livid, ash-colour'd, stringy, and when thrown into Fire it smells of roast-meat. Then a breaking and an emptying of the Vomica into the Cavity of the Chest, whence Breathing is rendered very difficult, and all the Symptoms of an Empyema do appear. Then is Breathing worst of all; all the Blood and Chyle is converted to Pus; The Preparation of the nourishing Juice (usually perform'd in the Lungs) is destroy'd, most all the Solids do entirely consume; a Hectic Fever with a small and languid Pulse, a troublesome sharp heat in the upper Parts, glowing Cheeks, an Hippocratic Face, an unexpressible Anguish chiefly towards evening, a great Drought, large overflowing Sweats in the Night, red Pustules in the Face, and about the Neck and Breast, a swelling of the Hand of the affected Side, a great Weakness, a Hoarseness, a falling of the Hair, an Itching all over, with watry Pustules; a Looseness with yellow, faetid, purulent, cadaverous Matter, pressing hard with almost a continual Motion to go to Stool, and spending the Spirits greatly; a supression of Spittle and Death. . . .

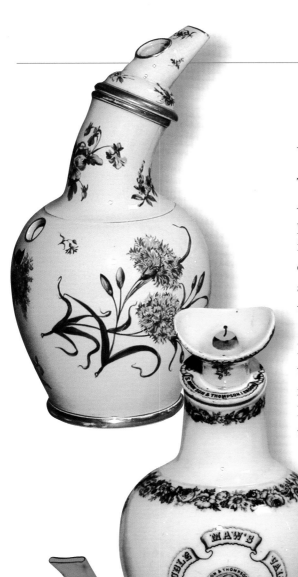

The early treatment of pneumonia was discussed by William Salmon in *A Compleat System of Physick* (1686):

The Air must be temperate, or rather enclining to heat. A cold Air is very bad in this case; because it sends its acid pointed particles through the Pores of the Body, which then associating themselves to the Blood coagulate it: it obstructs the lesser Blood-vessels, whereupon the volatile Spirits fly into Air, and the rest that remain fight with one another, coagulate and turn to Pus.

The meat must be light and thin, such as Chicken-broth, Barley-cream, and Oatmeal gruel. Lentils are held by Galen to be specifically bad. All Garden-fare are bad. The drink must be made of root of Licorace, Flowers of Poppy or Horse-dung because much alkali, which is good to imbibe the pleuritick Acid.

Immediate walking is bad. The Passions of the mind must be moderate, Anger must be forborn; for it is the greatest plague of a Man's Life, and is very dangerous to the Heart, as it does the highest violence to the mass of Blood, Grief, Care, and Fear, have all of them, as experience testifies, been the cause of this Disease.
Bleed the Basilick vein.
Cupping glasses to the Shoulder blades.
Take of the powder of volatile and fixt Salt of Vipers each half a Drachm, Peach Stone two Drachms, Bark of the Root of Cinnamon, Flowers of red Poppy each three Drachms, Root of Elecampane, lignum colubrinum each half an Ounce, Goats Blood three Drachms, Castor one Drachm, Spirit of wine camphorate, and impregnated with Crabs Eyes eight Drachms. Digest them, then let them be thrice separated according to art, and let it be tinged to redness with red Poppy flowers.

Boerhaave suggested more aggressive measures for the treatment of pneumonia: "In this Case therefore the Physician ought immediately to burn the affected Part to the quick with a red-hot Iron, and the Crusts ought afterwards to be cover'd over with strong Cleansers, and often be heated and constantly kept warm, with the most penetrant Fomentations; And the Patient ought besides to take inwardly Strong diluters, Openers, such things as are contrary to putrifactions and sweating Medicines in great Quantities. For these things, if any, will allay the fierceness of the Disease."

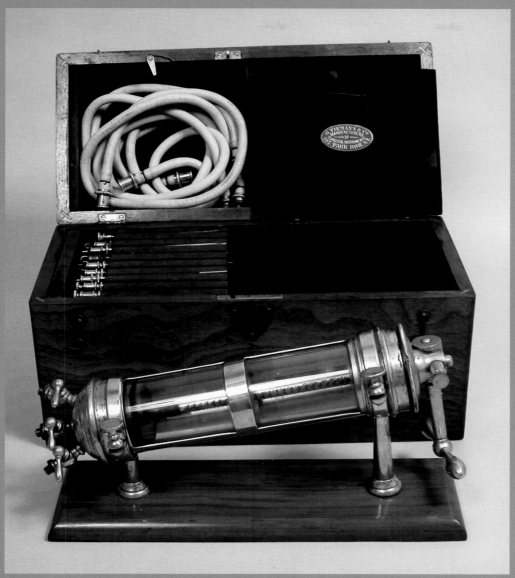

288. Opposite. Late eighteenth-century ceramic Inhalers: (top to bottom) hand-painted inhaler by Rorstrand, double valved earthenware inhaler by S. Maw, Son, and Thompson, Nelson-style earthenware inhaler by S. Maw and Sons

289. Above. Dieulafoy's Hospital aspirator (ca. 1880)

290. Potain's aspirator (ca. 1880) by Arnold and Sons

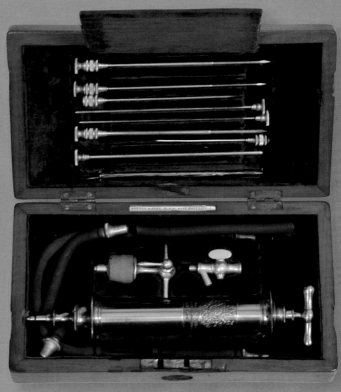

291. Early twentieth-century cigarette advertising: (top) armed services case and lighter: (bottom) medicated cigarettes for asthma by Cubeb and by Asthmador

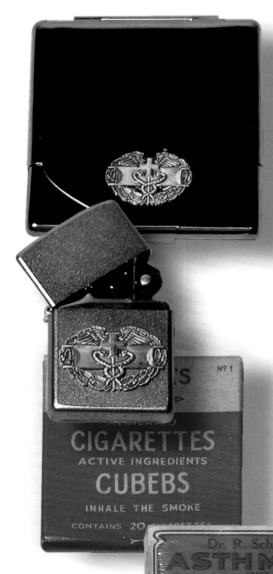

In the nineteenth century, medications for the treatment of respiratory disorders were given in a number of ways, including by mouth and clyster (or enema), as well as by inhaler (figure 288). Occasionally physicians removed fluid from the chest in order to improve ventilation, but chest surgery of any complexity was not available before the discovery of anesthesia later that century (figures 289, 290).

Tobacco

Physicians in the past paid little attention to preventive medicine, so many diseases unfortunately spread quickly in large populations. American Indians were the first recognized to use tobacco in the form of snuff. Smoking tobacco quickly became fashionable in the American colonies, and Christopher Columbus introduced it to Europe with his second voyage that ended in 1496. During the seventeenth century, ships' physicians employed tobacco enemas as a treatment for drowning, and in 1743, Laurence Heister described several other medical uses: "The Moderns have a new kind of Clyster, made of the Smoke of Tobacco, which appears to be of considerable Efficacy, and was introduced first by the *English*, after whom it has been used by several of the *European* Nations. It is used chiefly when other Clysters prove ineffectual, and particularly in the Iliac Passion, and in the *Hernia incarcerata*, though it may by used for other purposes, and is particularly serviceable in an obstinate Constipation of Obstruction of the Bowels." Physicians used a large syringe containing about a pint of tobacco, and instilled smoke into the recipient through a number of tubes and pumps.

Doctors recommended snuff for the treatment of colds, headaches, toothaches, and to protect against a number of contagious diseases including fairly common syphilis. Snuff was popular in the French court, though not all were in favor of its use and by the reign of Louis XIII, the practice was forbidden unless prescribed by physicians. Pope Urban XIII excommunicated anyone using snuff, and Tsar Michael I of Russia had offenders' noses cut off.

Tobacco use reached its zenith in the United States in the middle of the twentieth century. There was no recognition of any danger in smoking by manufacturers who were anxious to demonstrate the safety of their products, especially when used with filters. Medical logos appeared on cigarette cases and lighters, and a number of cures for respiratory conditions were marketed in the form of cigarettes (figure 291).

National magazines, including most prominently *Life,* ran advertising campaigns as early as 1930 (figure 292), and physician surveys could be found there for more than twenty years (figures 293–296). The "Lady with a Lamp" 1946 advertisement for Camel cigarettes was quite unusual with its effort to reach the female market (figure 297), and some tobacco companies were brazen enough to advertise in the *Journal of the American Medical Association* (figure 298). Athletes were eager to affirm that smoking was not detrimental to their performance, and, in fact, it improved their digestion (figure 299). Famous actors also got on the bandwagon, including Robert Young, who became Dr. Marcus Welby, America's favorite family physician on television from 1969 to 1976 (figure 300). Tobacco companies addressed a rising public concern regarding the potential health risks of smoking by introducing filtered cigarettes in the 1950s. Unfortunately for the P. Lorillard Company (and for many employees and smokers), the thirteen billion Kent filtered cigarettes they produced between 1952 and 1957 contained crocidolite asbestos fibers (figure 301). Thirty percent of each micronite filter manufactured for "extra protection" ironically contained a carcinogenic material that could produce mesothelioma, a difficult to treat tumor of the lining of the lungs. The health costs of tobacco use remain high.

GASTROENTEROLOGY

Artists turned their attention to the gastrointestinal tract as early as the fifteenth century, and fine representations can be found in a number of medical works over the last several hundred years (figure 302). Therapy for these diseases date back to the Ebers papyrus written about 1500 B.C., and since surgical intervention was not possible, medical therapy was prescribed:

> When thou examinest a person who suffers from an obstruction
> in his abdomen and thou findest that it goes-and-comes under
> thy fingers like oil-in-a-tube, then say thou: 'It all comes from his
> mouth like slime!' Prepare for him:
>> Fruit-of-the-Pompalm
>> Dissolve in Man's Semen
>> Crush, cook in Oil and Honey
>> To be eaten by the Patient for four mornings. Afterwards let
> him be smeared with dried, crushed, and pressed maqutgrain.
>> When thou examinest a person who has a hardening, his
> stomach hurts him, his face is pale, his heart thumps; when thou
> examinest him and findest his heart and stomach burning and his

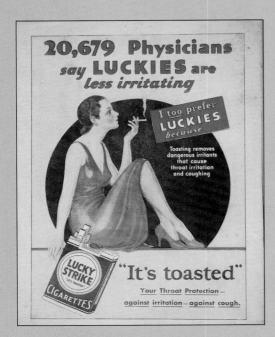

292. Lucky Strike cigarette advertising (1930)

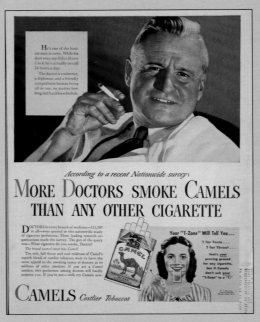

293. "Doctor's Smoke Camels" (ca. 1946) in *Life*

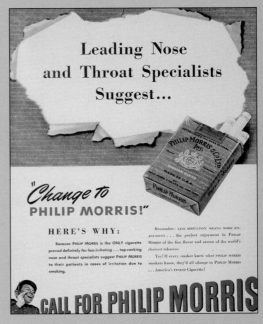

294. ENT specialists for Philip Morris (ca. 1940)

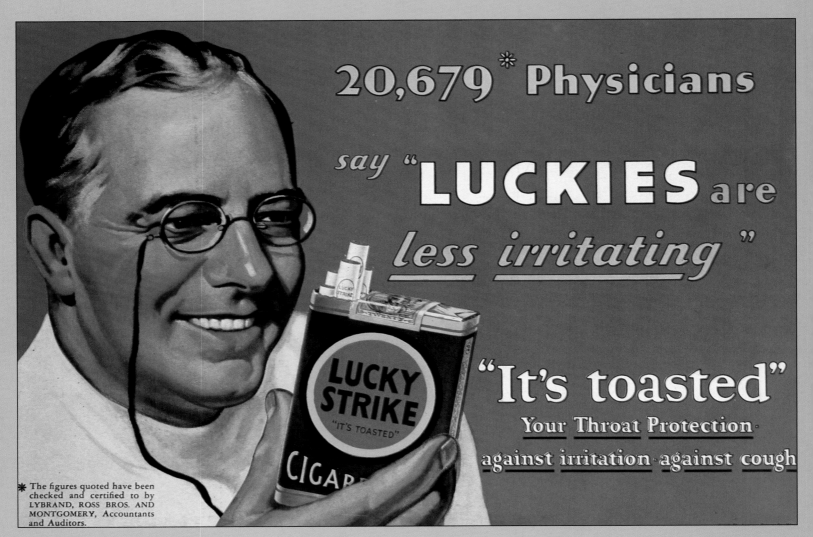

295. Physician advertising in *Hearst's International-Cosmopolitan* (1930)

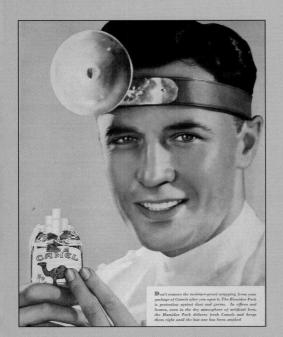

296. ENT advertising (1931) in *Collier's Magazine*

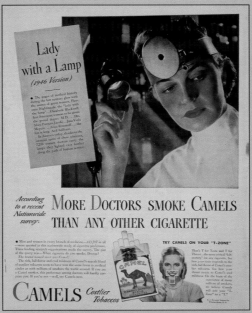

297. Lady ENT for Camel cigarettes (ca. 1946) in *Life*

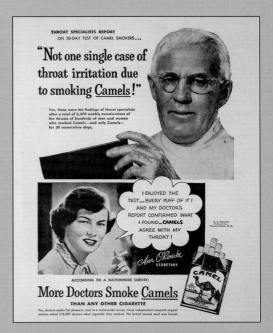

298. JAMA advertisement for Philip Morris cigarettes (1947)

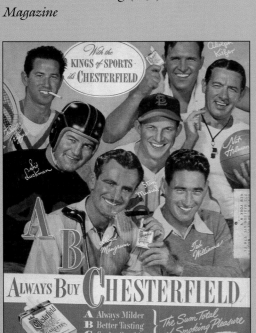

299. Athletes for smoking (ca. 1946)

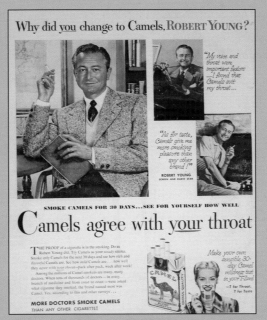

300. Robert Young (Dr. Marcus Welby) for Camels (ca. 1946)

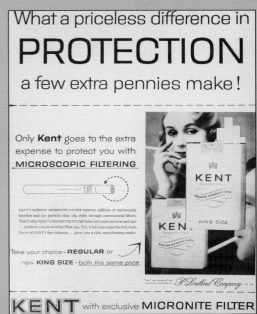

301. Kent micronite filter advertisement (ca. 1954)

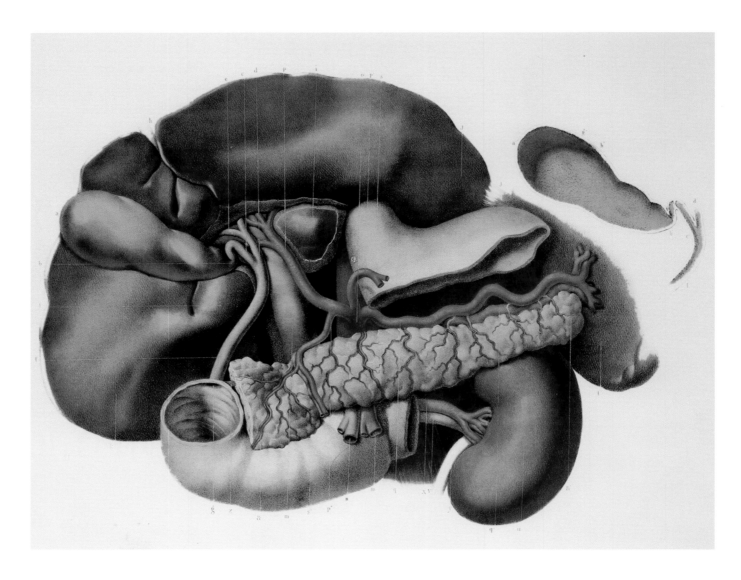

302. Pancreas and gall bladder in
Traité complet d'anatomie de l'homme,
2nd ed. (1866–1871) by J.M. Bourgery,
Claude Bernard, and N.H. Jacob

body swollen. . . . Make him a remedy that quenches the fire and empties his bowels by drinking Sweet-Beer-that-has-stood-in-dry-Dough. This is to be eaten and drunk for Four days. Look every morning for six days following at what falls from his rectum. If excrement fall out of him like little black lumps, then say to him: 'The body-fire has fallen from the stomach. . . .' If thou examinest him after this has come to pass and something steps forth out of him . . . make for him this remedy so that his face may cool. . . .

> To drive away the hardening in the abdomen:
>
> | | |
> |---|---|
> | Bread-of-the-Zizyphus-Lotus | 1 |
> | Watermelon | 1 |
> | Cat's dung | 1 |
> | Sweet Beer | 1 |
> | Wine | 1 |
>
> Make into one and apply as a poultice.

The treatment of colic remained unorthodox in the sixth century. Alexander of Tralles, who relied on the teachings of Galen, made this recommendation: "Remove the nipple-like projection from the caecum of a young pig, mix myrrh with it, wrap it in the skin of a wolf or dog, and instruct the patient to wear it as an amulet during the waning of the moon. Striking effects may be looked for from this remedy."

Later in eighteenth century, Hermann Boerhaave addressed the same problem in his *Aphorisms*:

> The Intestines, chiefly the thin Guts, are very often seized with the like acute Inflammation in their Membranes as the Stomach, from Causes common to all Inflammations carried thither; or from the matter of sharp Drink, Aliments, high Sauces, Medicines of Poisons reaching those Parts, detain'd in the Foldings of the Valvules and sticking to them; And also from a sharp, putrid and faetid purulent, ichorous, gangrenous, bilious, and atrabiliar Matter convey'd hither from the Gullet, Stomach, Liver, Spleen, Pancreas, and Gaul, which sticks also to them and gnaws them; Or lastly, from some strong preceding Convulsion, occasioning Flatusses, stopping the Motion, and thereby creating an Inflammation.
>
> When created in those Parts, it contracts the Guts, shuts up the Cavity, hinders the Passage of what presents it self, and occasions a very sharp, burning, fixed pain; Violent Convulsions when irritated by the Matter that is near and upon the affected Part; It stops the passage by Stool; excites a Vomiting of what is then taken, or approaches the Part, and that sooner or later after taking, according as its Seat is higher or lower; It creates painful Winds, most sharp gripping Pains, with great murmurings in the Guts, the Iliac Passion, twisting of the Guts, an Imposthume , Gangrene, Schirrus, Cancer; a very acute Fever, a very great Weakness from the fierceness of the Pain, and a very sudden Death.

Demonstrating that scientific investigation has no bounds, Boerhaave added the following in his *Of Belchings and Winds*:

> Belchings owe their birth to an Elastic Matter, which by the heat, effervescence and fermentation is made able to swell and dilate, which in one moment is retain'd, and in the next having loosen'd or broke its Prison, is push'd out with a loud and impetuous Noise.
>
> So that the Air, Salts of an opposite Nature, Summer Fruits, putrifying Humors, and such of the Vegetable Kind as are apt to ferment, supply the matter for Belches and Winds, whereof the

Noise and Stench doth differ according to the different Nature of its Producer.

Nor will all these occason any noisy sound, if they have a free passage to exhale at; Whence it appears, that the Contractions of the Sphincters of the Gullet, Stomach, of the superior and inferior Orifice of the Stomach and of the Intestines, do always meet together, and are again loosen'd together; Whence Belches, Winds, Farts, and the Frog-like croakings of the Guts.

If these two Causes do meet and act powerfully and last long, then both the Elastic Matter being by heat, motion, and its own proper Strength stirred up to a Dilatation, and imprison'd in a Cavity whose Fibres being by Convulsions contracted, do dilate the closing Membranes, stretch them, makes 'em painful, compresseth and squeezeth the adjacent Parts; whence arise intolerable Pain and Anguish, which cease instantly upon the letting out of the Winds. And if to this is joined a Fever, there ensue most inexpressible Torments.

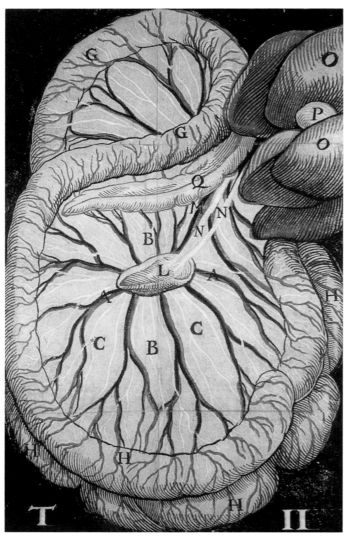

303. Normal colon in *De lactibus sive lacteis venis* (1627) by Gaspar Asellius

Boerhaave then suggested the following therapeutic approach:

As soon as it is known present by its Signs then ought the Cure to be attempted forthwith with all the most powerful Means whilst it is yet in this first state; Which is obtained, 1. By a large and repeated Bleeding as in the Pleurisie. 2. By the continual injecting of loosening, diluting, antiphlogistic Glysters repeated often to three or four or more times a Day. 3. By the drinking incessantly things of the same kind mixing Opiats with a due Caution; and also such things as are known to be contrary to the particular or singular Cause of the Disease. 4. By Fomentations of the like kind applied all over the Belly, and chiefly the Application of young, live, hot and found Animals; such as Puppies or Kittens. 5. And in the mean time prudently forbearing the use of any sharp things, or such as increase the Motion of the Blood, as are heating, whether Aliments, Drink, Medicines, Motion or Passions. 6. Continuing the Use of those, till the whole Evil be appeased, and doth not return in three Days after it.

Purging the System

Cathartics and enemas have always been a popular way of

cleaning the system in order to balance Galen's humors (figure 303). Greek historian Herodotus commented on Egyptian customs: "They purge themselves every month, three days in succession seeking to preserve health by emetics and clysters; for they suppose that all diseases to which men are subject proceed from the food they use." Several centuries later, Pliny justified the use of therapeutic enemas when he observed, "A bird called the Ibis uses his curved beak to purge himself through the part of his body which best controls his health, the anus, given the heavy bodily residues that are taken in and excreted." The Egyptians had, in fact, configured their enema tips in the shape of the Ibis' head though in reality, that bird uses oil excreted from its anal glands only to protect its feathers.

Avicenna (980–1037) pointed out the importance of emetics in his *Canon* (printed 1380):

Hippocrates advised vomiting to be induced monthly and for two consecutive days. On the second day the difficulty of the first day is obviated and that which has entered the stomach is fully emptied. To exceed this would be harmful.

Emesis carried out in this way gets rid of mucous and bile, and cleanses the stomach. For in the case of the stomach there is no cleansing secretion like that for the small intestine—where the bile cleanses the mucous membrane as it passes down the bowel.

Emesis clears heaviness of the head; clears the vision; removes nauseative dyspepsia. It benefits persons in whom bile is apt to pass into the stomach and decompose the food. For, if vomiting precedes the meal, the latter will always enter the stomach without being contaminated, and so the sense of loathing is removed which proceeds, from oiliness of food, as also the depraved appetite—namely, the longing for sharp, sour, or pungent things.

Emesis is also beneficial for flabbiness of the body, and for ulcers of the kidneys and bladder. It has a powerful effect in (anaesthetic) leprosy; in persons with an unhealthy colour of skin; in gastric epilepsy, jaundice asthma, tremor, hemiplegia. It is also an effective treatment in cases of impetiginous skin diseases in which there are ulcers covered with scabs.

It should be procured once or twice a month—after a heavy meal. It is well not to follow fixed time intervals.

Emesis is a great help for persons whose temperament is primarily bilious, and who are lean of habit.

Moses Maimonides (1135–1204) added his thoughts regarding the efficacy of enemas (figures 304, 305): "Galen mentions the fact that an

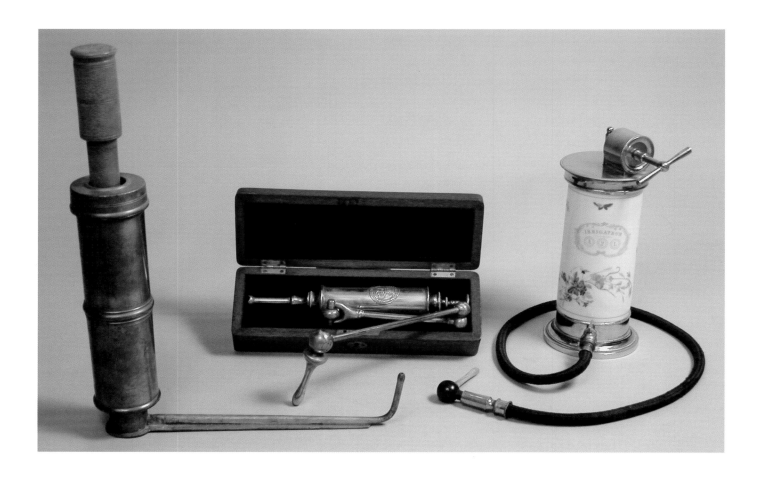

304. Personal enema instruments: (left to right) eighteenth-century French pewter set, mid nineteenth-century brass set, ceramic French irrigator eguisier (ca. 1880)

305. Large enema set with gastric tube (ca. 1860) by Maw and Son

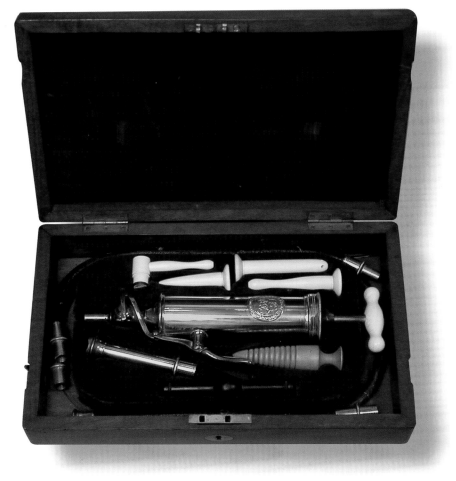

enema with liquid linseed is useful for tubercular patients, since it mitigates the bad juices. Note that the regular use of enema purifies the brain, liquefies intestinal matter, prevents premature aging, assists digestion and wards off many diseases and this is because it cleans and flushes from below and the upper organs get a clear way before them to dispose of the waste matter along the channels provided by very nature."

Samuel Gross was one of the preeminent surgeons of the nineteenth century and wrote the important *A System of Surgery* (1859) in which he reviewed several theoretical uses for this form of therapy: "Cathartics, considered as antiphlogistic agents, are employed for different purposes. In the first place, they may be administered simply to evacuate the bowels; secondly, to deplete the mucous membrane, and thus diminish the quantity of blood in the system; thirdly, to excite the action of the liver and mucous follicles; fourthly, to produce a revulsive effect, or to set up a new action at a distance from the original one; and finally, to stimulate the absorbents, thereby inducing them to remove inflammatory deposits."

The Therapeutic Clyster

Ancient Egyptians, Greeks, and Romans commonly used clysters for the rectal instillation of medications, usually milk and honey, and Hippocrates prescribed both liquid and air enemas for the treatment of fever. This practice appears to have been universal since references to a chamois bag attached to a tube made of either bamboo or ivory made for a similar purpose can be found in the Hindu *Sustra-samhita*. "Nutritive" enemas were not uncommon in the sixteenth century, and they contained a number of ingredients, including milk, olive oil, butter, and eggs. Whether or not this type of nutrition was appropriate during the holy fast of Lent was a heavily debated topic, though a physician named Montanus clarified the matter when he claimed that only nutrition taken by mouth was subject to Lenten laws.

Upper echelons of society embraced the use of clysters in the Renaissance after this instrument reportedly saved the life of Louis XI during a seizure in 1480 (figures 306, 307). This custom was then taken up by many members of the court, and even the royal dogs were treated with enemas. In one year alone, Louis XIII was reported to have self-administered over two hundred twelve enemas. After the king became ill, French Cardinal Richelieu directed the management of his care, which included three hundred twelve clysters, two hundred fifteen purgatives, and forty-seven phlebotomies over a six-month period. The cardinal himself was reported to have taken clysters with aphrodisiac properties, apparently keeping him in good stead for his third marriage at the age of eighty-five. These special treatments were called *restaurants*,

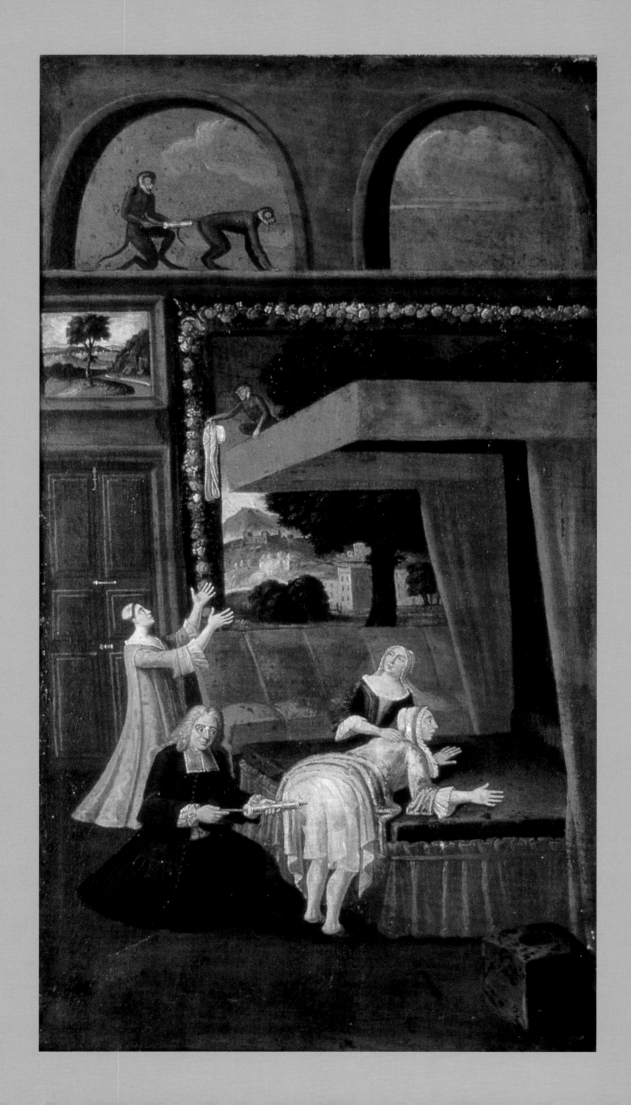

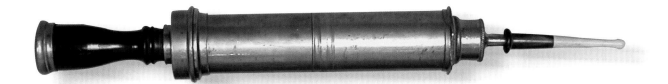

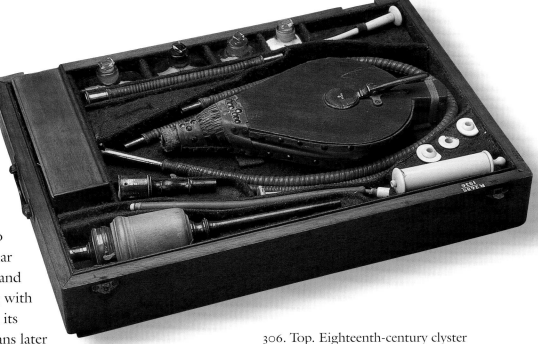

derived from the French word "to restore" and were probably popular because many contained tobacco and gave the user both the high along with the addiction of nicotine through its direct absorption. French physicians later developed the cylster pipe by which they could blow tobacco smoke directly into the rectum of the recipient, resulting in an enhanced effect (figure 308).

There was no decline in the popularity of therapeutic enemas in the court of Louis XIV, who received daily treatments for any number of digestive ailments. The therapeutic clyster was the fashion of the day to cleanse the system and to improve the complexion and psyche. *Limonadiers des posterieurs* ("lemonaders of the rear end") performed their service using the finest of fragrances with clysters personally fitted to each royal rump. Every morning, the limonadier carefully selected the proper clyster tip and chemical combination suitable for that day, whether it be rosemary, thyme, or orange blossom. The popularity of the therapeutic enema continued into the court of Louis XV, where ladies were required to take them on a regular basis. The king's medical consultant spent much of the day eating and taking enemas, sometimes both at the same time.

Since flexible tubing was not yet available, it has been suggested that the king's famous *fistula-in-ano* may have been partially caused by his

306. Top. Eighteenth-century clyster

307. Opposite. A clyster in use (ca. 1700), oil by an unknown French artist

308. Tobacco enema set by Evans and Co. of London (ca. 1780)

habitual use of three to four clysters a day. Ano-rectal fistulas resulting in an abnormal discharge of stool were fairly common at the time and cures were difficult to come by, thus driving many to the church for divine assistance. In the late seventh century, Fiacre moved from Ireland to France where he sat on a stone for several days while awaiting an audience with Bishop Faron. During that time, the stone softened and bore the imprint of his buttocks. St. Fiacre subsequently became the patron saint of proctology, and attained universal recognition for his treatment of diseases of the rectum. Any disease of the rectum was termed "fiacre," and since then, anyone with that problem who hoped for a cure has sat on that stone (figure 309).

309. (Left to right) American pewter bedpan (ca. 1777) and ceramic slipper bedpan (ca. 1870)

Early Forms of Intervention

Common problems of the gastrointestinal tract were often treated in unusual ways. Aretaeus suggested the following therapy for liver disease in the second century:

The formation of the blood is in the liver, and hence the distribution of it over the whole system. And the entire liver is, as it were, a concretion of blood. Wherefore the inflammations there are most acute; for nutrition is seated this place. If, therefore, inflammation from anywhere else, it is not remarkably acute; for it is an influx of blood that is inflamed; but in the liver there is no necessity for its coming from another quarter. For if any obstruction shut the outlets, the liver becomes inflamed by being deprived of its efflux, since the entrance of the food to the liver still continues patent; for there is no other passage of the food but this from the stomach and intestines to the whole body.

When you have soothed by these means, you must apply a cupping-instrument, unusually large, so as to comprehend the whole hypochondriac region, and make deeper incisions than usual, that you may attract much blood. And, in certain cases, leeches are better than scarifications; for the bite of the animal sinks deeper, and it makes larger holes, and hence the flow of blood from these animals is difficult to stop. And when the animals fall off quite full, we may apply the cupping-instrument, which then attracts the matters within. And if there be sufficient evacuation, we are to apply styptics to the wounds; but these not of a stimulant nature, such as spiders' webs, the manna of frankincense, and aloe, which are to

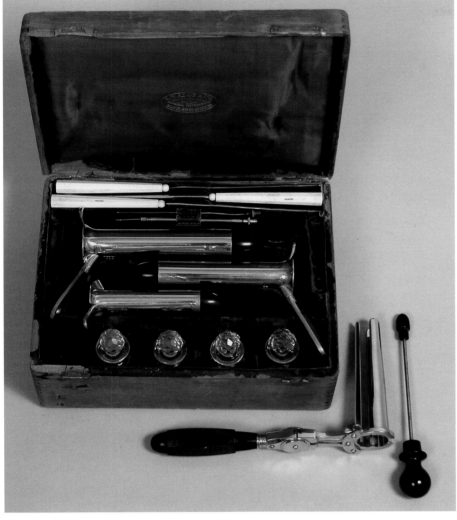

310. Rectal set by A.S. Aloe (ca. 1840), trivalve rectal dilator by Weiss (ca. 1880)

311. Ivory hemorrhoid clamp by Arnold and Sons (ca. 1860)

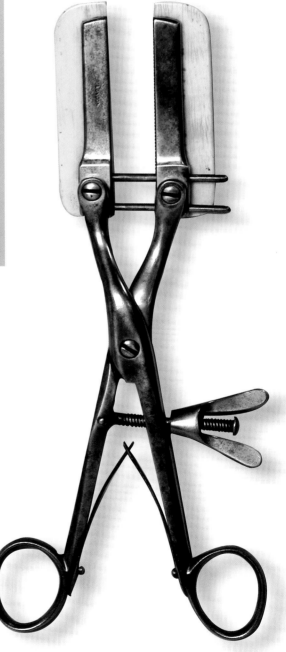

be sprinkled in powder on the part; or bread boiled with rue or melilot, and the roots of marsh-mallow; but on the third day a cerate, made with nut-ben, or the hairy leaves of wormwood and iris.

Nicholas Culpeper outlined a therapeutic approach for the very common problem of hemorrhoids in his *School of Physick* (1659): "*An Excellent remedy for the Piles.* Another remedy, the conceit of which pleases me very well, is this; Take a gray Cat, and cut her throat, then flea her and roast her, and save her grease, boil the blood and the grease together, and anoint the Piles with it as hot as you can endure it; this seems to me pretty rational, because a Cat is a Beast of *Saturn*."

Surgical intervention involving the gastrointestinal tract was unusual prior to the middle of the nineteenth century, though one exception was hemorrhoid surgery, which had been practiced for thousands of years (figures 310, 311). William Cheselden described a rare successful operation involving the gut in his 1768 *Case Studies*:

> The case of Margaret White, the wife of John White, a pensioner in the fishmongers alms-houses at Newington in Surry. In the fiftieth year of her age, she had a rupture at her navel, which continued till her seventy-third year, when, after a fit of the cholic, it mortified, and she being presently after taken with a vomiting, it burst. I went to her, and found her in this condition, with about six and twenty inches and a half of the gut hanging out, mortified. I took away what was mortified, and left the end of the found gut hanging out at the navel, to which it afterwards adhered; she recovered, and lived many years after, voiding the excrements through the intestine at the navel; and though the ulcer was so large, after the mortification separated, that the breadth of two guts was seen; yet they never at any time protruded out at the wound, tho' she was taken out of her bed, and sat up every day.

Despite occasional case reports like the above, surgical procedures involving the abdomen were not possible, and the agony endured by those suffering from what are now easily correctible conditions must have been almost beyond description. Swedish poet Esaias Tegnér (1782–1846) provided some insight into the horrors of recurrent cholecystitis, or gallstone attacks, in his poem *The Spleen*:

> I reached the summit of my life
> Where waters separate and run
> With frothy waves in different directions
> It was clear up there, and wonderful to stand.
> I saw the Earth, t'was green and wondrous
> And God was good and man was honest.
> Then, suddenly, a black, splenetic demon rose
> And sank his teeth into my heart.
> And see, at once the Earth was empty and forsaken
> And sun and stars went dark in haste . . .
> A smell of corpses runs through life,
> The air of spring and summer's glory poisoned . . .
> My pulse beats fast as in my youthful days
> But cannot count the times of agony.
> How long, how endless is each heartbeat's pain.
> O my tormented, burned-out heart!
> My heart? There is no heart within my breast;
> An urn there is, with ash of life enclosed.

Well after Sir William Harvey had written his epic *de Motu Cordis* (1628) that placed medicine on a scientific footing, pseudoscience continued to be a factor regarding decisions involving the advisability of surgical intervention. For example, John H. Kellogg, MD, LLD, founder of the famous sanitarium in Battle Creek, Michigan, where he developed a cold cereal that his brother parlayed into a breakfast-food empire, made the following observation: "Barclay Smith, the great English anatomist, first suggested the uselessness of the colon. Metchnikoff proved animals that possess the longest colons have the shortest lives, and announced that the colon bacillus is the germ of old age. Sir William Arbuthnot Lane, the eminent London surgeon, cites a long list of grave maladies, ranging from tuberculosis to rheumatism, cured by removal of this offending organ. The war still wages."

Élie Metchnikoff was a famous Russian biologist and 1908 Nobel Prize winner (in immunology) who had suggested that the colon was the cause of most illness since it was the source of toxic wastes that were resorbed back into the system. His argument of autointoxication is the same that had been used by physicians for centuries in defense of emetics and cathartics, and now with the possibility of anesthesia and aseptic surgery, the final solution was available: total colectomy. Sir William Arbuthnot Lane was the chief of surgery at Guy's Hospital in London and a well-respected surgeon because of his forceful personality and sharp powers of observation. After a review of the data, the conclusion of this eminent surgeon was to "take it all out." Lane made several initial trials at bypass, though finally resorted to complete colectomy as a treatment for everything from high blood pressure to tuberculosis to schizophrenia to depression to aging. By the beginning of the twentieth century, the procedure was widely accepted in Europe and in the United States, and Lane himself performed over a thousand operations.

312. Silver feeding implements: (top) silver sick siphon (1800–1830), Gibson's spoon, spoon with straw (ca. 1850)

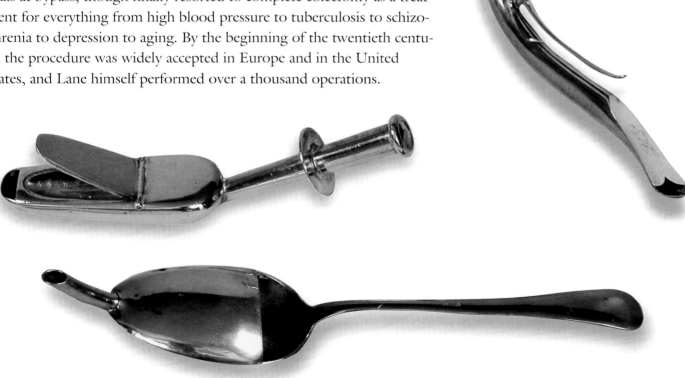

Others, however, were critical of this form of intervention, including writer George Bernard Shaw. In Shaw's *Doctor's Dilemma,* the character Dr. Cutler Walpole made the following statement: "Ninety-five per cent of the human race suffer from chronic blood-poisoning and die from it. It's as simple as A.B.C. Your nuciform sac is full of decaying matter—undigested food and waste products—rank ptomaines. Now you take my advice, Ridgeon. Let me cut it out for you. You'll be another man afterwards." Short of colectomy, the "colonic" and laxatives were the treatments of choice for almost any disease. Max Kiss added chocolate to his "Excellent Laxative" and named it Ex-Lax; fortunes were to be made.

Because of a significant need in the nineteenth century for devices to assist in the feeding and evacuation requirements of children and invalids, craftsmen produced a large number of wonderful nutritional aids out of pewter, silver, porcelain, and glass (figures 312, 313).

A CLASSIC DESCRIPTION

In some way, diabetes mellitus affects every organ system discussed in this chapter, and despite recent medical advances, this disease is unfortunately an approaching epidemic. Diabetes means "I pass through" in Greek, and the Romans added the term mellitus for "sweet" in order to differentiate this condition from the hypothalamic disorder, diabetes insipidus. The great Greek physician Aretaeus of Cappadocia wrote the following description in the second century, and it remains relevant today:

Diabetes is a strange affection, not very frequent among men, being a melting down of the flesh and limbs into urine. Its cause is of a cold and humid nature, as in dropsy. The course is the common one, namely, the kidneys and bladder; for the patients never stop making water, but the flow is incessant, as if from the opening of aqueducts. The nature of the disease, then, is chronic, and it takes a long period to form; but the patient is short-lived, if the constitution of the disease be completely established; for the melting is rapid, the death speedy. Moreover, life is disgusting and painful; thirst

unquenchable; excessive drinking, which, however, is dispropor-
tionate to the large quantity of urine, for more urine is passed;
and one cannot stop them either from drinking or making water.
Or if for a time they abstain from drinking, their mouth becomes
parched and their body dry; the viscera seem as if scorched up;
they are affected with nausea, restlessness, and a burning thirst;
and at no distant term they expire.

It took another 1,800 years to find a treatment for diabetes, and with the
availability of pancreas transplantation, a cure has finally become a reality.

The public criticism of physicians has always been a popular pastime,
and writers have rarely missed an opportunity to ridicule members of the
medical profession. Seventeenth-century French author Molière had
numerous personal medical problems and complained that he was hardly
strong enough to bear his own illnesses, much less the remedies offered
by his doctors. In Molière's play, *Love Is the Best Doctor,* Lysetta comments, "What will you do, sir, with four physicians? Is not one enough
to kill any person . . .?"

Despite the fact that Robert Louis Stevenson (1850–1894) survived
tuberculosis as a child, his character Billy Bones, in *Treasure Island* said,
"Doctors is all swabs."

313. Opposite. Nineteenth century
infant and invalid feeding vessels:
(top) porcelain teapot, silver pap
boat, boat-shaped earthenware bottle

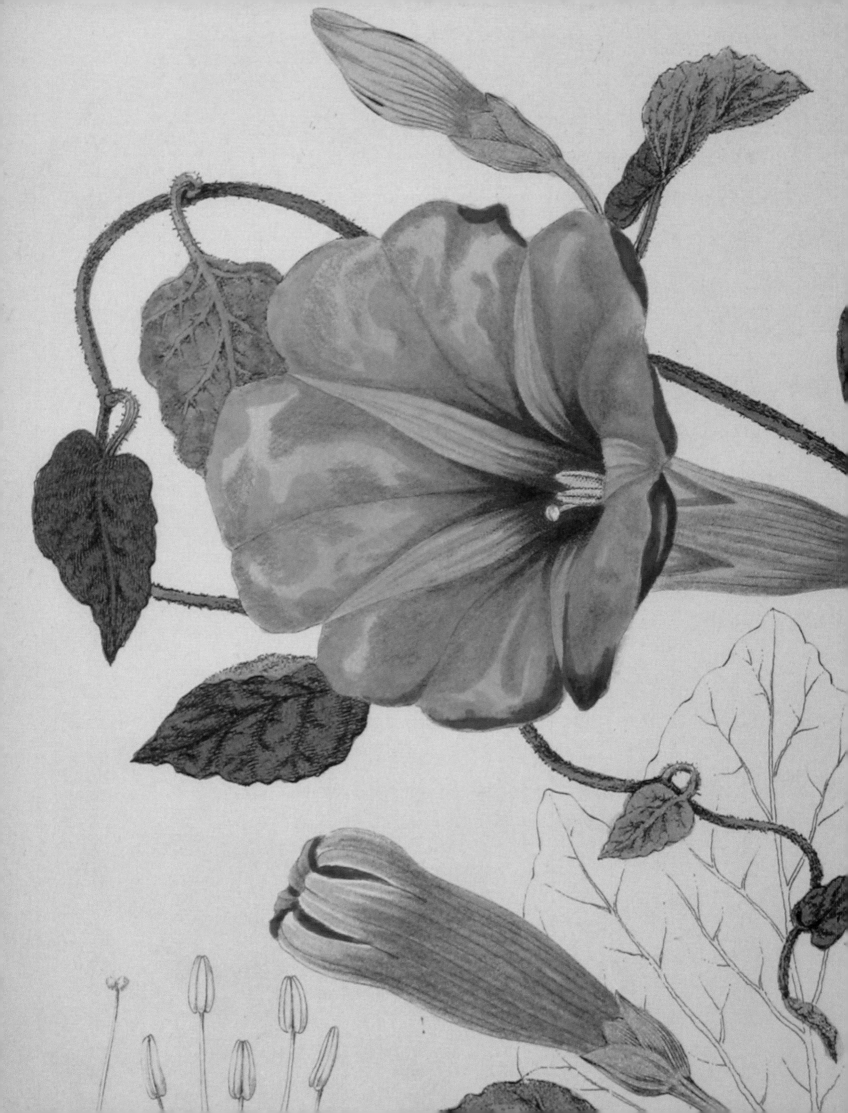

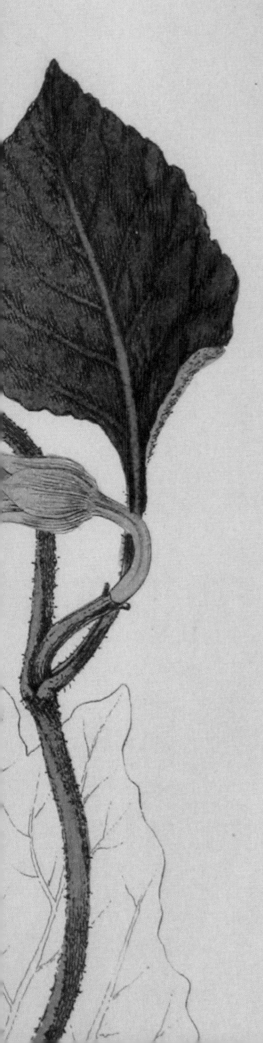

PHARMACY

The disgrace of medicine has been that colossal system of self-deception, in obedience to which mines have been emptied of their cankering minerals, the vegetable kingdom robbed of all its noxious growths, the entrails of animals taxed for their impurities, the poison-bags of reptiles drained of their venom, and all the inconceivable abominations thus obtained thrust down the throats of human beings suffering from some fault of organization, nourishment, or vital stimulation.

Oliver Wendell Holmes, MD
Border Lines of Knowledge in
Some Provinces of Medical Science, 1861

Detail, *Convolvulus Jalapa* (Jalap Bindweed) from *Illustrations and Descriptions of the Medicinal Plants of the London, Edinburgh, and Dublin Pharmacopoeias* (1828) by John Stephenson, MD and James Churchill, FLS

A recent "History of Medicine" was circulated over the Internet that reflects the frustration that many have endured throughout the ages regarding the delivery of medical care:

2000 BC	Here, eat this root.
1000 BC	That root is heathen, say this prayer.
1850	Prayer is superstitious, drink this potion.
1930	That potion is snake oil, swallow this pill.
1970	That pill is ineffective, take this antibiotic.
2000	That antibiotic is artificial, eat this root.

Long before recorded history, medical practitioners were treating patients with potions, herbs, and incantations. The earliest prescriptions found in Egyptian papyri (ca. 1500 B.C.) contained such varied substances as the biblical tree resins frankincense and myrrh, along with numerous herbs and the metals iron and lead. The use of animal products like blood, teeth, stool, and urine, was also quite common, and Egyptian physicians treated burns with "goat dung in yeast that is fermenting." Milk and honey was often used for the therapy of respiratory disorders, while for night blindness, "The liver of an ox, fried and mashed, should be taken; it is truly remarkable!" As we look back with scientific hindsight, some of these remedies had physiologic justification; night blindness, for example, is caused by vitamin A deficiency, a vitamin that is high in liver.

The customary symbol for a prescription is "Rx." This mark may have, in fact, had its origin as far back as ancient Egypt and the image of the left eye of Horus, the falcon-headed Egyptian god of health and prosperity (figure 314). Horus was the son of Isis, the nature goddess, and Osiris, the god of the underworld. Osiris was murdered by his brother, Seth, and in order to avenge his father's death, Horus confronted his uncle. In the ensuing battle, Horus lost his left eye, though Thoth, the god of wisdom and compassion, magically restored it. Horus then gave the eye to his father, Osiris, who experienced rebirth in the underworld.

The *udjat* ("Eye of Horus") had special meaning for the Egyptians, and they used each part of the symbol to measure not only food and land, but ingredients for their medical preparations. The entire eye accounted for one heqat, though for an unclear reason, adding the fractions together gives a total of only $^{63}/_{64}$. There was a great deal of symbolism attached to the Eye of Horus since in addition to representing a fraction, each section stood for a part of the body and one of the six senses:

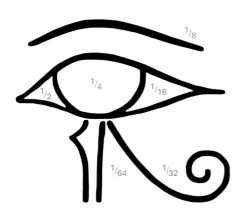

314. The Eye of Horus

315. Opposite. Manuscript page from *The Canon of Medicine* (fifteenth-century copy) by Avicenna (980–1037)

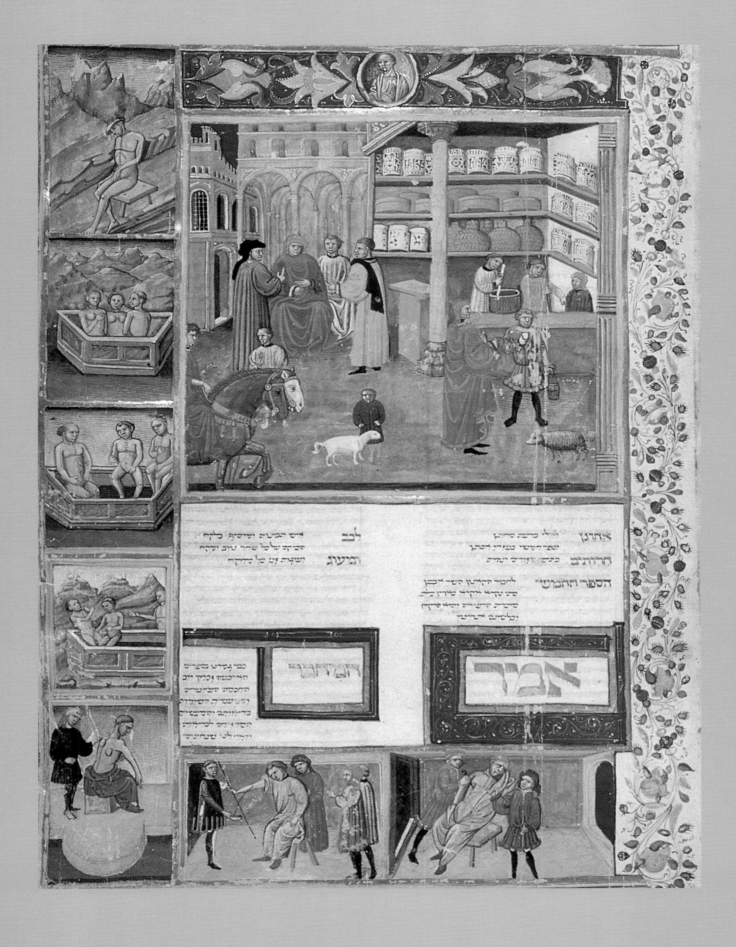

אהרון כלל מרבת שחוון לבב דיים הבמוות ודיוסיף בלקח
הספר מעשר בענייך וסרגן ונמך יצלצלו שהר נוב וסרקה
חרוותב כתם שזרר'ש יבהרת ומירעות ושענה זה כל ססקה

הספר והחבורש לוכתר תקלתון הסר יכבן
סני טחלא הרקייר סלרון שלל
מכזרבת דישעוזרה והכלייצעוה
הסהי זהגר לכלמיאהון
והלייבהם והריהזיב

רוב דיבור אמר

$^1/_{64}$ heqat: Planting a stalk in the ground (*touch*)

$^1/_{32}$ heqat: Grain became food (*taste*)

$^1/_{16}$ heqat: The ear (*hearing*)

$^1/_8$ heqat: A motion of an eyebrow (*thought*)

$^1/_4$ heqat: The pupil of the eye (*sight*)

$^1/_2$ heqat: The nose (*smell*)

Since the time of the ancient Egyptians, Horus' left eye has signified the restoration of health and may have evolved into the present Rx notation. There are other explanations, however, and the symbol may have come from the Latin word *recipere* ("recipe") meaning "take thou." "Rx" could be a descendant of the representation for the planet Jupiter as suggested by Sir William Osler in 1910: "In a cursive form it is found in mediaeval translations of the works of Ptolemy the astrologer, as the sign of the planet Jupiter. As such it was placed upon horoscopes and upon formula containing drugs made for administration to the body, so that the harmful properties of these drugs might be removed under the influence of the lucky planet." The Eye of Horus continues to represent healing and protective powers, and may have led American forefathers to include a similar figure, the Eye of Providence, on the reverse sides of both the seal of the United States and the one dollar bill. Both images stand above a thirteen-step pyramid.

The first recognized pharmacists practiced in the seventh century in the Middle East, and Arabian apothecary expertise subsequently influenced medical care in Europe for hundreds of years (figure 315). There was no clear division between physicians and pharmacists regarding the marketing of medications until Frederick III of Sicily officially separated pharmacy from medicine in 1240, leading to centuries of competition for the drug trade. Since formal training was not available to most, many providers involved in the delivery of health care, including barber-surgeons, tooth-pullers, midwives, and bleeders also entered the marketplace with their curatives (figure 316).

The apothecary trade was potentially lucrative, especially because all medications come with a significant placebo effect, placebo meaning "to please" in Latin. Studies have consistently shown that up to thirty percent of patients given an inactive substance report a positive outcome if given encouragement, a factor that has led to the promotion of a panacea of therapeutic agents over the centuries. In the fourteenth century, John of Mirfield wrote the following in *Breviarium Bartomolomaie*: "When Physick's dearly bought, it doth much healing bring. But when 'tis freely given, 'tis ne'er a useful thing." Dr. Thomas Sydenham (1624–1689), one of the greatest physicians in the history of medicine, expressed doubts regarding the efficacy of medications available to him when he wrote in *Medical Observations,* "The arrival of a good clown exercises a more beneficial influence upon the health of a town than of twenty asses laden with drugs."

STRANGE INGREDIENTS

Physicians and healers have used almost everything they could get their hands on for the treatment of internal and external diseases, with the approval of the customer often a primary goal. One of the earliest remedies was theriac, an ancient preparation containing numerous ingredients that varied depending on individual preference (figure 317). Legend has it that MithridatesVI (132–63 B.C.), King of Pontus, was interested in finding an antidote to snakebites and poisons, and, after much experimentation on his slaves, he discovered "mithridatium." Andromachus, physician to Nero, added the essential ingredient of viper's flesh, and the

316. *La Pharmacie rustique* (1775), an engraving by Barthelemi Hubner showing Michael Schuppach examining urine

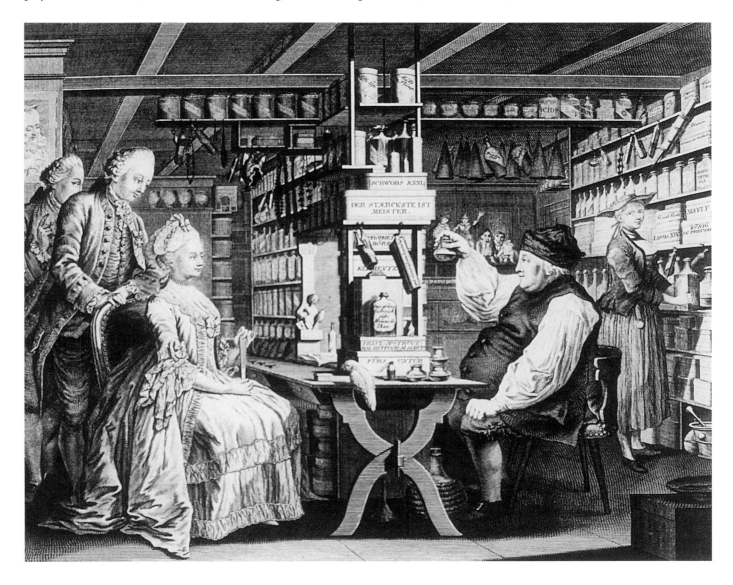

preparation became known as theriac, Greek for "wild beast." Under the direction of Galen, the number of ingredients reached seventy and he used it to treat the emperors he served. By the Middle Ages, theriac contained over one hundred ingredients, and its activity reached mythic proportions, often taking months to produce and years to age. It was used as an antidote for almost any medical condition, and was part of physicians' armamentaria to prevent the Black Death. Theriac was still available from pharmacists in France, Spain, and Germany into the latter part of the nineteenth century, much of its popularity probably related to the presence of opium.

Western physicians were not alone in their use of exotic ingredients. The Chinese added a variety of minerals to their medications, and one of the earliest and most unusual was a prescription composed of ground up "dragons' bones," or dinosaur fossils, for seizures. Master Ge Hong (A.D. 284–363?), was one of the foremost alchemists in the history of Chinese medicine, and employed numerous minerals in his role as a mythical guide to immortality. Cinnabar was the most important medication to be taken in order to reach that state, though it frequently contained the toxic materials mercury and arsenic. Six emperors of the Tang dynasty (A.D. 618–907) died seeking immortality by taking elixirs containing mercury and other metallic elements.

Gem therapy has been an important part of medical care for thousands of years and was used in the ancient Indian medical system, the Ayurveda. Western alchemists employed the medicinal properties of natural crystalline substances that were prepared in powdered form and mixed with water or honey for easy ingestion. Marbodus Redonensis, the twelfth-century Bishop of Rennes, recommended the use of topaz and green jasper for the treatment of fever and dropsy, and emerald for epilepsy. Paracelsus prescribed powdered jacinth for fever, and others depended on the red color of rubies and jasper to cure inflammation. Unfortunately, therapy with precious stones was sometimes risky, and in 1532, Pope Clement VII died after his fourteenth spoonful of a powdered mixture of diamonds and other precious minerals.

In 1693, *Salmon's English Physician* incorporated a number of animal parts in their therapeutic formulae:

The Toad.

A Toad dried in the sun, or an Oven and reduced to Pouder, and given inwardly is said to provoke urine, and cure the Dropsie, if curable: Others give the Ashes in the same Dose for the same purpose;

317. Italian tin-glazed earthenware jar, or albarello, containing theriac (ca. 1641)

outwardly applied (being mixt with a little Vinegar) it draws out the Poison of Carbuncles. Blown up the nostrils it stops their Bleeding; so also the whole Toad dryed and smelt to, or hung about the neck in a silk Bag. Laid upon the Navel, or so hung as to touch the upper part of the Belly, it is profitable against the Diabetes, and cures pissing a Bed; and yet laid to the Reins, it brings forth the Hydropick water by Urine; and applied to the soles of the Foot, it draws away distempers from the Head, helps Frenzies, and Fevers. The pouder is good against old Ulcers and Fistulaes, and biting of Serpents.

The Rat.

Their Flesh

I conceive the flesh to be antiparalitick, and therefore beneficial to those who have a resolution of the nerves.

The Fat

It is good against all manner of pains and aches.

The Ashes of the whole Rat

Strewed upon ulcerations, it heals them; blown into the eye, it clears the eyesight.

The Dung

It helps the alopecia and other fallings of the hair . . . mix for a dose against the Worms.

In the absence of available and satisfactory medical care, "folk medicine" has been popular across all cultures. The following are a few examples from the seventeenth through the nineteenth centuries:

A child afflicted by whooping cough can be cured by thrusting the head of a living fish into the child's mouth for a few moments.

To cure convulsions, take parings from the sick man's nails, hair from his eyebrows and head 'bound up in a clout, with a halfpenny.' Whoever found this package would inherit the disease.

Physicians in Lancashire recommended "for warts rub them with a cinder, and this tied up in paper, and dropped where four roads meet, will transfer the warts to whoever opens the parcel." Alternatively, one could rub the warts with dust from under a stone at the intersection of the four roads and repeat:

A'm ane, the wart's twa,
The first ane it comes by
Tacks the warts awa.'

An Assyrian proverb:

Take a white cloth. In it place the mamit.
In the sick man's right hand;

And take a black cloth,
Wrap it round his left hand.
Then all the evil spirits
And the sins which he has committed
Shall quit their hold of him
And shall never return.

Cataracts were cured by cutting out the tongue of a live fox and then setting him free. "Dry the tongue, tie it in a red bag, and hang it around the affected man's neck for a cure." A common belief was that paralysis resulted from a shrewmouse crawling over the affected limb, and a cure could be accomplished only by plugging up the mouse in a hole in the trunk of a tree. Deafness was certain to be cured by dropping ants' eggs mixed with onion juice into the affected ear. To cure a stye in England or Scotland, one must pluck one hair from the tail of a black tomcat, and rub the pustule nine times the first night of the new moon.

Urine has been used as a medication from the earliest recorded history, and it continues to be an ingredient in substances that are used therapeutically today. Early Egyptians applied urine topically for the treatment of burns, and urine has played an important part in wound and skin care in cultures throughout the world, including those in ancient China, India, Africa, and the Americas. In *Naturalis Historia* (A.D. 77), Gaius Plinus Secundus (A.D. 23–79), or Pliny the Elder, listed some of the ways in which urine was used: "The ashes of burnt oyster shells, mixed with old urine, yield a remedy against all sorts of running sores and skin rashes on children. Corrosive sores, burns, anal trouble, cracked skin, and scorpion bites are also treated with urine. The greatest midwives have asserted that no better washing-medium exists for skin diseases. With an addition of soda, urine cures head wounds, dandruff, and spreading sores, particularly on the genitals. Every individual benefits most from his own urine, if I may say so." Recent studies suggest that some of the constituents of urine may indeed be helpful in wound care, including urea that may act as a dessicant, and urokinase is an anticoagulant to debride diseased tissue.

According to some, ingesting urine in the pursuit of health dates back as far as the Bible (Proverbs 5:15): "Drink waters out of thine own cistern, and running waters out of thine own well." In ancient Hindu Ayurvedic medicine, the practice of urine therapy was called "shivambu," and the *Damara Tantra* stated, "A sensible man gets up early in the morning when three quarters of the night has passed, faces east and passes urine. The initial and concluding flow of urine is to be discarded. The intermediate flow is to be consumed. This is the most suitable method." French physicians in the eighteenth century recommended that their patients drink preparations containing urine for many medical conditions, and offered this therapy under the more acceptable name *l'eau de mille fleur* ("water of a thousand flowers"). Nicholas Culpeper suggested another use for urine in his *School of Physick* (1659): "Take all the Urine the party makes at one time that hath the Quartain Ague, and knead flour, and make a cake with it, and when it is baked, give it to a Dog of the house; do so twice or thrice, and in so doing the party will be well and the Dog sick. Chuse a Dog for a Man, but a Bitch for a Woman."

Artifacts from the departed were sure to provide mysterious and powerful cures. In the twelfth century, Western physicians prescribed mummy powder for nausea, seizures, headaches, paralysis, and as an antidote to poisoning (figure 318). Some French physicians boiled mummies and used the oil that rose to the top, though French surgeon Ambroise Paré disagreed with the use of mummies when he said, "not only does this wretched drug do no good, but it causes great pain to the stomach, gives foul-smelling breath, and brings on serious vomiting."

A sure Scottish cure for epilepsy was produced from the burned skull or bones of a buried man, and one could cure a headache by using the dried and powdered moss growing on a human skull in snuff. Another unusual custom took place in 1752 at the hanging of notorious highwayman, Nicholas Mooney, in Bristol. As reported in *Popular Antiquities,* "after the cart drew away, the hangman very deservedly had his head broke for attempting to pull off Mooney's shoes; and a fellow had like to have been killed in mounting the gallows to take away the ropes that were left after the malefactors were cut down. A young woman came fifteen miles for the sake of the rope from Mooney's neck, which was given to her, it being by many apprehended that the halter of an executed person will charm away the ague and perform many other cures."

MEDICAL BOTANY

Healers have always made use of easily available resources, so the central role played by plants and plant products in the history of medicine is not surprising. Many herbs used in ancient Egypt continue to be recommended by physicians throughout the world today with some familiar examples, including castor oil (cathartic), aloe vera (skin restorative), colchicum (joint pain relief), garlic (stimulant, digestive aid), honey (antibiotic), parsley (diuretic), mint (digestive aid), and poppy (pain control). The biblical birthday gifts of frankincense (*boswellia carterii*) and myrrh (*commiphora myrrha*) are derived from the gums of trees, and though they were used for incense, they were also employed medically as stimulants and astringents. Additionally, frankincense was a popular remedy for vomiting and respiratory infections, while myrrh was used to treat head and neck pain, along with loose stools. According to Ovid, King Cinyrus' daughter, Myrrh, desired her father and conceived a child

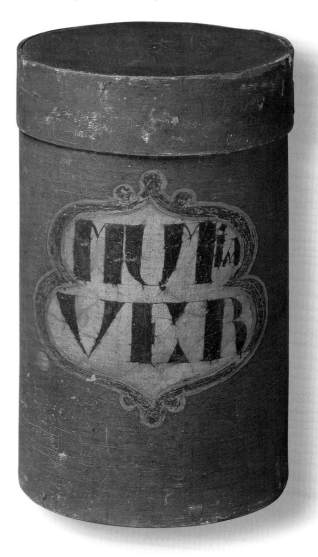

318. European powdered mummy container (ca. 1600–1800)

413

after she had seduced him. The king banished his daughter to the desert where the gods turned Myrrh into a tree that bore her name and produced a therapeutic sap to represent her tears of remorse.

Herbs have been an important part of Chinese medical care for thousands of years, beginning with what is the considered the earliest and most important medical work, the *Nei Ching* ("Canon of Medicine"). It is said to reflect medicine as practiced during the reign of Huang Ti, or the "Yellow Emperor," in the twenty-seventh century B.C., though the book was published much later in the third century B.C. Shen Nung is generally accepted as the father of Chinese medicine, and, in about A.D. 500, he authored the *Shen-nung pen ts'ao ching* ("Devine Husbandman's Materia Medica"). Considered the earliest known Chinese pharmacopoeia, it contained the first reference to the properties of herbs, which were divided into three major categories: superior herbs for nourishment, middle herbs to balance bodily systems, and inferior herbs for the treatment of disease. This text contains 365 medications, many of which remain in use today. It is a long-held belief that Shen Nung tested each plant on himself and then viewed the effects through a window that he had made in his abdomen. The high point of Chinese medicine was reached during the Ming dynasty (1368–1644) when Li Shih-chen wrote the *Pen ts'ao kang mu* ("The Great Herbal"), where he summarized the medical uses of over eighteen hundred herbs, minerals, and animal products.

For centuries, physicians in China decided which plants were appropriate for each disease according to their yin and yang properties. Yin herbs were cool, sour, bitter, and salty with the American variety of ginseng an example. This herb has been in use for thousands of years and remains popular for its restorative, aphrodisiac, and sedative properties, though some types of ginseng act as a stimulant. Yang herbs, on the other hand, were hot, sweet, and pungent, a good example being *ma huang*, or ephedra, which has been used since antiquity as a stimulant and a bronchial dilator for asthma and colds, though recently it has become a major ingredient in diet pills. In addition to the use of herbs, four other important categories of medical therapy in traditional Chinese medicine were trees, insects, stones, and grains.

Western physicians have used herbs and plants from China, India, and Southeast Asia for treating a number of medical conditions for centuries. An active trade in spices began in ancient Greek communities and was continued well into the Renaissance. The food was bland, so in addition to using spices for therapy, many used them as taste additives, perfumes, and cosmetics. It was the search for an alternate route by sea to capture the spice trade and bypass the slow and expensive Arab overland caravans that led Columbus to set sail westward for the Indies, mistakenly to discover the New World. The transport of spices was extremely lucrative, and the only ship of Magellan's five that returned safely carried enough cargo in cloves to pay for the entire voyage of all five ships. Europeans continued to purchase spices for their presumed therapeutic properties into the Middle Ages. One of the oldest was cinnamon from China and Burma, which was used both as an antiseptic and a carminative (for the relief of gas). Cloves from the Spice Islands (Ternate and Tidore) were considered a good stimulant, while pepper from India was a popular tonic, stimulant, and aphrodisiac.

Physicians believed that planets influenced the color of plants, and they thus gave those colors great significance in their choice of therapy. For example, those who suffered from smallpox were frequently given drinks with dissolved red ingredients, including the extracts of pomegranate seeds, burnt purple, and mulberries. Patients were also surrounded by red in hopes that the color would bring the red pustules to the surface of the body. According to John Gaddeson, physician to Edward II, "When the son of the renowned King of England lay sick of the smallpox I took care that everything around the bed should be of a red colour; which succeeded so completely that the Prince was restored to perfect health, without a vestige of a pustule remaining."

Pedacius Dioscorides, a Greek surgeon under Emperor Nero, wrote the earliest "formulary" in the first century. *De Materia Medica Libri Quinque* contained more than five hundred plants and remained popular for sixteen centuries. Herbal texts are available today, and a number of useful medications had their origins in these books, including atropine, cocaine, digitalis, ergot, morphine, salicylate, and quinine. In 1558, German physician and botanist Leonard Rauwolf was the first to describe Rauwolfia, though it had already been used as a sedative in India. It was one of the earliest antihypertensive agents and, up until a few years ago, was in use under the name of reserpine.

Medications were largely uncontrolled for safety and efficacy, so physicians regularly prescribed a number of potentially dangerous substances. In his classic first-century text *De Medicina,* Celsus described the method of preparation of a still popular drug:

Take a handful of poppy when it is ripe for taking its tears, put it into a vessel, add enough water to cover it, and cook it. When it is well cooked, squeeze out the mass of poppy into a vessel before discarding it, and mix with the fluid an equal quantity of raisin wine. Boil it until it thickens, then cool it and make it into pills about the size of domestic beans.

They have many uses. They induce sleep, whether taken alone or dissolved in water. Added, in small quantity, to the juice of rue, or to raisin wine, they stop ear-ache. Dissolved in wine, they stop colic.

Mixed with beeswax and attar of roses, and with a little saffron added, they cure inflammation of the vulva; and dissolved in water which is then applied to the forehead, they stop running of the eyes.

Other potentially dangerous medications that were "over the counter" included:

arsenic (rat's bane): used to treat intermittent fever after it cured disease in workers at a copper smelting plant. Likely the arsenical fumes had killed the malaria bearing mosquitoes.

aconite (wolfsbane): a diaphoretic or sedative, though fatal if the leaves were not well-cooked.

belladonna (atropine, deadly nightshade): a diaphoretic, cathartic, and anticholinergic that caused convulsions and death if too much was taken. The three fates in Greek mythology were Clotho, Lachesis, and Atropos, and it was Atropos who cut the thread of life at the time of death. The name *belladonna* is derived from the Italian "beautiful woman," and may have been used by the ancient Assyrians to dilate pupils. (In fact, modern surveys suggest that men uniformly prefer women with larger pupils.) Though belladonna, or atropine, has been employed as a poison in the past, it is useful today in treating cardiac dysrhythmias. It may have been atropine that Dr. Roger Chillingworth gave to the Reverend Dimmesdale after he had impregnated his wife in Hawthorne's *The Scarlet Letter* (1850).

mercury (calomel, quicksilver): a cathartic and anti-inflammatory. Mercury was popular in ancient times as an antiparasitic and was found in topical ointments. It was also an ingredient in tattoos, including those of Egyptian Queen Nefertiti. Mercury was the Roman messenger of the gods, but also the god of alchemy, and it was his speed (along with the metal's liquid nature) that led to the use of the term *quicksilver* for that metal. The Greeks named the same god Hermes, and early alchemists "hermetically sealed" their potions. Mercury was later used in the treatment of syphilis, though it was found to be toxic when some leaked out of its wrappings on a ship and killed all the rats. Side effects of mercury ingestion include salivation, bleeding from the gums, bloody stools, lost teeth, slurred speech, depression, irritability, neuropathy, and renal failure. "Mercurial trembling" was noted in those who silvered mirrors, while British hat makers developed personality disorders with the use of mercury, and thus the genesis of the expression "mad as a hatter." The hatter in Lewis Carroll's *Alice in Wonderland* exemplified this bizarre behavior.

strichnine: a laxative, diuretic, diaphoretic, and also a respiratory suppressant.

antimony (tartar emetic): "Stibium" was given to several monks in the fifteenth century as a treatment for cachexia, though unfortunately, they all died. The name of the medication was changed to antimony (meaning "antagonist to monks"), and since it caused nausea and vomiting, its medicinal use was banned for many years until it was credited with curing the French King Louis XIV of typhoid fever in 1657. Antimony was then used into the nineteenth century for the treatment of typhoid fever and several tropical parasitic infestations.

lead: The ancient Greeks classified lead as one of the basic seven metals. It represented the planet Saturn, and so lead poisoning became known as "Saturnism." The Romans fermented their wine in lead-containing vats because of its sweet taste, and some historians attribute the decline of the Roman Empire to subsequent lead encephalopathy in Roman leaders. Sweet tasting lead continues to cause lead paint poisoning in children.

The origin, properties, and medicinal use of a number of plants were beautifully illustrated and colorfully described in *Medical Botany: or, Illustrations and Descriptions of the Medicinal Plants of the London, Edinburgh, and Dublin Pharmacopoeias* (1828), by John Stephenson, MD. and James Churchill, FLS (figures 319–331):

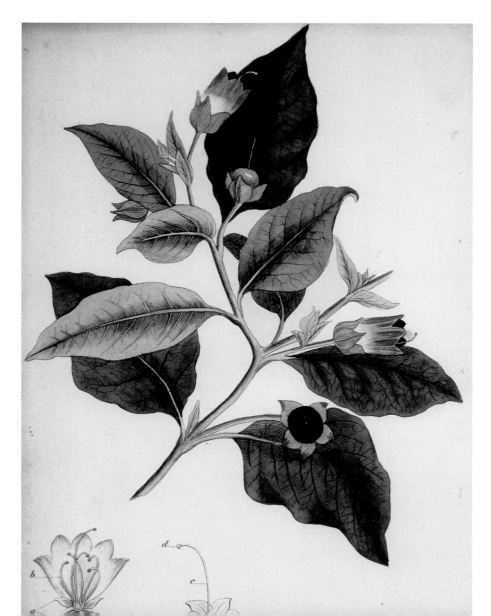

319. *Atropa Belladonna* (Deadly Nightshade)
The poisonous qualities of Belladonna reside in every part of the plant; but chiefly predominate in the fruit: and we possess but too many well-attested narratives of the fatal effect of its berries; which in appearance are very alluring to children. . . . It possesses anodyne and antispasmodic virtues; in small doses, relieving pain; and has a direct action on the brain and nervous system: but in larger doses, according to Dr. Bostock, it exerts its influence on the alimentary canal. Like Digitalis, Nicotiana, and some other narcotics, it sometimes operates as a diuretic; and in a few rare instances, has been known to excite the action of the salivary glands, and to produce salivation.

320. *Spigella Marilandica* (Maryland Worm-grass, or Carolina Pink)
This plant was first used by the Cherokee Indians, as an anthelmintic. . . . If it proves purgative it is said to be most effective: and should it not, it must be conjoined with cathartics; which prevent the narcotic symptoms, such as stupor, headache, dilated pupil, flushings of the face, stiffness of the eyelids, that so frequently follow its administration.

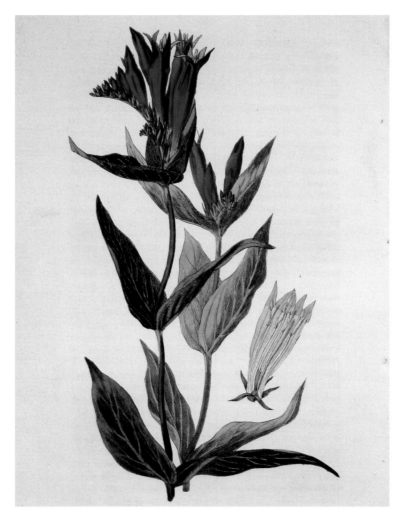

321. *Hyoscyamus Niger* (Common Henbane)
Henbane is one of our most valuable narcotics. The principal use which is made of it, is as a substitute for opium, when the latter disagrees, or is contraindicated by particular symptoms. It appears to be free from the constipating qualities of opium, especially if exhibited in large doses. Like digitalis and other narcotics, it often operates as a diuretic, and sometimes increases the cuticular discharge.

Wepfer relates, that several monks made a repast on the roots of wild endive, among which were mixed by mistake two roots of henbane. In a few hours, some experienced vertigo; others a burning of the tongue, lips and throat. Severe pains were also felt in the iliac region, and in all the joints. The intellectual facilities and organs of vision were perverted, and they gave themselves up to actions that were mad and ridiculous. They however recovered.

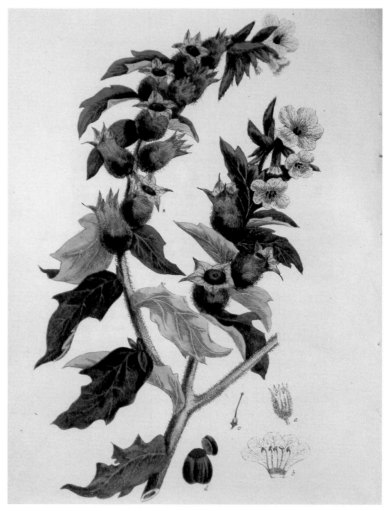

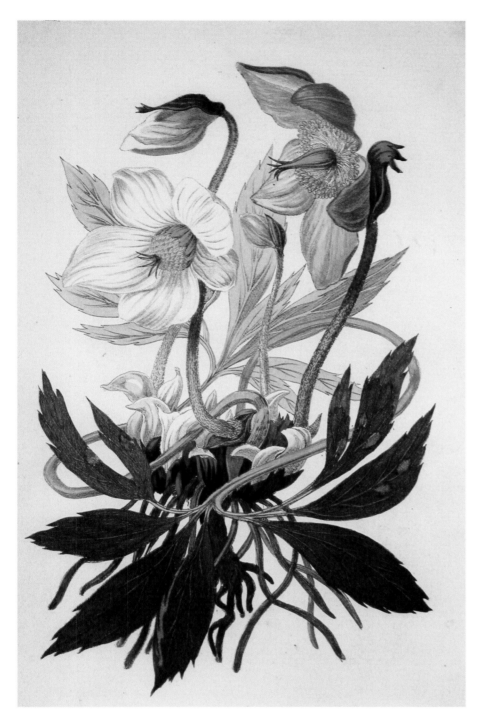

322. *Helleborus Niger* (Black Hellebore)

Before the grand discoveries, which chemistry has made on the attributes of metallic substances, the most violent vegetable medicines were boldly administered, and this plant has been highly extolled by Avicenna, Gesner, Klein, Milman, and many others, in mania, dropsy, cutaneous diseases, and worms.

Two persons took a decoction of this root in cider. . . . Three quarters of an hour after taking it, alarming symptoms were developed, without exciting suspicion of the real cause. One of the men, therefore, took another dose, when vomiting delirium, horrible contortions, accompanied with immediate coldness supervened, and death at last ensued. On dissection, sixteen hours afterwards, the appearances in each were found precisely similar, except that in the one who took the largest quantity they were more strongly marked. The lungs were gorged with blood. The mucous membrane of the stomach was considerable inflamed, of a blackish brown colour, and reduced almost to a gangrenous state. The oesophagus and intestines were natural.

323. *Solanum Dulcamara* (Woody Nightshade, or Bitter-sweet) Chemical Properties and Uses— Chronic rheumatism, gout incipient phthisis, asthma, jaundice, and several other diseases, are said to have been benefited by the use of this plant. . . .

In 1825, a child of Mr. Simmons, four years old, residing in Camden's Place, swallowed some of the berries. He was a fine, stout, healthy boy. The symptoms were . . . attended with violent vomiting and purging, with contraction of the abdominal muscles. There was also a profuse secretion of saliva. I took five ounces of blood from the arm; gave twelve grains of calomel in a little sugar, and ordered the oily mixture with four drops of laudanum in each dose. Leeches were also applied to the abdomen. In the evening, I found that the bowels had been freely acted on, and the breathing was much improved. I continued my attendance for several days, and consider that his recovery was probably protracted from my not having seen him, till three hours after he had taken the berries.

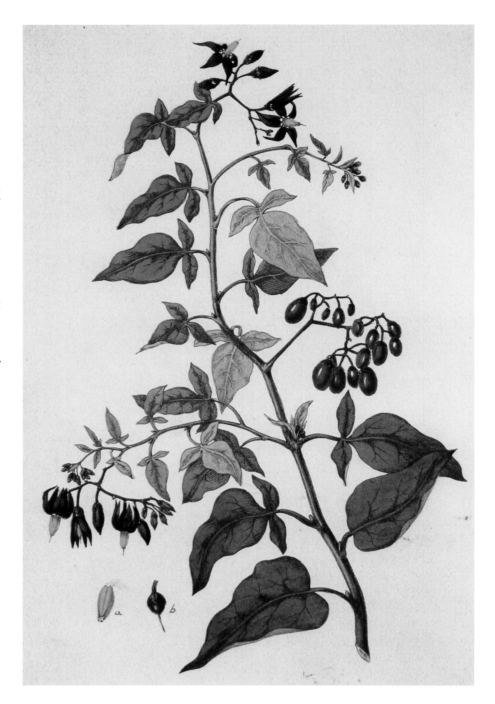

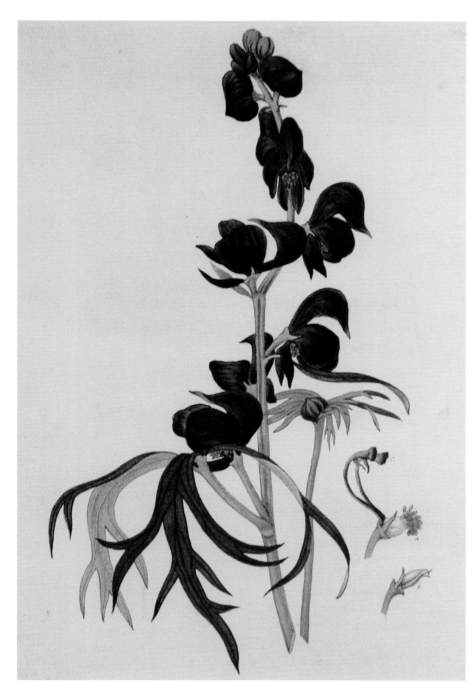

324. *Aconitum Napellus* (Common Monk's-hood, or Wolf's-bane)
It is to Baron Stöck that we are principally indebted for our knowledge of this powerful remedy; which, according to his account, is diuretic, as well as diaphoretic, and narcotic. He administered it for intermittent fevers, chronic rheumatism, gout, exostosis, paralysis, and scirrhus, and narrates many well-marked cases of these diseases, in which it was eminently successful.

John Crumpler, at eight in the evening, ate some salad, in which had been put by mistake a certain quantity of *A. napellus*. He felt immediately a burning heat on the tongue and gums, and a great irritation in the cheeks. He thought that the blood no longer circulated in his limbs; he had however no inclination to vomit.

Perceiving the symptoms to increase, he drank about a pint of oil, and a great quantity of tea, which produced vomiting. The symptoms far from disappearing were aggravated. At ten o'clock, Vincent Bacon, a surgeon, was called in, and found him in bed, with his eyes and teeth fixed, his hands and feet cold, the body, for the most part, covered with a cold perspiration, and the pulse scarcely perceptible, and the breathing so short, that it could with difficulty be perceived. He made him swallow two spoonsful of spirit of hartshorn, which occasioned coughing and vomiting: he then administered an infusion of *Carduus Benedictus*, until several vomitings were procured. The patient shortly had a stool, and vomited afresh. The pulse became a little raised, but was intermitting, and extremely irregular. Some stimulating medicines were given; the next morning he was a great deal better, and the cure soon completed. . . .

A person having eaten some of the leaves of the *A. napellus*, became maniacal, and the surgeon who was called to his assistance declared, that the plant was not the cause of his disorder; and to convince the company that it was perfectly innocent, he ate freely if its leaves, and soon after died in great agony.

325. *Ncotiana Tabacum* (Virginia Tobacco)

Dr. Fowler, in a distinct treatise, has adduced many cases in which an infusion of Tobacco was advantageously administered in dropsy: but as digitalis is more easily managed, and appears to exert the same kind of effects, it is generally preferred. He also recommends it is *dysuria*, and as that disease is sometimes connected with spasmodic action, Tobacco frequently proves useful; acting both as a diuretic and antispasmotic.

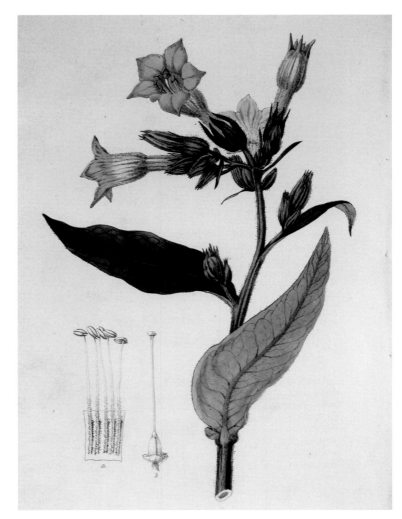

326. *Anthemis Nobilis* (Common Chamomile)

Chamomile is a powerful tonic and stomachic, and inferior to no other, when properly administered. It is an excellent and popular remedy for a weakened state of stomach, attended by the ordinary symptoms of indigestion, as heartburn, loss of appetite, flatulency, &c.

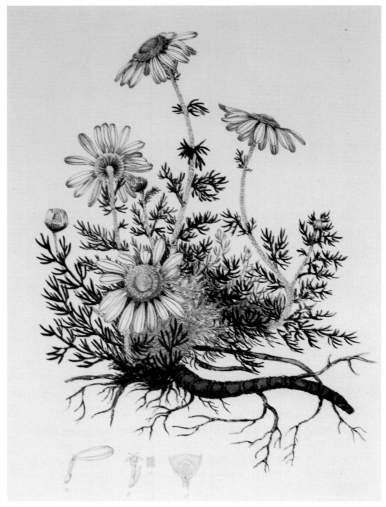

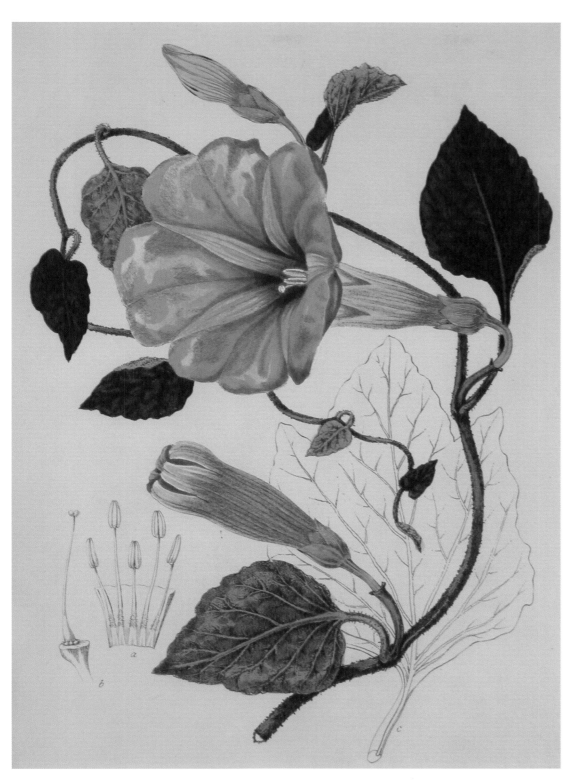

327. *Convolvulus Jalapa* (Mexican or Jalap Bindweed)

Jalap is an active purgative, and one on which we can rely. It produces copious evacuations from the small and large intestines, and would be administered much oftener, were it not for the griping and distressing nausea that often arise from it. It is, notwithstanding, a safe medicine . . . to be of eminent use in typhus, scarlatina, cynanche maligna, marasmus, chorea, and tetanus.

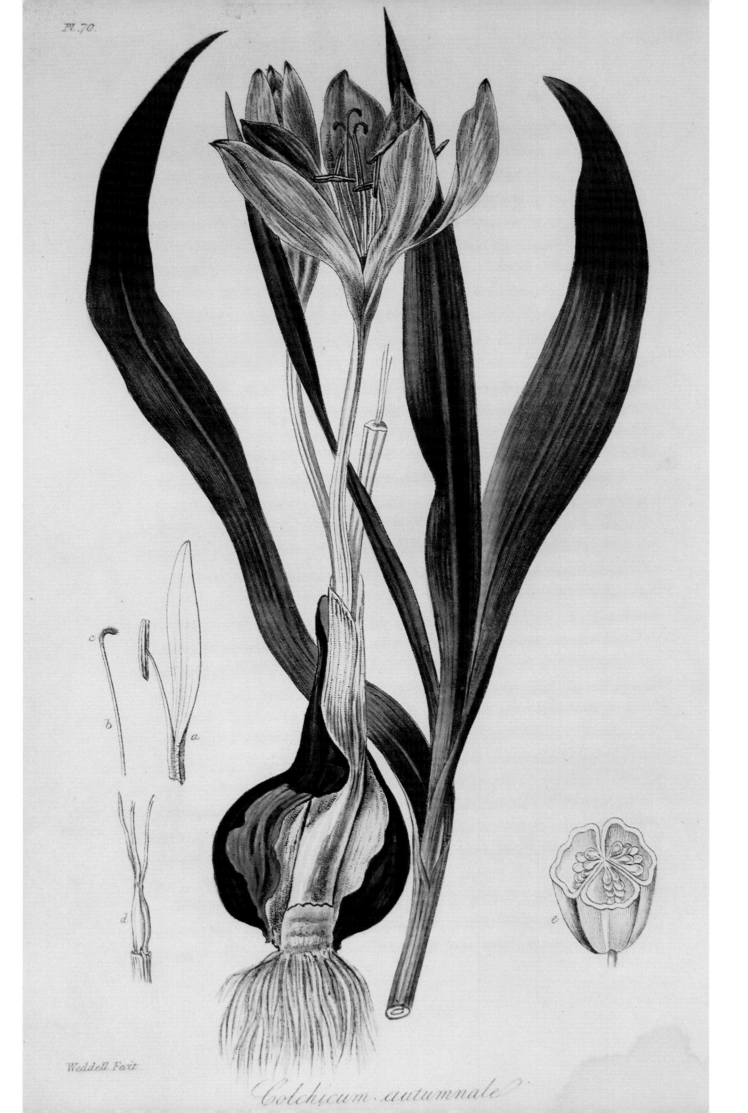

Pl. 70.

Weddell Fecit

Colchicum autumnale

328. *Colchicum Autumnale* (Common Meadow-saffron)

Colchicum is one of the most powerful remedies we are possessed of, in consequence of the direct action it is capable of exerting over the heart, and arteries. On the continent it has been chiefly used in the treatment of hydrothorax, and asthma . . . and in a few hours, generally succeeds in destroying the paroxysm of gout. Poisonous Effects . . .

Susan Lang was about thirty years of age, and of good health and constitution; she was about two months gone in pregnancy of a bastard child, and, having read in a newspaper, that a woman was taken up for causing abortion by taking Meadow-safforn, she determined on getting rid of her burthen by a similar measure. She accordingly bought twopenny worth, and made an infusion of it, which she took on an empty stomach, early in the morning of the 10th of March, 1827. I was called to her about four o'clock on the afternoon of the 11th, and on enquiry learned that she had miscarried the proceeding evening. I found her in a very hopeless state; her extremities were quite cold, and the whole of her body, particularly the hands, feet, and face, livid; the glossy stare of impending death was in her eyes; the respiration was hurried, and the pulse could not be felt at the carotids, and but faintly at the heart. Notwithstanding, the sensorium was undisturbed, and she gave me a clear account of what she had done, her motives for so doing, and the effects the poison had on her. She said, that in about half an hour after she had taken it, her stomach became sick, gripes came on, and a violent purging, which continued with great severity. She had had no medical assistance, and had past a most wretched time from the morning before, and was so tormented with pain and purging, that she had not a wink of sleep in the course of night. I administered to her large draughts of brandy and spices, but to no effect, as she died in two hours after I was called in. The body was opened the next day, and all the viscera were found perfectly sound, with the exception, that the mucous membranes of the stomach and bowels was dreadfully inflamed, throughout its course.

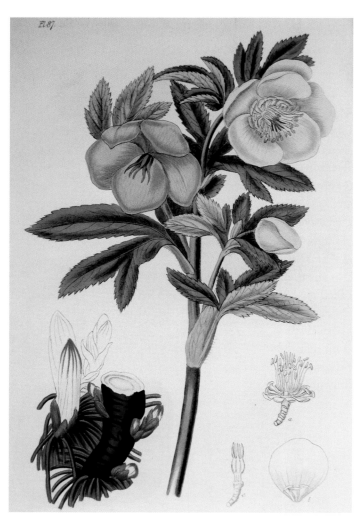

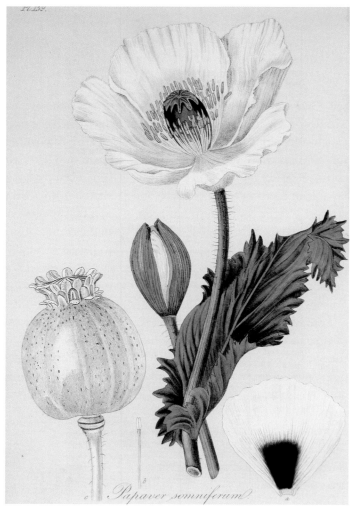

329. *Helleborus Orientalis* (Oriental, or True Hellebore)

The roots of this species of Hellebore, formerly called *Melampodium*, from their black colour, are acrid and violently cathartic. They have been supposed to be useful in maniacal cases, epilepsy, paralysis, hypochondriasis, dropsies, and a variety of other diseases. . . .

330. *Papaver Somniferum* (White Poppy)

Opium has been employed for ages as the most active and efficient means we possess to support the powers of the system, mitigate pain or irritation, induce sleep, relieve inordinate action, check morbidly increased evacuations, and diminish morbid sensibility.

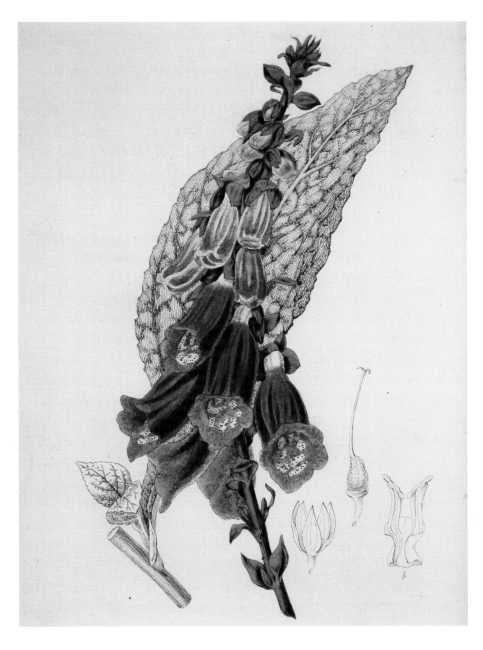

331. *Digitalis Purpurea* (Purple Foxglove)

Were all that has been written on Digitalis to be collected, a ponderous volume of contradictions would be the result, for although the known virtues of the plant may be stated in a very small compass, it was at one time held forth as a never failing remedy in the worst and most common of diseases—pulmonary consumption. It was of course prescribed by almost every practitioner throughout the united kingdom; but in time, which settles down the minds of men to a just appreciation of the truth, has proved that it is only in the incipient stages of consumption, when indurated tubercles are producing their irritative effects on the lungs, in which the constitution is beginning to participate, that the sedative effects of Digitalis, which are so benign and truly valuable, can be advantageously produced. . . . As a diuretic, it is much used and highly prized, being more powerful and certain in its effects than any other.

Case 1st.—Dr. W. Henry was called in October 1809, to assist a female, an out-patient of the Manchester Infirmary, labouring under dropsy, who had taken an overdose of decoction of Foxglove. It was prepared by boiling two handfuls of the leaves in a quart of water, and then pressing the mass, so as to expel the whole of the liquor. Of this, at seven A.M. she drank two tea-cups full, amounting in the whole to not less than ten ounces by measure. Before eight, she began to be sick and vomited part of the contents of her stomach. Enough, however, was retained to excite vomiting and retching throughout the whole of that and the following day, during which, every thing that was taken was instantly rejected. In the intervals of sickness she was excessively faint, and her skin was covered with a cold sweat. The tongue and lips swelled, and there was a constant flow of viscid saliva from the mouth. Very little urine was voided on the day she took the Digitalis, and on the following days, the action of the kidnies was entirely suspended. When Dr. Henry saw her, which was forty-eight hours after she had taken the poison, the tongue was white, the ptyalism continued, though in a less degree, and the breath was foetid. The pulse was low, irregular, (not exceeding forty,) and after every third or fourth pulsation, an intermission occurred for some seconds. She complained also of general pains in the limbs, and cramps in the legs. By the use of effervescing draughts, and aether with ammonia, she gradually recovered her imperfect health.

THEORIES OF THERAPY

Aureolus Philip Theophrastus Bombastus von Hohenheim (1493–1541) boastfully named himself Paracelcus after the famous Roman medical historian Celsus, though his name meant "better than Celsus." He was one of the most controversial figures in the history of medicine, considered by some a great medical reformer though by many others a quack. Paracelsus was of Swiss descent and spent much of his time wandering about the countryside, characteristically using the common vernacular rather than Latin as his form of medical communication. According to Fielding Garrison, "by his relations with barbers, executioners, bath keepers, gypsies, midwives, and fortune tellers, he learned a great deal about medical practice, and incidentally acquired an unusual knowledge of folk-medicine and a permanent taste for low company."

Prior to Paracelcus, physicians had remained faithful to the teachings of Galen by attempting to maintain a balance between natural humors with leeches, diuretics, emetics, and cathartics. Paracelcus changed all that, and for the first time relied on the use of chemicals, or "alchemy," to treat his patients. He regarded sulphur, mercury, and salt as elements of fundamental importance in regulating bodily functions and emphasized the spiritual aspects of disease by using astrology along with heavy metals in his therapy. To the chagrin of other faculty members, he advanced to become a professor of medicine at the university in Basil after he had cured the long-standing leg ulcers of famous Renaissance publisher John Froben. It did not take long for Paracelcus to antagonize the faculty. "All the universities have less experience than my beard," he said, and to fellow professors, "You must follow in my footsteps; I shall not go in yours. Not one of you will find a corner so well hidden but that the dogs will come and lift their legs to defile you. I shall become monarch. . . . You will eat dirt." On June 24, 1527, Paracelsus burned the books of Galen and Avicenna in a public bonfire commenting "thus the realm of medicine has been purged."

Paracelcus believed that medicine and surgery were part of the same profession and that any intervention should only be in a conservative and reasoned manner. In *Grosse Wundartznei*, he wrote, "The surgeon must also know that nature cannot be converted or changed, but that he must follow nature, not nature him. If he uses remedies contrary to nature, he will ruin everything. Now you cannot replace a limb that has been cut off and it is ridiculous to attempt it. In Veriul I saw a barber surgeon replace an ear that had been cut off and stick it back with mason's cement. He was given great praise and a loud cry of 'miracle.' However, the next day the ear fell off since it was undermined with pus. The same thing happens with limbs if one tries to stick them back on again, but what glory is there is such chicanery?" Paracelsus described an ideal surgeon in the same work:

> The basis of medicine is love, and not everyone can be a physician. Every surgeon should have three qualities, first as regards his own *person*; second, as regards the *patient*, and, third, as regards his *art*. As regards his own person, the surgeon should not think he knows everything or is competent to handle all things. Not the outlay of money, nor the attendance at school, nor the reading of books will make a surgeon. The surgeon should not run a house of ill-fame, he should not be a hangman, or apostate, nor belong to the priesthood, or be an actor or poet. The barbers, bathers, and others of their ilk think they have learned it all by the menial work of their trade. But you must learn daily from your own experience and from the experiences of others for no matter how experienced or wise you may be, the time comes when your knowledge fails you and the patient suffers. Be modest and mild; do not praise yourself but give credit to others where credit is due. Think more of the patient than the money you may gain from him.

Paracelcus employed natural cures, though perhaps some of his success could have been related to his "secret ingredient" laudanum, or opium.

CONTROLLED SUBSTANCES AND SELF-EXPERIMENTATION

Medications were sold to the public with little if any testing for safety or efficacy. In 1534, Antonio Brasalova, physician to Pope Paul III, suggested that condemned prisoners be used as subjects in the clinical evaluation of new medications. Because of the difficulty in finding willing subjects, physicians not infrequently experimented on themselves, as was the case in the discovery of anesthesia and the early use of many narcotics.

One example is found in *An Inquiry into the Nature and Properties of Opium* (1793) by Samuel Crumpe, MD:

> Experiment I
> I poured a small quantity of a strong watery solution of Opium into my left eye; it immediately occasioned considerable pain, which continued for about ten minutes, and a smart degree of inflammation both in the tunica adnata and palpebrae, which remained very observable for many minutes after the pain had ceased; the pain and inflammation were likewise attended with an effusion of tears.

Experiment II

Having reduced a small quantity of Opium to powder, I drew it up my nose: it produced the same effects as weak snuff would have done. This experiment was made with similar event by Dr. Alston: Opium, he says, heats and irritates the nose, and creates an inclination to sneeze.

Experiment III

I injected some of the same solution above mentioned into the urethra, which was immediately followed by a sense of heat and pain. The result of this experiment I have indeed seen verified in several instances, wherein a simple aqueous solution of Opium was used by way of injection in gonorrhea. . . .

Peruvian natives have been chewing coca leaves for thousands of years because of their presumed properties in extending life. Coca was also considered useful as a stimulant, an aid to digestion, and even as an aphrodisiac. Robert Louis Stevenson wrote *The Strange Case of Dr Jekyll and Mr. Hyde* while on a six-day binge of cocaine. Arthur Conan Doyle's character Sherlock Holmes remarked that cocaine was "so transcendentally stimulating and clarifying to the mind that its secondary action is a matter of small moment." Famous psychoanalyst Sigmund Freud was also an advocate and wrote *On Cocaine* in 1884:

A few minutes after taking cocaine, one experiences a certain exhilaration and feeling of lightness. One feels a certain furriness on the lips and palate, followed by a feeling of warmth in the same areas; if one now drinks cold water, it feels warm on the lips and cold in the throat. On other occasions the predominant feeling is a rather pleasant coolness in the mouth and throat.

During the first trial I experienced a short period of toxic effects, which did not recur in subsequent experiments. Breathing became slower and deeper and I felt tired and sleepy; I yawned frequently and felt somewhat dull. After a few minutes, the actual cocaine euphoria began, introduced by repeated cooling eructation. Immediately after taking the cocaine I noticed a slight slackening of the pulse and later a moderate increase.

I have observed the same physical signs of the effect of cocaine in others, mostly people my own age. The most constant symptom proved to be the repeated eructation. This is often accompanied by a rumbling which must originate from high up on the intestine; two of the people I observed, who said they were able to recognize movements in their stomachs, declared emphatically that they had repeatedly detected such movements. Often, at the outset of the cocaine effect, the subjects alleged that they experienced an intense feeling of heat in the head. I noticed this I myself as well in the course of some later experiments, but on other occasions it was absent. In only two cases did coca give rise to dizziness. On the whole the toxic effects of coca are of short duration, and much less intense than those produced by effective doses of quinine or salicylate of soda; they seem to become even weaker after repeated use of cocaine.

Freud concluded his treatise on cocaine with a recommendation for its appropriate use as a mental and appetite stimulant, an aphrodisiac, a local anesthetic, a treatment for asthma and digestive disorders, and, ironically, as an aid for the withdrawal from both morphine and alcohol addictions. All this and "exhilaration and lasting euphoria, which in no way differs from the normal euphoria of the healthy person" and "no craving for further use of cocaine appears after the first, or even after repeated taking of the drug. . . ."

Perhaps the greatest surgeon of the nineteenth century was William Halsted, who helped bring surgery to prominence around the world with his surgical training program while at the Johns Hopkins University. He also became dependent on cocaine after self-experimentation and required hospitalization for an extended period of time, never fully recovering.

John Smyth Pemberton (1831–1888) was an Atlanta, Georgia, druggist whose obsession was to earn a fortune by inventing a beverage that could be used as a medication. He was aware of the properties of coca, and he wanted to produce a drink containing alcohol that competed with Vin Mariani, a popular coca product invented by Corsican chemist Angelo Mariani that was sold in both Europe and the United States (figure 332). Vin Mariani had received numerous testimonials from the rich and famous, including Thomas Edison, Queen Victoria, British Shakespearean actor Sir Henry Irving (the first actor ever to be knighted), and three popes. Pope Leo XIII awarded the coca containing Vin Mariani a gold medal "in recognition of benefits received from the use of Mariani's tonic." French sculptor Frédérick-Auguste Bartholdi commented that had he used Vin Mariani earlier in his life, the Statue of Liberty would have been a few hundred meters higher. Pemberton's French Wine Coca was marketed in 1885 in Atlanta chemists' shops as an "intellectual beverage" and an "invigorator of the brain," additional ingredients including kola nut and the purported aphrodisiac damiana. His wine was also intended to be a nerve tonic for the relief of morphine

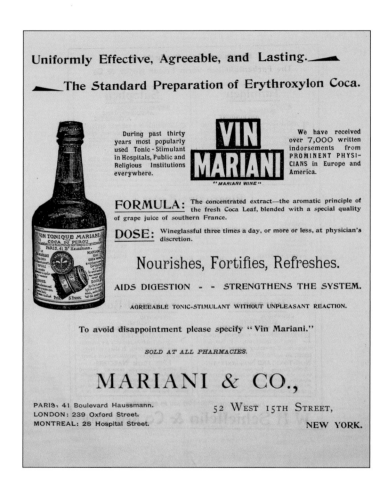

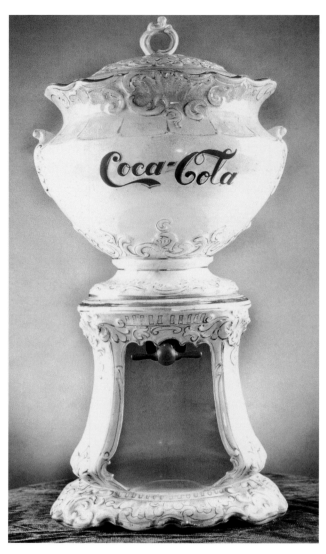

332. Advertisement for Vin Mariani, *New York Medical Journal* (November 1895)

333. Early twentieth-century ceramic Coca Cola dispenser

addiction, a problem he struggled with himself.

Pemberton produced his wine at a time when the temperance movement was gaining momentum in America, and he was forced to modify his formula to be a temperance drink "offering the virtues of coca without the vices of alcohol." After some experimentation, citric acid was added to coca leaf and kola nut, and the Pemberton Chemical Company was born. A contest to name the new product followed, and was won by Frank Robinson, who created the now famous name "Coca-Cola" and designed the script trademark. Coca-Cola was introduced in 1886 as "a valuable brain-tonic and cure for all nervous afflictions" (figure 333).

As is often the case in stories of great discovery and wealth, John Pemberton's personal success was short lived, however. His morphine addiction progressed, and he developed cancer from which he died on August 16, 1888. Before his death, Pemberton sold two-thirds of the

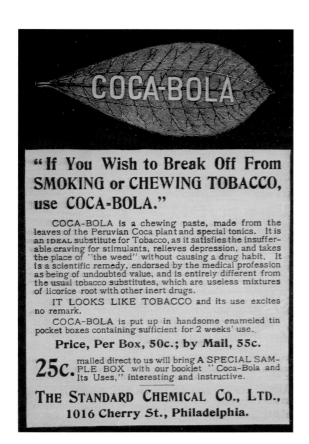

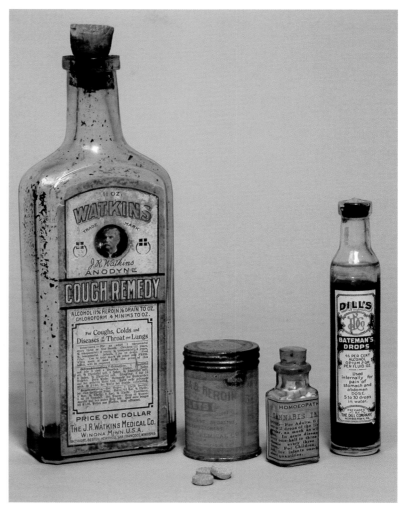

stock in his corporation, leaving one third for his son so that he "will always have a living." Pemberton's son, Charley, died six years later from a morphine overdose, and John Pemberton's wife died penniless. To this day, Coca Cola yearly imports several tons of inactive coca extract from South America for their beverages.

Over the next several decades, medications containing what are now controlled substances, including heroin and opium, found instant success in pharmacies when sold over the counter (figures 334, 335).

HOMEOPATHY

Samuel Hahnemann (1755–1843) was born in Meissen, Germany, and studied in Leipzig and Vienna. He briefly practiced medicine, though became disenchanted and retired after only a few years. Hahnemann was persuaded to return to the field of therapeutics, however, after an interesting observation related to malaria. He obviously was unaware of the

334. Coca Bola advertisement (ca. 1900)

335. Over-the-counter controlled substances (ca. 1900): heroin cough remedy, cannabis for children's diseases, opium for abdominal pain

relation that malaria had to the disease-producing mosquito, though he did know that malaria could be successfully treated by quinine obtained from Peruvian bark. He also noted from self-experimentation that small quantities of quinine could produce the same symptoms as malaria: "My feet, my fingertips, at first became cold. I grew languid, and drowsy; then my heart began to palpitate, and my pulse became hard and small; intolerable anxiety, trembling, prostration through all my limbs. Then pulsation in my head, flushing of my cheeks. . . ." Hahnemann concluded that drugs causing the original symptoms of a disease could be curative if given in smaller amounts, an idea he expressed in his hallmark phrase *similia similibus curantur* ("like cures like"). According to Hahnemann, "The only really salutary treatment is that of the homeopathic method, according to which the totality of symptoms of a natural disease is combated by a medicine in commensurate doses, capable of creating in the healthy body symptoms most similar to those of the natural disease."

An example of this form of therapy is offered in the preface to the first British edition of Samuel Hahnemann's *Organon of Homoeopathic Medicine* (1833):

> Mercurial preparations, when administered internally, produce symptoms local and constitutional, so closely resembling the poison of lues venerea that medical practitioners, who have spent many years in the investigation of syphilis, find it very difficult—nay, in some instances impossible (guided by appearances)—to distinguish one disease from the other. Of all the medicines used in the treatment of lues, Mercury is the only one that has stood the test of time and experience. Let us then compare the effects of syphilis with those of Mercury. The venereal poison produces on the skin pustules, scales, and tubercles. Mercury produces directly the same defoedations of the skin. Syphilis excites inflammation of the periosteum, and caries of the bones. Mercury does the same. Inflammation of the iris from lues is an every-day occurrence; the same disease is a very frequent consequence of Mercury. Ulceration of the throat is a common symptom in syphilis; the same affection results from Mercury. Ulcers on the organs of reproduction are the result of both the poison and the remedy, and furnish another proof of the doctrine *similia similibus*.

Hahnemann borrowed some of his ideas from Hippocrates, who had said, "Through the like, disease is produced, and through the application of the like, it is cured." Additionally, Paracelsus had provided Hahnemann with the principle of "signatures," which was the astrological concept that stars impart an effect on plants reflected in their form

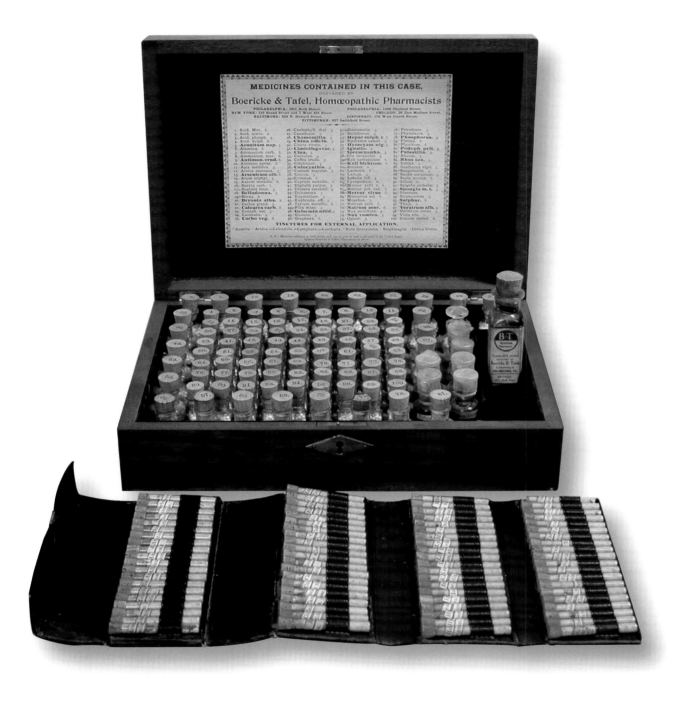

and color. The root of the orchid is shaped like a testicle and thus should be used for diseases affecting the male genitals; the Latin word for *orchid* is testicle and is the genesis of such related terms as *orchitis,* which refers to an inflammation of that organ. Other examples include the black spot in the flower euphrasia resembling an eye and the nutmeg a brain. Extracts of those substances, according to Hahnemann, should therefore be used to treat diseases of those organs. According to his "law of infinitesimals," the more diluted the dose, the more powerful was the effect, though Hahnemann had difficulty in getting pharmacies to stock his diluted medications since small amounts were not profitable (figure 336).

336. Homeopathic sets, top one by Boericke and Tafel (ca. 1890)

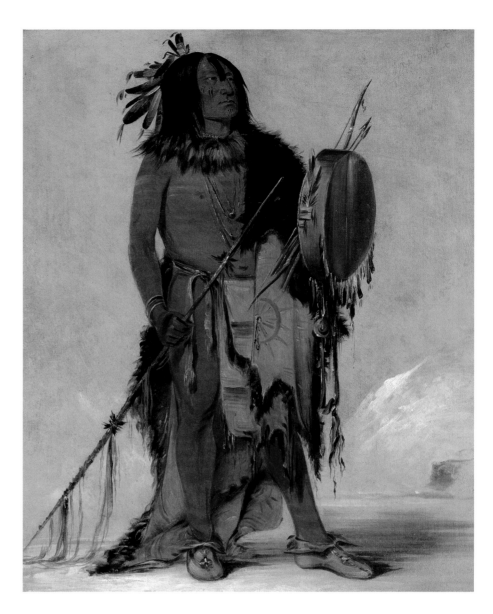

337. *White Buffalo, an Aged Medicine Man (Blackfoot)* (1832), oil on canvas by George Catlin

THE DRUG TRADE

Most medications in the United States prior to 1880 came from England and Europe, where heads of state regularly gave patents to their favorite manufacturers. This practice was so widespread in England that in 1624, Queen Elizabeth passed the Statute of Monopolies, which gave Parliament the power to authorize patents. Prescriptions were always written in Latin since, according to the dean of the faculty of medicine at Montpellier, Laurence Joubert, "if prescriptions are published in the simple tongue the mob will take them and trade in them." There was no requirement to disclose the ingredients until the reign of Queen Anne, and the first patent for a medication was granted to Nehemiah Grew for Epsom Salts.

"Patent medicines," those with disclosed ingredients, were initially exported to America from England with great success since production in the colonies was limited to home remedies and Indian cures (figure 337). In 1708, Nicholas Boone of Boston advertised a number of patent medicines he imported from England, the first of which was Daffy's Elixir. Though most of the early drugs came from overseas, a few were "home grown" folk remedies, including those from Benjamin Franklin's mother-in-law, the Widow Read, who sold "her well-known Ointment for the ITCH." The popularity of imported drugs led to the development of local drug wholesalers, though it was not until the Revolutionary War that the first laboratory in the United States was established in Carlisle, Pennsylvania, marking the beginning of the American pharmaceutical industry. This also marked the official separation between medicine and pharmacy.

The first American patent for a medication was awarded to Samuel Lee Jr. of Windham, Connecticut, in 1796 for his "bilious pills" for the treatment jaundice, dysentery, dropsy, and worms. The industrial race was on, and it didn't take long for the competition to begin. Samuel H.P. Lee was another Connecticut physician who also obtained a patent for "bilious pills" several years later in 1799. A dispute raged between the two for ten years, Lee warning, "If people incautiously purchase his pills for mine, I shall not be answerable for their effect."

338. *Lydia Pinkham's Vegetable Compound* (ca. 1890)

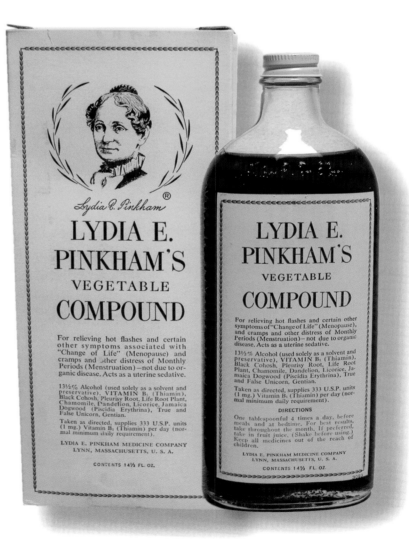

Thomas Dyott of Philadelphia was the first to produce medications that were distributed nationally, while Lydia Pinkham aggressively advertised her vegetable compounds, making Ms. Pinkham's face the most recognized in the United States in the late nineteenth century (figure 338). According to advertising accompanying the bottle, "In tests with their own patients, doctors found that Pinkham's Compound and Tablets relieved 63% and 80% (respectively) of functionally-caused 'hot flashes' in the cases tested. Most women also found they were less irritable and jittery. Instead of the 'edgy,' moody feelings so frequently associated with menopause, they enjoyed a more cheerful sense of 'well-being.'" Lydia Pinkham was responsible for advertising her own product, and at times, that promotion could be quite vivid: "A FEARFUL TRAGEDY, a Clergyman of Stratford, Connecticut, KILLED BY HIS OWN WIFE, Insanity Brought on by 16 Years of Suffering

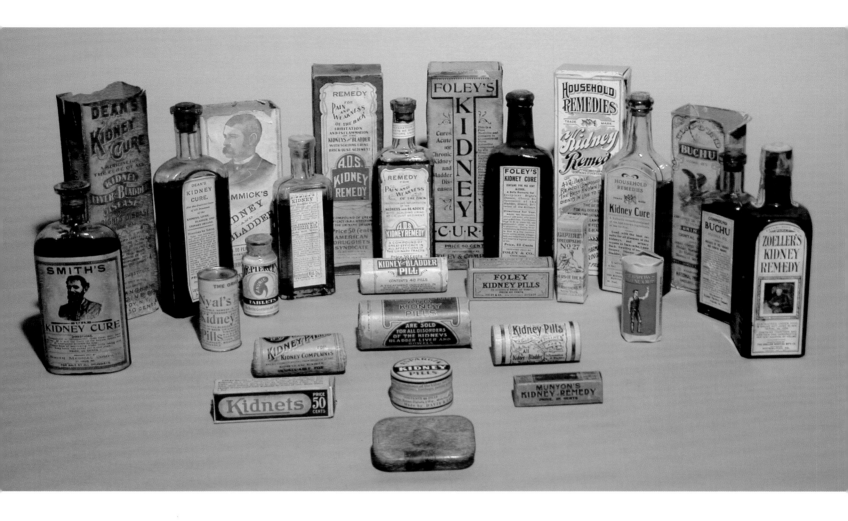

339. Late nineteenth-century patent medications related to diseases of the kidney

340. Opposite above. Late nine-teenth-century testimonial for the cure of kidney disease from the Alpha Medical Institute

341. Opposite below. Trade card for *Horsford's Acid Phosphate* (late nine-teenth century)

with FEMALE COMPLAINTS THE CAUSE. Lydia E. Pinkham's Vegetable Compound, The Sure Cure for These Complaints, Would Have Prevented the Direful Deed."

The use of patent medications was widespread, and their popularity increased throughout the latter part of the nineteenth century for a number of reasons. The growth of cities set the stage for the spread of communicable diseases like tuberculosis, yellow fever, and typhoid fever, while advertising in home newspapers made quick fix remedies almost irresistible. Religious leaders tended to publicly support patent medicines to a point that the Connecticut Medical Society felt impelled to pass a resolution in the 1840s that said, ". . . the clergy, who have been recipients of free medical attention seem to be turning a penny by endorsing quack medicines." The society supported only medical groups that had agreed "to discontinue free attention unless clergymen withdrew their endorsement of patent medicines." An increase in the number of local drugstores improved their availability, and the public tended to embrace over-the-counter medicines to avoid popular aggressive treatments like bleeding and purging recommended by respected physicians of the day, including Benjamin Rush. There was no difficulty in finding

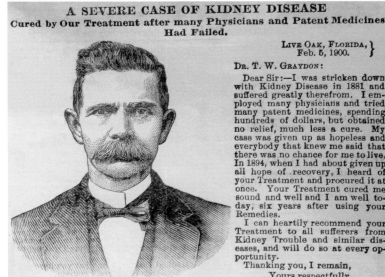

someone willing to write a prescription, and, in 1835, Lemuel Shattuck of Massachusetts complained, "Any one, male or female, learned or ignorant, an honest man or a knave, can assume the name of physician, and 'practice' upon any one, to cure or to kill, as either may happen, without accountability. It's a free country!" In *Humbugs of New-York* (1838), David Reese spoke about new physicians "whose chief mission appear to be to open men's purses by opening their bowels."

The number of manufacturers quickly multiplied, and according to the *Portsmouth Journal* in Ohio, "how easily a mechanic can become an entrepreneur . . . he finds that mercury is good for the itch, and old ulcers; that opium will give ease; and that a glass of antimony will vomit. Down goes the hammer, or saw, razor, awl, or shuttle— and away to make electuaries, tinctures, elixirs, pills, plasters, and poultices" (figure 339). Drug producers employed a variety of advertising techniques, including testimonials and beautiful trade cards with outrageous claims suggesting that their products were both safe and effective (figures 340–343).

Many of the most popular drugs were almost certainly addictive since they contained a significant amount of alcohol. For example, the alcohol content of some of the most popular remedies were Hostetter's Bitters, 44 percent, Burdock's Blood Bitters, 25 percent, and Hood's Sarsaparilla, 18 percent. In addition to herbs and unregulated chemicals, many bizarre ingredients were sold with great fanfare and promise (figure 344). The whole era is represented by the now famous snake oil (figure 345). This liniment was popularly used for musculoskeletal complaints with the advertised expectation that the reptile's flexible nature could be transferred to the patient by topical application. The effectiveness of these medications can still be debated, though there is no dispute regarding some of the marketing blunders that continued into the late twentieth century (figure 346).

THE APOTHECARY SHOPPE

Apothecary shops became a recognized part of most communities during the eighteenth century. The Roman god Janus was regarded as the guardian of doorways, and

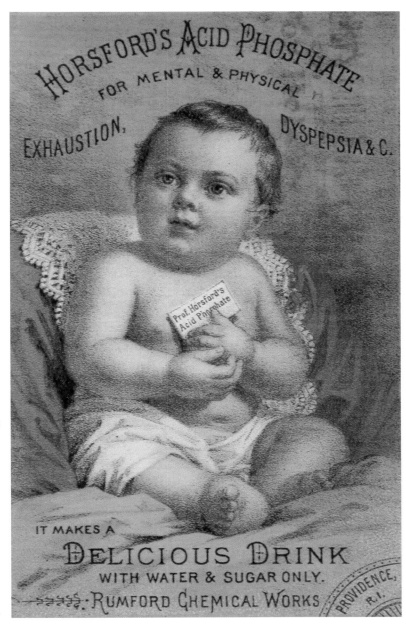

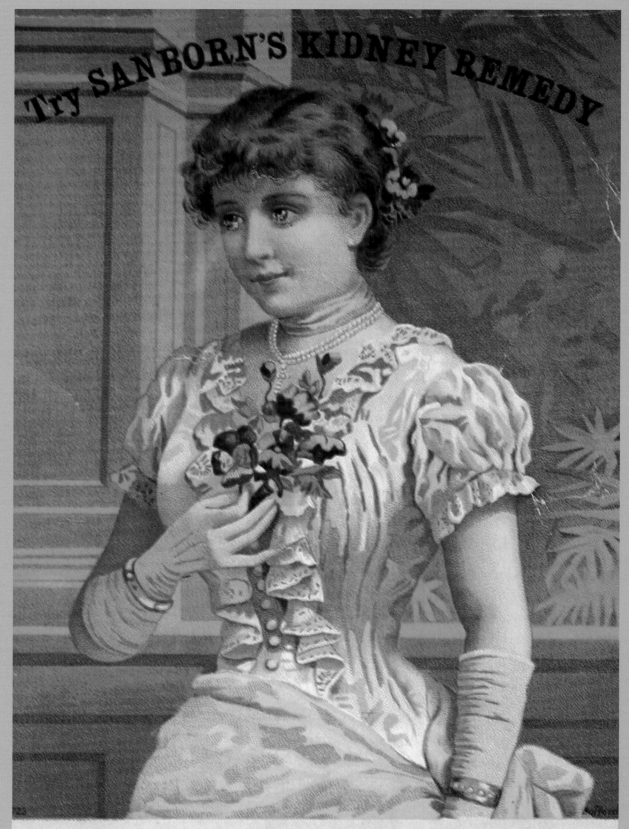

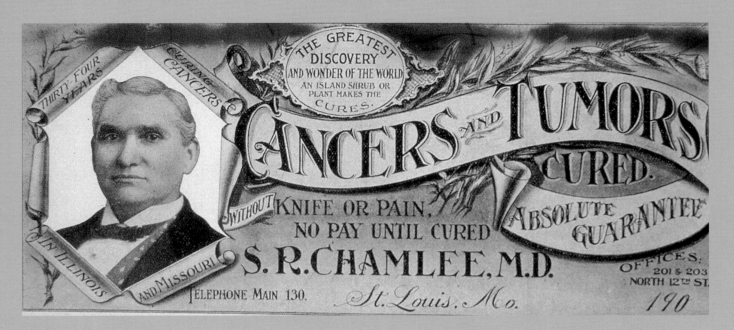

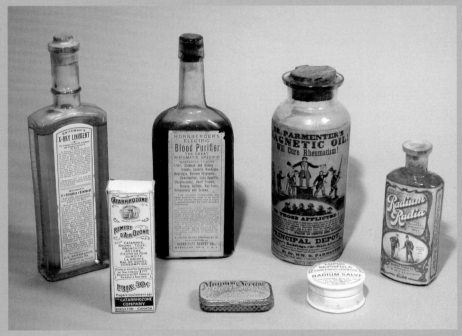

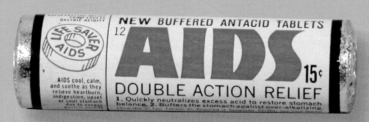

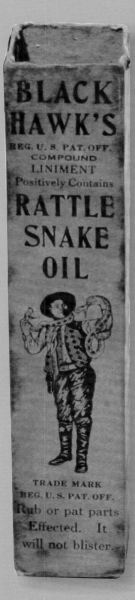

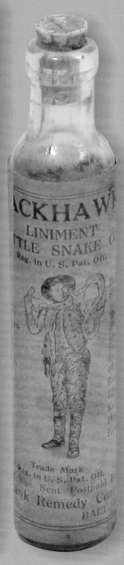

342. Opposite. Trade card for *Sanborn's Kidney Remedy* (late nineteenth century)

343. Top. Late nineteenth-century cancer cure

344. Unusual early nineteenth-century ingredients: (top) X-ray liniment, electric blood purifier, magnetic oil, radium radia; (bottom) ozone, magnetic pills, radioactive salve

345. Right. Blackhawk's Rattlesnake Oil (ca. 1880)

346. AIDS, a buffered antacid (ca. 1980)

347. Early nineteenth-century earthenware Janus

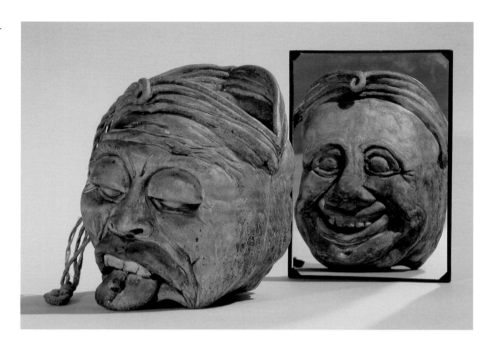

could often be found hanging outside, his two faces used to demonstrate
the before and after effects of the powders, lotions, and ointments inside
(figure 347). Incidentally, Janus was also the god of beginnings and was
the genesis of the name of the first month of the year, January.

Apothecary show globes have been associated with the pharmacy
trade for centuries. They appear to have originated in the British Isles,
but their purpose remains open to much speculation, some believing
that sixteenth-century alchemists placed strangely colored liquids in glass
containers to lend an air of mystery and magic in order to attract customers. Others speculate that the red color in show globes was displayed
in apothecary shops to warn passersby of plague or other diseases inside
the city, while green was a sign of safety. The red and blue colors may
also have represented arterial and venous blood. These wonderful works
of art were available in either standing (figures 348) or hanging styles
(figure 349–351). A potential customer could also be first attracted to a
pharmacy by an apothecary jar, though these intricate ceramics were not
likely affordable to the average pharmacist (figure 352).

The mortar and pestle remain modern symbols of the apothecary
shop, and pharmacists have used them for grinding and mixing medications for hundreds of years. Composition varied and included vessels
made of wood, stone, bronze, Wedgwood, porcelain, and glass. At the
turn of the last century, pharmacists rightfully stopped using metal for
fear that some of the material might be escaping into the medications
(figure 353).

Scales used for weighing medications were first seen in Egypt in
about 1500 B.C., and, by the nineteenth century, those found in apothe-

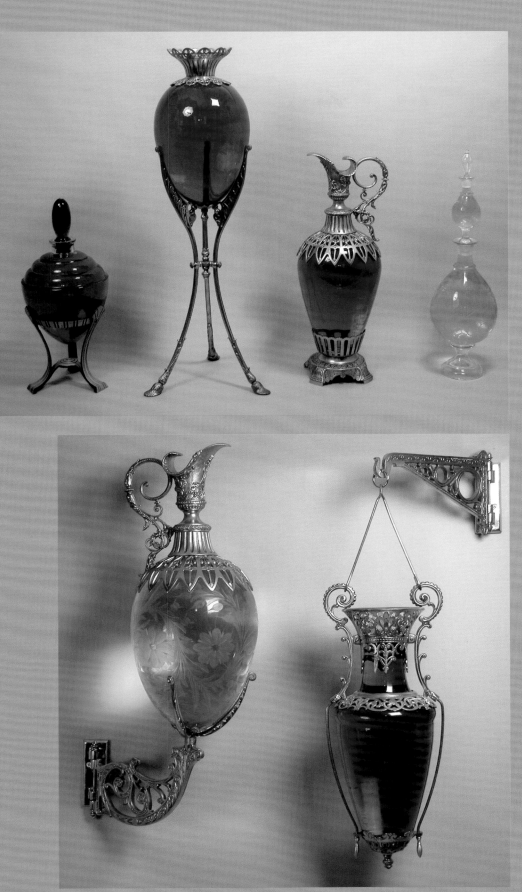

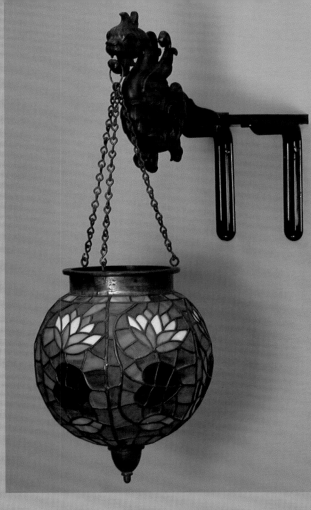

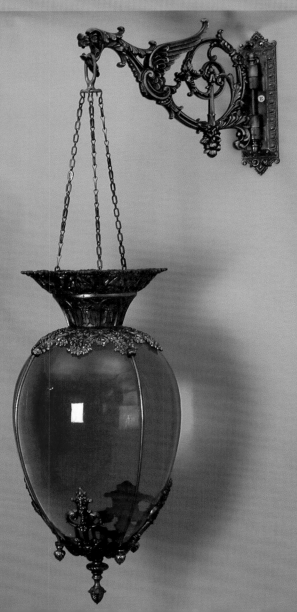

348. Top. Standing Show Globes; (left) "art deco" (ca. 1930), others late nineteenth century, probably by Whitall, Tatum, and Co.

349. Above. Hanging show globes: (left) by Whitall, Tatum & Co.; and (right) by Clark, Woodward, and Co. (ca. 1909)

350. Top right. Stained glass hanging show globe with gargoyle bracket by Banks Druggist's Fixtures, Co.

351. Bottom right. Hanging show globe by Whitall, Tatum, and Co. with lion bracket (ca. 1880)

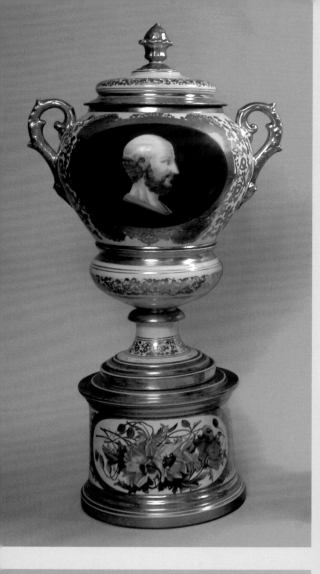

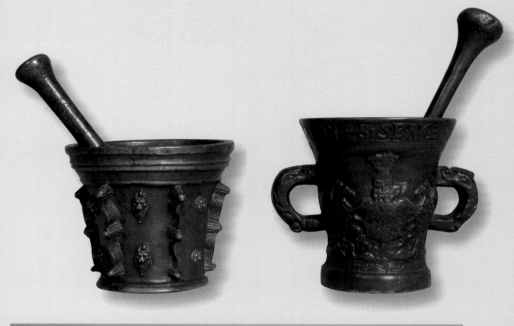

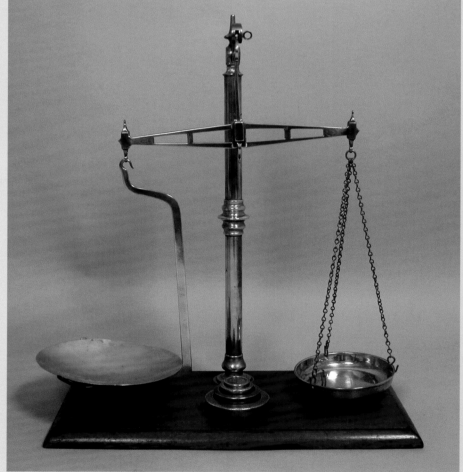

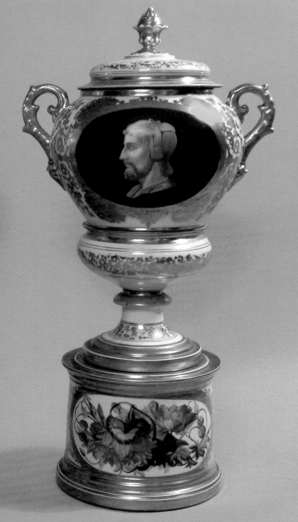

352. Left. Two Paris porcelain portrait *vases a devanture* (ca. 1850) with portraits of Hippocrates (top) and Galen (bottom)

353. Top. (left) Late fifteenth-century bronze mortar and pestle in the Gothic style with ribbed handles; (right) Burgundian mortar and pestle (1638)

354. Large British beam scale (ca. 1880) by W. and T. Avery

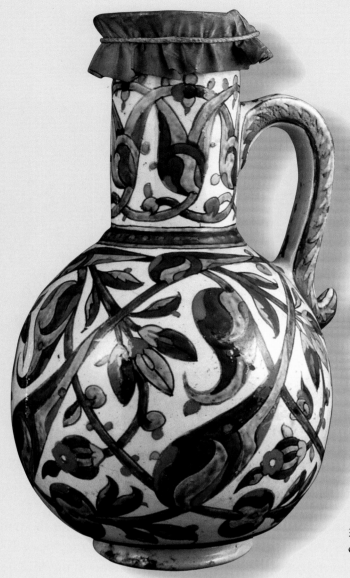

355, 356. Sixteenth to seventeenth-century earthenware jars

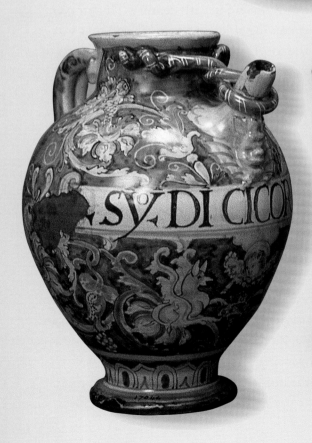

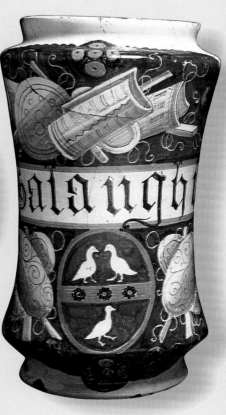

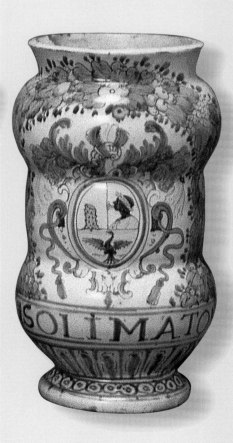

445

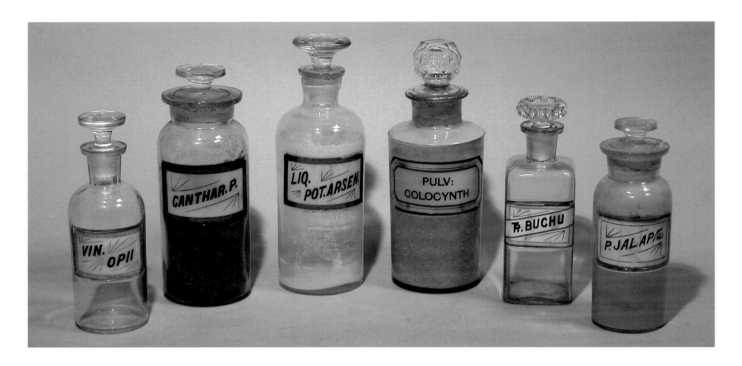

357. Late nineteenth-century variety of labeled glass pharmacy bottles

cary shops were often quite large and ornate (figure 354). Physicians also carried small sets of scales to individually measure medications in their offices or at the bedside.

Drug jars were used to store pharmaceuticals for thousands of years. Shapes varied, and the popular *albarello* ("little tree") jars date back to the eleventh century when they were common in the Middle East, remaining popular in Europe into the eighteenth century. This jar was cylindrical in shape with inner curving sides and an open top that was covered with parchment. In the fourteenth century, containers began to be made with a mixture of tin, lead, and potash though porcelain was popular for the manufacture of drug jars, particularly in France at the end of the eighteenth century. Different countries used various terms for the fashionable tin glaze container: Italians (majolica), the Dutch (delftware), and the French (faience). Though quite fragile, many have survived (figures 355, 356). Most chemicals were stored in glass (figure 357), while medications could also be found in treen or ceramic ointment pots. A number of "drug pots" were manufactured in England in the nineteenth century to hold topical preparations. Earlier types were called "gallipots" since they were brought to England from the Mediterranean in ships or galleys.

There were many ways to store medications at home throughout the eighteenth and nineteenth centuries. Medicine chests came in many shapes and were used to hold liquids and powders in labeled bottles and canisters, with an occasional secret compartment in the rear to hold poisons. Drawers in the front held all the necessary accessories, including a mortar and pestle, graduated cylinder, medicine spoon, and scales (figures 358, 359). These medications could also be carried by physicians in small apothecary cases or even on horseback in saddlebags (figures 360, 361). By the beginning of the twentieth century, however, beautiful chests went out of style since preformed pills and mass-produced packaging took the place of individually measured powders and ointments (figure 362).

PUT ON THE BRAKES

The number and variety of dangerous drugs grew out of control, and Samuel Hopkins Adams brought that fact to the public's attention in 1905 with a landmark article published by *Colliers* entitled "The Great American Fraud." Adams said, "Gullible America will spend this year some seventy-five million dollars in the purchase of patent medicines. In consideration of this sum it will swallow huge quantities of alcohol, an

358. Genoese medicine chest of governor Vincenzo Giustiniani (ca. 1565)

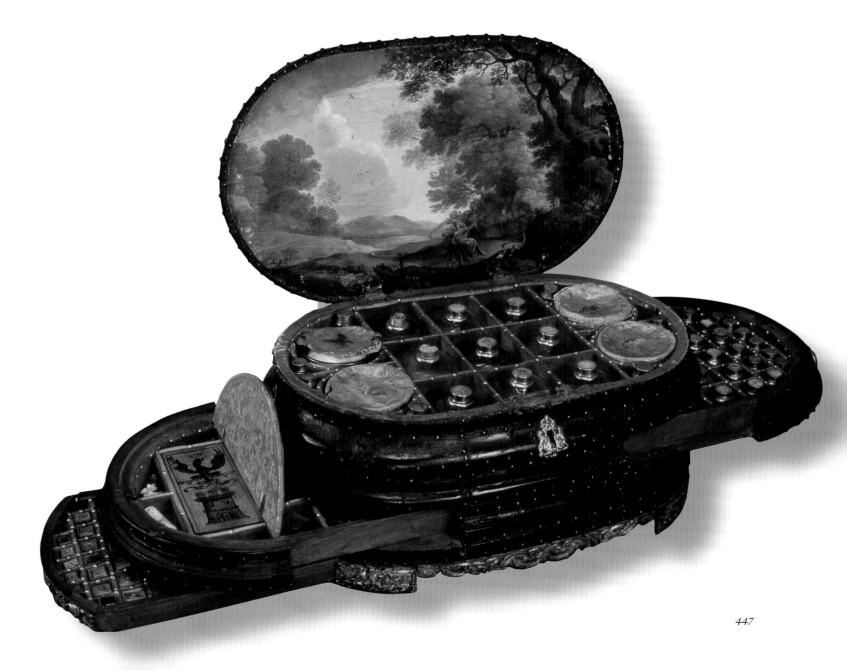

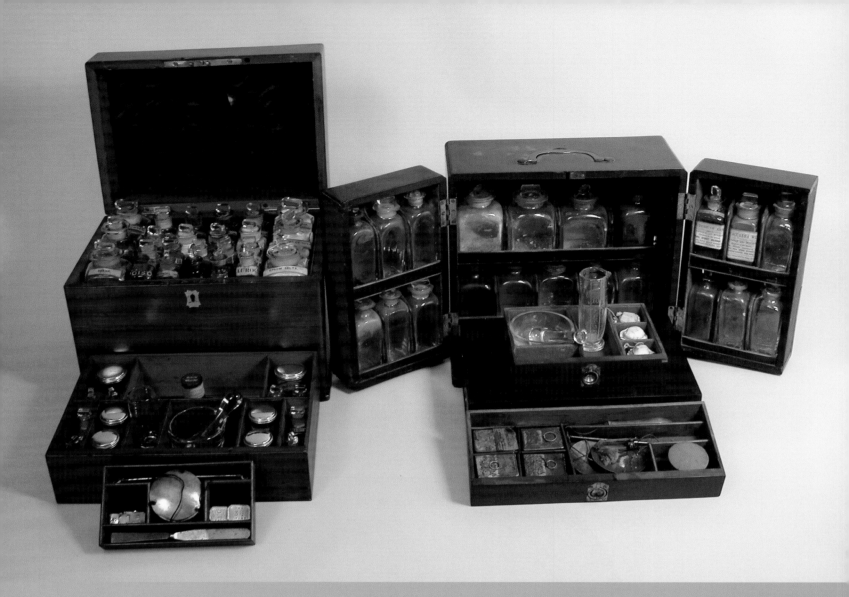

359. Above. (left to right) English medicine chest with hand scales (ca 1860); late nineteenth century British triptych style apothecary chest

360. Portable Buggy Bag (ca. 1875)

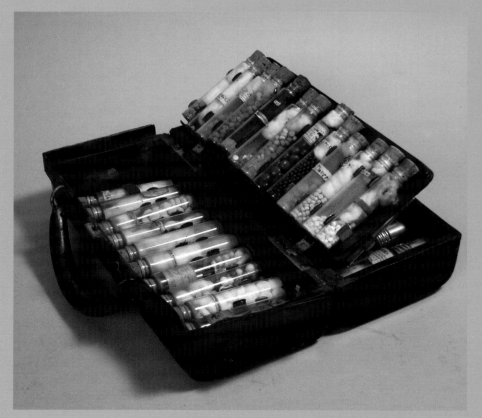

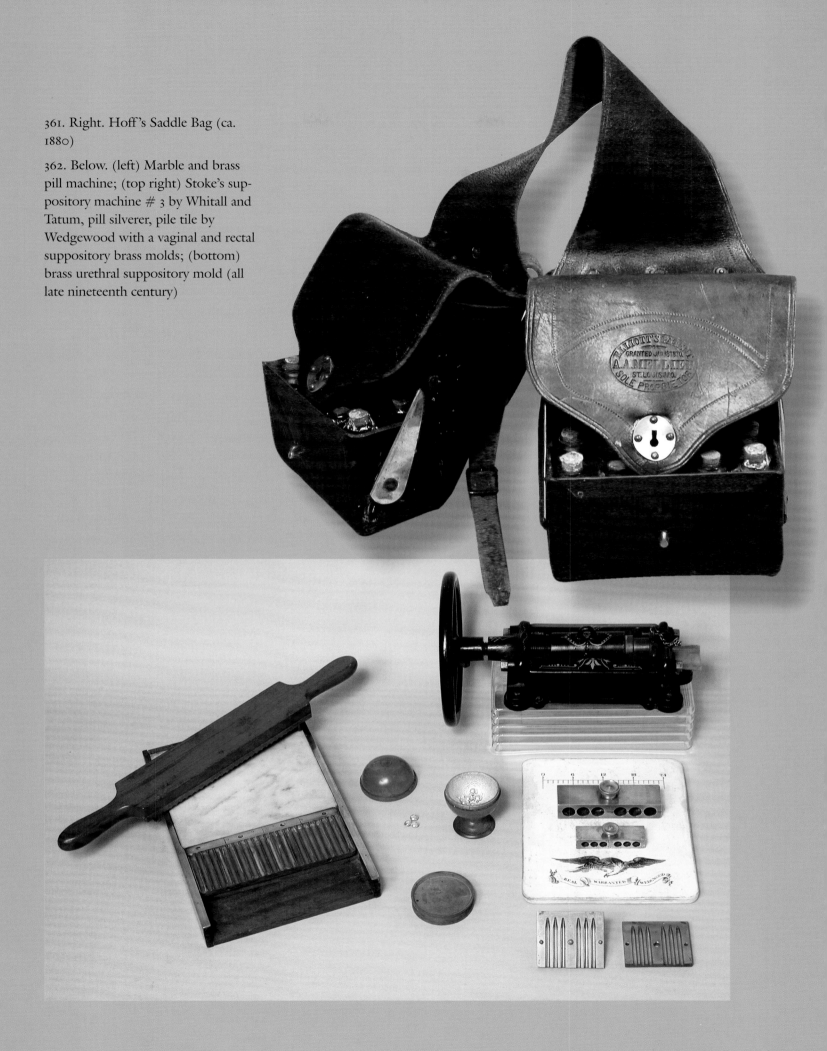

361. Right. Hoff's Saddle Bag (ca. 1880)

362. Below. (left) Marble and brass pill machine; (top right) Stoke's suppository machine # 3 by Whitall and Tatum, pill silverer, pile tile by Wedgewood with a vaginal and rectal suppository brass molds; (bottom) brass urethral suppository mold (all late nineteenth century)

appalling amount of opiates and narcotics, a wide assortment of various drugs ranging from powerful and dangerous heart depressants to insidious liver stimulants; and, far in excess of other ingredients, undiluted fraud. For fraud, exploited by the skilfulest of advertising bunco men, is the basis of the trade." The sale of catarrhs and syrups containing narcotics "is a shameful trade that stupefies helpless babies and makes criminals of our young men and harlots of our young women."

The federal government became involved in the pharmaceutical industry with the passage of the Federal Pure Food and Drug Act a year later in 1906. This law established a ban on the interstate commerce of mislabeled drugs, though many medications remained ineffective and sometimes harmful. The law only addressed medications that were "false or misleading in any particular," and the first drug to be tested under the new regulation was Cuforhedake Brane-Fude in 1908. This medication was manufactured in Washington, DC (adding to the ease of prosecution), and was a headache remedy that contained potentially toxic acetanilide along with caffeine and was twenty-four percent alcohol. This "most wonderful, certain and harmless relief" was produced by Robert N. Harper, who had been a leader in the community at the time, serving as commissioner of pharmacy for the District, president of a bank, and president of the Chamber of Commerce. Cuforhedake Brane-Fude was accused causing twenty-two deaths, and since there was no evidence that it contained "brain food," Harper was found guilty. President Theodore Roosevelt had been especially interested in this case and summoned the prosecutor, Dr. Harvey Washington Wiley, to his office after the conviction, reminding him: "It is your duty to make an example of this man, and show to the people of the country that the pure food law was enacted to protect them. He has been convicted after a fair and impartial trial, and you should use every argument in your power to convince the judge to impose a jail sentence. To a man of his wealth, a fine as a penalty . . . would be little less than ridiculous." The president and Wiley were not pleased with a sentence that included no jail time, and Wiley later commented that Harper "had made two million in the product. He was fined $700 . . . and was just $1,999,300 ahead." The new law remained a poor deterrent since the fines were small and transgressors were rarely sent to prison.

Drug companies were quite powerful, and it usually took a crime of high public visibility to provide enough impetus for the passage of legislation. Dr. Johnson's treatment for cancer had no therapeutic value, and the case against its manufacturer eventually reached Oliver Wendell Holmes' Supreme Court. To the surprise of many, the makers of Dr. Johnson's prevailed, affirming the illegality of false labeling but not of

untrue therapeutic claims. Most angered was Congressman Swagar
Sherley of Kentucky, whose subsequent Sherley amendment to the food
and drug law was passed in 1912, declaring that a medication was unlaw-
ful "if its package or label shall bear or contain any statement, design, or
device regarding the curative or therapeutic effect of such article or any
of the ingredients or substances contained therein, which is false and
fraudulent."

One of the first to feel the weight of this new regulation was William
Radam's Microbe Killer, an oral medication that supposedly released
healing gases to disinfect the entire body and cure such diverse diseases
as malaria, leprosy, small pox, measles, headache, and constipation. Its
creator, William Radam, was a former Texas gardener who was described
by R.G. Eccles in an 1889 edition of the *Druggists' Circular* as "out-
quacking the worst quacks of this or any other age." The government
seized 539 boxes of Radam's Microbe Killer that had a retail value of
$5,166. Chemists determined that it contained ninety-nine percent tap
water and one percent sulfuric acid, the cost of production a mere
$25.82. At best, it acted as a mild laxative, though testimonials by satis-
fied customers in court documented cures of any number of serous conditions such as diphtheria and cancer. In this case, however, the defense
was unsuccessful in establishing a convincing argument, and the prosecution prevailed.

Despite occasional victories, medical fraud and deceit continued, and
the US Postal Service became an unwilling partner since much of the
drug commerce and advertising took place through the mail. Privacy
laws were quite strict, and officials from the post office were not allowed
to open mail under any circumstance, making prosecution for mail fraud
almost impossible. To sidestep the issue, post office officials elected to
use rather unusual methods in order to entrap the manufacturers of suspicious medications. In 1913, the postal inspector sent the following letter to the Interstate Remedy Company regarding a normal anatomic
finding: "There is something wrong with my testicles and I don't know
what to make of it. I noticed for some time that they don't hang even
and that the left one hangs lower. I ain't got the nerve to ask out doctor
about it. Please use plain envelope."

Federal law did not mandate the testing of drugs for safety and efficacy, a flaw that was corrected with the passage of the Food, Drug, and
Cosmetic Act in 1938. Once again, it took a major disaster to focus
national attention on the problem before legislation could be passed.
Sulfanilamide was a potent antibiotic active against streptococcus and
staphylococcus. Physicians for Franklin Delano Roosevelt Jr. had successfully prescribed it for a strep throat, and sulfanilamide had been fre-

quently used to treat gonorrhea. In 1937, the solvent diethylene glycol was added, and the combination was tested only for appearance, fragrance, and flavor. One hundred and seven died, many of them children, and it was determined that the drug broke the law because it was mislabeled as an elixir, and did *not* contain alcohol. The fine was a staggering $26,100, and the discoverer of the drug took his own life. Commenting on the verdict, however, the physician owner of the company spun the court's finding in a different direction: "I do not feel that there was any responsibility on our part."

Passage of the 1938 Food, Drug, and Cosmetic Act was a result of that tragedy, and the first case to be filed related to the use of Marmola tablets, a thyroid extract recommended for weight loss. As the pharmaceutical industry watched, the government prevailed, and ninety-seven percent of all drug labels on the market at the time were quickly modified. In 1943, a federal court referred to the 1938 legislation: "The purpose of the law is to protect the public, the vast multitude which includes the ignorant, the unthinking, and the credulous who, when making a purchase, do not stop to analyze." Ironically, federal regulations probably went too far with the prohibition of alcohol (1920–1933) — except for "medicinal" use only (figure 363).

The passage of legislation was one way in which consumers were protected from the dangers of useless and sometimes harmful patent medications (figure 364). The clever have, however, always been able to take advantage of the unsuspecting, and loopholes in the law have always rewarded ingenuity. As a consequence, mistrust of physicians and their prescriptions has been a popular pastime going back to the beginning of the practice of medicine. Shakespeare reflected these misgivings in *The Life of Timon of Athens* (act 4, scene 3):

Trust not the physician;
His antidotes are poison, and he slays moe than you rob.

In 1905, American humorist Mark Twain responded to an advertisement for a patent medicine that was touted to be a "miracle cure" for acne, appendicitis, corns, diabetes, dandruff, diphtheria, measles, mumps, pneumonia, tapeworm, and whooping cough for a life "without disease, death and always in youthful tonic." Twain wrote, "The person who wrote the advertisements is without doubt the most ignorant person now alive on the planet, also without doubt he is an idiot, an idiot of the 33rd degree and scion of an ancestral profession of idiots stretching back to the

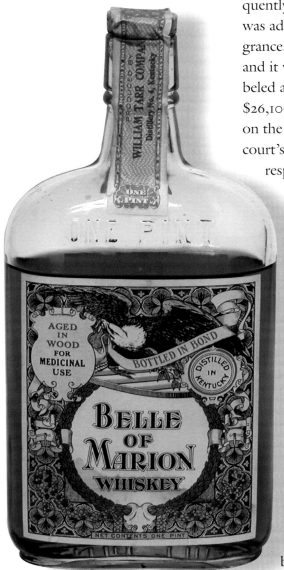

363. Prescription whiskey (ca. 1930)

Missing Link. . . . A few moments from now my resentment will have faded and passed, and I shall probably even be praying for you; but while there is yet time I hasten to wish that you may take a dose of your own poison by mistake and enter swiftly into the damnation which you and all other patent medicine assassins have so remorselessly gamered and do so richly deserve."

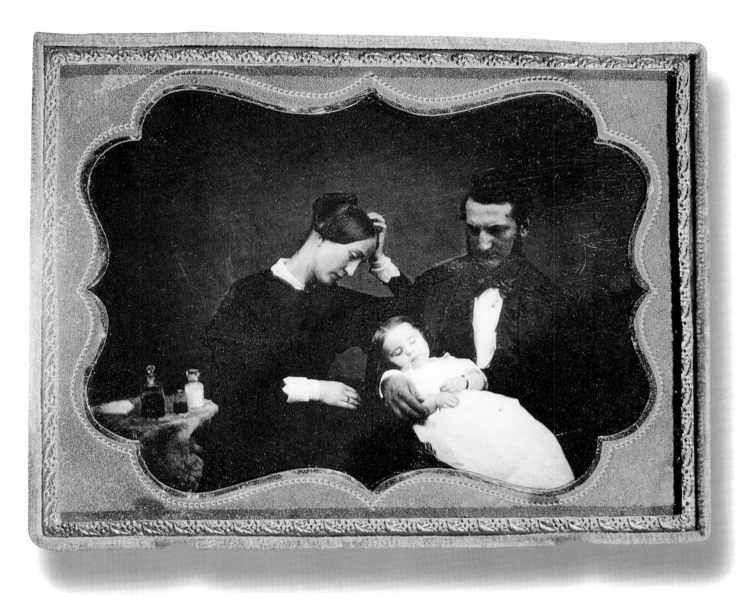

"If the whole materia medica as used, could be sunk in the bottom of the sea, it would be all the better for mankind and all the worse for the fishes."

Oliver Wendell Holmes, MD

364. Nineteenth-century daguerreotype reflects the grief suffered by parents as they mourned the loss of their daughter, the useless medications at their side (ca. 1848)

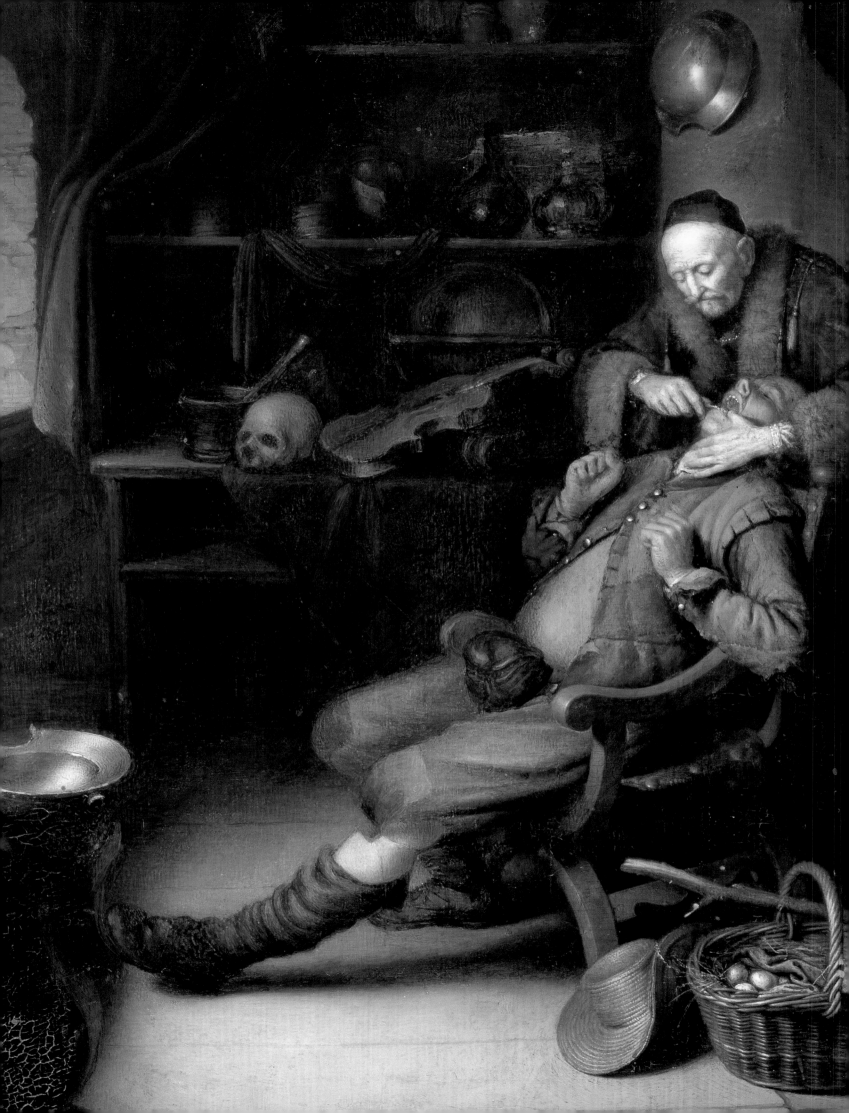

DENTISTRY

"For there was never yet philosopher
That could endure the toothache patiently"

William Shakespeare
Much Ado About Nothing, Act 5, Scene 1

"The Dentist" by Gerrit Dou (1613–1675)

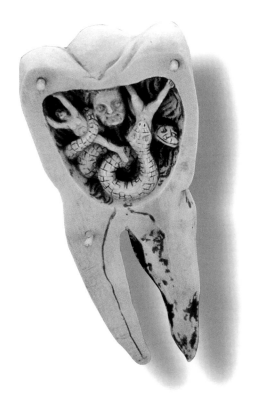

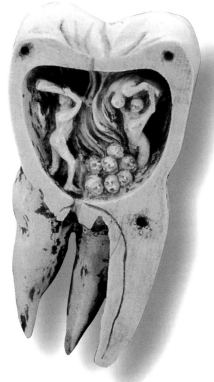

365. Ivory teeth with images of a tooth worm and suffering in Hell (ca. 1780), from southern France

366. The martyrdom of Saint Apollonia, oil on canvas by Jacob Jordaens (1593–1678)

Physicians and healers of all sorts have always been interested in the diagnosis and treatment of disorders of the teeth and gums because of the ubiquitous and pressing nature of the problem. Dental disease has been found in human remains from as early as the Stone Age, and it was in the seventeenth century that teeth began to show a significant increase in the rate of decay as the importation of inexpensive sugar from the New World increased. Soon after, dentistry began to evolve into the profession that it is today.

THE TOOTH WORM

For centuries, the "tooth worm" played a mythical role as the primary cause of dental disease and discomfort (figure 365). "The Legend of the Toothworm" can be found on an ancient tablet from Nineveh, now at the British Museum:

> After Anu had created the heavens,
> The heavens created the earth,
> The rivers created the brooks,
> The brooks created the swamps,
> The swamps created the worm,
> Then came the worm before Shamash [Sun God]
> Before Ea [God of the Deep] came her tears:
> "What willst thou give me to eat and destroy?"
> "Ripe figs will I give thee."
> "What good are ripe figs to me? Take me up and let
> me reside between the teeth and the gums, so that I may
> destroy the blood of the tooth and ruin their strength;
> the roots of the tooth I will eat."
> "Since thou hast said this, Worm, May Ea strike thee
> with the power of her fist; This is the magic ritual:
> Mix together beer, the sa-kil-bir plant, and oil.
> Then repeat the magic formula thrice and place
> the mixture on the tooth."

Belief in the tooth worm survived well into the eighteenth century and may have had as its origin the maggots that can sometimes be found in decaying tissue. The nerve inside a decayed tooth could also have been mistaken for a worm that caused the destruction. In the past, adequate dental care was difficult to come by, and, according to the Greek physician Galen (A.D. 120–200), many used the tooth worm as a way to take advantage of unsuspecting sufferers. This excerpt is from Galen's *On Diseases Hard to Cure* (ca. A.D. 180): "I came upon a man surrounded by

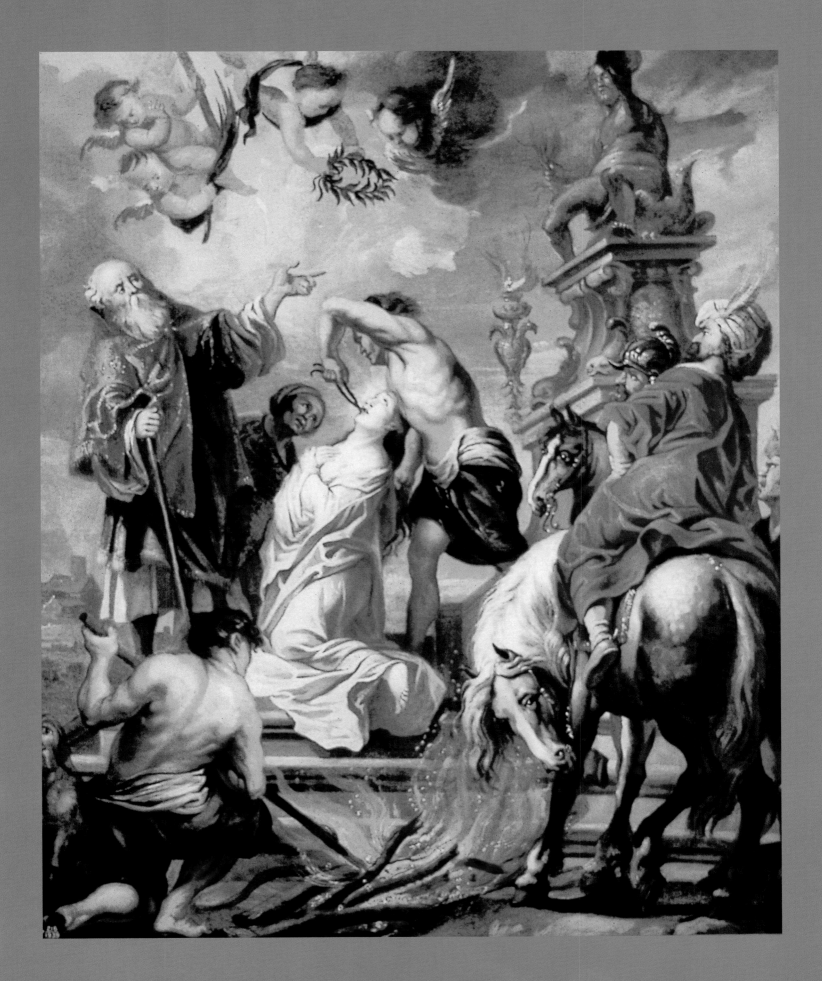

a crowd of fools. 'I have met Galen,' he declared, 'who has taught me all he knows. Here is a remedy for worms in the teeth.' The quack had prepared a ball of pitch and tar, lit it, and held it smoking in the open mouth of the patient, who could not bear to keep his eyes open. As soon as they were shut, he slipped into the patient's mouth worms he had concealed in a little pot, and pretended to draw them out. The fools offered him all they had. He even went so far as to try venesection on the wrong side of the elbow. I immediately revealed myself to the crowded, saying 'I am Galen, and he is a swindler.' I then warned him, asked the authorities to summons him, and they had him flogged."

Another popular method used by thirteenth-century "dewormers" was to introduce several fruit worms into a piece of cake, which they would then place in the cavity of a diseased tooth. The cake softened when the patient bit down, the worm was released, and the quack removed the "tooth worm" to the admiration of onlookers.

More reputable physicians were also concerned about this problem. This is an eleventh-century cure for dental worms from an English version of *Regimen Sanitatis Salernitanum* (1607):

> If in your teeth you hap to be tormented
> By meane some little wormes therein do breed,
> Which pain (if need be tane) may be prevented,
> Be keeping cleane your teeth, when as you feede;
> Burne Francomsence (a gum not evil sented),
> Put Henbane unto this, and Onyon seed,
> And with a tunnel to the tooth that's hollow,
> Convey the smoke thereof, and ease shall follow.

A PATRON SAINT

For centuries, the pathophysiology of dental disease was a mystery, providing an opportunity for those dealing in superstition and the occult to explain the unexplainable. Many turned to religion, and as a result St. Apollonia became the patron saint of dentistry after her execution in A.D. 249. Her image is found in churches throughout the world, and she is usually pictured carrying pincers holding a tooth in her right hand and a martyr's palm in her left (figures 366, 367). Apollonia was the daughter of a magistrate in Alexandria. Her conception followed her mother's prayers to the Blessed Virgin for help in having a child, and upon finding this out, Apollonia decided to become a Christian. The timing of this conversion was unfortunate, however, since it took place during the reign of Nero when Christians were persecuted, and Apollonia found herself in the midst of a bloodthirsty mob. The first victim was an elderly gentleman named Metranus who was beaten with staffs, splinters of reeds were

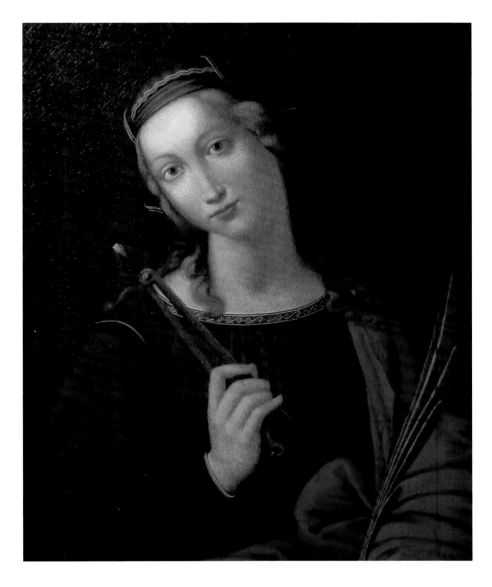

367. Nineteenth-century reproduction (?) of Saint Apollonia, oil on canvas by Sassoferrato (Giovanni Battista Salvi) (1609–1685)

thrust into his eyes, and he was stoned to death. Soon to follow was Cointha, a Christian woman who was executed after being tied to the tail of a horse and then dragged over sharp stones. The next was holy man Serapion whose bones were broken, and then he was dropped off the roof of his house. It was then Apollonia's turn, and according to Dionysius, the bishop of Alexandria, "They seized that marvelous aged virgin Apollonia, broke out all her teeth with blows on her jaws, and piling up a bonfire before the city, threatened to burn her alive if she refused to recite with them their blasphemous sayings." Apollonia prayed and then leapt into the flames, while pronouncing that those who invoked her name would be relieved of tooth pain. Because of the prevalence of dental disease at the time, St. Apollonia was worshiped by many, and a number of holy places claim to have one of her original teeth. As suggested in the following Bavarian prayer, pain and suffering were looked on by many in the church as a punishment for bad behavior:

St. Apollonia
A poor sinner I stand here,
My teeth are very bad.
Please be soon reconciled
And give me rest in my bones
That I forget the toothache soon.

Apollonia, Apollonia
Though the holy saint in heaven
See my pain in yourself,
Free me from evil pain
For my toothache may torture me to death.

Apollonia of Bayerland,
I raise to thee my right hand
And promise thee ten candles
If thou takest my toothache from me.

A great many superstitions surrounded diseases of the teeth both because they were the cause of so much discomfort and because they survived long after the death of the owner. In primitive societies, witch doctors wore necklaces of teeth to signify longevity and to help in healing, a custom still popular in many in parts of the world where animal teeth are worn as protective amulets. Off the southern tip of India in Sri Lanka (formerly Ceylon) now resides the Sacred Tooth of Buddha in the Dalada Maligarva. The tooth is about three inches long and is one of the most important relics in the Buddhist religion. In about A.D. 360, Princess Kalinga commandeered the sacred artifact from its home in India and took it to Ceylon, setting the stage for about 1,200 years of violence between the two countries as the tooth was restolen and then returned once again. Finally, in order to control the bloodshed, the Portuguese took possession of the tooth following their conquest of Ceylon, and they promptly destroyed it. Wikrama Ahu built a magnificent castle around the current religious artifact (which is actually an animal replacement). Another "tooth of Buddha" is regularly viewed by many thousands of pilgrims in China.

Spanish painter Francisco José de Goya y Lucientes (1746–1828) recognized the fabled power of teeth when he sketched a woman protecting her face with a scarf as she reached up to remove a tooth from a hanged man still on the gallows. In regard to his work, *A caza de dientes* (Out Hunting for Teeth), Goya wrote, "Teeth from the hanged are singularly effective in the art of witchcraft, as without these one cannot make anything rational" (figure 368). Nails from a coffin and moss from the skull of a corpse were also collected for use by those suffering the agony of painful teeth and gums.

368. Opposite. *A caza de dientes* (*"Out Hunting for Teeth"*), sketch by Francisco José de Goya y Lucientes (1746–1828)

460

EARLY THERAPY OF DENTAL DISEASE

The first physician known to have specialized in dental care was Hesi-Re, who practiced in ancient Egypt in 2650 B.C. and was "the greatest of those who deal with teeth." The direct approach was to remove the tooth, since, short of extraction and analgesia, little could be offered to those in pain. There has never been a shortage of noninvasive remedies, however, and some were indeed bizarre by modern standards. The mouse was revered in ancient Egyptian medicine as a magical treatment for many diseases, and undigested mice have been found in the mummified remains of children dating back to 5000 B.C. One Egyptian treatment for tooth decay consisted of dividing a live mouse and then rubbing one sectioned piece along the diseased tooth or gum. Mouse therapy continued into ancient Rome where Caius Plinius Secundus (Pliny the Elder, A.D. 23–79) recommended that a mouse be eaten twice a month for the prevention of dental disease.

The famous Roman physician and historian Cornelius Celsus (25 B.C.–A.D. 50) offered this treatment for a toothache: "It may be numbered amongst the worst tortures, the patient must abstain entirely from wine, and at first even from food; afterwards, he may partake of soft food but very sparingly, so as not to irritate the teeth by mastication. Meanwhile by means of a sponge he must let the stream of hot water reach the affected part and apply externally, on the side corresponding with the pain, a cerate of cypress or of iris on which he must then place some wool and keep the head well covered up." Another Roman physician, Archigenes (54 B.C.–A.D. 17), was the first to recommend drilling out the pulp of a diseased tooth. He would then place any number of different materials into the hollowed cavity, including turpentine, iron sulfate, the burnt slough of a serpent, roasted earthworms, and crushed spiders' eggs. A red-hot cautery was the treatment of choice for pain control.

In addition to acupuncture, the ancient Chinese treated dental pain in the following way: "Roast a bit of garlic and crush it between the teeth, mix with chopped horseradish seeds or saltpeter, make into a paste with human milk; form pills and introduce one into the nos-

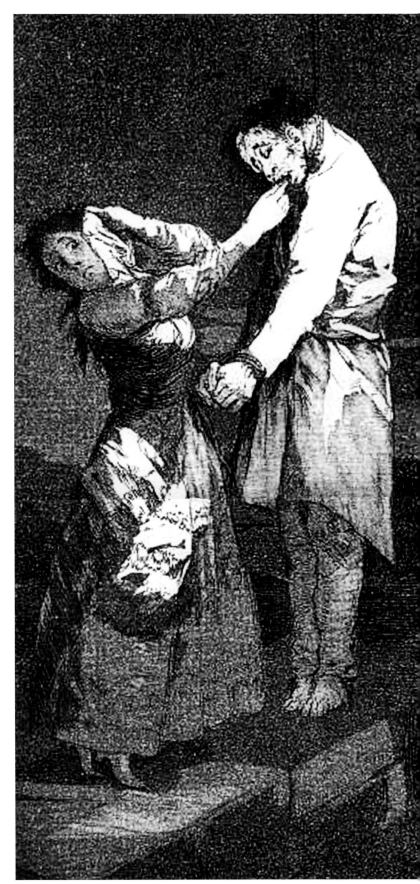

tril on the opposite side to where the pain is felt." If unsuccessful, arsenic pills were placed near the offending tooth for analgesia.

The great physician Galen recommended that painful teeth be treated by rubbing the gums either with the milk of a bitch or the brains of a hare. A later medieval custom was to place a piece of bread or meat in a bag to be hung around the neck with the prospect that the toothache would subside as the material decayed. Inhabitants of Friedrichshagen in Germany thought they could find relief from dental disease with prayers followed either by walking around a pear tree three times or by spitting into the mouth of a frog.

In his *School of Physick* (1659), Nicholas Culpeper wrote: "To rub the Teeth and Gums every morning, and after meat too, if you please, with Salt, is the best way under the sun to preserve the teeth sound and clean, from rotting and aking." His suggestion for toothache: "If a Hog-louse or Wood-louse be pricked with a needle, and any aking tooth presently touched with that needle, the pain will instantly cease." He also proposed a method for dental extraction: "To draw a Tooth without pain, fill an earthen Crucible full of Emmets, Ants, or Pismires (call them by which name you will) Eggs and all, and when you have burned them, keep the ashes, with which if you touch a Tooth, it will drop out." Other formulae from the past include pitch mixed with raven or mouse manure, juice from a plant grown in a human skull, or the fat of a green frog.

Lazare Rivierè was a seventeenth-century professor of medicine at Montpellier, and gave the following advice:

Where the pain was occasioned by hot humors, the treatment began by bleeding the arm. The following day an aperient was administered. Afterward, if the pain still persisted, the sufferer was cupped in the region of the neck; resinous plasters were placed at the temples. In addition to this, various remedies were introduced into the ears, various operations were performed on the aching part itself. And this was followed by extracting the offending tooth.

Pseudoscience always remained an option for the creative. Mark Twain presented an example in his autobiography: "We had the 'faith doctors,' too, in those early days—a woman. Her specialty was toothache. She was a farmer's old wife and lived five miles from Hannibal. She would lay her hand on the patient's jaw and say, 'believe,' and the cure was prompt. Mrs. Utterback. I remember her well. Twice I rode out there behind my mother on horseback, and saw the cure performed. My mother was the patient."

PULL A TOOTH, CURE A PATIENT

When all else failed, dental extraction was the last resort, and this was a common procedure since dental disease was so widespread. Early Chinese tooth pullers removed teeth with their fingers, and spent hours strengthening their hands by removing nails from wooden planks. The practice of pulling teeth was passed from one practitioner to another much like any other trade well into the seventeenth century. The tooth was first loosened either by placing a small amount of arsenic under the gum or by shaving the gum with a scalpel. It was then rocked back and forth with a crude instrument, being careful not to break it off. Tooth pullers and barber-surgeons, who also practiced minor surgery and bleeding, spent most of their time out-of-doors and traveled from one town to another, often in a carnival atmosphere with music, jugglers, and magicians (figure 369). J. Menzies Campbell described a seventeenth-century scene in Scotland:

> They glibly promised cures for every disease including toothache. There was always a zany who, in a droll manner, sang lewd yet amusing songs riveting the attention of disorders which his master could cure. The entourage also included dancers with curious antics and performers on the tight rope. The bedizened quicksilver enlivened the proceedings with comic orations, while perched on a well-appointed chariot drawn by four (sometimes six) elegantly caparisoned horses. Not infrequently, he reinforced his claims by quoting scripture or by prayers to saints. Although never averse to superstitious cases which he had miraculously cured, he remained profoundly silent on the array of persons he had caused to suffer grievously or even liquidated. Tooth-drawing was always one of the most popular sidelines to entertain the crowd of ignoramuses, who besieged his stage.

It is not surprising that those who practiced dentistry were not held in high esteem. In France there is an old adage "*Mentir comme un arracheur des dents*" ("to lie like a snatcher of teeth") (figures 370, 371). Great eighteenth-century dentist Pierre Fauchard described one of the slight of hand techniques used by early quack dentists (with an accomplice) in order to attract customers at the Pont-Neuf Bridge in Paris: ". . . pretended paid sufferers come up from time to time to the operator who holds in his hand a tooth all ready wrapped in a very fine skin with blood of a chicken or some other animal, introduces his hand in the mouth of the pretended sufferer, drops into it the tooth hidden in his

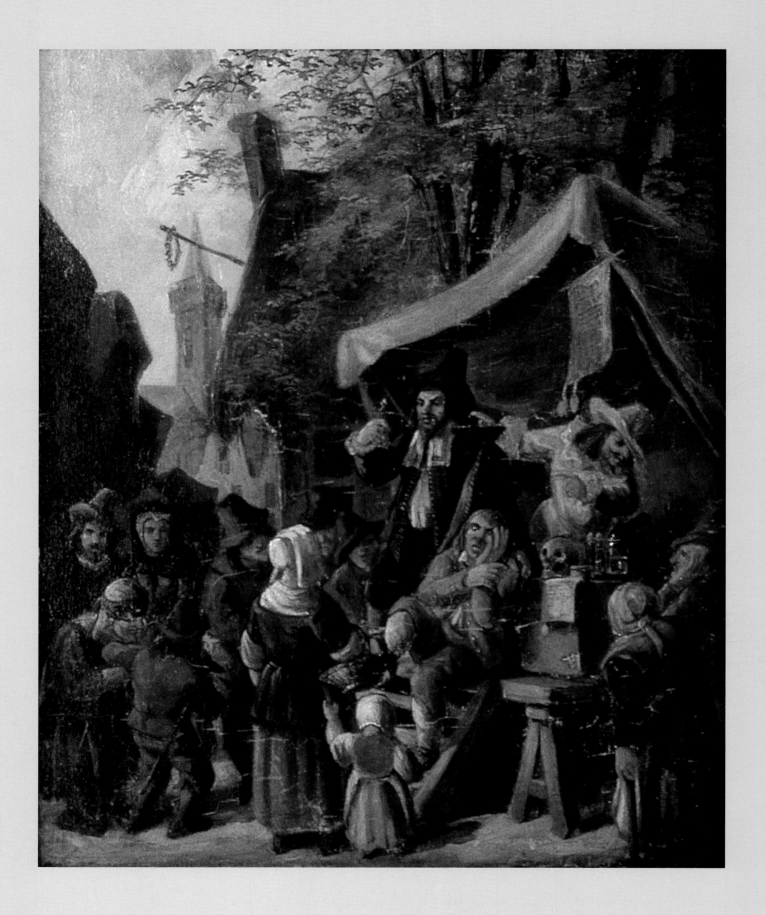

hand. Then he has only to touch the tooth or do something of the sort with a powder or a straw or the point of his sword, he has only if he wishes to ring a bell in the ear of the pretended patient, who spits during this time that which he has in his mouth. One sees him spit out the blood and the bloody tooth, which is only the tooth which the impostor or the patient has introduced into the mouth."

Dental extraction was frequently the treatment of choice for dental disease even into the eighteenth century, though it remained universally feared and almost always postponed. Queen Elizabeth spent many days and nights in pain, agreeing to an extraction only after the Bishop of London allowed a surgeon to pull one of his own teeth in 1578 "and she was hereby encouraged to submit to the Operation herself." All teeth were at risk, except perhaps the canine, or eyetooth, since cavernous sinus infections extending into the orbit and eye after extraction made physicians reluctant to venture there. These particular teeth, however, were often removed as a punishment, and those who considered breaking the law were forced to weigh whether or not they would "give their eye-tooth" for the object of their desire.

Benjamin Rush, MD, was America's preeminent physician in the eighteenth century, and he believed that tooth decay was an important cause of many systemic diseases. Rush was a strong proponent of dental extraction and wrote the following in his *Medical Inquiries and Observations* (1809):

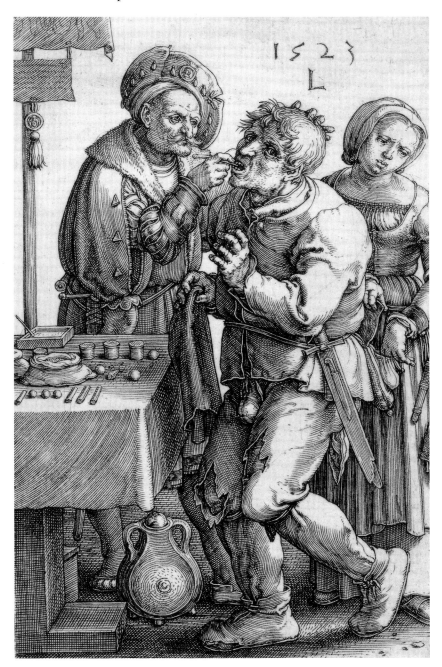

When we consider how often the teeth, when decayed, are exposed to irritation from hot and cold drinks and ailments from pressure by mastication, and from the cold air, and how intimate the connection of the mouth is with the whole system, I am disposed to believe they are often the unsuspected causes of general, and particularly of nervous diseases. When we add to the list of

369. Opposite. Quacks on stage, oil on wood attributed to a painter from the Netherlands

370. *The Dentist* (1523), copperplate engraving by Lucas van Leydon

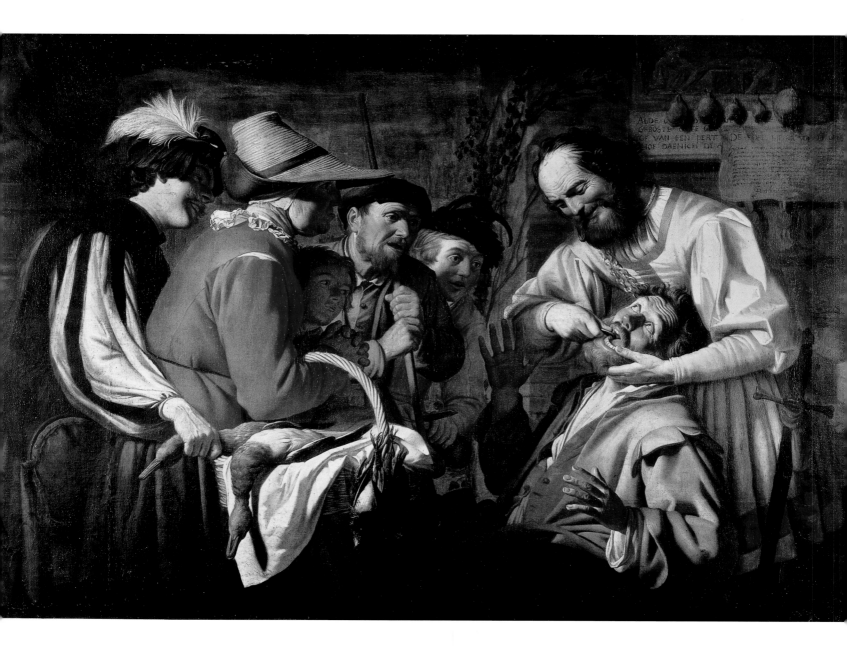

371. *The Tooth Puller* by Gerrit van Honthorst (1590–1656)

those diseases the morbid effects of the acrid and putrid matters, which are sometimes discharged from the carious teeth, or from the ulcers in the gums created by them, also the influence which both have in preventing perfect mastication and the connection of that animal function with good health, I can not help thinking that our success in the treatment of all chronic diseases would be very much promoted, by directing our inquiries into the state of the teeth in sick people, and by advising their extraction in every case in which they are decayed. It is not necessary that they should be attended with pain, in order to produce disease, for splinters, tumors, and other irritants before mentioned, often bring on disease and death, when they give no pain, and are unsuspected causes of them. This translation of sensation and motion into parts remote from the place where impressions are made, appears in many instances, and seems to depend upon an original law of the animal economy.

DENTISTRY BECOMES A PROFESSION

Early physicians interested in diseases of the mouth and gums finally began to gain respectability with the publication of *Le Chirurgien Dentiste, ou Traite des Dents* in 1728 by Pierre Fauchard. Fauchard was concerned not only with surgical technique but with dental anatomy and pathophysiology, discounting the long-held belief that tooth decay was caused by tooth worms. Additionally, he directed a great deal of time to the study of preventive dentistry and periodontal disease, all important steps in differentiating dentistry from medicine. Fauchard is now recognized as the "Father of Dentistry" and was the first to use of term *surgeon-dentist,* forever changing dentistry from a trade of tooth pullers to a true profession of specialists.

Bartolomeo Eustachio was a pupil of Vesalius in the sixteenth century and is considered to be the first dental anatomist, though dental anatomy was included only as a part of more comprehensive medical anatomy texts prior to the eighteenth century (figures 372, 373). An early description of the teeth can be found in *Orthopaedia: or, the Art of Correcting and Preventing Deformities in Children*, by Nicholas Andry (1743):

Along the Gums of the upper and lower Jaw there is a Row of small while hard Bones, of a middling Length and Thickness, which not only serve as an Ornament to the Mouth, but assisting out Pronunciation. They are called the Teeth. In Adults they are commonly thirty-two in number, *viz.* sixteen in each Jaw. Of these thirty-two there are eight fore Teeth, *viz.* four above, and as many below. These are called *Incisores* or Cutters, upon account of their Office, which is to cut or break the solid Aliments. They are likewise called the glad Teeth, because they chiefly appear when one laughs.

Next to the *Incisores* are four very sharp Teeth, called the

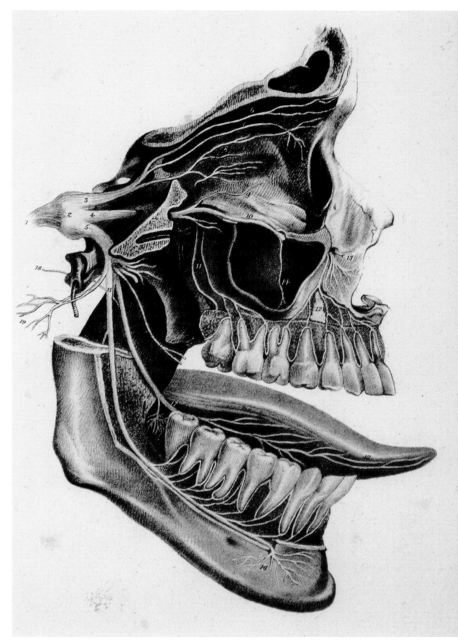

372. *The Anatomy, Physiology, and Pathology of the Human Teeth* (1844) by Paul B. Goddard

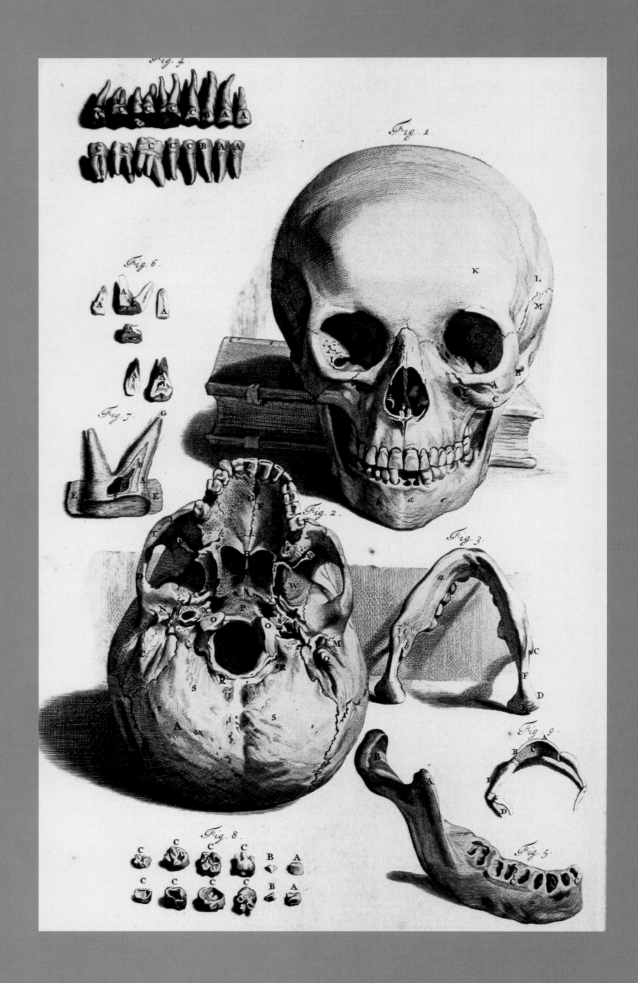

Caninae, two above, and two below. They are called *Caninae* because they are pointed like Dogs Teeth. The upper ones are called the Eye Teeth, because they are situated under the Eyes. The *Caninae* are followed by twenty other Teeth, ten above, and ten below, five on each side of the Jaws, and these are called the *Molares, viz.* the last on each side of the Jaws, are commonly called the Wisdom Teeth, because they do not push out till one and twenty.

Fortunately, some accurate anatomic models survived from the nineteenth century and can be appreciated today (figures 374, 375).

A number of obstacles needed to be overcome before the survival of dentistry as a profession could be secured. Standards of practice had not been established, and friction developed between those who attended their patients at different levels of professional care. Concern over the quality of dental treatment and the need for a regulatory body is evident in this quote by Shearjashub Spooner in *Guide to Sound Teeth, or, A Popular Treatise on the Teeth* (1836):

> One thing is certain, this profession must either rise or sink. If means are not taken to suppress and discountenance the malpractices of the multitude of incompetent persons, who are pressing into it, merely for the sake of its emoluments, it must sink—for the few competent and well-educated men, who are now upholding it, will abandon a disreputable profession, in a country of enterprise like ours, and turn their attention to some other calling more congenial to the feelings of honorable and enlightened men.

Training in dentistry finally became formalized when the Baltimore College of Dental Surgery was chartered in the United States in 1840, becoming the first dental school in the world. Two dentists contributed to this remarkable accomplishment, and they were the only two dental faculty members at the opening of that institution. Horace H. Hayden was a geologist from Connecticut who was initially a patient of the famous American dentist John Greenwood and then became his student. In 1810, Hayden received a license to practice dentistry from the Medical and Chirurgical Faculty of Maryland, the first person ever to receive that honor anywhere. He taught a regularly scheduled course on dentistry at the University of Maryland School of Medine in 1837, lectures that had first been offered earlier in 1821. Chapin A. Harris was born in New York and practiced both medicine and dentistry in Ohio before moving to Baltimore, where he studied under Hayden. In 1839, Harris published a book that became a foundation of dentistry for the next seventy years,

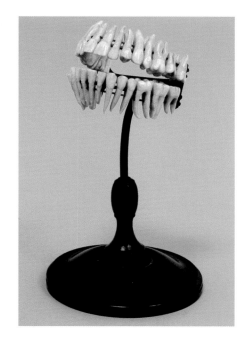

373. Opposite. *The Anatomy of Humane Bodies* (1698) by William Cowper

374. Hand-carved ivory teeth (ca. 1840)

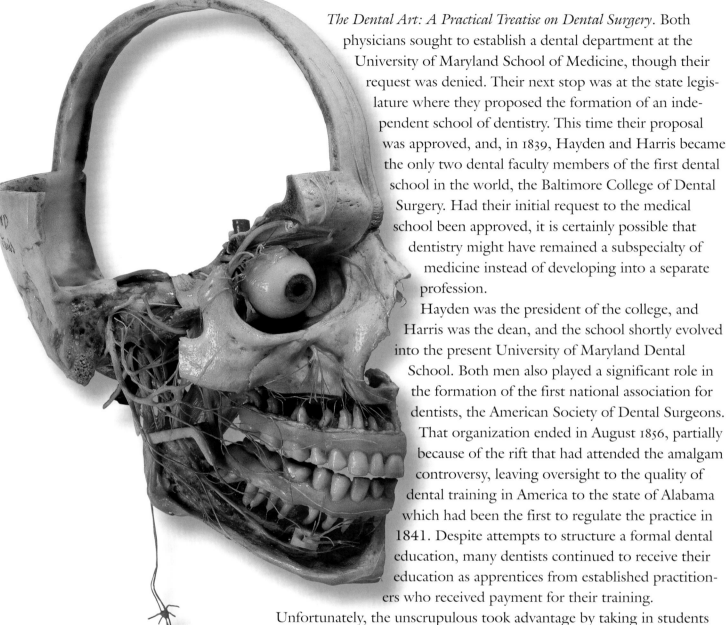

375. Prepared anatomical skull (ca. 1870–1900) by Tramond, Paris

The Dental Art: A Practical Treatise on Dental Surgery. Both physicians sought to establish a dental department at the University of Maryland School of Medicine, though their request was denied. Their next stop was at the state legislature where they proposed the formation of an independent school of dentistry. This time their proposal was approved, and, in 1839, Hayden and Harris became the only two dental faculty members of the first dental school in the world, the Baltimore College of Dental Surgery. Had their initial request to the medical school been approved, it is certainly possible that dentistry might have remained a subspecialty of medicine instead of developing into a separate profession.

Hayden was the president of the college, and Harris was the dean, and the school shortly evolved into the present University of Maryland Dental School. Both men also played a significant role in the formation of the first national association for dentists, the American Society of Dental Surgeons. That organization ended in August 1856, partially because of the rift that had attended the amalgam controversy, leaving oversight to the quality of dental training in America to the state of Alabama which had been the first to regulate the practice in 1841. Despite attempts to structure a formal dental education, many dentists continued to receive their education as apprentices from established practitioners who received payment for their training.

Unfortunately, the unscrupulous took advantage by taking in students merely for their tuition, leaving the population exposed to a generation of incompetent operators that preyed on an unsuspecting public. An 1845 editorial of the *American Journal of Dental Science* pointed this out: "We know of one who has the unblushing effrontery to promise to fit them for the profession in one month—to teach them the whole art and science of dentism, both surgical and mechanical, in 26 days; and this, not requiring their constant attendance, but two hours twice or three times a week."

Chapin Harris continued to personally fund the first dental journal, the *American Journal of Dental Science*, until his death in 1860. His personal efforts at keeping the dental school's journal alive, however, had plunged his widow into great debt. Harris' colleagues organized a benefit in his honor, and they were delighted to total the donations for the event at $1,000, though had to later subtract the cost of the fund-raising event, which was $915. Mrs. Harris was at first indignant at the offer, though subsequently grateful to accept the remaining sum as an honorarium.

In England, training in dentistry was considered to be part of a general medical education until 1858 when the Royal Dental Hospital was recognized as a branch of the University College in London. The Royal College of Surgeons did not issue a dental diploma until 1880 when a four-year course of study was necessary to meet the requirement.

THE AMALGAM WARS OF 1840–1850

Diseased teeth had always been treated by extraction until advances in the sixteenth century allowed some the option of trying to save the tooth by filling the cavity with various materials. The great surgeon Ambrose Paré (1510–1590) used either lead or cork, though by the beginning of the eighteenth century, little had changed as Pierre Fauchard packed dental cavities with lead or tin foil. Philip Pfaff (1715–1767), the dentist to Frederick the Great of Prussia, improved the quality of dental filling material, though at the same time, significantly increased cost by using the gold foil.

In 1803, English dentist John Fox invented a more affordable alternative metallic filling that was composed of bismuth, lead, and tin, which he called "Fusible Metal." This mixture liquefied at a temperature of 212 degrees Fahrenheit and could be poured directly into the cavity where it would harden and preserve the tooth. Unfortunately, the fusing temperature was much too high to be clinically useful, though the later addition of mercury made the requirement a more acceptable 140 degrees Fahrenheit. Combinations of metals containing mercury have since been called amalgams, though early formulas had only marginal commercial success since they had to be melted with a red-hot iron cautery. It was not until 1826 that a clinically useful mixture was discovered when August Taveau of Paris and Thomas Bell of England independently created an amalgam of coin silver filings mixed with mercury. This new combination was obviously quite attractive to dentists since it would be soft when poured into the cavity, and would harden quickly at a temperature comfortable to the patient without the use of a cautery. Additionally, the cost was much less than that of gold, though some of the early amalgams would sometimes either expand or shrink shortly after the patient had left the dentist's office.

Several years later in 1833, the Crawcour brothers immigrated to the United States from France and brought with them the use of amalgam fillings, causing one of the most significant controversies in the history of dentistry, the so-called "Amalgam Wars." They used a mercury-based amalgam that they called "Royal Mineral Succedaneum" instead of the "royal mineral" gold that had been popular in America. This raised numerous ethical, economic, and political questions that divided the dental community into two groups: the craftsmen who employed amalgam for its ease of use and low cost, and the physician-dentists with a medical degree who favored the use of gold leaf. Physician-dentists accused the craftsmen-dentists of profiteering and malpractice by their disregard for the potential medical risks related to the use of mercury, while the latter took exception to any interference in their freedom to practice as they saw fit.

The American Society of Dental Surgeons was organized in 1840, and the controversy immediately surfaced. The new organization took the medical high ground, fearing that mercury caused depression, indigestion, paralysis, and death, and declared "the use of amalgam to be malpractice." The Crawcour brothers were "swindling villains," according to Shearjashub Spooner. On December 5, 1843, in Boston, Josiah Flagg commented:

> This mercurial compound is still in use in our City, and the country about it, I will not say by dentists, but by a host of imposters, 'operators on teeth,' whose advertisements fill a part of almost every newspaper; some of whom, perhaps, are even ignorant of its deleterious effects, but many of whom know well its qualities, and too well to trust it in their teeth. It is an article which can be applied by any one who can stop a hollow tooth with wax or putty, and if it could be retained no longer than these its evils would be very greatly diminished.
>
> I am fully aware that these *cements* or *amalgams* have been used in some cases, when they *seem* to be of service; but here, still, is deception; for in all such cases that have come under my observation, (and these are very numerous,) it can be demonstrated, by an examination of them, that great mischief is going on beneath such fillings, and that a different and better treatment might have been adopted.

In Dr. Chapin A. Harris' address to the first graduating class of the Baltimore College of Dental Surgery, he spoke of amalgam, stating that "it is one of the most abominable articles for filling teeth that could be employed." The society demanded that all its members sign the following or be expelled:

> *I hereby certify it to be my opinion and firm conviction that any amalgam whatever . . . is unfit for the plugging of teeth or fangs and I pledge myself*

never under any circumstance to make use of it in my practice, as a dental sur-
geon, and furthermore, as a member of the American Association of Dental
surgeons, I do subscribe and unite with them in this protest against the use of
the same. Given under my hand and seal the _____day of____, 184_.
    Signed_____

Many refused to sign, so many were expelled. Economic and political pressures increased over the years, and members continued to drop
out as more used amalgam. The requirement to sign the pledge was
rescinded in 1850, but that was too late to save the American Society of
Dental Surgeons, and it disbanded on August 1, 1856. Three years later in
1859, craftsman organized themselves to form the American Dental
Association, dropping many of the course requirements demanded by
the physician-dentists.

The argument was taken up again in 1880 with the studies of Dr.
Eugene Talbot, who demonstrated the toxicity of mercury vapor, though
he didn't prove any increased levels of mercury from dental amalgams.
Debate over the safety of amalgam and its relation to the development
of chronic disease continues today.

PROSTHETICS

The art of producing replacement dentures began with the Etruscans
when they designed false teeth skillfully crafted of ivory and bone as
early as 700 B.C. (figure 376). Not until the eighteenth century did dentures regain the same level of sophistication.

Settlers in the New World were dependent on British and European
dental expertise for the manufacture of prostheses well into the eighteenth century. In 1749, Sieur Roquet emigrated from Paris to Boston
where he advertised his wares in the *Independent Advertiser*: "He also

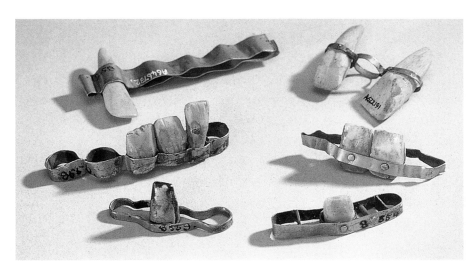

376. Etruscan bridges (seventh century B.C.)

cures effectually the most stinking Breaths by drawing out, and eradicating all decayed Teeth and Stumps, and burning the Gums to the Jaw Bone, without the least Pain or Confinement; and putting in their stead, an entire Set of right African Ivory Teeth, set in a Rose-colour'd Enamel, so nicely fitted to the Jaws, that People of the first Fashion may eat, drink, swear, talk, Scandal, quarrel, and shew their Teeth, without the least Indecency, Inconvenience, or Hesitation whatever." American dentists also recognized the popular demand for dentures, and one of the first to respond was the famous American patriot and silversmith Paul Revere. He was a practicing dentist for at least four years, and in 1790 placed an advertisement in the *Boston Gazette,* which illustrates some of the defiant character that led him to his famous ride several years later in the American Revolution: ". . . he still continues the Business of a Dentist, and flatter himself that from the Experience he has had these Two Years (in which time he has fixt some Hundreds of Teeth) that he can fix them as well as any Surgeon, Dentist who ever came from London. . . ."

The well-documented trials and tribulations of George Washington attest to the difficulties early physicians had in the preparation of dental prostheses. Washington had suffered from diseases of the teeth and gums since the age of twenty-two, when he lost his first tooth. Though he was known to be fond of sweets, periodontal disease may have been the major cause of Washington's tooth loss since original teeth that had been included in one of his dentures were cavity free. Another possible cause of his loss of teeth may have been the fact that physicians in the mid 1760s had given Washington large quantities of mercury in the form of mercurous chloride, or calomel. This was a common treatment for any number of inflammatory diseases, including pneumonia, pleurisy, rheumatism, and was the classic treatment for syphilis in the eighteenth century. Calomel was also a purgative, and the loss of teeth was a frequent side effect.

Washington continued to lose teeth on a regular basis until he was down to only one tooth, a premolar on the left side of his jaw when he took the oath of office as the first president of the United States in 1789 at the age of fifty-seven. Washington visited most of the dentists in colonial America, though his favorite was Dr. John Greenwood, who produced almost all of the dentures worn by the first president. They were constructed of various combinations of hippopotamus ivory, cow teeth, elephant tusk, natural teeth, and gold (though none were made of wood as legend would have it). James Gardette manufactured one set for Washington in 1796, and John Greenwood produced others in 1789, 1791, 1795, 1797, with the last one in 1798 (figure 377). President Washington was never totally comfortable with his dentures, and on

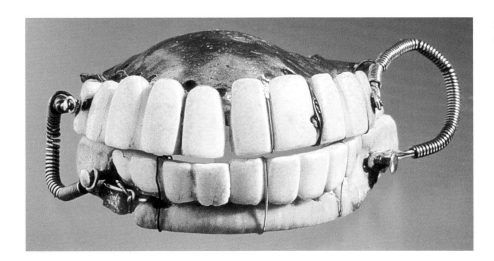

377. President George Washington's
dentures (1795)

returning a set to Greenwood for repair in 1797, he commented that
they were "both uneasy in the mouth, and bulge my lips out in such a
manner as to make them appear considerable swelled." Washington's
1795 set (his most complete) was stolen in 1981 while on loan to the
Smithsonian Institution in Washington, DC. It contained springs to
keep the teeth apart, so that if Washington relaxed his facial muscles, his
mouth popped open, which might have been the reason for the stern
visage he seemed to always maintain in his paintings and on the one dollar bill. According to one observer in 1790, "His mouth was like no
other I ever saw; the lips firm and the under jaw seemed to grasp the
upper with force, as if the muscles were in full action when he sat still."
Another commented, "His mouth was his strong feature, the lips being
always tightly compressed. That day they were compressed so tightly as
to be painful to look at."

Carved ivory dentures tended to stain, decay, and often retained an
unpleasant odor, so alternative prostheses were always in demand. Major
battlefields provided a rich source of teeth from fallen soldiers for use in
dentures, including "Waterloo" teeth that were popular in France after
that famous battle. During the American Civil War, many waited near
battlefields for the fighting to conclude, sending thousands of teeth back
to England after they had finished their gruesome harvesting. Prostheses
made from these artifacts were really not satisfactory, however, and the
breakthrough in the development of removable dentures finally came in
the latter part of the eighteenth century when French Chemist Alexis
Duchâteau became uncomfortable with his own ivory denture. He
began to experiment with various types of porcelain with Parisian dentist
Nicholas Dubois de Chémant, who went on to be honored throughout
France and the world as the inventor of the first artificial teeth constructed from only inorganic material. In 1808, Giuseppangelo Fonzi, an
Italian dentist living in Paris, developed individual porcelain teeth with

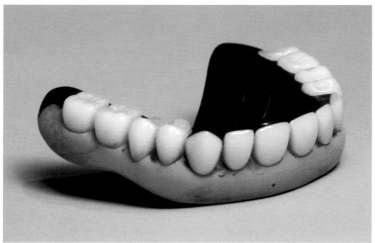

378. Vulcanite denture with porcelain teeth and gold inlay (ca. 1880)

platinum pins soldered into a thin metal base. The teeth in his "terro-metallic corruptibles" were easier to wear than those of ivory and were more natural since they could be individually shaded. Fonzi's new technique spread quickly all over Europe, and he became the dentist to royal families in Bavaria, Russia, and Spain. Unfortunately, his dentures were difficult to manufacture in quantity, and natural tooth replacements remained popular into the middle of the nineteenth century.

The demand for dentures dramatically increased in the mid nineteenth century when the discovery of anesthesia made relatively painless extractions possible. There followed a need for a material to form the base of dentures that was less expensive than gold or ivory. In 1839, Nelson Goodyear responded with the discovery of a hardened rubber material that he called vulcanite. Dental prostheses at last became available to the masses since dentures with vulcanite bases and porcelain teeth were easy to manufacture, affordable, and quite comfortable (figure 378). Goodyear allowed its patent for vulcanization to lapse in 1861, but for an inexplicable reason, it was reassigned to Boston dentist John A. Cummings in 1864 (after twelve years of denied requests). Cummings immediately sold those rights back to the Goodyear Dental Vulcanite Company (GDVC) where they were aggressively enforced by their treasurer, Josiah Bacon. Bacon charged a yearly royalty of up to $100 per dentist for the right to use his vulcanite product (in addition to a fee per denture), and he spent the next ten years prosecuting anyone who refused to pay. He was despised by all in the profession and was known as "the active and engineering Mephistopheles of this whole skinning raid upon the dentists." Bacon was successful, and his legal status was affirmed after an appeal to the Supreme Court, though the court later reversed itself for the first time in its history after finding out that Bacon had himself engineered the appeal for his own purposes.

The story, however, came to an abrupt end in San Francisco in 1879. Rather than capitulate and pay the GDVC licensing fees following losses in previous legal actions, Dr. Samuel P. Chalfant had closed his practice twice, moving to the west coast to again set up shop. Josiah Bacon followed him there in order to include Chalfant on a long list of defendants, and he once again prevailed over a tearful Chalfant. The now fully defeated dentist took the law into his own hands the following day and ended Bacon's reign of terror on the dental community with a pistol shot. Dentures finally became affordable when GDVC mercifully allowed their vulcanite patent to expire two years later in 1881.

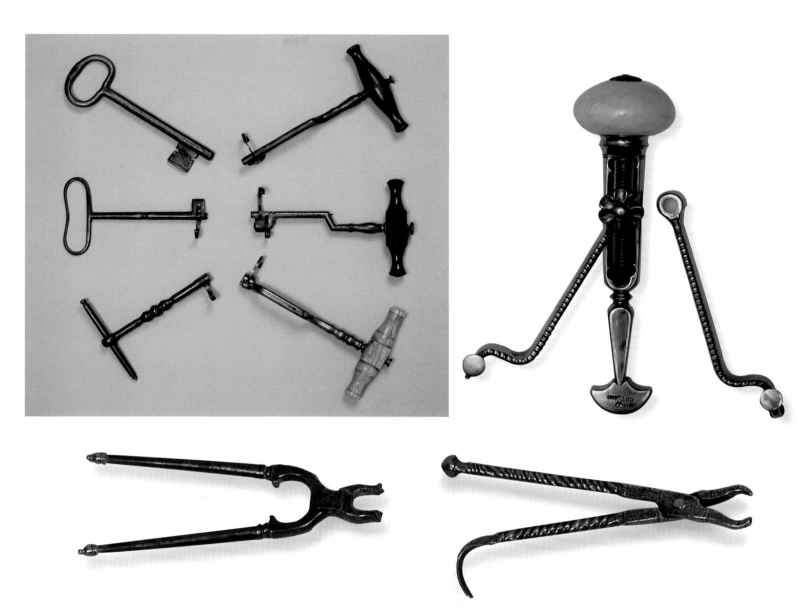

DENTAL EQUIPMENT AND FURNITURE

The first to illustrate dental instruments was Albucasis of Cordova (936–1013) in his *Altasrif* where he described the use of scalers: "Sometimes on the surface of the teeth, both inside and outside, are deposited rough ugly-looking scales, black, green, and yellow; this corruption is communicated to the gums, and the teeth are in process of time denuded. Lay the patient's head on your lap and scrape the teeth and molars." Other early dental instruments were simple pliers-like tools made by blacksmiths for the extraction of teeth (figure 379). In 1826, Cyrus Fay designed and constructed the first dental forceps that was produced for different types of teeth, though they were not universally accepted until they were used by Sir John Tomes several years later.

In the early fourteenth century, Guy de Chauliac invented an instrument that continued to be used into the late eighteenth century called a dental pelican because it resembled the beak of that bird (figure 380).

379. Dental extraction forceps (ca. 1600 and 1690)

380. Top right. Dental pelican with endless screw mechanism (ca. 1800) by Cotzand

381. Top left. Tooth keys: (left) eighteenth-century door key with dental keys below; (right) nineteenth-century dental keys of wood, ebony, and ivory

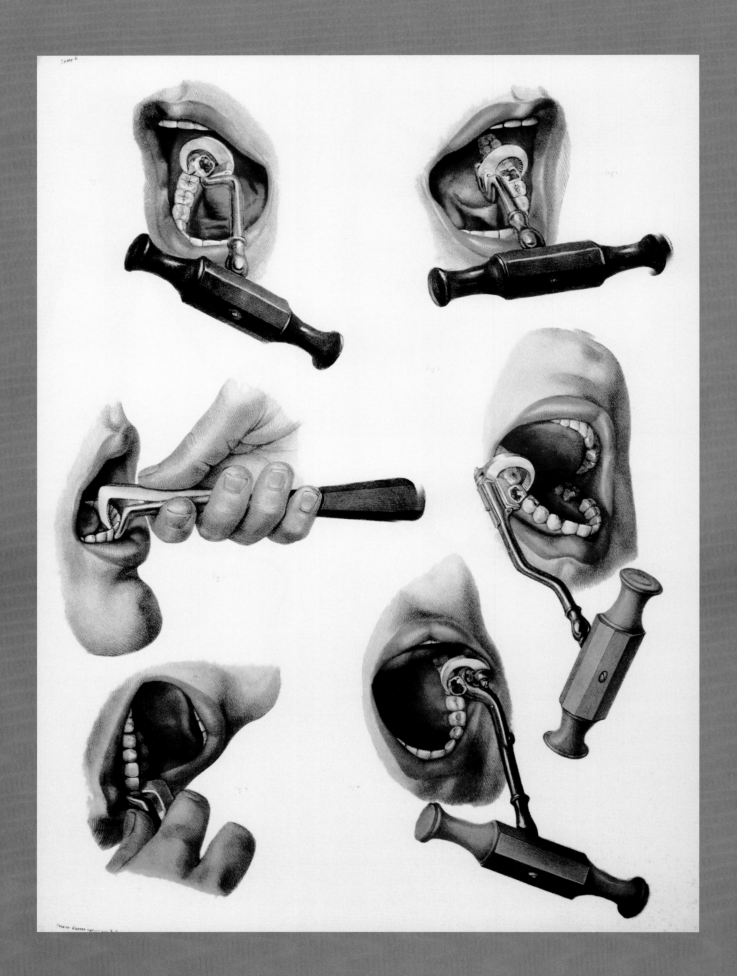

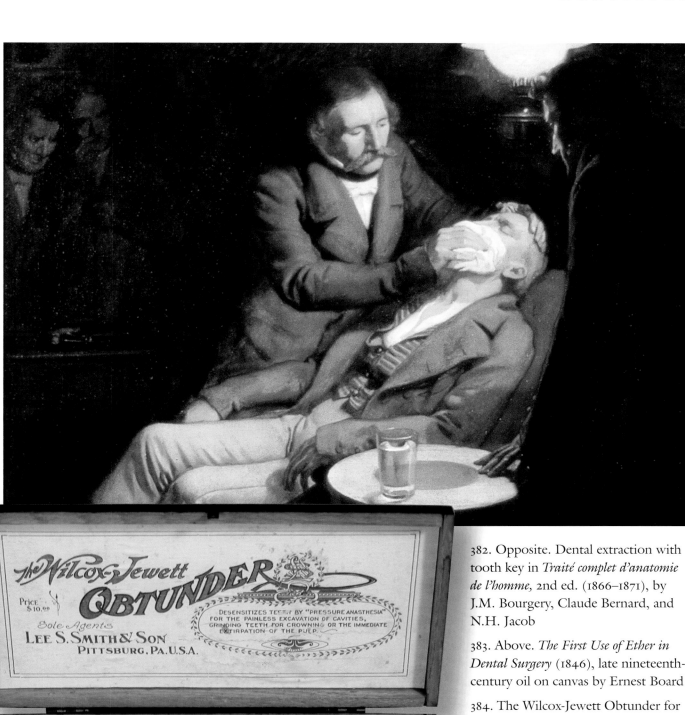

382. Opposite. Dental extraction with tooth key in *Traité complet d'anatomie de l'homme,* 2nd ed. (1866–1871), by J.M. Bourgery, Claude Bernard, and N.H. Jacob

383. Above. *The First Use of Ether in Dental Surgery* (1846), late nineteenth-century oil on canvas by Ernest Board

384. The Wilcox-Jewett Obtunder for cocaine injection (ca. 1915)

With it, the operator could apply extreme leverage to loosen the tooth out of the socket, and according to John Woodall in *The Surgeon's Mate* (1617), "If it bee the furthest tooth of the jaw either above or below, or that it be a stumpe, except it be of the foremost teeth, the pullicans are the fittest instruments to draw with." Pierre Fauchard added, "Of all the instruments used for drawing the teeth, a pelican, such as the one I have described, appears to me the most useful. Its effect is more prompt, more sure that that of any of the others when one knows how to handle it, without which the pelican, however, perfect it may be, is the most dangerous of all instruments for drawing teeth." Door keys became the models for the next generation of extraction instruments. They were appropriately called tooth keys, and were popular into the twentieth century (figures 381, 382).

As the population in the United States grew, so did the need for dentists and dental equipment. John D. Chevalier began to specialize in the manufacture of dental instruments when he opened the first dental supply house in 1833 in New York City. Samuel W. Stockton was a Philadelphia jeweler who was the first to find success in producing porcelain teeth in quantity and invited his nephew, Samuel S. White, to train as an apprentice. In 1844, White began making dental equipment on his own and continued that vocation following the Civil War. After his death in 1881, the Samuel S. White estate merged with the Johnson brothers to form the S.S. White Dental Manufacturing Company, which became the largest manufacturer of dental equipment in the world.

After the discovery of anesthesia in the mid nineteenth century (figures 383, 384), dental techniques and the variety of surgical procedures increased dramatically. That led to a need for more advanced equipment, and resulted in the production of the finest instruments ever made featuring such exotic materials as ebony, ivory, tortoise shell, and mother of pearl, with handles containing inset ruby, amethyst, topaz, emerald, and sapphire (figures 385–388). These instruments could not be adequately sterilized, so ironically they may have actually contributed to the morbidity of those operated on. Manufacturers, however, were interested in sales, and, despite the well-known risk of sepsis without sterilization, many dentists were anxious to impress patients with their wonderful instrumentation. Regardless of that fact, however, much of the

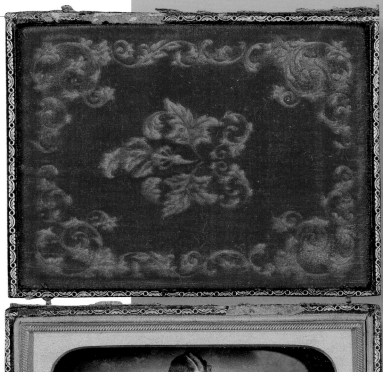

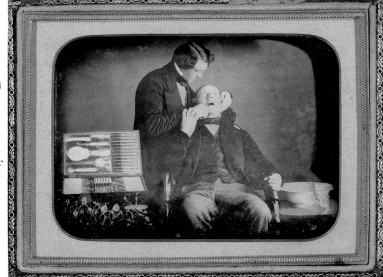

385. Opposite. Bow drill (mid nineteenth century)

386. Opposite. Late eighteenth- and nineteenth-century dental instruments: (top) two ivory file carriers, two dental cauteries, goat's foot elevator, chisel, split-shaft punch elevator by Benjamin Bell, ebony dental screw; (bottom) ivory Archimedes drill, ivory hand drill

387. Above. Daguerreotype of a dentist with his instruments (ca. 1855)

388. Opposite. Large cased dental set of ivory and mother-of-pearl (ca. 1860) by John D. Chevalier

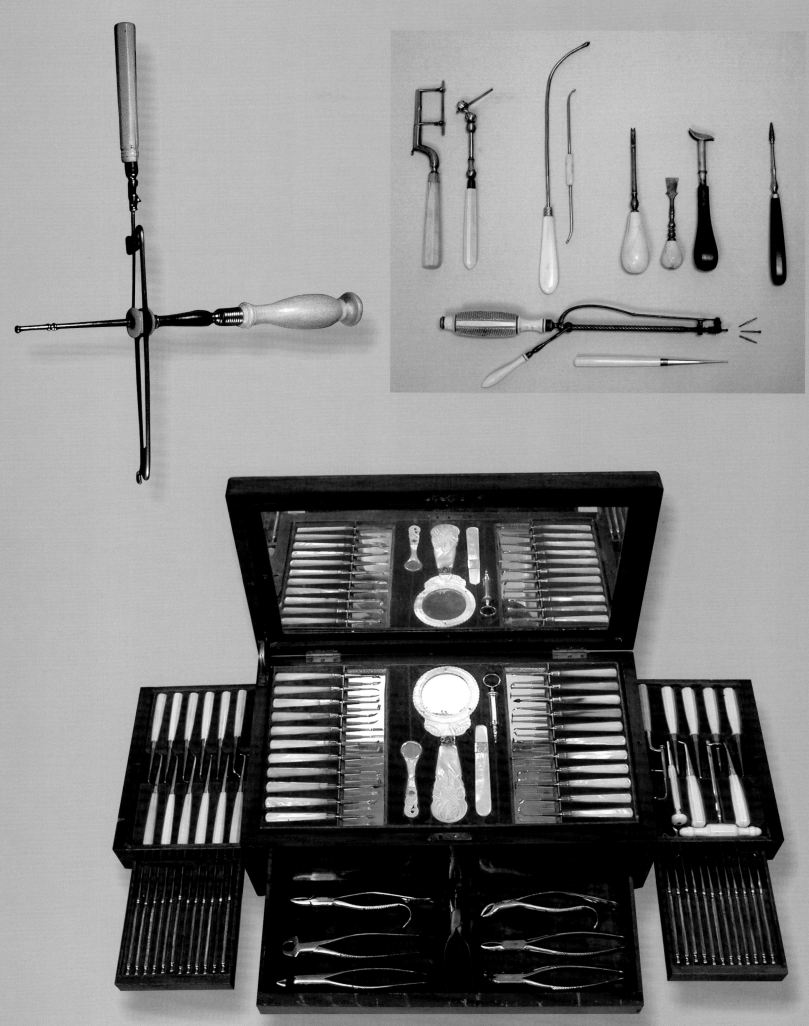

481

equipment found in dentists' offices remained intimidating, as this early article from the *Chicago Herald* suggests:

> His instruments of torture, called by courtesy dental tools, were many and varied. He was very skillful in his profession and when he took a job he did it in first-class style. The dental tools are simply copies in miniature of articles used in the Spanish inquisition and on refractory prisoners in the Tower of London. There are monkey wrenches, raspers, files, gouges, cleavers, pickes, squeezers, drills, daggers, little crowbars, punches, chisels, pincers, and long wire feelers with prehensile, palpitating tips, that can reach down through the roots of a throbbing tooth and fish up a yell from your inner consciousness. When a painstaking dentist cannot hurt you with the cold steel, he lights a small alcohol lamp and heats one of his little spades red hot, and hovers over you with an expectant smile. Then he deftly inserts this into your mouth and when you give a yell he says, 'Does that hurt?'

In 1790, George Washington's dentist, John Greenwood, invented the foot-operated dental engine as a modification of his mother-in-law's spinning wheel. His design did not catch on for another eighty years since dentists preferred to use smaller finger, bow, and hand-held rotating drills. Finally, on February 7, 1871, James Beall Morrison (1829–1917) of St. Louis provided an important advance in the progress of dental surgery with his patent for a foot-operated dental engine. Morrison was quite proud of his invention when he commented on ". . . some quite nervous ladies, for whom I have removed caries previously by manual excavation. Their judgment was unanimous that this type of operation, that is with the aid of this machine, is completely painless and relatively more pleasant than any other method of resection." Morrison's foot engine was mass-produced and remained popular in dental offices around the country until electricity became generally available thirty years later. The only drawback to the foot engine was the challenge faced by dentists of spending many hours a day pedaling while concentrating on the accuracy of a drill—without losing balance.

During the nineteenth century, great craftsmen turned their attention to the production of dental furniture as manufacturers attempted to meet the needs of a growing population that was more able to afford dental care. The use of a chair specifically designed for the dental patient is a rather recent practice, and prior to the eighteenth century, a patient simply placed his head between the knees of the operator. Pierre Fauchard commented that "the patient must be seated in an armchair which is steady and firm, suitable and comfortable, the back of which should be of horsehair or with a soft pillow raised more or less according to the stature of the patient and particularly to that of the dentist." The first chair to be used specifically in the dental office was designed by Josiah Flagg in 1790 when he added a headrest to an armchair, that chair now considered to be the oldest dental chair in the United States (figure 389). James Snell designed the first chair for use by other dentists in 1832, and the industry rapidly matured with the production of the all-metal frame dental chair by James Morrison, manufactured by the Johnston brothers of New York in 1872. This chair had great range, and could be easily raised with a hand crank. The Johnson brothers also produced the Wilkerson Dental Chair, which was invented by former Confederate prisoner of war M.B. Wilkerson, and was the first chair to replace cranks with levers (figure 390).

The manufacture of dental furniture became an art as cabinets were made of beautifully hand-carved mahogany, oak, walnut, and rosewood with nickel-plated swinging doors, mother-of-pearl drawer pulls, and beveled mirrors. Other fixtures found in the late eighteenth century dental office included wonderfully crafted spittoons, ornate bracket tables, and brass- or nickel-plated lamps (figure 391).

389. Josiah Flagg dental chair (1790)

390. "High-Low" Wilkerson dental chair (1886)

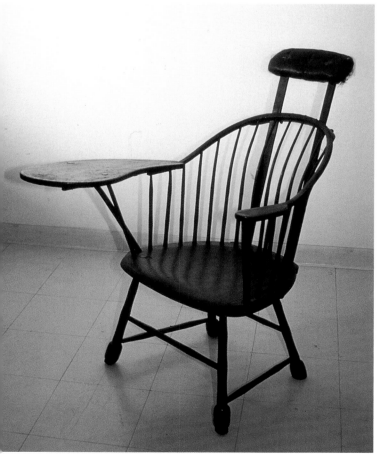

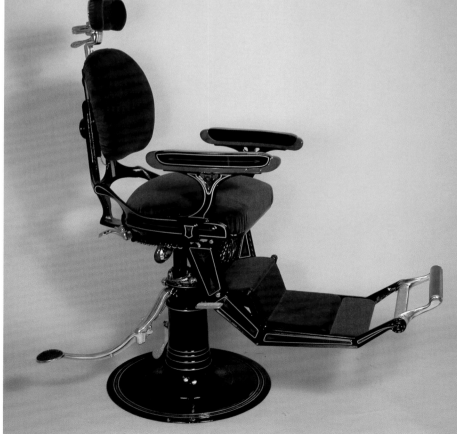

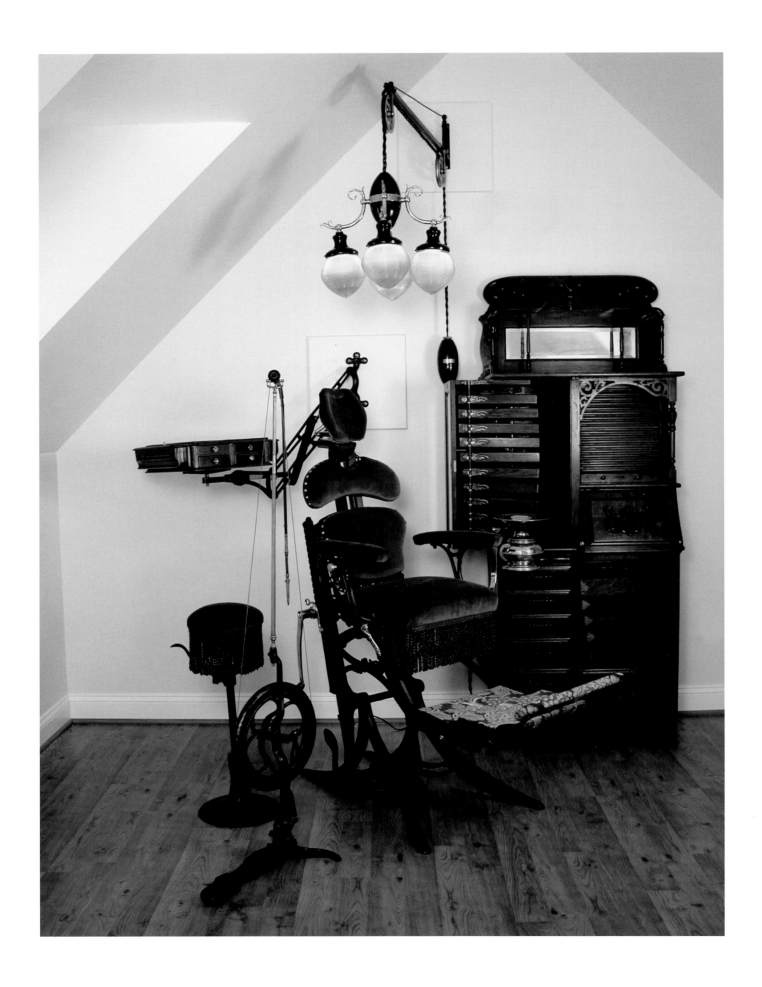

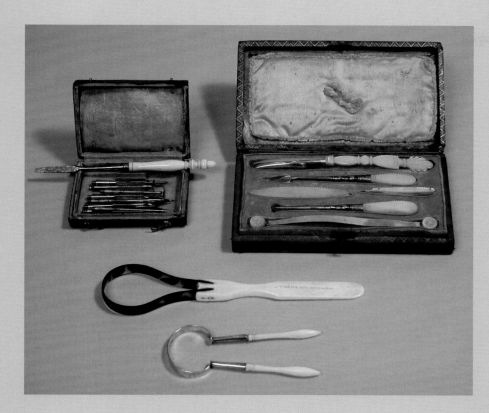

391. Opposite. Nineteenth-century dental office: Morrison dental chair with spittoon by S.S. White, dentist's stool by Smith, foot dental engine by S.S. White, Holmes bracket table with S.S. White bracket, Electro-Dental MFG. Co. Rhein cluster light (ca. 1911), quarter-sewn oak dental cabinet (ca. 1902) by The Harvard Co.

392. Nineteenth-century dental hygiene sets: (top left) ivory with multiple blades; (top right) mother-of-pearl with toothbrush; (bottom) tooth scrapers (upper) by Prout and (lower) silver and ivory (ca. 1780)

393. Queen Victoria's oral hygiene instruments

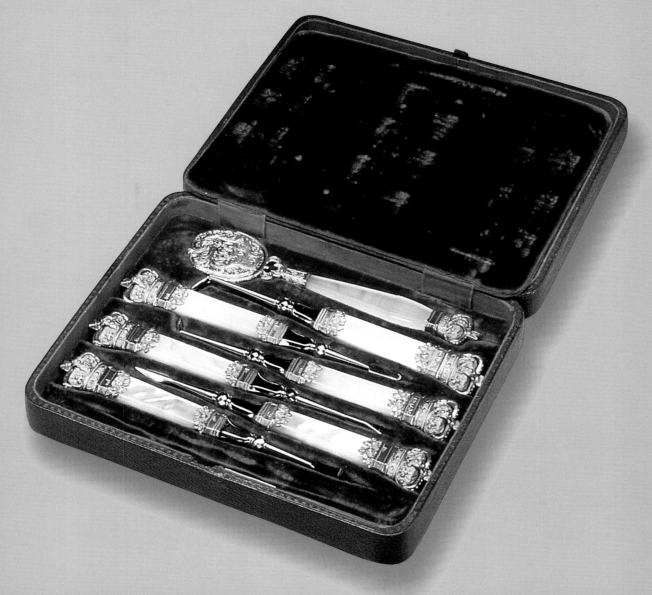

PERSONAL DENTAL HYGIENE

An interest in personal dental hygiene dates back to the ancient Chinese and Babylonians, who cleaned their teeth with chewsticks. The Romans also used small fibrous wood sticks for dental care, as do many today in Africa and some Islamic countries. In his *History of Medicine* (1860), Francesco Puccinotti reviewed several medieval recommendations that included references to dental hygiene:

> When you get up each morning, stretch your limbs; nature is comforted thereby, the natural heat is stimulated, and the limbs strengthened. Then comb your hair, as the combing removes uncleanliness and comforts the brain. Wash your hands and face also with cold water to give your skin a good colour and to stimulate the natural heat. Wash and clean your nose and your chest by expectorating, and also clean your teeth, because the stomach and the chest are aided thereby, and your speech becomes clearer. Clean your teeth and your gums with the bark of some odoriferous tree. From time to time fumigate your brain with precious spices; in hot weather use cold things like sandalwood; when it is cold, use hot things like cinnamon, cloves, myrrh, the wood of aloes, and similar articles. This thorough fumigation will open your nostrils and your brain, will keep your hair from degenerating and becoming white, and will keep the face plump. Adorn

394. Dental Powders: Royal Tooth Powder (ca. 1900), Allen Pharmaceutical Co., New York and Plainfield, NJ, Dr. Huff's Tooth Powder (ca. 1921), Hot Springs, AR; Dr. Lyon's Ammoniated Tooth Powder (licensed by the University of Illinois Foundation, 1951), Sterling Drug, NY, Dr. VC Bell's Tooth Powder (ca. 1890), American Dentifrice Co., NY, Smith's Rosebud Tooth Powder, Rosebud Perfume Co., Woodsboro, MD (ca. 1910)

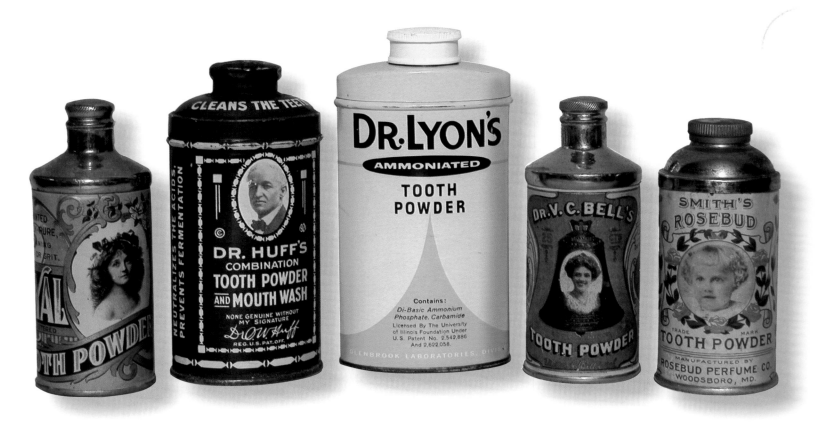

your body with fine clothing as the spirit is rejoiced thereby; and chew fennel, anise, cloves, because this strengthens the stomach, gives a good appetite, and sweetens the breath. . . .

With advances in mass-manufacturing techniques came a number of instruments produced for personal use (figures 392, 393). The Chinese may have been the first to utilize urine as a mouthwash, though it has been used in many cultures for that purpose probably because of the ammonia. The great French surgeon-dentist Pierre Fauchard advised that his patients use their own urine in cleaning their mouths and quickly added, "What would one not do for the sake of one's health?" Ammoniated tooth powders remained popular into the twentieth century (figure 394).

THE END OF AN ERA

In the latter part of the nineteenth century, Greene Vardiman Black (1836–1915) organized, classified, and expanded the techniques of dental care, and is now known as the "Father of Modern Operative Dentistry." Fine materials and craftsmanship yielded to the standard bactericidal materials of steel and chrome that we see in modern dental offices today, and dentistry became based on scientific principles to take its place as a legitimate branch of medicine.

". . . no one can excel whose loss of teeth, or rotten livid stumps, and fallen lips and hollow cheeks, destroy articulation, and the happy expression of countenance; whose voice has lost its narrative tone, and whose laugh, instead of painting joy and merriment, expresses only defect and disease.

The foulness of the teeth by some people is little regarded; but with the fair sex, with the polite and elegant part of the world, it is looked on as a certain mark of filthiness and sloth; not only because it disfigures one of the greatest ornaments of the countenance, but also because the smell imparted to the breath by dirty rotten teeth, is generally disagreeable to the patients themselves, and sometimes extremely offensive to the olfactory nerves in close conversation."

Dr. Benjamin Fendall, *Maryland Gazette*, August 15, 1776

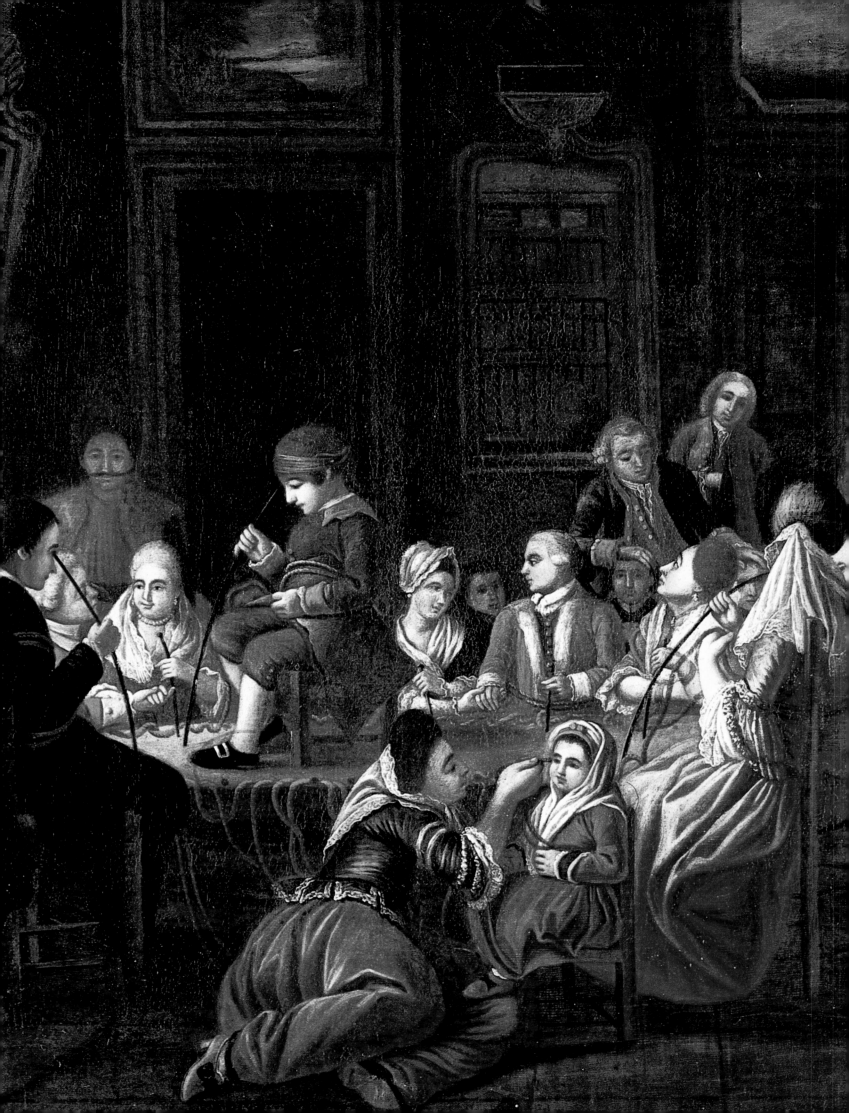

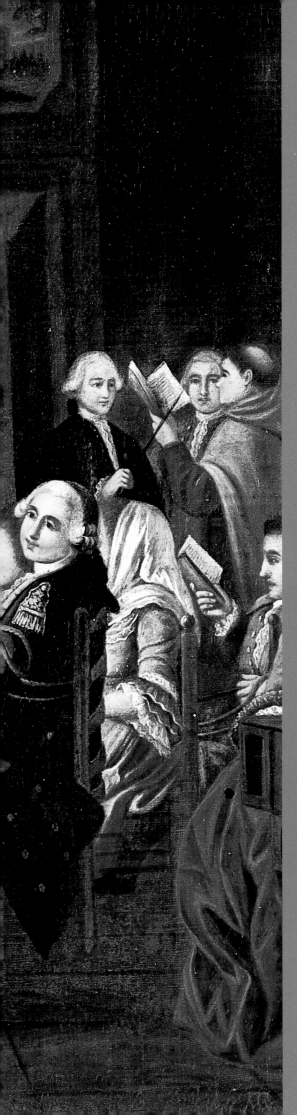

QUACK MEDICINE

"The philosophies of one age have become the absurdities of the next, and the foolishness of yesterday has become the wisdom of tomorrow…"

William Osler, MD
Chauvinism in Medicine, 1902

Detail. A group of mesmerised
French patients (1778/1784), oil on
canvas, artist unknown

As long as there has been suffering, there have been those who have taken it upon themselves to provide relief, whether it be by herbs and incantations or by the latest genetically engineered and scientifically proven therapies. Sorcerers and charlatans have always found success in marketing their wares since there was (and is) disagreement regarding what is efficacious (figure 395). Mercury was a foundation in the treatment of syphilis well into the nineteenth century and "quicksilver," which was another name for this metal, became the genesis for the term *quack* to represent the unethical or incompetent physician. Dr. Oliver Wendell Holmes provided us with a good definition of quack medicine in *The Professor at the Breakfast Table* (1892): "A Pseudo-science consists of a *nomenclature*, with a self-adjusting arrangement, by which all positive evidence, or such as favors its doctrines, is admitted, and all negative evidence, or such as tells against it, is excluded. It is invariably connected with some lucrative practical application." The line between quackery and cure has always been blurred—and remains so today.

One of the reasons for confusion regarding the efficacy of various therapeutic regimens in the past has been the fact that many patients improve spontaneously no matter what therapy they choose. Additionally, the healed often falsely attribute curative powers to the medication or event that had just preceded their improvement. A well-known philosophic fallacy applies: *Post hoc, ergo propter hoc* ("after it, therefore because of it") or the assumption that because one event precedes another, the first event must be the cause of the second. That logic has led to the acceptance by many of the bizarre medical customs and home remedies to which we are still accustomed.

"Placebo affect," or the power of belief in the therapy, also helps to determine clinical outcomes. This factor was noted by Sir Humphrey Davy (1778–1829) while evaluating the use of the anesthetic nitrous oxide as a possible treatment for paralysis. Dr. Paris wrote the following in his *Pharmacologia*:

> Previous to the administration of the gas, [Davy] inserted a small thermometer under the tongue of the patient, as he was accustomed to do upon such occasions, to ascertain the degree of animal temperature, with a view to future comparison. The paralytic man, wholly ignorant of the nature of the process to which he was to submit, but deeply impressed . . . with the certainty of its success, no sooner felt the thermometer under his tongue than he concluded the talisman was in full operation, and in a burst of enthusiasm declared that he already experienced the effect of its benign influence throughout his whole body: the opportunity

395. "The Quack Doctor" in *Every Saturday* (January 14, 1871) by F.O.C. Darley

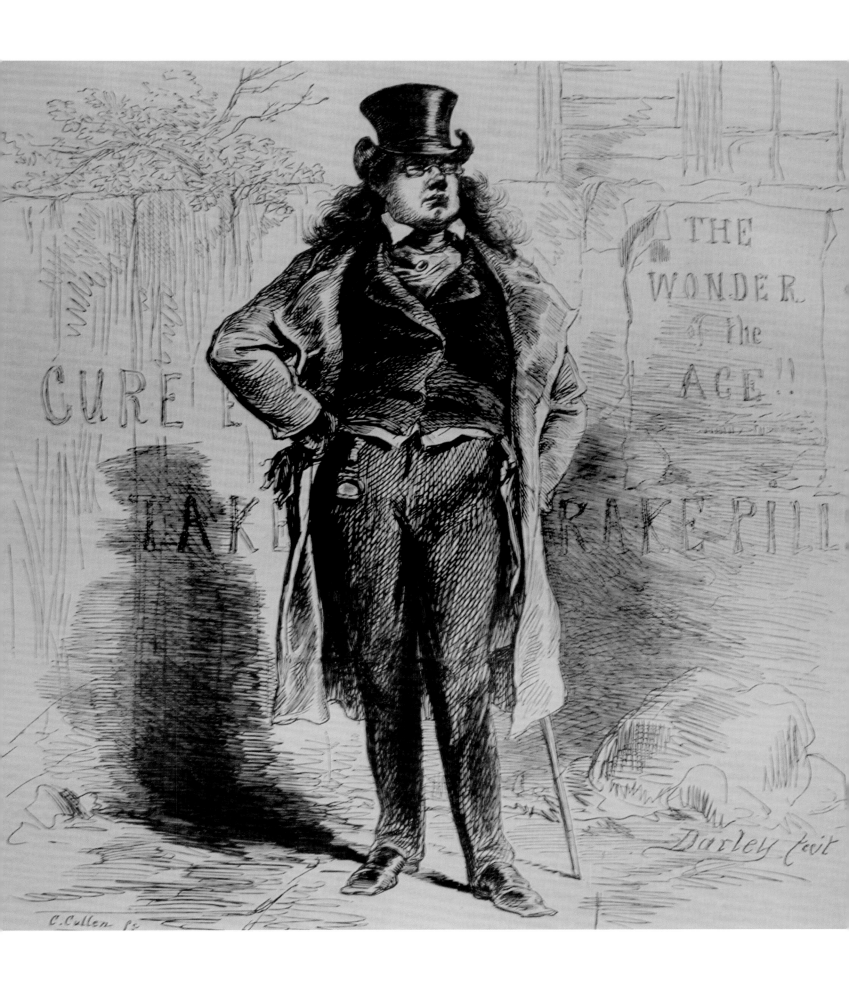

was too tempting to be lost; Davy . . . desired his patient to renew his visit on the following day, when the same ceremony was performed, and repeated every succeeding day for a fortnight, the patient gradually improving during that period, when he was dismissed as cured, no other application having been used.

Mark Twain (1835–1910) commented on the placebo effect in his *Christian Science and the Book of Mrs. Eddy*: "No one doubts—certainly not I—that the mind exercises a powerful influence over the body. From the beginning of time, the sorcerer, the interpreter of dreams, the fortuneteller, the charlatan, the quack, the wild medicine-man, the educated physician, the mesmerist, and the hypnotist, have made use of the client's imagination to help them in their work. They have all recognized the potency and availability of that force. Physicians cure many patients with the bread pill; they know that where the disease is only a fancy, the patient's confidence in the doctor will make the bread pill effective. Faith in the doctor. Perhaps that is the entire thing. It seems to look like it." In *The Wonderful Wizard of Oz*, published by L.F. Baum in 1900, the wizard noted: "It was easy to make the Scarecrow and the Lion and the Woodman happy, because they imagined I could do anything."

Prior to the advent of the scientific method, both physicians and charlatans had a fairly high success rate for a number of reasons. Perhaps one-third of their patients improved by placebo effect, a large percentage improved spontaneously, while those who worsened or died did so only because they had waited too long to seek medical attention (and take the medications offered to them). In the opinion of many, the latter group had indeed deserved punishment and could not have been saved by any human hand since they surely had sinned. After observing the way in which medicine was practiced in the eighteenth century, Benjamin Franklin perhaps properly came to the conclusion that "God heals and the doctor takes the fee."

Physicians have only been regulated and licensed within the last few hundred years. Before that, anyone could and did practice medicine. Caspar Stromayr discussed some of his concerns related to the provision of medical care in the preamble to his manuscript *Practica copiosa* (1559):

I cannot omit but must show you how such vagrants and destroyers of people acquire their masterships, obtain diplomas and seals. Namely, when an unsuccessful bather, barber, cobbler or tailor or whatever tradesman he may be when he does not know what to do, to provide himself in sloth and have a full belly every day and have something left over besides and become rich. If he has perhaps watched a surgeon once, twice, three or even four times, then he dares to move away one, three or four miles away from those who know him to a place where he is not known. Then he injures the inhabitants of the new location. He pretends to be a surgeon whom one would not trust at home with a sow and who could not open a vein.

He dares and does not ask afterward how it turned out. Now someone comes to him with a plea for help with an aqueous rupture. He talks him into believing it to be a rupture. He wishes and knows how to help him but the patient must submit to an operation. Then the patient says 'Dear Master I don't understand it. I came to you for that reason so as to get advice and help from you.'

He cuts into it undaunted. The water runs out. He either shells out or removes the testicle, assuming and saying that he had helped. And after recovery he says to the patient 'I will reduce my fee by one guilder and give it to you as a present. Give me a letter and your seal that I am a good surgeon and that I have helped you well.' The patient is happy, does it gladly. He would rather give him a letter than a guilder.

Now what does the surgeon do with it?

He takes the letter and shows it to everyone, hangs or nails it on all church towers or courthouses, preens himself as one who has cured a large rupture. He knows this skill and is a Master as is the custom among such tramps, and he is known full well that an empty keg gives out a louder sound than a full one. If he knows half as much as he pretends and claims, he would not have to wander around the country as a parasite to defraud people of their money. He could well be found at home and then the simple minded common people would believe and run to him. . . .

Again he cuts for a rupture. The patient recovers to the extent that he does not die. However, what does he do for him? Namely that he has him lie on his back for three or four weeks and does not permit him to get up at all. The patient believes that things are going well and that he has been cured. For as long as he is lying on his back his rupture lies within and does not protrude. . . He forbids him things which are impossible to keep, takes his money and departs. When then the patient gets up and believes himself cured, his rupture comes out as large as before.

A later example of some of the specific techniques employed by quacks and charlatans is here outlined by J. Friend in his book *The History of Physick* (1726):

There are so many little arts used by Mountebanks and

Pretenders to Physick, that an entire treatise, had I a mind to write one, would not contain them: but their impudence and daring boldness is equal to the guilt and inward conviction they have tormenting and putting persons to pain in their last Hours, for no reason at all. Now some of them profess to cure the Falling-Sickness, and thereupon make an issue in the hinder part of the head, in form of a cross, and pretend to take something out of the opening, which they hold all the while in their hands. Others give out, that they can draw snakes or lizards out of their patients' noses, which they seem to perform by putting up a pointed iron probe, with which they wound the nostrils, 'till the blood comes: then they draw out the little artificial animals composed of liver, etc. Some are confident, they can take out the white specks in the eye. Before they apply the instrument to that part, they put a piece of fine rag into the eye, and taking it out with the instrument, pretend it is drawn immediately from the eye. Some again undertake to suck water out of the ear, which they fill with a tube from their mouth, and hold the other end to the ear; and so spurting the water out of their mouths, pretend it came from the ear. Others pretend to get out worms, which grow in the ear, or roots of the teeth. Others can extract frogs from the under-part of the tongue; and by lancing make an incision, into which they clap in the frog, and so take it out. What shall I say of bones inserted into wounds and ulcers, which, after remaining there for some time, they take out again? Some when they have taken out a stone from the bladder, persuade their patients, that still there's another left; they do this for this reason, to have it believed, that they have taken out another. Sometimes they probe the bladder, being altogether ignorant and uncertain, whether there be a stone or no. But if they don't find it, they pretend at least to take out one they have in readiness before, and show that to them. Sometimes they make an incision in the anus for the piles, and by repeating the operation often bring it to a fistula, or an ulcer, when there was neither before. Some say they take phlegm, of a substance like unto glass, out of the penis or other part of the body, by the conveyance of a pipe, which they hold with water in their mouths. Some pretend, that they can contract and collect all the floating humors of the body to one place, by rubbing it with winter-cherries; which causes a burning or inflammation, and then they expect to be rewarded, as if they cured the distemper; and after they have supplied the place with oil, the pain presently goes off. Some make their patients believe that they have swallowed glass:

so, taking a feather, which they force down the throat, they throw them into vomiting, which brings up the fluff they themselves had put in with that very feather. Many things of that nature do they get out, which these imposters with great dexterity have put in; tending many times to the endangering the health of their patients, and often ending in the death of them. Such counterfeits could not pass with discerning men, but they did not dream of any fallacies, and made no doubt of the skill of those who they employed: till at last when they suspect, or rather look more narrowly into their operations, the cheat is discovered. Therefore no wise men ought to trust their lives in their hands, nor take any more of their medicines, which have proved so fatal to many.

The practice of medicine was considered to be a trade in the United States until medical schools appeared in the late eighteenth century, allowing (and forcing) governmental licensing agencies the responsibility of setting standards for the profession. This, however, did not stop those eager to make a profit at the public's expense, and diploma factories sprang up to offer medical degrees from fictitious colleges for only a small fee. The most notorious of these was St. Luke's Hospital in Niles, Michigan, where authentic-looking certificates were distributed "with your name handsomely engrossed in an old round style of letters, with two pieces of dark blue ribbon and a large corporate gold seal affixed thereto." The documents had "the general appearance of a regular Hospital Medical Diploma," and the cost was $5 in "Heavy Royal Linen Paper," $7.50 on "Imitation Parchment," and $10 on "Genuine Sheepskin." No patient had ever stayed at St. Luke's Hospital, and the doors closed in about 1900 following the passage of legislation restricting this type of activity by the Michigan State Government. The main reason that the hospital closed, however, probably was because of a report by the Michigan Board of Health regarding the president and cofounder, Dr. Charles Granville, when "one of his numerous wives found him out and, after being put under $500 bond, he left for parts unknown."

Granville soon turned up on the medical staff of the Christian Hospital in Chicago with a former partner from Michigan, Dr. Arthur Probert. Their modus operandi was the same, though their statement of purpose was very compelling: "For the Care and Cure of the afflicted (of any Creed or Nationality) according to the Ethics of the Golden Rule, using to that Noble end all the combined wisdom afforded by Modern Medical and Surgical Science, with an association of Expert Specialists, representing every school, branch and system of the healing art, all working harmoniously together for the Cure of the Sick, with the Golden

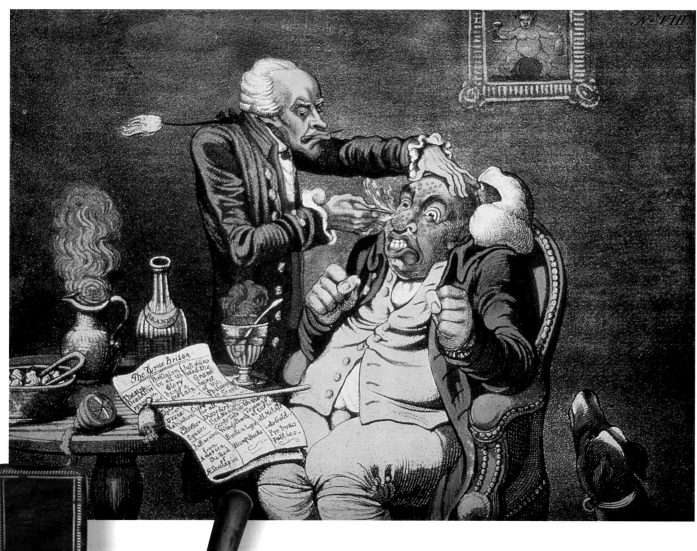

Rule as their code of moral and professional ethics." This ruse did not last long, nor did other diploma mills like the Metropolitan Medical College ("Collegium Medicinae Metropolitanium") in Illinois where the two founders were successfully prosecuted for fraud.

QUACKS BECOME LEGIT—PERKINS TRACTORS

Dr. Elisha Perkins (1741–1799) was a prominent New England physician who trained at Yale and practiced in Norwich, Connecticut, during the latter part of the eighteenth century. He observed a contraction of muscles that had been touched by a metal instrument during surgery, and also noted a relief of pain when a dental probe separated tooth from gum. On February 19, 1796, he patented the first medical quackery device in the United States after creating two metal probes that supposedly "drew out" disease and pain when drawn across the skin on any part of the body. His Perkins Tractors were two rods of brass and iron, though one tractor was supposedly made of copper, zinc, and gold, and the other iron, silver, and platinum (figures 396, 397).

Enthusiastic over the early success of his invention, Perkins took his discovery to Philadelphia, where he was received with great fanfare. According to Dr. Walter Steiner, "Diseases of the most obstinate nature, which had baffled medical art, were removed by the metallic tractors, and many persons of advanced age, who had been crippled for years with chronic rheumatism, were, in several instances, perfectly cured." At Perkins' arrival in Philadelphia, Congress was in session, and many were fascinated with this miracle cure, including George Washington who purchased a set for his family. The chief justice of the United States, the Hon. Oliver Ellsworth, commented in a letter to his successor, John Marshall: "In some cases the effects wrought are not easily ascribable to imagination, great and delusive as is its power."

Perkins had faith in his invention, though was eventually expelled by the same Connecticut medical society that he had helped form, after being called "a patentee and user of nostrums." In May 1796, the following resolution was passed:

> VOTED. It having been represented to the Society, that one of their members had gleaned up from the miserable remains of animal magnetism, a practice of stroking with metallic Instruments, the pained parts of human bodies, giving out that such stroking will radically cure the most obstinate pain to which our frame is incident, causing false reports to be propagated of the effects of such strokings, especially where they have been performed on some public occasions, and on men of distinction; also that an excursion has been made abroad and a patent obtained from under the authority of the United States, to aid such delusive quackery; that under such auspices as membership of this Society announce to the public, that they consider all such practices as barefaced imposition, disgraceful to the faculty, and delusive to the ignorant; and they further direct their Secretary to cite any member of this Society, practicing as above, before them, at their next meeting, to answer for his conduct, and render reasons why he should not be expelled from the Society, for such disgraceful practices.

Unfazed by this and other rebukes, Perkins continued marketing his invention. He traveled to New York in order to cure an epidemic of yellow fever with his tractors, and died there in 1799 from the disease that he had hoped to treat.

Elisha's son, Benjamin, however, persisted and opened the Perkinsean Institute in 1803. As a way of justifying his father's invention

396. Opposite. Perkins Tractors from the Perkins family (ca. 1796)

397. *Metallic Tractors* (1801), aquatint with watercolors on paper by James Gillray

in 1795, Benjamin was quick to point out the findings of Luigi Galvani when he said that "they act on the Galvanic principle." He also noted the experiments of Galvani's nephew, Giovanni Aldini, by inferring that Galvanism could perhaps be instrumental in reviving the dead. Following his London experiments involving the application of electrical currents given to a recently executed criminal, Aldini stated, "On the first application of the arcs the jaw began to quiver, the adjoining muscles were horribly contorted, and the left eye actually opened." Mary Shelly wrote her classic horror story of reanimation by electricity just a few years later in 1818, and the introduction of her second edition of *Frankenstein* included the comment that reanimation of the dead is "not of impossible occurrence." The idea for her novel may have come in part from the work of Aldini.

Benjamin Perkins manufactured these small rods in a home furnace and made a handsome profit by selling them for many times the cost of production. They were also aggressively marketed in England: "The true Briton theatre. Dead alive. Grand exhibition in Leicester Square. Just arrived from America, the rod of Aesculapius. Perkinism in all its glory, truly a certain cure for all disorders, red noses, gouty toes, windy bowels, broken legs, humpbacks. Just discovered, the grand secret of the philosopher's stone, with the true way of turning all metals into gold, pro bono publico."

The following testimonial was published in the *Proceedings* of the Perkinean Institute by the Rev. John Trusler of Bath in 1803:

Last Sunday evening, three eminent physicians of Bath drank tea at my house in company of another gentleman and Mr. Parks, who is here giving lectures on the Ptolemaic System, and showing, as he is pleased to express it, the absurdity of the Copernican. Our conversation was on what he called the *solar fluid*, or, as others term it when combined, *electric matter*—Parks was saying, that it pervaded all substances, even the human body, and was constantly in motion on every necessary occasion to produce an equilibrium in nature. At this instant one of the medical gentlemen complained of a coldness in his forehead, attended with a nausea in his stomach, and asked if any of the company present had a pair of Tractors. I produced mine. One of his medical brethren applied them together in all directions in the other's forehead, and ere five minutes had elapsed, he cried out 'I am well! Feel gentlemen my forehead, it is become quite warm, nay, hot, the nausea also left me.'

We then reasoned on the cause of this cure, and it was supposed and believed, that the Tractors being good conductors of

this solar fluid, had restored, in the part affected, the equilibrium
before lost.

In 1803, Benjamin Perkins left England with a 10,000-pound profit
from his efforts at the institute. He became a successful publisher in
New York, though died soon thereafter in 1810. According to Dr. Oliver
Wendell Holmes, the tractors were forgotten by the next year, though
not the "magical" effects of galvanism.

PHRENOLOGY

The assessment of character and intelligence by the the examination of
physical appearance is comical in one respect, though offensive regarding
both race and gender in another (figure 398). This "science" was taken
seriously in the nineteenth century and was referred to as either phrenology or physiognomy.

Viennese physician Dr. Franz Gall (1758–1828) created the study of
phrenology, which is a description of personality based on facial characteristics. He subdivided the brain into thirty-seven separate "organs,"
and felt that each was responsible for a different character trait. Though
Gall was totally wrong in the pseudosience he developed, he was the
first to consider the possibility that separate areas of the brain could have
different functions. One of his students, Joseph Spurzheim, brought his
teachings to the United States in 1832 where he expanded that theory.
According to Spurtzheim, as we grow in utero, dominant areas grow
faster, and thus result in the development of a variety of facial features
and personality characteristics (figures 399–401). Appearance was thereby a direct predictor of behavior to those practicing phrenology, and this
discipline captured the attention of many in the United States.
Prominent phrenologists viewed their profession as an important science, ironically warning the public against charlatans. A. Boardman
wrote the following in his 1851 edition of *A Defense of Phrenology*: "We
look upon phrenology as among the first human sciences in interest and
importance—as a science which not only furnishes us with the true physiology of the brain, but of a science pregnant with more important influences than the revelations of Galileo."

In 1905, Henry C. Lavery of Superior, Wisconsin, invented his complex psychograph to evaluate personality by determining an individual's
head measurements (figure 402). The psychograph contained 1,954 parts,
and the cost to lease one was $2,000 with an additional $35 a month. In
only five minutes, the operator was able to describe a patient's personality
in thirty-two different categories that included constructiveness, secretive-
ness, caution, friendship, dignity, combativeness, and wit.

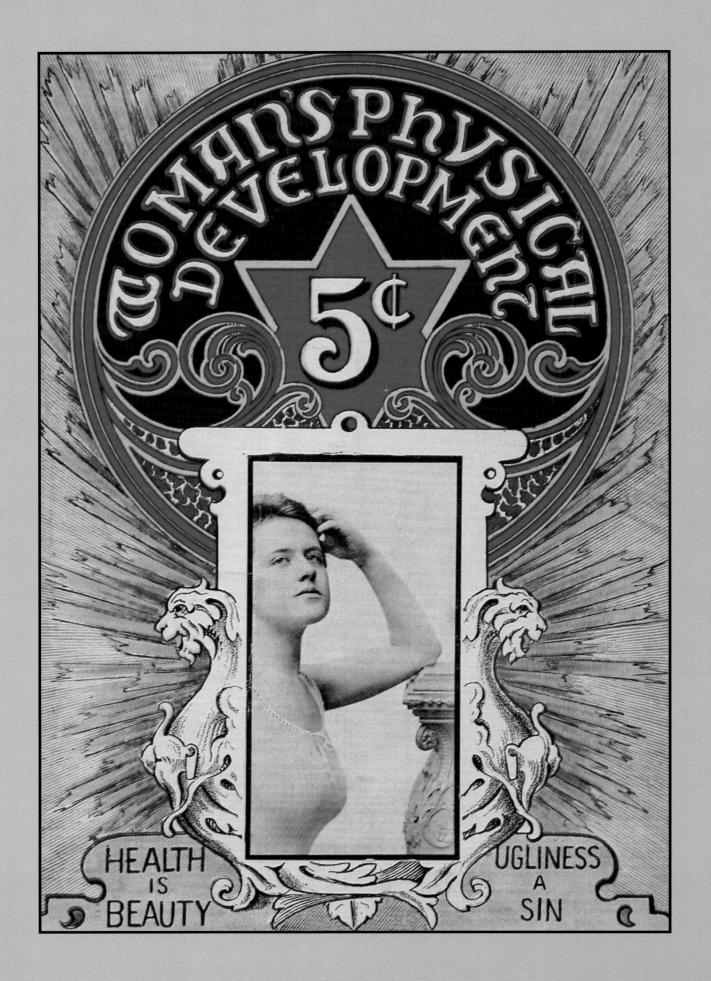

WOMAN'S PHYSICAL DEVELOPMENT

5¢

HEALTH IS BEAUTY

UGLINESS A SIN

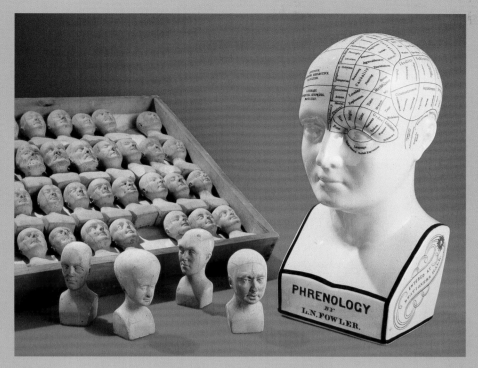

398. Opposite. *Woman's Physical Development* (1901) by the Physical Culture Publishing Co.

399. A case of sixty phrenology heads (1831) by William Bally, Dublin, ceramic phrenology head by Lorenzo Fowler (1860–1896)

400. Below left. *The Phrenological Journal* (October 1867)

401. Below right. "The Melancholy Nose" in *New Physiognomy, or, Signs of Character as Manifested through Temperament and External Forms* (1880) by Samuel R. Wells

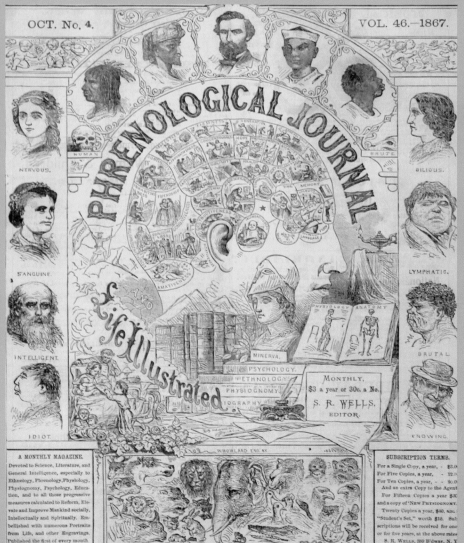

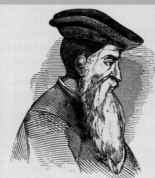

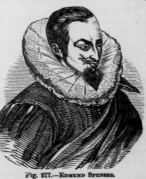

THE MELANCHOLY NOSE, which indicates a tendency to despondency and dark forebodings of the future.

A person with this excessively elongated nasal protuberance is liable to be unnecessarily fearful of dangers (often imaginary), and to make himself miserable by "borrowing troubles," and indulging in "the blues." With such persons the future is allowed to overshadow and darken the present as with a cloud of sorrow. Calvin,

Fig. 276.—STEPHEN GARDINER.

John Knox, Bishop Gardiner, Spenser, and Dante had noses of this character.

The Melancholy nose is often seen in clergymen, who dwell more on fear than on hope in their discourses.

THE INQUISITIVE NOSE.

The horizontal length of the nose from the lip outward (fig. 275, *c d*), indicates the faculty of *Inquisitiveness.* When

Fig. 277.—EDMUND SPENSER.

The same reasoning was true regarding the study of physiognomy, a "science" that related physical traits and body habitus to behavior. For example, a broad-chested individual was more likely to be interested in sensual pleasure, while someone with muscular features would have had a strong character. A well-coordinated person was intelligent; and a short, slight individual was considered impulsive. Comparative physiognomy, or a demonstration of the similarity between animal and human traits, was also popular at the turn of the last century. Physiognomists noted the similarity between owners and their pets as we sometimes do today (figure 403).

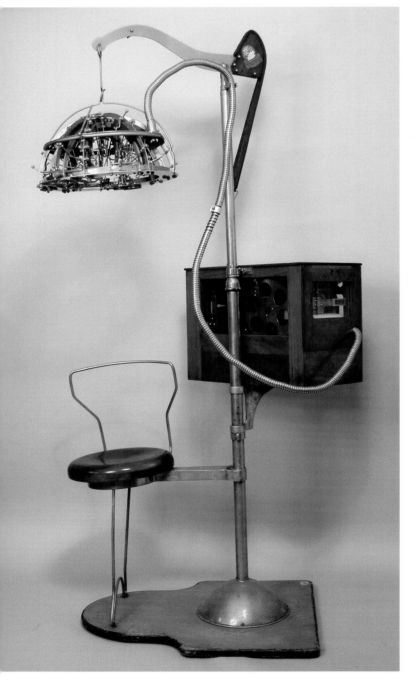

402. Psychograph (ca. 1935) by the Psychograph Co., Minneapolis, Minnesota

In the United States, two brothers, Lorenzo and Orson Squire Fowler, were only too happy to apply the new "science" of phrenology to an eager and credulous population. They were responsible for a large number of readings at the Phrenological Institute in New York City and published many works related to the subject, including the *Phrenological Journal*. The breadth of their publishing interests was indeed wide and included the first edition of Walt Whitman's *Leaves of Grass* and *Life Illustrated*, a new photography magazine. Lorenzo Fowler gained great fame through his readings and moved to London in 1863. It was there that he met up with the famous American writer and humorist Mark Twain, who had developed a healthy distrust for medicine in general and for phrenology in particular after an early exposure while growing up in Hannibal, Missouri. He visited Lorenzo on two occasions, the first under a pseudonym in order to test the validity of this science. In his autobiography, Twain made the following observation:

Fowler received me with indifference, fingered my head in an uninterested way, and named and estimated my qualities in a bored and monotonous voice. He said I possessed amazing courage, and abnormal spirit of daring, a pluck, a stern will, a fearlessness that were without limit, I was astonished at this, and gratified too; I had not suspected it before; but then he foraged over on the other side of my skull and found a hump there which he called 'caution.' This hump was so tall, so mountainous, that it reduced my courage-hump to a mere hillock by comparison, although the courage hump had been so prominent up to that time—according to his description of it—that it ought to have been

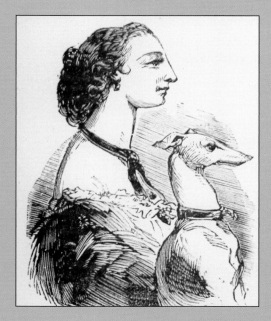
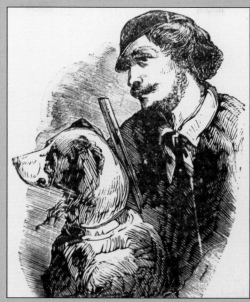
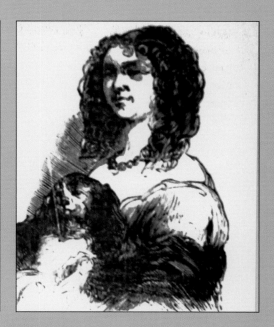
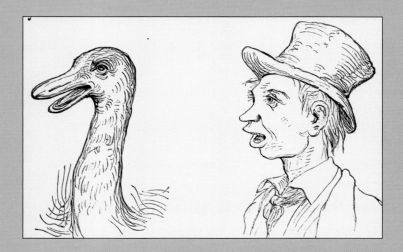
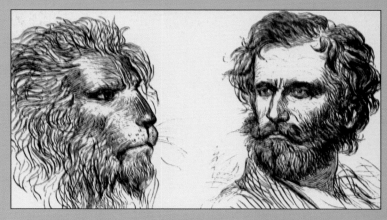
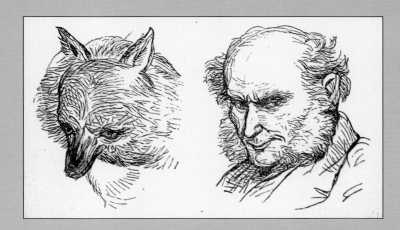
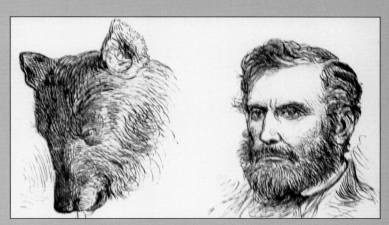

403. Comparative Physiognomy in
*New Physiognomy, or, Signs of Character
as Manifested through Temperament
and External Forms* (1880) by Samuel
R. Wells

a capable thing to hang my hat on; but it amounted to nothing, now in the presence of that Matterhorn which he called my Caution. He explained that if that Matterhorn had been left out of my scheme of character I would have been one of the bravest men that ever lived—possibly the bravest —but that my cautiousness was so prodigiously superior to it that it abolished my courage and made me almost timid. He continued his discoveries, with the result that I came out safe and sound, at the end, with a hundred great and shining qualities; but which lost their value and amounted to nothing because each of the hundred was coupled up with an opposing defect which took the effectiveness all out of it. . . . [He] gave me a chart which I carried home to the Langham Hotel and studied with great interest and amusement—the same interest and amusement which I should have found in the chart of an imposter who had been passing himself off for me and who did not resemble me in a single sharply defined detail. I waited for three months and went to Mr. Fowler again, heralding my arrival with a card bearing both my name and my *nom de guerre*. Again I carried away an elaborate chart. It contained several sharply defined details of my character, but it bore no recognizable resemblance to the earlier chart.

HEALING AND THE ELEMENTS

Before technology provided healers with sophisticated bells and buzzers, most were content to use the elements they had at hand, such as water, light, and temperature. One common goal was to increase circulation, and thus the oxygen supply to various diseased parts of the body. Because they felt that light was the source of life, some Egyptian cults worshipped the sun and the healing ability of light, and many Egyptians wore colored amulets to channel those healing rays. In 1876, Augustus Pleasanton used blue light to stimulate endocrine glands and the nervous system, while Seth Pancoast used red and blue to treat the autonomic nervous system in 1877. In 1910, J.H. Kellogg, MD, wrote in *Light Therapeutics*: "The classic experiments of Finsen, some of which the writer had the opportunity to witness, having twice visited the Light Institute at Copenhagen to see the work of this ingenious investigator and become acquainted with his methods, clearly demonstrated that the actinic rays are a powerful excitant of vital activity, and hence promote to the highest degree all the processes of animal life and energy. . . . To be able to harness this force, to control it, and to focus it upon any desired organ or function of the body, is one of the newest and greatest triumphs of modern therapeutics (figures 404–407).

Col. Dinshah Ghadiali was a "metaphysician" and the president of
the Spectro-Chrome Institute. According to his theories, most diseases
could be treated by shining lights of differing colors and intensity on
the ill and disabled. The foundation of Ghadiali's therapy rested on the
assumption that colors projected on the skin were effective in treating
various diseases, both internal and external, by altering abnormal physiology. Since ninety-seven percent of the body is composed of the four
elements oxygen, hydrogen, nitrogen, and carbon, the human body
was responsive to the four "color wave potencies" of those elements:
blue, red, green, and yellow. Disease resulted when these colors were
unbalanced, and the treatment consisted of creating the correct color
combination. Diseased organs produced a particular abnormal "auric"
energy that could be either stimulated or suppressed by the appropriate
color. The instrument he used allowed colors to be mixed and projected
on the patient, and a six-pointed star was found on his devices that contained all of the primary and secondary color combinations. For the full
effect, patients were to sit in front of the color projector while nude
and facing north during certain phases of the moon. The following is
from Ghadiali's *Spectro-Chrome Therapeutic System*: "From this we learn
that Green light is a pituitary stimulant, a germicide and a muscle tissue
builder. Yellow light is a digestant, and antihelmintic and a nerve
builder. Red is a liver energizer, a caustic and a haemoglobin builder.
Violet is a cardiac depressant; Blue is a vitality builder; Indigo is a
hemostatic; Turquoise, a tonic; Lemon, a bone builder; Orange, an
emetic; Scarlet, a genital excitant; Magenta, a suprarenal stimulant, and
Purple an anti-malarial." Ghadiali justified the use of his invention by
the fact that light had already been employed as a therapeutic agent in
treating neonatal jaundice, and it also was shown to play a significant
physiologic role in the activation of vitamin D.

This notice appeared on the plate of Ghadiali's Spectro-Chrome
Color Machine (figure 408):

> Spectro-Chrome Metry, Measurement and restoration of the
> human radio-active and radio-emanative by attuned color
> waves. The science of automatic precision, no diagnosis—no
> drugs—no manipulation—no surgery, conceived, originated,
> developed, applied & copyrighted 1920 by Colonel Dinshah P.
> Ghadiali, MD, ME, DC, PHD, LLD. Metaphysician and
> Psychologist. . . . Understanding: As the proper use of this
> Spectro-Chrome requires special training and technical knowl-
> edge in the user and also necessitates the production of the
> attuned color waves by means of the genuine, Dinshah attuned
> color wave slides, this apparatus is sold without any liability

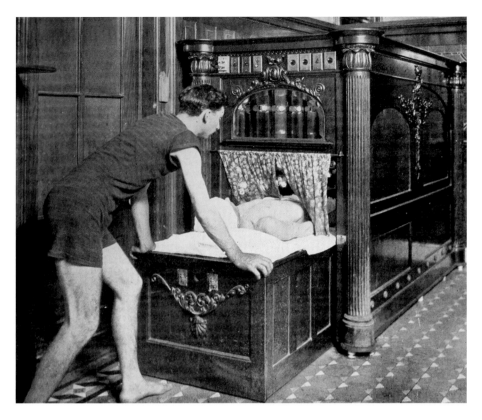

404. The Horizontal Electric-Light Bath from *A System of Instruction in X-Ray Methods and Medical Uses of Light, Hot-Air, Vibration and High-Frequency Currents* (1902) by S.H. Monell, MD

405. Hot-air application to the lower half of the body

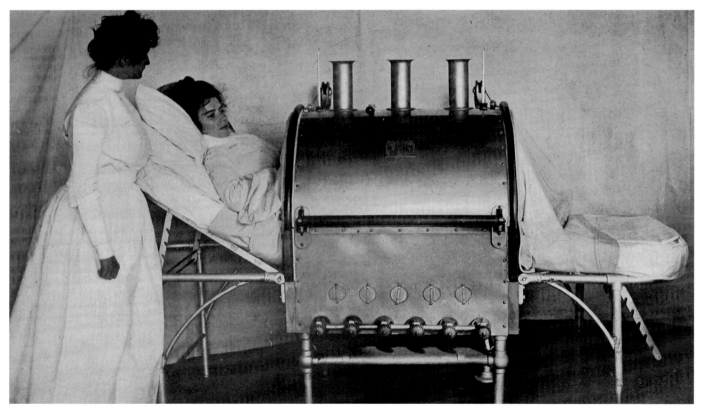

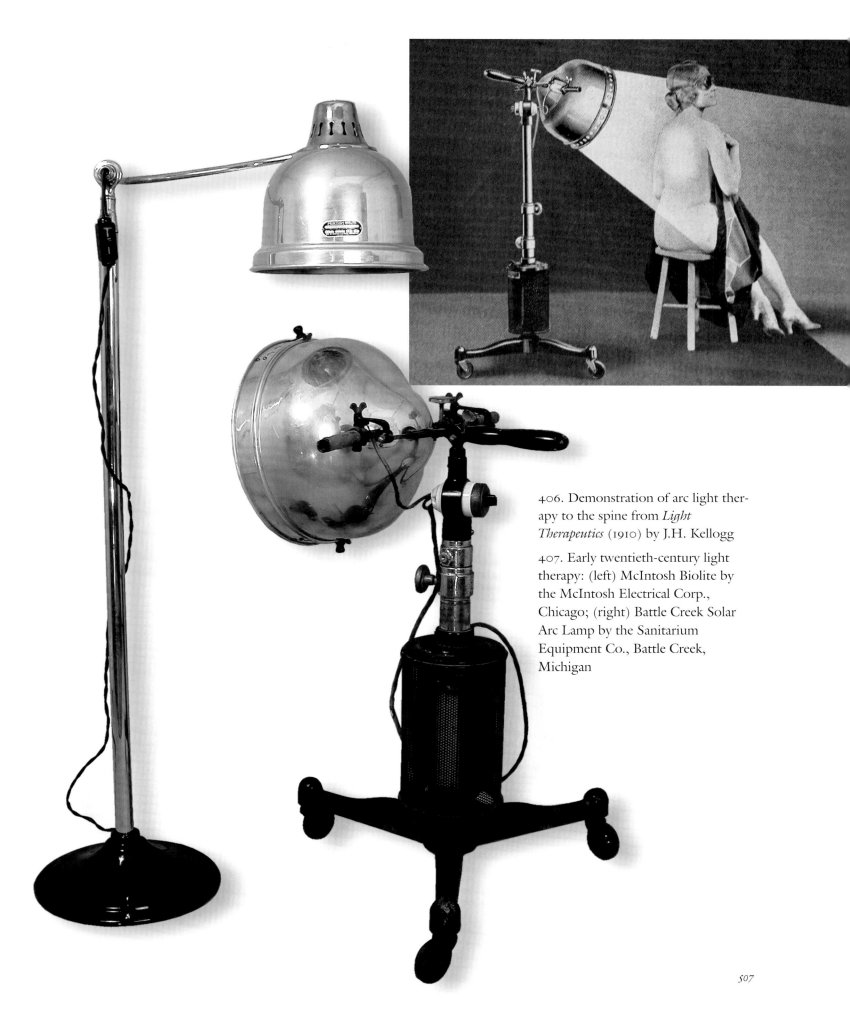

406. Demonstration of arc light therapy to the spine from *Light Therapeutics* (1910) by J.H. Kellogg

407. Early twentieth-century light therapy: (left) McIntosh Biolite by the McIntosh Electrical Corp., Chicago; (right) Battle Creek Solar Arc Lamp by the Sanitarium Equipment Co., Battle Creek, Michigan

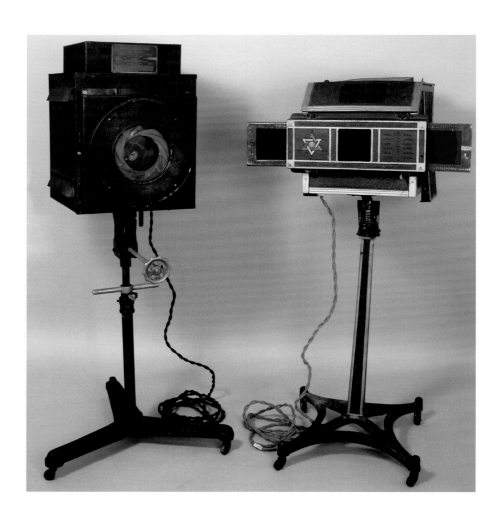

408. Early twentieth century Dinshah Spectro-Chrome Metry devices by the Spectro-Chrome Institute, Malaga, New Jersey

guarantee or warranty, expressed or implied, regarding the results attainable and its purchase or possession does not confer on the purchaser or possessor any title, designation or degree pertaining to the practice of spectro-chrome metry or obligate the spectro-chrome institute in any manner.

Ghadiali's devices were quite popular early in the twentieth century, and their use was supported by testimonials from those in many branches of the medical community. This is the introduction to the *Spectro-Chrome Metry Encyclopaedia* (1939):

KATE W. BALDWIN, Medical Doctor, Fellow American College of Surgeons, Fellow American Academy Of Ophthalmology And Oto-Laryngology, Fellow American Medical Association, Member American Academy Of Political and Social Science, Life Member Maryland Academy Of Sciences, Honorary President Scientific Order Of Spectro-Chrome Metrists, Former Senior Surgeon, Women's Hospital Of Philadelphia, Pennsylvania, United States Of America.

To All Those Who Are Really Interested In The Best For

Securing And Maintaining Sound Body In Which To
Function:—

I talk from personal experience of the System, having used it
for over 12 years in my practice as a Physician and also as a
Surgeon.

Spectro-Chrome is by far the best that has ever been given to
the science of reconstructing and maintaining the Physical Body
in normal condition.

The Best should be the aim of all and we must not be satisfied
until it is found.

As there is nothing better than the best, why multiply words?
Investigate for yourself, with an open mind.

I would close my office today, if I were deprived of Spectro-
Chrome.

KATE W. BALDWIN

According to records of the American Medical Association, Col.
Dinshah Ghadiali was never licensed to practice medicine in the United
States, despite having held a number of titles, including "Doctor of
Chiropractic, Philosophy, and Legal Law." He was also a member of the
following prestigious organizations: Fellow and Ex-Vice-President of the
Allied Medical Association of America, President of the All Cults
Medical Association, President of the American Association of Spectro-
Chrome Therapists, President of the American Anti-Vivisection Society,
Member of the American Association of Orificial Surgeons, Member
and Ex-Vice-President of the National Association of Drugless
Practitioners, and Member Anti-Vaccination League of London.

As one might expect, Ghadiali sooner or later ran afoul of the law.
His legal troubles began in 1925 after a pistol fight in Portland, Oregon,
and he was sentenced to five years in federal prison for violation of the
Mann Act after transporting a nineteen year old across state lines for
immoral purposes. The president commuted the doctor's sentence after
several years in prison because of his behavior during a riot, though
Ghadiali returned to the Spectro-Chrome business and, in all, sold
about 10,000 devices. With the establishment of skeptical regulatory
agencies, Ghadiali came under more rigid scrutiny, and an avalanche of
indictments and court battles followed. During one trial, he called sixty-
five witnesses, though the case did not go well after one of his patients
suffered a seizure while on the witness stand requiring the attention of
several doctors in the audience just after having claimed to be cured of
epilepsy. Ghadiali was found guilty of twelve criminal counts in 1947,
fined $24,000, given five years probation, and was subsequently
required to burn his entire collection of personal printed material. He

restructured his institute for educational rather than therapeutic purposes, and, in 1959, a permanent injunction was issued against Ghadiali and his Spectro-Chrome. He died in 1966.

WATER THERAPY

Water therapy is one of the most ancient forms of treatment, and was popular in ancient Egyptian cultures probably because water was so readily available, and was capable of producing so many easily recognizable physiological effects. The word *spa* is an abbreviation of the Latin "salus per aquam," or "health through water," and hydrotherapy continued to be useful in Italy where the afflicted could receive treatment at various temperatures in the famous Roman baths. Soldiers found relief from their injuries through water therapy in bathhouses at their garrisons, while the public also attended similar structures in order to bathe, exercise, and socialize. The interiors of early spas were made of the finest marble and mosaic, while larger houses included gardens, a library, or a theater where various forms of entertainment were presented. Slaves tended furnaces in the basement from which heat flowed through a system of ducts, the heat so intense at times that the Romans had to wear sandals and walk on raised floors. A typical day at the bathhouse might begin with an exercise program of weightlifting or wrestling at the palaestra followed by a visit to the caladarium, or steam room, and then on to the frigidarium for cold-water therapy. The visit might then end with a perfumed oil massage, a discussion with friends, and then attendance at a play.

The influence of the Roman Empire spread to England where natural hot springs in the city of Bath provided a perfect location for the creation of a temple and a series of spas to honor the goddess Sulis Minerva. The mineral water there contained magnesium, sulfur, and calcium, and was considered so curative that the King's Bath was built on the ruins of the temple later in the eleventh century well after Roman control had ended. The popularity of the natural springs continued to grow, and Bath was visited by Queen Elizabeth I in 1574, to be followed later by Charles II, James II, and Queen Anne.

In 1747, John Wesley, MA, founder of the Methodist Church, wrote *Primitive Physic* in which he included a number of medical applications for the use of hydrotherapy:

> *For ague or intermittent fever*: "go into the cold bath just before the cold fit" or "drink a quart of cold water just before the cold fit, and then go to bed and sweat."
> *For asthma*: "take a pint of cold water every morning, washing the head therein immediately after . . . vomit with a quart or more of warm water. The more you drink of it the better."

To prevent swelling from a bruise: "immediately apply a cloth five
or six times doubled, dipped in cold water, and new dip when it
grows warm."
For hysteric colic: "Using the cold bath two and twenty times a
month has entirely cured hysteric colic fits and convulsive
motions."
For chronic headache: "keep your feet in warm water a quarter of
an hour before you go to bed, for two or three weeks."
For mania: "apply to the head, cloths dipped in cold water, or
pour cold water on the head out of a teakettle, or let the patient
eat nothing but apples for a month."

The use of hydrotherapy began to gain widespread popularity in
Western medicine as a result of the observations of a ship's surgeon, Dr.
William Wright. When many members of his crew fell ill, he moved
them from the overheated lower compartments of the ship to the deck.
There they were cooled with water and recovered faster than those who
had remained below. During an August 1, 1777 trip to Liverpool, the
doctor himself fell ill and did not improve with the usual opiates and
"gentle vomits." Dr. Wright ordered that three buckets of cold water be
thrown on him, and "I felt immediate relief. The headache and other
pains instantly abated and a fine glow and diaphoresis succeeded.
Towards evening, the febrile symptoms threatened a return and I had
again recourse to the same method as before with the same good result."

These findings were published in the *London Medical Journal*,
though the water cure only became popular after it appeared in the 1797
book by James Currie, MD, *Medical Reports on the Effects of Water, Cold
and Warm, as a Remedy in Fever and Other Diseases*. Signer of the
Declaration of Independence and prominent eighteenth-century
American physician Benjamin Rush recommended the use of cold water
therapy to "wash off impurities from the skin, promote perspiration,
drive the fluids from the surface to the internal parts of the body, brace
the animal fibers, stimulate the nervous system, and prevent the 'diseases
of warm weather.'" He also suggested that cold water be used for the
treatment of such diverse conditions as epilepsy, tetanus, whooping
cough, cardiac dysrhythmias, and psychosis.

Nineteenth-century Austrian farmer Vincenz Priessnitz (1799–1851)
further focused international interest on hydrotherapy after a "miraculous" self-cure of fractured ribs by the use of wet bandages and large
water intake. Word spread until soon he was treating all in his home-
town of Graefenberg for almost every medical condition. In time, thousands of patients from all over the world in every social stratum made
the trip to Austria for therapy. Priessnitz's "Graefenberg Cure" included
specialized douches, sitz baths, water streams, and cold plunges to cure

such diverse conditions as smallpox, syphilis, hernias, and tumors. America's first woman physician, Elizabeth Blackwell, visited the Graefenberg Clinic for therapy, though the treatment was unsuccessful, and she eventually lost vision in one eye.

Early Native Americans in the New World also enjoyed the presumed healing benefits of hydrotherapy. The earliest known water treatments were used by the Mohawk Indians at the Saratoga hot springs in New York, and spas became commercially available there as early as 1790. Soon after, another leading health resort achieved success in Hot Springs, Arkansas, because of the warm water that flowed underground. Spanish explorer Hernando de Soto had, in fact, visited there three centuries earlier in 1541 while looking for El Dorado, the City of Gold, and initially hoped that he had found the mythical "fountain of youth." The significance of Arkansas' natural resources were later recognized by the US government in 1832 when the town of Hot Springs was established as the nation's first federal reservation. (The term *reservation* initially meant "land which was set aside—or reserved—for later use," though as the country moved westward, it referred to territory given to Native Americans.) The healing waters in Hot Springs, Arkansas, became commercialized in 1854 when John and Sarah Hale constructed the first bathhouse there. This is one of their early advertisements:

> Here nature calls from fortune's frown, for children of disease,
>   And bids them throw their crutches down, and go where e'er
> they please.
>   Let each come here, for here alone exists the power to save,
>   Here tottering forms but skin and bone are rescued from the
> grave.

Those suffering from any number of complaints, including rheumatism and muscular weakness or pain, traveled to Arkansas to discover the miraculous healing powers of the hot springs, and included veterans from the Civil War through World War II.

In 1902, Dr. John Kellogg outlined physiological bases for the medical uses of water in his *Rational Hydrotherapy*:

> There is no more powerful means of exciting increased activity of the heart than hydriatic applications. Short, very hot fomentations over the heart, the application of large, very hot or very cold compresses over the entire chest and trunk or to other large areas, hot and cold applications to the spine, hot water drinking, and the hot enema are all efficient means of stimulating a flagging heart to increased action. . . . Cold water is a physiologic tonic, and has the advantage over medicinal tonics of all sorts, in

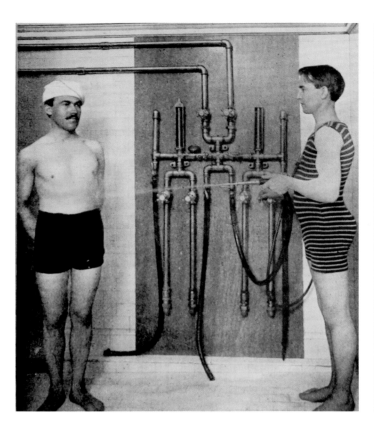

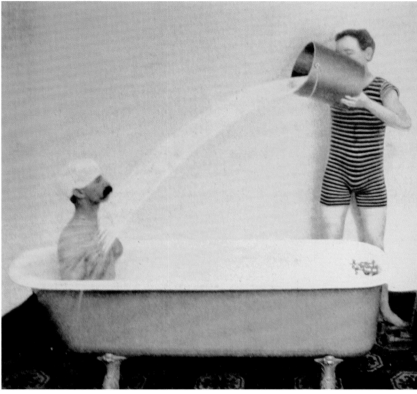

that it awakens nervous activity without the imposition of any
extra burden upon any vital organ, and without hampering the
activity of any function. The cold bath employed in such a manner as to produce tonic effects accomplishes its results by increasing vital resistance to the causes of pathological processes, by
making the wheels of life run more smoothly, by lifting the
whole vital economy to a higher level (figures 409, 410).

409. Splenic douche from *Rational
Hydrotherapy* (1902) by J.H. Kellogg

410. "Affusion" as a form of
hydrotherapy from *Rational
Hydrotherapy* (1902) by J.H. Kellogg

VIBRATION AND MESSAGE THERAPY

Massage therapy is an ancient practice that has remained popular theoretically by improving circulation and increasing oxygen to diseased tissues.
According to more modern proponents of vibration, treatment at the right
location and frequency could also be therapeutic in other ways. Maurice
Pilgram, MD, in *Mechanical Vibratory Stimulation* (1911), wrote, "The general theory upon which this treatment is based is that all the functions and
organs of the body are controlled by certain nerves or nerve centers, located principally in the spinal cord, and that in the course of disease, if these
centers are reached and treated, restoration to normal action may be
expected in most cases to take place." He further added:

Treatment by mechanical-vibratory stimulation has been found
by practical experiment to be capable of:

1) Increasing the volume of the blood and lymph flow to a given area or organ;

(2) Increasing nutrition;

(3) Improving the respiratory process and functions;

(4) Stimulating secretion;

(5) Improving muscular and general metabolism, and increasing the production of animal heat;

(6) Stimulating the excretory organs and assisting the functions of elimination;

(7) Softening and relieving muscular contractures;

(8) Relieving engorgement and congestion;

(9) Facilitating the removal through the natural channels of the lymphatics, of tumors, exudates, and other products of inflammation; relieving varicosities, and dissipating eruptions.

(10) Inhibiting and relieving pain.

Small hand-operated home devices were fashionable in the early twentieth century (figures 411–413), and they were touted to cure almost any disease. One of the more popular was the Macaura Pulsocon, invented by the "vibrotherapist" Gerald Macaura, who established his therapeutic institute in Manchester, England, in 1908. Renal failure was one of the diseases purportedly (and preposterously) cured by the Pulsocon:

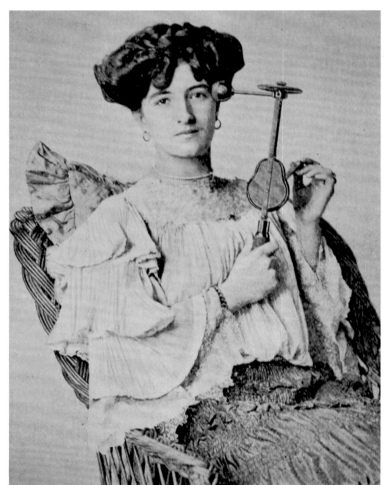

411. Demonstration of the VeeDee (ca. 1910) used for headaches

This disease may be either functional or organic. Functional derangements of the kidneys respond very readily to Mechanical Stimulation. Organic disease (Bright's Disease) is, however, more difficult to deal with, and was formerly considered incurable. Bright's Disease of the kidneys is principally characterized by swelling, watery deposits in the lower extremities, and puffiness underneath the eyes. Such patients must be treated gently along the spine and over the groin and kidneys. Deeper treatment may be applied to the backs of the legs, and also the abdomen. Dr. J.W. Williams states that 'Vibration is really a splendid treatment for the kidneys. It arouses them into action, and enables them to draw off the watery deposits from the system.' What we say is: 'It is the most efficacious treatment known for the kidneys.'

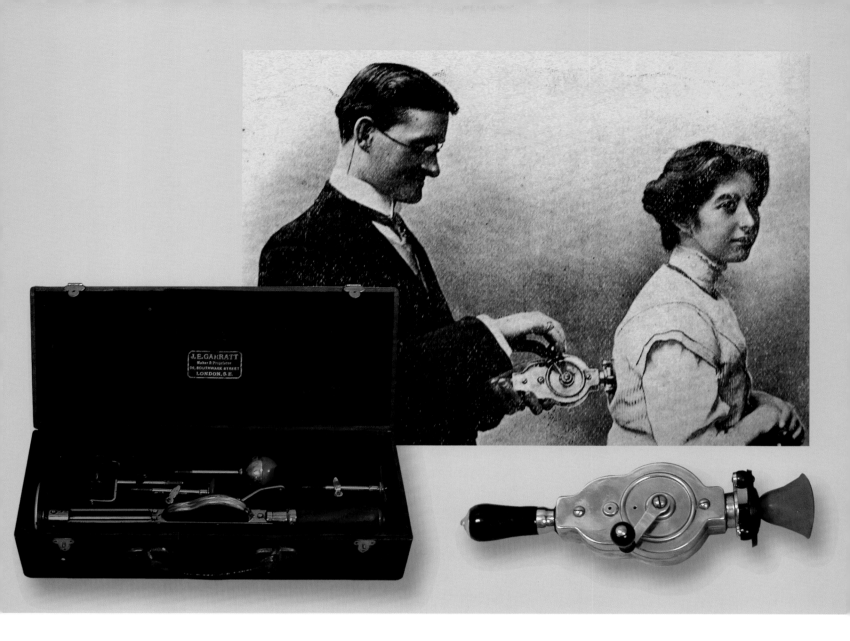

Members of the Macaura Institute issued this warning regarding the treatment of deafness:

From the number of advertisements and its cure by electrical appliances, patent medicines, etc., together with the misleading statements of people who claim to cure what they know absolutely nothing about, it seems difficult for the ordinary individual to distinguish between the genuine and the bogus article. . . . It is a well known fact, even by those who suffer from chronic Catarrhal Deafness, that the little chain of bones in the inner ear are more or less bound together (ankylosed) by a catarrhal deposit. What could be more reasonable than to expect Mechanical Pulsation to loosen up these little bones? This is what actually happens when the Pulsocon is applied. It produced elasticity in this apparatus of the inner ear. It tones up and strengthens the drum of the external ear also. And now, when I claim that this is a rational common-sense method of treating Deafness, I'm sure you will agree with me. Of course it goes without saying that if there is any nerve-deficiency existing, the Pulsocon treatment is the only pos-

412. Vibration of the "internal organs" with the Macaura's Pulsocon (ca. 1920)

413. Early twentieth-century hand-held vibrators: (left) VeeDee by J.E. Garratt, London; (right) Macaura's Pulsocon by the British Appliances and Manufacturing Co., Glasgow

sible remedy, because it is the one thing which arouses dormant nerves and muscles into action.

As is the case in quack medicine, the argument is reasonable and compelling, though the device is absolutely worthless in providing the advertised cure. Macuara was convicted of swindling in Paris and given a sentence of three years.

Exercising increases strength, so certainly the logical treatment for "weak eyes" would be to exercise those muscles. Physicians jumped to that conclusion, coming up with a variety of eyeball massagers since their production and sale was perfectly legal without a requirement for the guarantee of safety or efficacy (figures 414, 415).

From the time of Hippocrates, the term *hysteria* ("womb disease") has been considered a female disorder. The symptoms were many, including anxiety, insomnia, swooning (or perhaps petit mal seizures), and almost any abdominal discomfort. Aretaeus of Cappadocia was a second-century Greek physician who believed that an inflamed uterus was the culprit, and Pieter van Foreest wrote in *Observationem et Curationem Medicinalium ac Chirurgicariom Opera Omnia* (1653): "When these symptoms indicate, we think it necessary to ask a midwife to assist, so that she can massage the genitalia with one finger inside, using oil of lilies, musk root, crocus, or similar. And in this way the afflicted woman can be aroused to the paroxysm. This kind of stimulation with the finger is recommended by Galen and Avicenna, among others, most especially for widows, those who live chaste lives, and female religious, as Gradus proposes; it is less often recommended for very young women, public women, or married women, for whom it is a better remedy to engage in intercourse with their spouses." In the early twentieth century, vaginal stimulation with vibratory devices for the treatment of female hysteria was a common and lucrative part of many physicians' office practices, and small electric vibrators were frequently found in homes throughout America for personal use (figures 416, 417).

Larger pieces of vibrating equipment, including beds and chairs, could be found in hospitals and sanitariums for the treatment of a variety of systemic disorders, as well as for an improvement in cell nutrition, body secretion, elimination, peristalsis, blood and lymph flow, and general metabolism to name just a few of the purported benefits (figures 418–422).

MESMER AND HIS MAGNETS

The magnetic property of bits of amber, which are the fossilized resin of the pine trees, has been a source of wonder to many throughout the ages. In the sixteenth century, alchemist Paracelsus also observed that

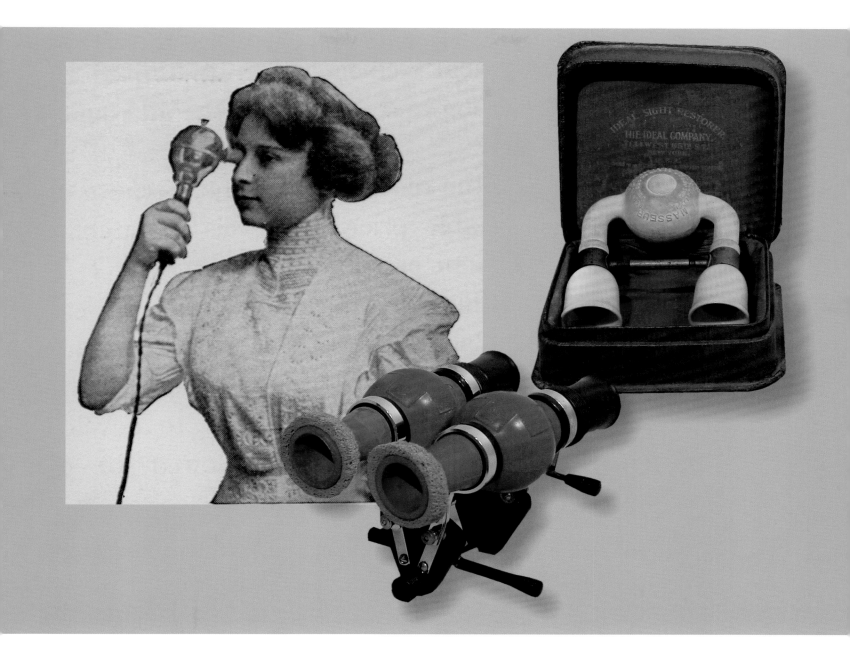

414. Early twentieth-century eyeball massagers: (left to right) the Ideal Company and the Neu Vita massager

415. Vibratory treatment of the eye

lodestones containing magnetite were attracted to iron. It did not take long for some physicians to recognize this phenomenon as an opportunity to incorporate mysterious forces in the care of their patients. According to early proponents, magnetic therapy applied to diseased tissues promoted health by attracting iron in the blood, and thus improved circulation. Additionally, magnets dilated blood vessels and "aligned" all elements of the body to promote a better relationship with the earth's magnetic field. The first to bring international attention to the possibility that imbalanced magnetic life forces (termed "animal magnetism") could be an important cause of disease processes was the German physician Franz Anton Mesmer (1734–1815).

The charismatic Mesmer was a firm believer in astrology and main-

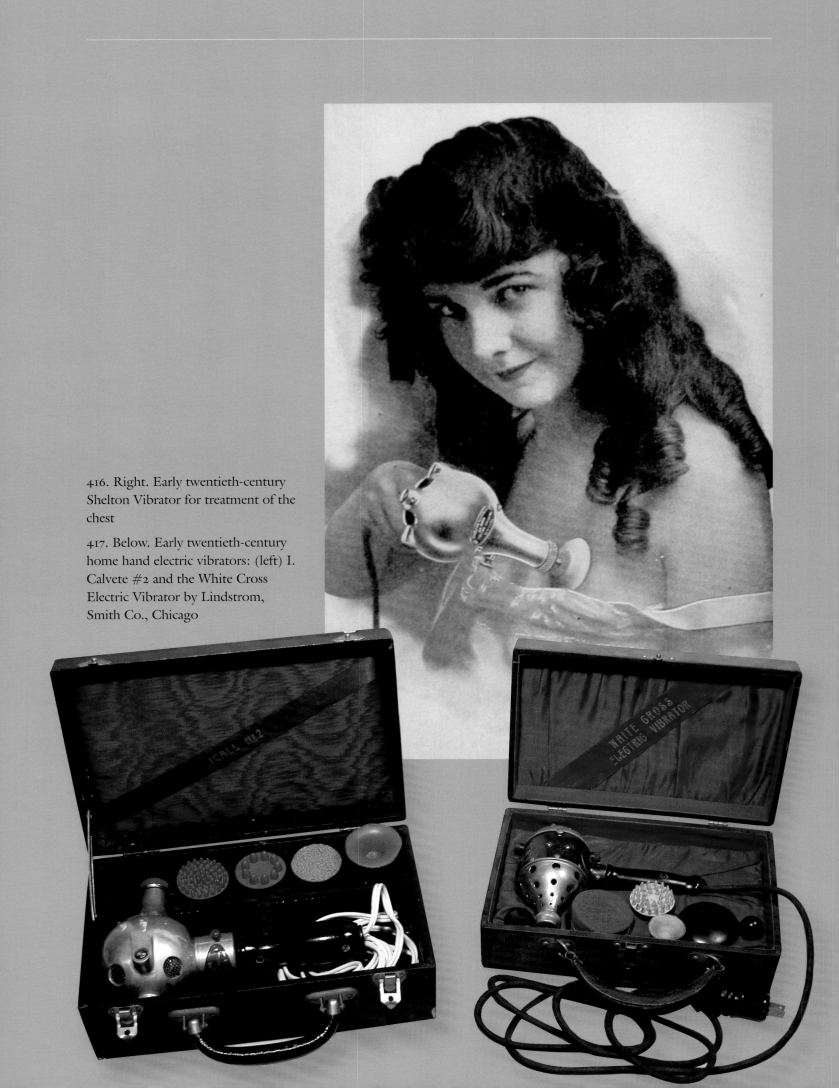

416. Right. Early twentieth-century Shelton Vibrator for treatment of the chest

417. Below. Early twentieth-century home hand electric vibrators: (left) I. Calvete #2 and the White Cross Electric Vibrator by Lindstrom, Smith Co., Chicago

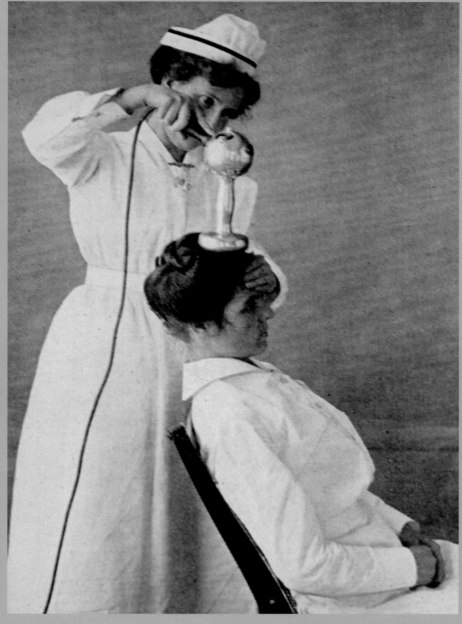

418, 419. Vibratory treatment for the head and stomach from *The Value of Vibrotherapy as a Therapeutic Measure* (1913) by J.H. Kellogg

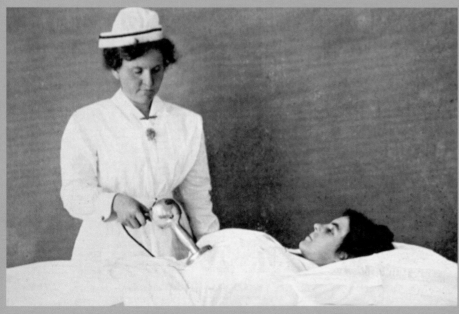

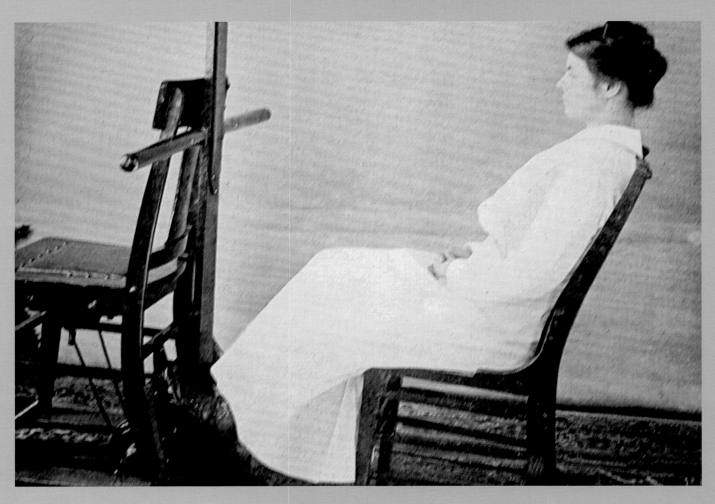

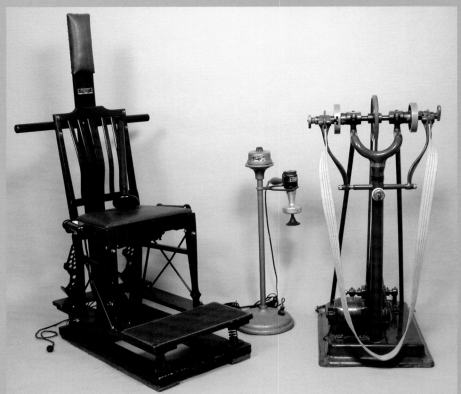

420. Using the foot attachment of the Vibratory Chair from *The Value of Vibrotherapy as a Therapeutic Measure* (1913) by J.H. Kellogg

421. Early twentieth-century "Professional" vibratory devices: Battle Creek Vibratory Chair by the Sanitarium and Hospital Equipment Co., Massage Vibrator by the Battle Creek Equipment Co., and the Battle Creek Health Builder Oscillo-Manipulator by the Sanitarium and Hospital Equipment Co.

tained that health could only be achieved by the flow of animal magnetism in channels throughout the body. By applying magnets over diseased tissues, the free flow of animal magnetism could be re-established, and health could be restored. Though Mesmer's methods varied, he was famous for playing a glass harmonica during many of his "magnetic séances." The following encounter was related by one of Mesmer's neighbors, Heinrich Schreiber: ". . . Mesmer sat directly opposite me, knee to knee, his flashing and deeply penetrating gaze fixed incessantly on me, stroking downwards, fairly near me, with both hands, or only with the right hand or the thumb thereof. He also pressed both thumbs together directly on the pit of the stomach. Gradually sweat appeared on my chest and back. I felt a burning in the pit of the stomach, then an inclination to vomit. There followed strong coughing with plentiful expectoration, and an extraordinarily powerful, and quite involuntary respiration. . ." (figure 423).

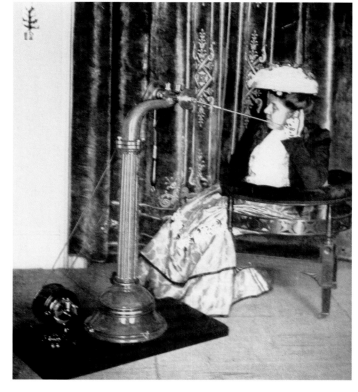

422. Vibration for ear disease by a tissue oscillator (ca. 1920)

Charles Mackay was a British attorney who described one of Mesmer's more famous techniques of using a large wooden tub, or magnetic baquet:

> In the centre of the saloon was placed an oval vessel, about four feet in its longest diameter, and one foot deep. In this were laid a number of wine bottles, filled with magnetized water, well-corked-up, and disposed in radii, with their necks outwards. Water was then poured onto the vessel so as just to cover the bottles, and filings of iron were thrown in occasionally to heighten the magnetic effect. The vessel was then covered with an iron cover, pierced through with many holes, and was called the baquet. From each hole issued a long movable rod of iron, which the patients were to apply to such parts of their bodies as were afflicted. Around this baquet the patients were directed to sit, holding each other by the hand, and pressing their knees together as closely as possible, to facilitate the passage of the magnetic fluid from one to the other.
>
> Then came the assistant magnetizers, generally strong, handsome young men, to pour into the patient from their fingertips fresh streams of the wonderous fluid. They embraced the patients between the knees, rubbed them gently down the spine

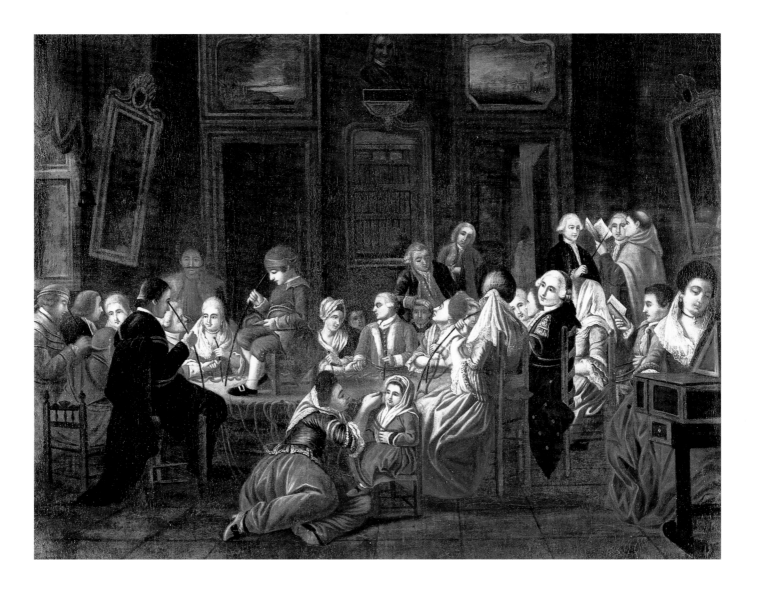

423. A group of mesmerized French patients (1778–1784), oil on canvas by an unknown artist

and the course of the nerves, using gentle pressure upon the breasts of the ladies, and staring them out of countenance to magnetise them by the eye. All this time the most rigorous silence was maintained, with the exception of a few wild notes on the harmonica or the piano-forte, or the melodious voice of a hidden opera-singer swelling softy at long intervals. Gradually the cheeks of the ladies began to glow, their imaginations to become inflamed; and off they went, one after another, in convulsive fits. Some of them sobbed and tore their hair, other laughed till the tears ran from their eyes, while others shrieked and screamed and yelled till they became insensible altogether.

This was the crisis of their delirium. In the midst of it, the chief actor (Dr. Mesmer) made his appearance, waving his wand, like Prospero, to work new wonders. Dressed in a long robe of lilac-colored silk richly embroidered with gold flowers, bearing in his hand a white magnetic rod, and with a look of dignity which would have sat well on an eastern caliph, he marched with solemn strides into the room. He awed the still-sensible by his eye, and the violence of their symptoms diminished. He stroked the insensible with his hands upon the eyebrows and down the spine; traced fingers upon their breast and abdomen with his long white wand, and they were restored to consciousness. They became calm, acknowledged his power, and said they felt streams of colour or burning vapour passing through their frames, according as he waved his wand or his fingers before them.

Following his graduation from the University of Vienna, Mesmer soon became a patron of the arts, and it was in Vienna that he met the young Wolfgang Amadeus Mozart. Mesmer invited the twelve-year-old prodigy to present his first opera, *Bastien und Bastienne*, on his splendid estate, and Mozart later reciprocated by representing his benefactor in the first act of *Cosi Fan Tutti*. In that comic opera, Despina disguised herself as a physician and passed a magnet over Ferrando and Guglielmo, who had feigned their death, while singing, "This is the magnet, the Mesmeric stone that originated in Germany and became so famous in France."

In 1778, Dr. Mesmer unsuccessfully attempted to restore eyesight to eighteen-year-old pianist Maria Paradis, and the scandal that followed resulted in his departure for Paris where he achieved great fame. Mesmer became the physician to Marie Antoinette and attended Lafayette, though his popularity was noted by King Louis XVI, who appointed a four-member committee from the Paris Medical Society to investigate Mesmer's discovery of animal magnetism. At their request, five others were added from the Royal Academy of Sciences. Included in that group were Antoine Lavoisier, the father of modern chemistry, the American ambassador to France, Benjamin Franklin, and Dr. Joseph Guillotin, whose name tragically became all to familiar to both Lavoisier and the king himself at a later date. The commissioners concluded that Mesmer was a charlatan who had made no contribution to either the scientific or medical communities and whose only attribute was an impressive power of suggestion. Mesmer left Paris shortly after the revolution and ultimately spent the rest of his life quietly practicing medicine in Switzerland where he died at the age of eighty-one.

Though Dr. Franz Mesmer is recognized as an early pioneer of hypnosis, credit for that discovery went to James Braid, who refined the technique in 1842 and popularized the term *hypnosis* (from the Greek word for sleep, *hypnos*). Mesmer's legacy in the English language remains the term *mesmerize*, which means "to cast a spell."

ELECTRICITY

From the time of the ancients, electricity was always an astonishing and almost miraculous phenomenon. Any number of superstitions and myths attended the natural occurrence of lightening, and early Vikings believed that this marvel originated from a magic hammer thrown to earth by Thor, the god of thunder. In the latter part of the eighteenth century, Benjamin Franklin established the relationship between lightening and electricity with his famous kite experiment, and Liugi Galvani discovered the electrical basis for muscular activity in his experiments on frogs' legs. Christian A. Kratzenstein (1723–1795) received credit for the first therapeutic use of electricity when he replaced "bad" with "good" electricity in the treatment of rheumatism and the plague. In 1745, a statue of the goddess of health, Hygeia, could be viewed outside of John Graham's "temple of health" for free, though the cost was 250 pounds to go inside for the cure of sterility by sleeping on a bed connected to electric coils. Several universities in the United States offered courses on electrotherapy and conferred graduate degrees in this new specialty (figure 424).

Electricity could be produced in a number of ways, and entrepreneurs were eager to capitalize on a growing and unregulated industry. Faradic, galvanic, wet and dry cell batteries, and static electricity produced direct current for home devices before indirect current was available to power larger machines in doctors' offices. One of the more popular devices was the Boyd's galvanic battery in which electricity was purportedly produced by the "amalgamation" of several different metals (figures 425, 426). When hung around the neck, this device cured by "electrifying the entire system." In his 1879 handbook, Boyd was not restrained in guaranteeing the efficacy of his Miniature Battery, claiming that it cured almost any condition, including "Rheumatism, Gout, Swollen Joints, Neuralgia, Dyspepsia, Lumbago, Aches and Pains, Pain in the Bones, Sciatica, Scrofula, Ulcers and Sores, Tumors, Boils, Carbuncles, Chills, Vertigo, Nervous and General Debility, Loss of Manhood, Impotency, Seminal Weakness, Female Complaints, Barrenness, Liver Complaints, Fever, Kidney Disease, Diabetes, Jaundice, Pleurisy, Diphtheria, Cerebro-Spinal Meningitis, Constipation, Hysteria or Fits, Heartburn, Weak Stomach, Flatulence, Piles, Deafness, Disease of he Heart, Dropsy, Gravel, Spinal Diseases, Paralysis, Weak Back, and Wasting." Testimonials were (and are) a popular way of promoting a product. That was cer-

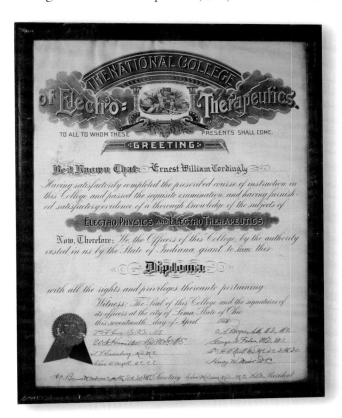

424. Diploma from the National College of Electro-Therapeutics (1928)

tainly true in the case of the Boyd's Battery. The following is an example:

Trafalgar, Ind., Jan. 25, 1880

Mr. J.C. Boyd, Esq.:

I have tried your batteries, and to my satisfaction and surprise I am compelled to give them the greatest of praise. I have been troubled with the itching piles, and it is doing me much good. I think in a few weeks more I will be entirely cured. My wife has also worn one, and it has done her more good than all the doctors in the land could do. She was troubled with many female complaints, cold feet, etc.; it has warmed up her feet so that she can sleep with her feet out from under the cover part of the time now. My little boy is wearing one for rheumatism. It has set him up so that he is able now to go to school. An old lady friend of ours is wearing one since we have for heart trouble, a fluttering around the heart, and it entirely cured her. So, great praise to the battery.

Now I will send for six more, as there are others here wanting them.

Yours truly, J.M. Cook

Consumers were offered many ways in which to utilize the new marvel of electricity at home. In 1854, Davis and Kidder patented a magneto-electric machine that became one of the earliest and most popular home electric devices of the nineteenth century (figures 427, 428). It generated an electric current from spinning magnets, which sent a small shock to surprised and delighted patients suffering from any number of nervous disorders.

Another option was the electric belt, which contained a copper disc in the front with two to four chrome-plated nickel discs at the rear. The "copper-nickel interaction" supposedly created a healing electromagnetic field to treat almost any disease by magnetizing iron in the blood, thus improving oxygenation to all tissues (figures 429-433). A belt was available for each sex, the male belt containing an attachment for improved potency. According to the *Perfect Organ Developer,* "It is impossible for a woman to love a man who is sexually weak. To enjoy life and be loved by women you must be a man. A man who is sexually weak is unfit to marry. Weak men hate themselves. Upon the strength of the sexual organ depends sexual strength, in both men and women, furnishing the ambition and energy for all the advancement in life. It is a well established scientific fact that the musicians, financiers and pugilists are men of exceptionally strong sexual power. Well developed sexual organs manifest themselves in the clear ringing voice, the glossy hair, the sparkling eye, the personal magnetism and force of character."

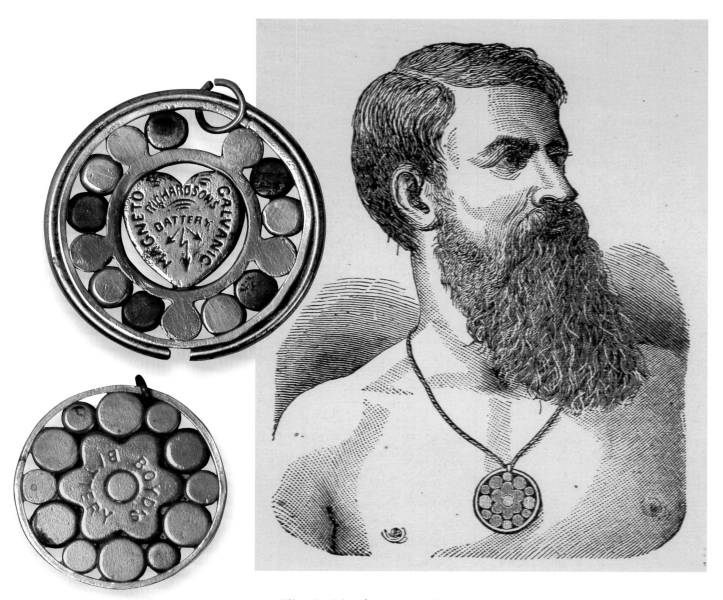

425. Above right. *Boyd's Battery* (1879)

426. Late nineteenth-century "magnetic" pendants by Richardson and Boyd

427. Opposite above. Magneto-Electric machine by Green (ca. 1880)

428. Opposite below. Magneto-Electric machines (ca. 1880): left unmarked, right by Joseph Gray and Son, Sheffield

Elias Smith of Normal, Illinois, was the first to produce electromagnetic body coils in 1869. The most commercially successful body coil, however, was the I-ON-A-CO (I Own A Company) body coil, an eighteen-inch insulated coil of wire connected to house current and worn around the neck or waist (figures 434, 435). It was nicknamed the "magic horse collar" and was shown to be effective when an accompanying light attached to a smaller coil glowed as it was passed within the field. Gaylord Wilshire of Los Angeles developed the I-ON-A-CO and charged $55 each, though he never reaped the financial benefit of his "discovery" since he died of kidney failure in New York not long after its production. Wilshire was a multifaceted individual and for a time was involved in real estate speculation just outside of Los Angeles, now remembered today by his famous namesake the Wilshire Boulevard. Booklets accompanying the belts always contained testimonials with the following an example written for the Theronoid belt, an imitation of

Wilshire's invention: "New York. My father was very sick with high blood pressure and a very weak heart. The doctor told him he would have to lie in bed or he would not live long. You know how an old man of 72 is. He would not stay in bed, so I told him to try the Theronoid. Thank God he can walk around and has no more pains. He attends to the furnace and walks up and down the stairs without any trouble. The Thernoid is a wonderful treatment and I recommend it to anybody who wants to get well. Yours truly, Mrs. S. Schlesinger."

Large electrostatic generators, sometimes referred to as friction machines, could produce a high-voltage current when spinning glass plates or cylinders were in contact with pads of various materials (figures 436–440). The resulting charge was then stored in Leyden jars, which acted as capacitors, and the current was used therapeutically in any number of ways the imagination could conceive. Despite the fact that these devices were without any proven merit, many were found in physicians' offices in the early twentieth century. Electrostatic generators also provided a good source of electricity for early X-ray machines, though the early use

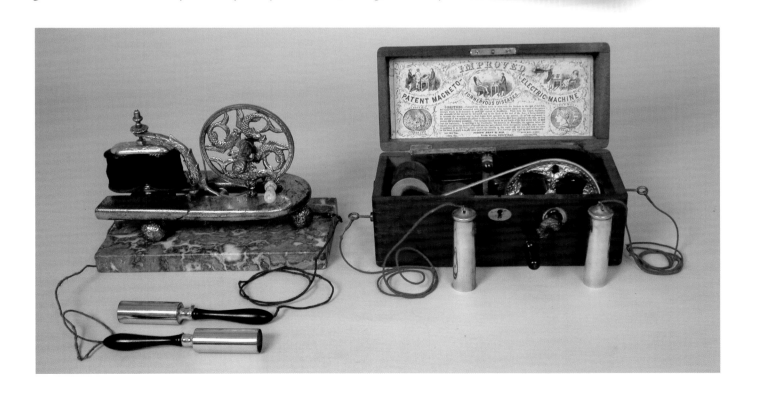

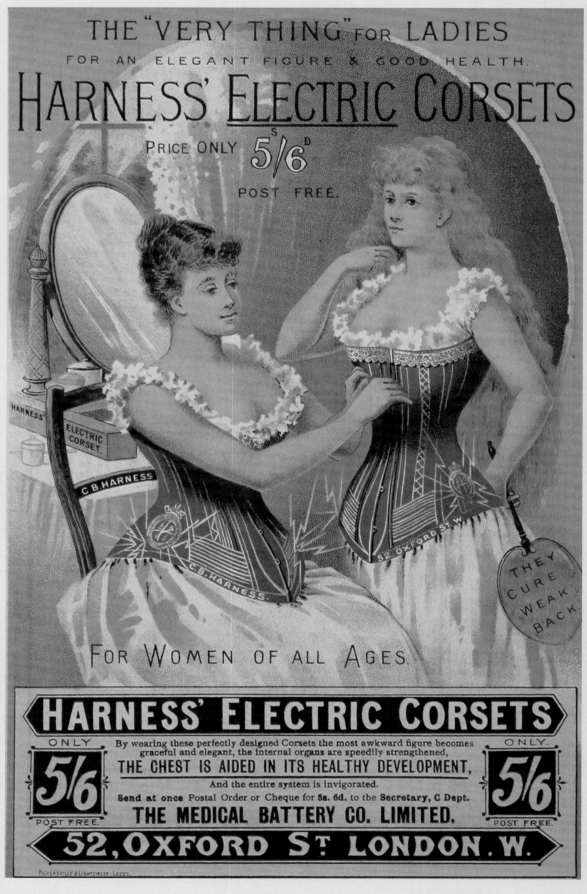

429. Early twentieth-century trade card for Harness' Electric Corsets

430, 431. Opposite above. Advertisements for Pulvermacher's Electric Belts (ca. 1920)

432. Opposite. Advertisement in *The Cosmopolitan* (1903)

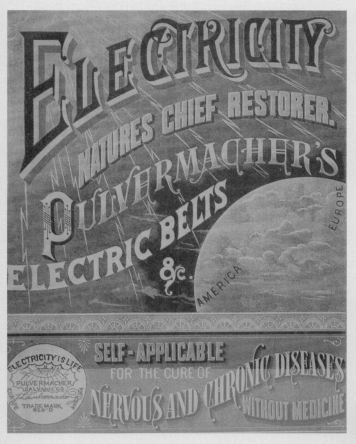

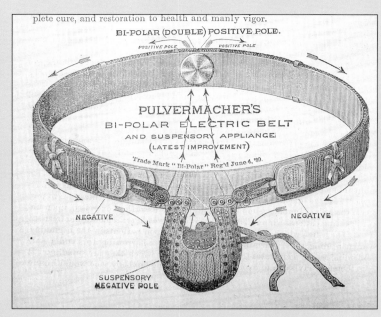

433. Below. Male and female magnetic belts by Mioxrls (ca. 1920)

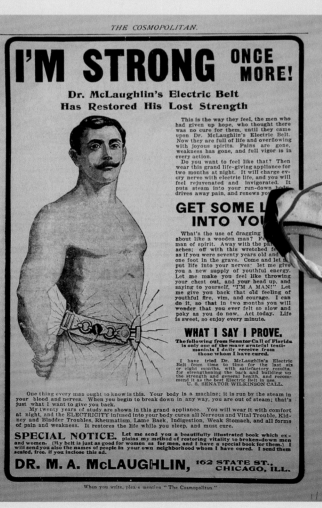

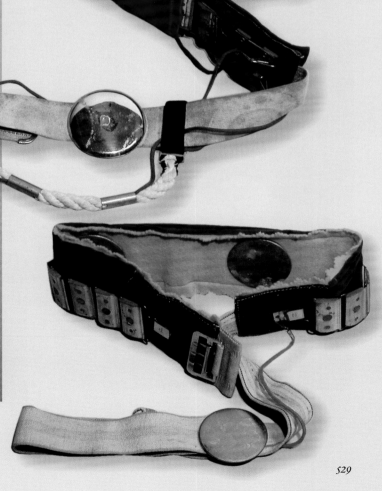

of X-rays was not universally accepted. This is a quote from the *Pall Mall Gazette* soon after Wilhelm Conrad Röntgen's important discovery:

> We are sick of the roentgen rays. It is now said, we hope untruly, that Mr. Edison has discovered a substance—tungstate of calcium is its repulsive name—which is potential, whatever that means, to the said rays. The consequence of which appears to be that you can see other people's bones with the naked eye, and also see through eight inches of solid wood. On the revolting indecency of this there is no need to dwell. But what we seriously put before the attention of the Government is that the moment tungstate of calcium comes into anything like general use, it will call for legislative restriction of the severest kind. Perhaps the best thing would be for all civilized nations to combine to burn all works on the roentgen rays, to execute all the discoverers, and to corner all the tungstate in the world and whelm it in the middle of the ocean. Let the fish contemplate each other's bones if they like, but not us.

434. Theronoid coil with small demonstration light (ca. 1930)

435. Demonstration of the Theronoid Coil (ca. 1930)

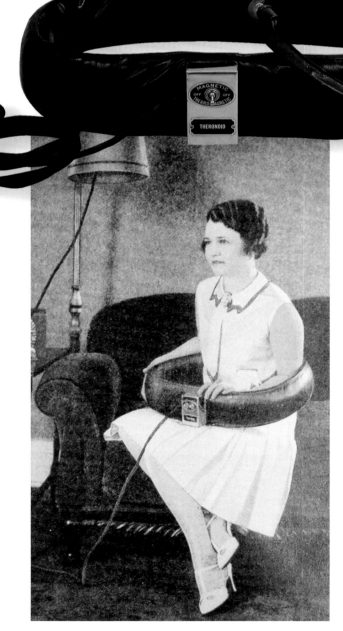

At the beginning of the nineteenth century, physicians used both wet and dry cell battery-powered devices in a number of ways. Diagnostically, there was a need to be able to differentiate between nerve and muscle disorders, while therapeutically, physicians hoped to increase strength by the stimulation of muscle groups (figures 441–443). Guillaume B.A. Duchenne, MD (1806–1875), was one of the pioneers of electrotherapy and a founder of modern neurology. In 1862, he published two atlases demonstrating various expressions that could be produced by stimulating different facial muscle groups (figure 444). In fact, Charles Darwin used some of those illustrations in his 1872 text, *The Expression of the Emotions of Man and Animals*.

The Electreat was a hand-held, battery-powered apparatus for home use that was to be drawn across the body to relieve pain and strengthen the heart. This instrument was first manufactured in Peoria, Illinois, in 1919 and has the distinction of being the first device seized by the government under the Food, Drug, and Cosmetic Act of 1938 (figures 445, 446).

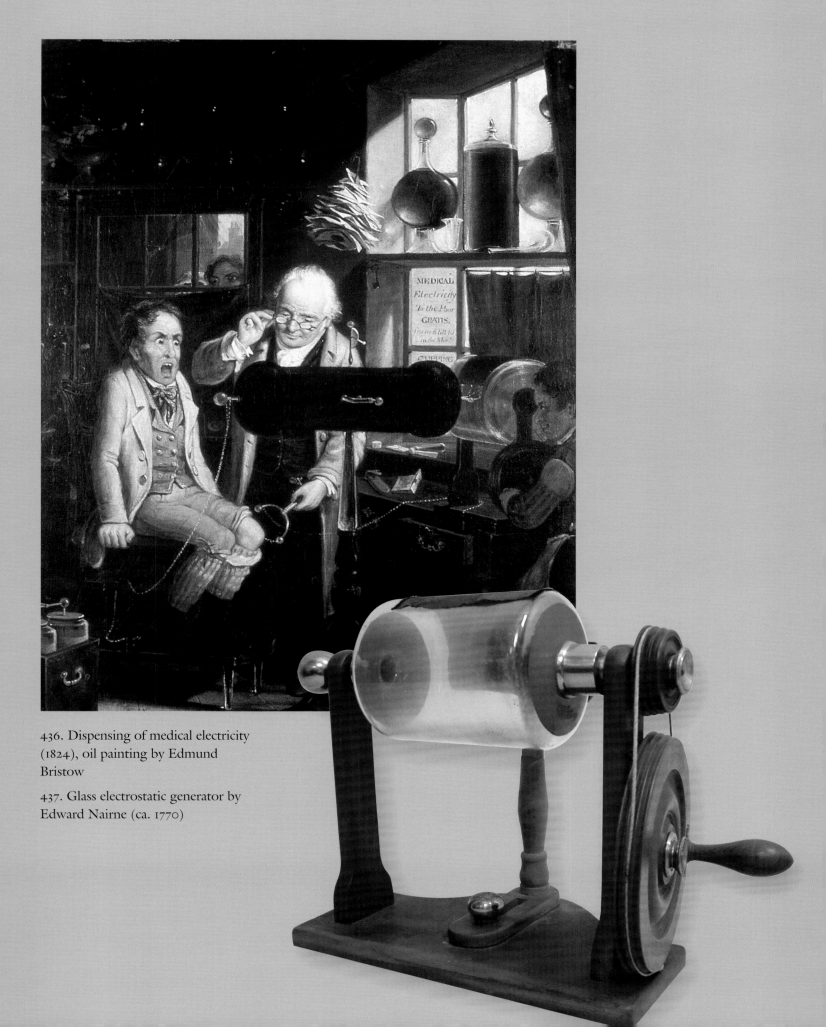

436. Dispensing of medical electricity
(1824), oil painting by Edmund
Bristow

437. Glass electrostatic generator by
Edward Nairne (ca. 1770)

Carnival sideshows often had a place in their penny arcades for electrotherapy (figure 447). Entrepreneurs saw a commercial opportunity as they advertised their Electric Battery Slot Machine in the *Western Druggist*:

> It's simplicity makes it possible for the weakest individual to use the current without the aid of an assistant, regulating the quantity of current desired with perfect ease. For an amusement it cannot be excelled. One can use it alone with a great degree of satisfaction and benefit, or a group of from two to six persons can use it jointly and regulate the current to suit themselves, shutting same off at will simply by releasing the knob. Many afflicted persons use this machine as a cure for disease and a

438. Ramsden electrostatic generator by Pixii of Paris (ca. 1780)

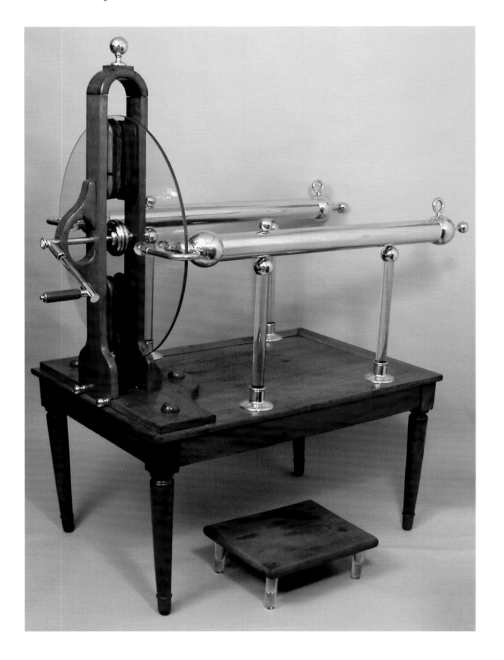

benefit to the human system, using it constantly from day to day, thereby making it a profitable investment. A battery runs from two to six months, and used for a penny would earn an average to $10.00, and for a nickel, $40.00, battery only costing 25 cents each. It is an excellent treatment for rheumatism, headache, nervousness, neuralgia, and all nervous disorders.

Nikola Tesla was one of the greatest inventors of modern times, and his early landmark discoveries include the radio and alternating current. He was able to transform household electricity into high-voltage, high-frequency,

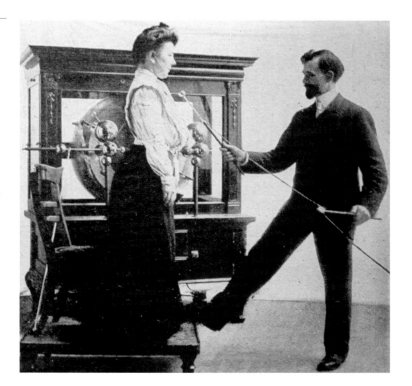

439. Chest treatment with an electrostatic generator from *Practical Electro-Therapeutics* (1908) by Franklin Gottschalk, MD

440. Early twentieth-century twenty-four-plate electrostatic generator (by Wagner?) with glass legged table and hand electrodes

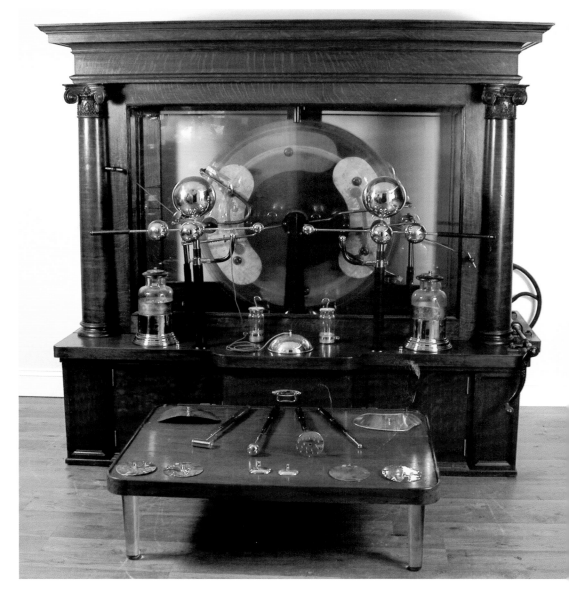

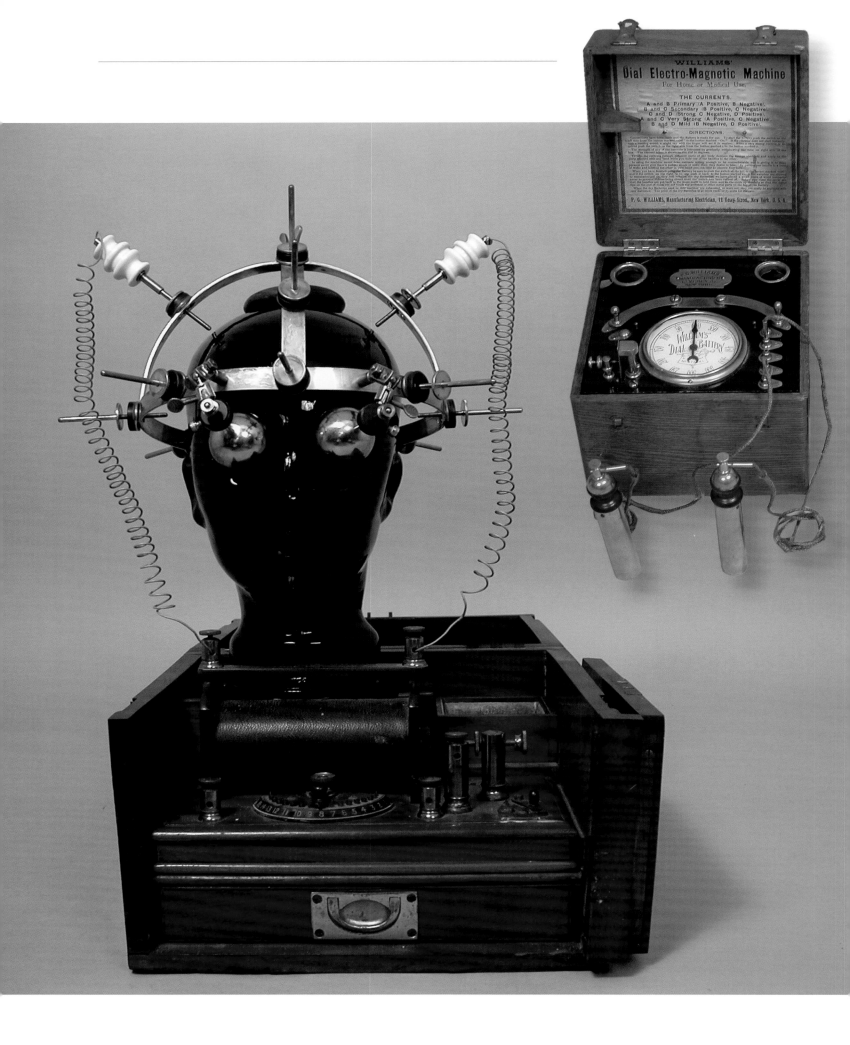

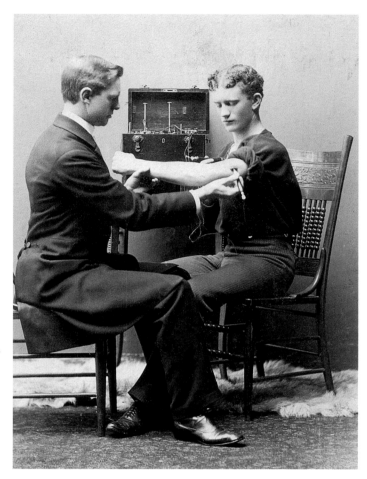

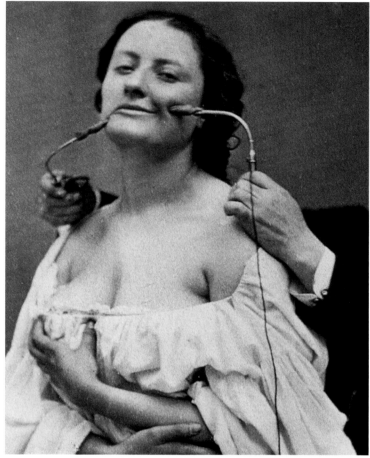

and low-amperage energy. His development of high-frequency current in 1891 was picked up by the medical community very quickly, and a variant—the "violet ray" machine—became one of the most popular health devices of the early twentieth century (figures 448–454). Cased sets using Tesla's disruptive discharge coil design were sold as late as the 1950s, and contained numerous annealed glass tubes that were designed to spark when touched to various parts of the body. The tubes were constructed under low vacuum and glowed with different colors, depending on the gas within. The most popular was argon that glowed purple, the next being the same red neon that is seen in modern neon signs. The high frequency of the electrical charge was between 400–500 khz and is not felt by human nerves, though it was the production of a high-frequency current, ultraviolet light, ozone, and a magnetic field that gave physicians a basis on which to make claims for medical cures. Theoretically, these devices resulted in an increased oxygen supply to diseased tissues by "ozonation" of the blood resulting in increased strength and vital energy. In *A Working Manual of High Frequency Currents* (1916), Noble Eberhardt, MD, PhD, claimed that "violet ray" vacuum tubes increased local blood supply, oxidation, nutrition, secretions,

441. Opposite, right. Battery-powered Williams' Dial Electro-Magnetic Machine and the Electraply by the Electraply Laboratories, Inc., Philadelphia (ca. 1910)

442. Electric helmet by Energo of Turin, Italy; Faradic Battery by S. Maw Son and Thompson, London (ca. 1930)

443. Above left. Neurological exam (ca. 1884), gelatin silver print by Charles Lanier

444. Above right. Electrostimulation by Guillaume B.A. Duchenne, MD (1862), albumin print by Adrien Tournachon

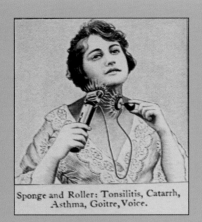

Sponge and Roller: Tonsilitis, Catarrh, Asthma, Goitre, Voice.

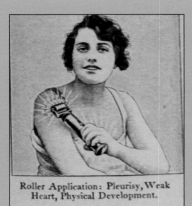

Roller Application: Pleurisy, Weak Heart, Physical Development.

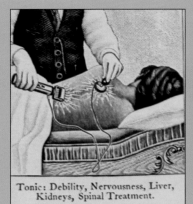

Tonic: Debility, Nervousness, Liver, Kidneys, Spinal Treatment.

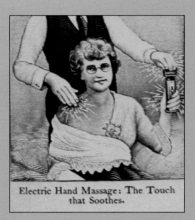

Electric Hand Massage: The Touch that Soothes.

445. Above. Demonstration for the use of the electreat hand-held device (ca. 1925)

446. Right. Electreat device with external and internal attachments (ca. 1925), Electreat Mfg. Company, Peoria, Illinois

447. Below. Penny arcade device (ca. 1930) by the Midland Manufacturing Company

448. Opposite. Catalog cover for the Vi-Rex Electric Company (ca. 1930)

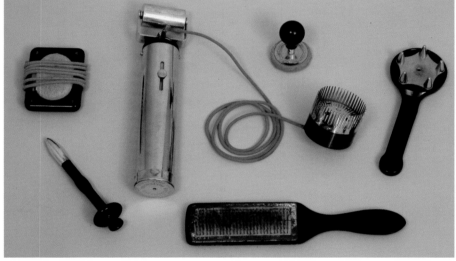

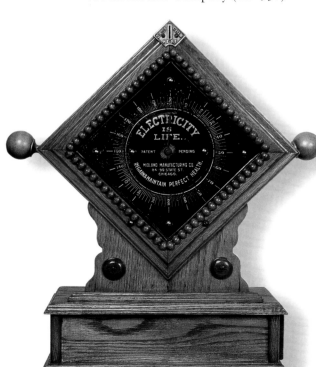

ozone, and metabolism. Larger sets were manufactured for doctors' offices, and some electrodes were made that produced ozone to be inhaled for the cure of all respiratory complaints. In 1951, the US Food and Drug Administration banned violet ray devices, with an allowance for dermatologists to use them for their antibacterial properties.

Heat by way of shortwave diathermy was another popular way in which physicians stretched the limits of early discoveries in electricity (figures 455–463). According to a catalog accompanying a United Short Diathermy Unit:

The story of how Short Wave Diathermy was developed is an interesting one. It begins some years ago in a high-powered short wave radio station. At that time a group of men were busy installing transmitters for broadcasting Short Waves. While they were testing the transmitters, the men began to

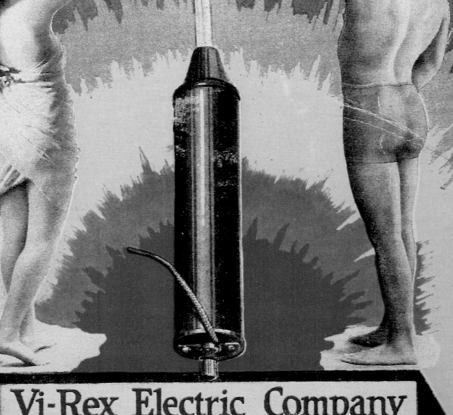

Violet Rays

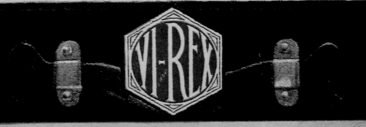

Vi-Rex Electric Company
326 W. Madison St.   Chicago, Ills.

VI-REX

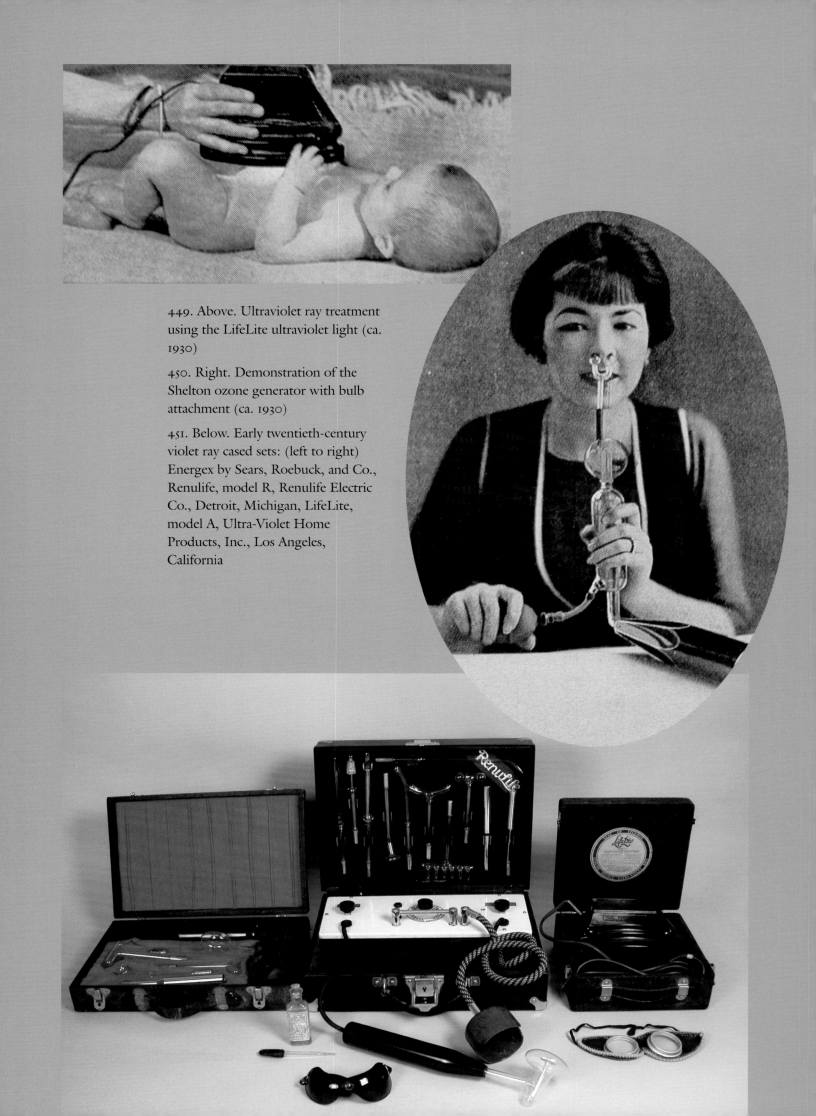

449. Above. Ultraviolet ray treatment using the LifeLite ultraviolet light (ca. 1930)

450. Right. Demonstration of the Shelton ozone generator with bulb attachment (ca. 1930)

451. Below. Early twentieth-century violet ray cased sets: (left to right) Energex by Sears, Roebuck, and Co., Renulife, model R, Renulife Electric Co., Detroit, Michigan, LifeLite, model A, Ultra-Violet Home Products, Inc., Los Angeles, California

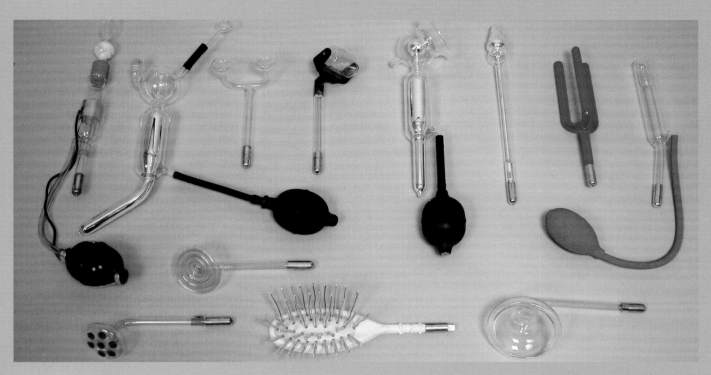

452. Above. Early twentieth-century violet ray attachments: (top) two ozone generators, ophthalmic attachment, body roller, ozone-cocaine wound electrode, insulated rectal electrode, penile applicator, insulated vaginal applicator; (bottom) radium electrode, body coil, head and hair brush, breast attachment

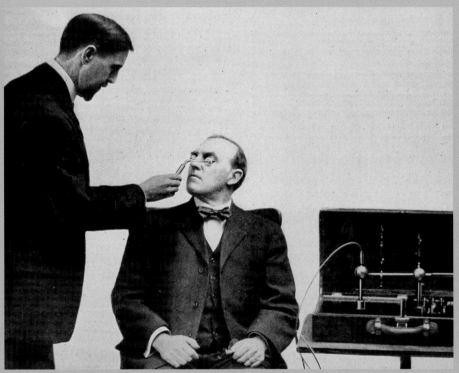

453. Left. Demonstration of the bifurcated eye vacuum tube from *High Frequency Electric Currents in Medicine and Dentistry* (1910) by S.H. Monell, MD

454. Below. Treatment of the chest with the violet ray from *High Frequency Electric Currents in Medicine and Dentistry* (1910) by S.H. Monell, MD

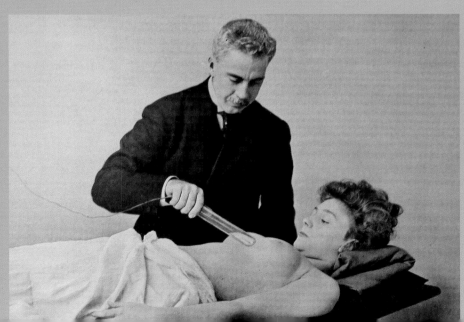

feel unusually warm. . . . Laboratory workers became interested in this unusual occurrence and investigated. After a long period of research, they came to the following conclusions. First, that people working in that particular room in the short wave radio station retained the heat of those short wave transmitters in their bodies. Second, that as a result of retaining this heat, their resistance to all common forms of colds, rheumatic pains, and general muscular discomforts was greatly strengthened. . . . Doctors became interested and used this new method to help ease the pain of those suffering from rheumatism and general muscular discomforts. The results were astounding!

Medical improvement resulted from the development of so-called "converted heat" defined as "that form of heat which is the result of converting energy into heat via chemical or mechanical means. In this type of heat (Short Wave Diathermy) electro magnetic waves (radio waves) are converted into heat that is able to penetrate deeply into the body. The resistance that bone, muscles, nerves, and tissues offer to the passage of the waves creates heat by molecular friction." S.H. Monell, MD, justified high current Tesla coils for diathermy in his *High Frequency, Electric Currents in Medicine and Dentistry* (1910): "Thus we can make high frequency currents increase metabolism, allay sensibility, stimulate the sympathetic nervous system, increase or diminish the functions of the glands, tone up muscular fibre, and act as a general tonic. . . These currents produce a general vitalizing and invigorating effect without undue stimulation. Speaking broadly, we have in them the closest approach to artificial vital force that has yet been produced."

Harry Eaton Stewart, MD, supervisor of physiotherapy for the US Public Health Service, felt that diathermy was beneficial to the health of all organ systems. He wrote the following in his book, *Diathermy and its Application to Pneumonia* (1923):

There is no question however, but that diathermy through the heart will improve the coronary circulation and minimize the effect of toxins on its muscular structure. A current of absolute steadiness derived from an even current supply and applied through a machine with a clean spark gap is absolutely essential. From 500 to 800 ma. is the maximum current strength that should be used and nearly double the usual time should be consumed in raising and lowering the current strength. There is undoubtedly after cardiac diathermy a decrease in muscle tone persisting for a short time after the treatment, similar to that obtained and too often regarded, in the body cabinet, electric light bath. For this reason the patient's activity during the first few hours after the treatment should be distinctly restricted. Rest in the horizontal position for at least an hour is especially desirable.

Brain. Diathermy has been successfully used in the treatment of a number of cerebral conditions. The electrodes may be applied anteroposteriorly on forehead and occiput, about 3 by 5 inches in size, or they may be used laterally through the parietal region. With the employment of sufficient lather the hair offers no obstacle to the application of the plates. The cautions just cited as to the steadiness of current and the careful grading of its rise and fall apply with especial emphasis to the treatment of the brain. Moreover, because of the resistance of the double thickness of the skull, lower amounts of current should be employed. Regardless of the size of the electrodes, not over 500 ma. should ever be used through the brain. To accelerate the absorption of the clot after hemiplegia and to improve the nutrition of surrounding neurons that may receive pressure-injury without destruction, this current has a special value.

In those conditions when general cerebral degeneration sets in due to arteriosclerosis, this current is a rival to galvanism in its effect on improving the nutrition of brain cells. Occasionally remarkably good results have followed its careful application. Every patient receiving cerebral diathermy should be constantly and carefully watched. They should be told to report the slightest feeling of nausea or vertigo, and because these symptoms at times appear but with slight warning, they should be under uninterrupted observation.

While generally safe, these electrical devices could be lethal if not used properly. Hugh Morris, MD, DMRE, included the following admonition in the appendix to his *Medical Electricity for Massage Students* (1953): "It is essential that the iron bedstead should by no possibility be in such a position as to act as a means of 'earthing' the patient, that is, it should not be in contact with any earthed metal, *e.g.*, heating or water pipes, radiators, or even an 'earthed' wireless receiver. The increasing use of radiant heat baths, resuscitation cradles, thermal pads for eye and ear work, and similar appliances receiving current in direct connection with the main current supply, necessitates increased precautions lest the patient be accidentally 'earthed'; patients undergoing treatment should be out of range of accidental contact with 'earthed' metal, such as radiators." Morris goes on to describe an unfortunate accident: "A patient, in bed in a hospital ward, was receiving treatment to the leg from a radiant heat bath of the ordinary metal type. In this a metal frame carried metal

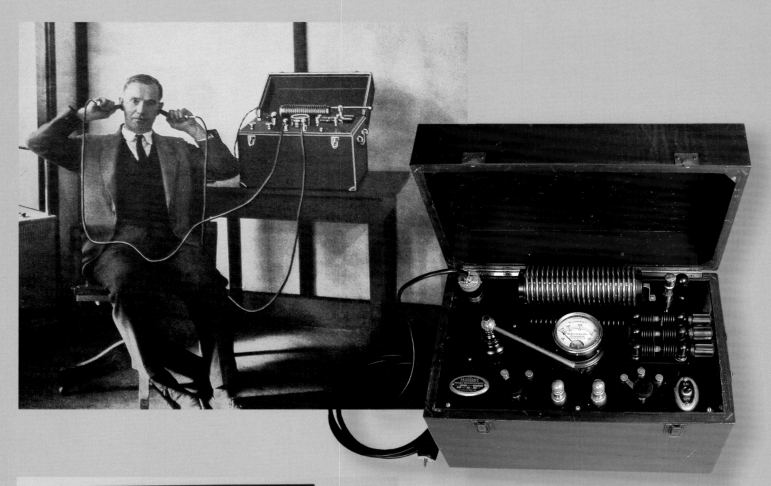

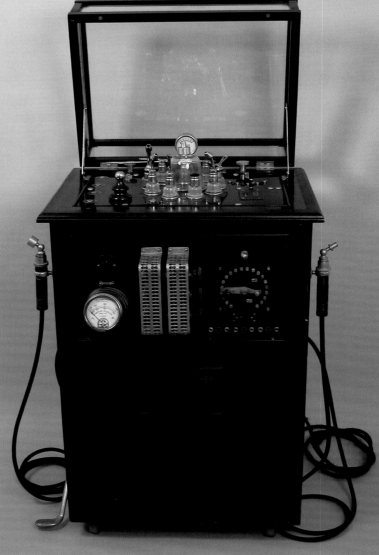

455. Above, left. Diathermy for deafness using two terminals of the D'Arsonval from *Practical Index to Electro-Therapy* (1925) by Joseph Waddington, MD, CM

456. Above, right. The Portable Diathermy Apparatus by the McIntosh Electric Corporation, Chicago (ca. 1930)

457. Left. Thompson-Plaster "Neurisco" by the Thompson-Plaster X-Ray Co., Inc., Leesburg, Va. (ca. 1930)

458. Opposite above, left. Diathermy treatment of the knee from *Diathermy and Its Application to Pneumonia* (1923) by Harry Eaton Stewart, MD

459. Opposite above, right. D'Arsonval type high-frequency machine with Oudin Resonator (ca. 1930)

460. Opposite below, left. Diathermy with treatment of the knee with pads (ca. 1920)

461. Opposite below, right. Diaathermy unit by the United Diathermy Co. of Pittsburgh, Pa.

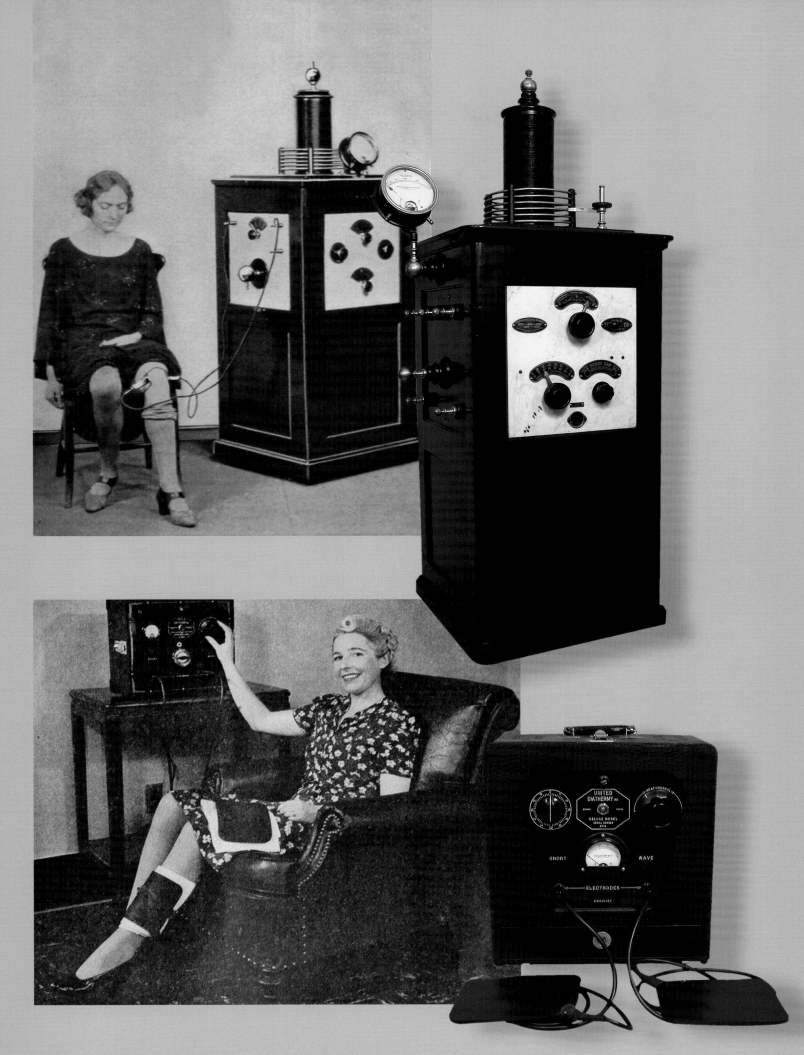

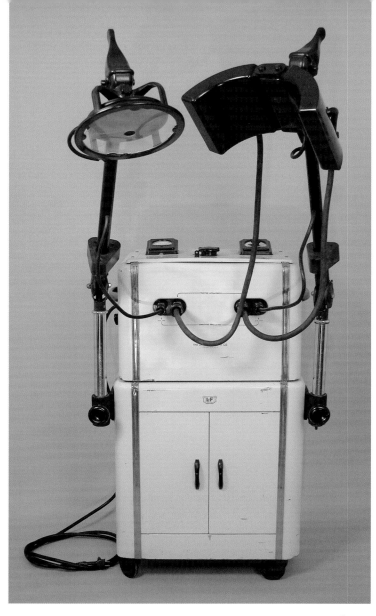

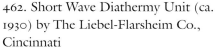

462. Short Wave Diathermy Unit (ca. 1930) by The Liebel-Flarsheim Co., Cincinnati

463. Above right. Long-path Air-Spaced Plate application to the sinuses with the Liebel-Flarsheim Diathermy Unit (ca. 1930)

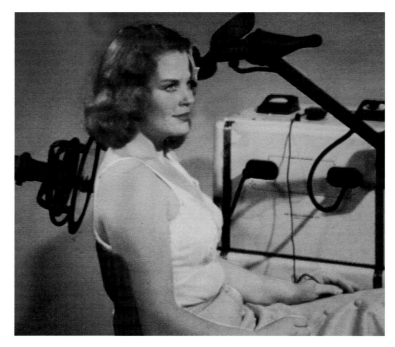

lamp-holders on metal brackets, and moreover these were fixed in such a way that by long use or accident the fastenings of seven out of eight brackets had become loose, causing failure of insulation and rendering the metal case 'live.' No shock was felt, however, until the patient, sweating from the effect of the treatment, grasped the iron bedstead, which happened to be in contact with a hot-water pipe, and was electrocuted. The current was alternating, 50 cycles and 230 volts."

KING OF THE QUACKS

Albert Abrams, AM, MD, LLD, FRMS, was born in San Francisco in 1864, and eventually became the king of American charlatans. He was trained as a pathologist, though his proprietary career really began when he became a neurologist and studied spinal diseases and spondylotherapy. Abrams believed that the diagnosis and treatment of a number of illnesses started with the percussion of reflex centers in the spine, and he was happy to provide courses on the subject for up to $200 apiece. Early in his career, Abrams prophetically commented, "The physician is only allowed to think he knows it all, but the quack, ungoverned by conscience, is permitted to know he knows it all; and with a fertile mental field of humbuggery, truth can never successfully compete with untruth." In 1922, Abrams became interested in the more lucrative field of electricity in medicine.

Albert Abrams' electric devices were termed ERA for Electronic Reactions of Abrams (later to be called "radionics"), and he was responsible for the production of a generation of quack machines that flooded the market in the first part of the twentieth century (figure 464). Abrams began by placing a drop of blood from one of his patients onto a "dynamizer," which was a remarkable combination of coils and wires that used radio waves in order to determine the vibration frequency that he attributed to each disease. The medical assistant would turn the patient westward in a dim light, affix an electrode to his forehead, and then tap his abdomen in various areas in order to arrive at a diagnosis. It was by estimating the degree of dullness during this percussive phase that the operator could differentiate between such diseases as cancer, syphilis, tuberculosis, malaria, and typhoid fever. Later, Abrams found that he could make the same diagnoses by using a patient's signature alone (and at the same time, determine the sex and religion of that subject). The treatment method recommended by Abrams involved an "oscilloclast," which was a machine that supposedly duplicated the vibrations characteristic of each disease in order to neutralize that disorder. Abrams described the principles behind the operation of his devices:

1. Physiologic phenomena are manifestations of electronic energy.

464. Abrams dynamizer and reflexo-phone (ca. 1920)

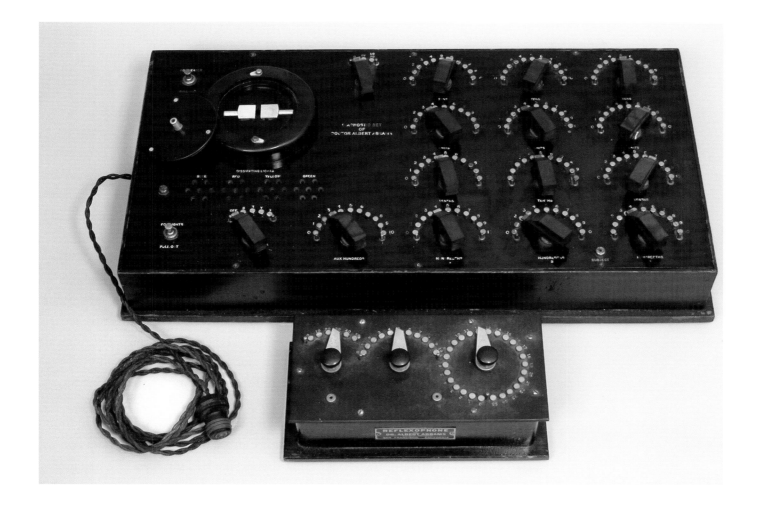

2. Pathologic phenomena are manifestations of perturbed electronic energy.

3. The energy in health and disease has an invariable and definite rate of vibration (determinable by the electronic reactions).

4. Specific drugs possess a like vibratory rate as the diseases for which they are effective. These like vibratory rates (homovibrations) of drugs owe the efficiency to their inherent radioactivity. Thus, an obsolete drug like gamboge painted on the chest in incipient tuberculosis will effect a symptomatic cure within a few weeks. Gamboge possesses the same vibratory rate as tuberculosis. Our conception that drug action is dependent on direct cellular contact is thus demolished . . .

5. All forms of energy whether derived from heat, electricity or magnetism may be made to yield different rates of vibration and these rates corresponding to diseases are utilized for their destruction.

Testimonials poured in, and this was a typical clinical note from Abrams' own *Physico-Clinical Medicine*: "Cancer of the uterus. Inoperable. Severe uterine hemorrhages. Electrode of Oscilloclast to cervix and hemorrhage ceased after second treatment. After 14 treatments the patient declared she was well. Another case of the same character was followed by equally good results." and "Cancer of the pylorus and pylorectomy executed at the Mayo Clinic. Later, vomiting, severe pains, loss in weight, etc. After the third treatment pains ceased and, after 14 treatments, she was well and continued so when I last saw her."

This testimonial from W.P. Meyers, MD (Cal), was printed in the *Journal of the American Medical Association* on March 25, 1922: "We are swamped with work and our three cord Oscilloclast is working to full capacity. We are still astonishing the incredulous and keeping busy. We must have another Oscilloclast at once for there are so many here who demand treatment." The oscilloclast contained simple radio tubes, and a shortwave tuner, rheostats, condensers, and other components, all of which were not meaningfully connected. It could not be purchased but was for lease at about $200, with an additional $5 monthly rental fee. The device was carefully sealed, and the lessee had to sign an agreement that he would never open it for inspection. Abrams had thus fulfilled two of the most important rules of quackery: 1) There must be a logical basis for the treatment or procedure, and 2) The patient must either see or feel the "cure" in action. Meaningful results, however, remained a problem, and his devices were finally put to the test as a result of a court challenge. They were inspected by Prof. R.A. Millikan, head of the California Institute of Technology and winner of the Nobel Prize in physics. His impression was that this device was the kind of a machine that a ten-year-old boy would build to fool an eight year old. The American Medical Association collected rather damning evidence when blood samples from many unusual sources were sent to unsuspecting Abrams practitioners for analysis and preposterous results were reported. For example, a blood sample from a male guinea pig was sent to a laboratory in Albuquerque, New Mexico, where the diagnosis of an infection of the left fallopian tube was made. Abrams died a wealthy man on January 13, 1924, leaving funds for his Abrams College, along with a blizzard of lawsuits and many imitators of his devices (figures 465, 466).

Since electricity was more available in the twentieth century, manufacturers felt free to use their imagination. They aggressively promoted devices that used indirect current in the home as well as in doctors' offices where large equipment such as cages and chairs could be found (figures 467–470). Some physicians even ventured into the dangerous practice of mixing water and electricity in their treatment regimens (figures 471, 472).

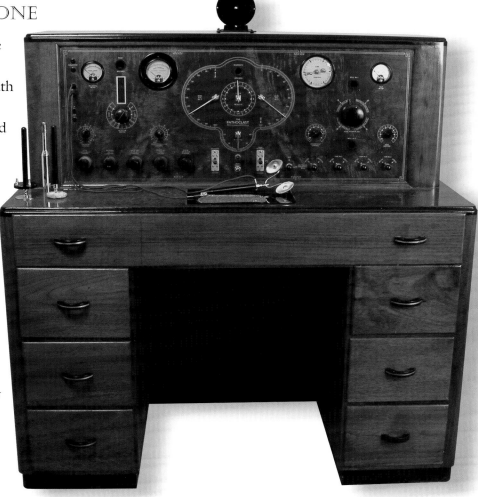

465. The Pathoclast, Model IX-C by Pathometric Laboratories, Chicago (ca. 1930)

RUTH DROWN: A QUEEN ASCENDS THE THRONE

In the early part of the twentieth century, there were many eager to take the mantle of Albert Abrams, the most prominent of whom was Ruth B. Chase, born in Greeley, Colorado, in 1892. She was later known as Dr. Ruth B. Drown and became America's greatest radionics innovator. At the age of nineteen, Drown married a farmer and had two children, though it was not long before she left her family and moved to California to work in a gas station. She then took a job at the Southern California Edison Company, and, in 1923, had a life-altering experience when she attended a lecture by Dr. Frederick F. Strong on the use of radio waves for the treatment of various diseases.

Ruth Drown subsequently trained to become a chiropractor, and, over the next forty years, she and her daughter, Dr. Cynthia Chatfield (also a chiropractor), amassed a fortune by treating over 35,000 patients from all over the country. Drown developed a medical

466. Short Wave Oscilloclast with accessories, College of Electronic Medicine, San Francisco; RDK, or Radio Disease Killer, by the RDK Corporation of America, New York (ca. 1930)

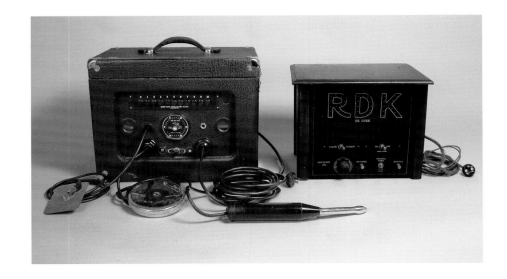

empire based on techniques similar to those of Albert Abrams, and employed the generation of vibrations presumably to neutralize the abnormal ones produced in various diseases. After being admitted to the Drown Laboratories for diagnosis and treatment, attendants seated patients next to a large console that contained nine dials and positioned their feet on footpads made of German silver. Dr. Drown placed an electrode on the patient's body, and, following a manipulation of the dials, she could diagnose almost any medical condition. For therapy, the doctor used a similar machine or sometimes placed the patient in a large hollow coil. The presence of a subject, in fact, was not necessary, and given a dried sample of blood, Dr. Drown could diagnose and treat a patient from any part of the world. Later in her career, she invented a revolutionary "radio-vision" device through which she was supposedly able to photograph internal organs. Drown taught that magnetic fields surround each of us, and, according to her *Drown Atlas of Radio Therapy*, "Any patient who is weak and depleted should never take shower baths and stand in the water over the drain, because the patient's magnetism is washed down with the water through the drain, leaving him depleted."

Though Drown's treatments remained popular for many years, the medical community questioned her methods on numerous occasions. In 1949, the University of Chicago supplied Drown with a blood sample from a patient with tuberculosis, and the diagnosis that was returned suggested widely metastatic carcinoma of the breast and blindness in one eye. After reviewing her devices, a committee from that institution reported, "It is our opinion that the machine is a sort of Ouija board in which the operator develops the audible end point by the amount of pressure applied to the stroking finger without any causal relationship to the position of three potentiometer dials. In the three patients she attempted to diagnose, Mrs. Drown registered spectacular failures. It is our belief that her alleged successes rest solely on the noncritical attitude

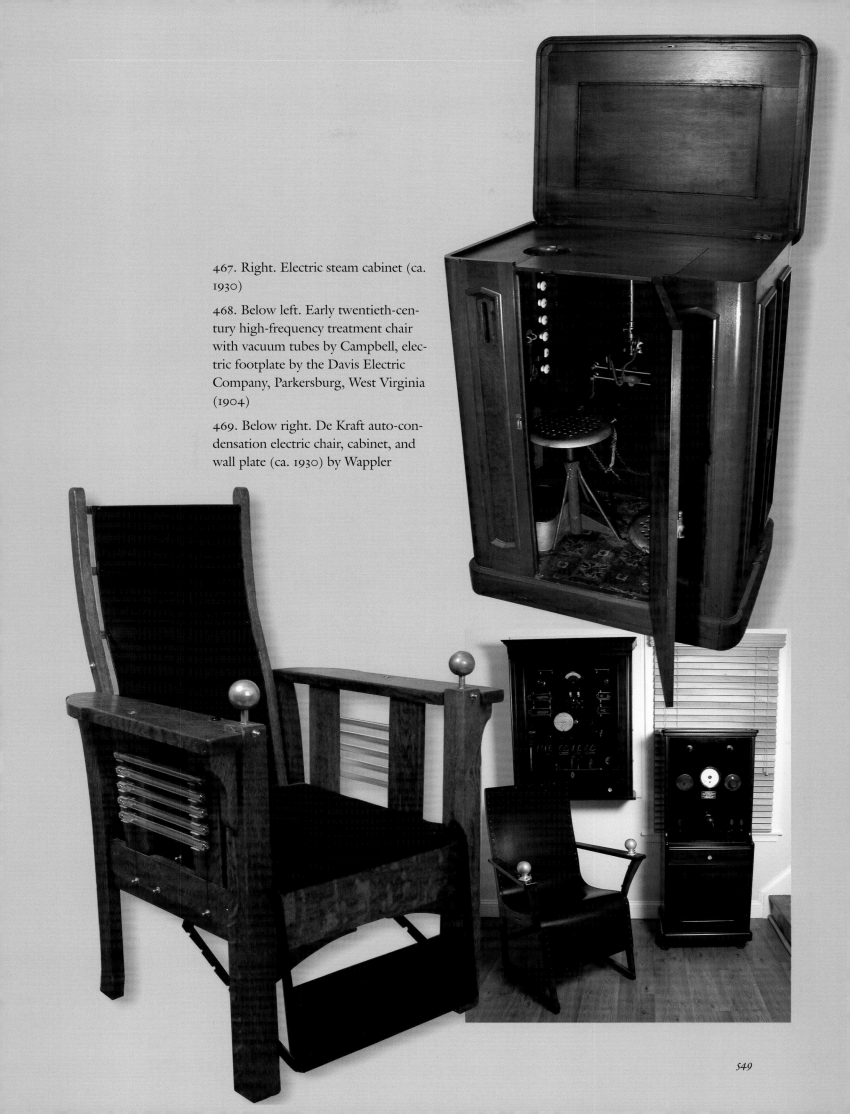

467. Right. Electric steam cabinet (ca. 1930)

468. Below left. Early twentieth-century high-frequency treatment chair with vacuum tubes by Campbell, electric footplate by the Davis Electric Company, Parkersburg, West Virginia (1904)

469. Below right. De Kraft auto-condensation electric chair, cabinet, and wall plate (ca. 1930) by Wappler

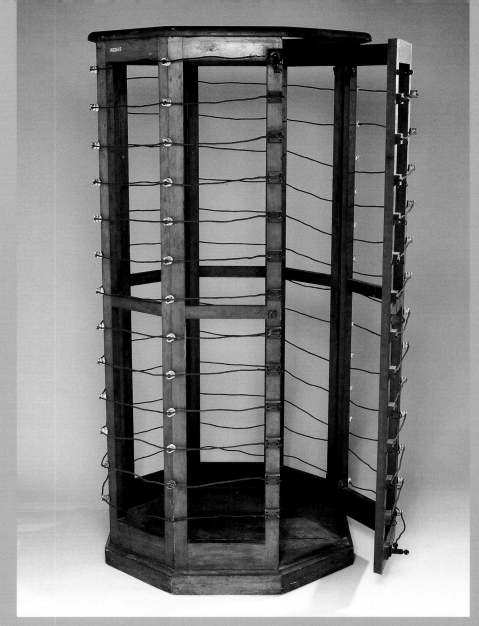

470. Right. Electrotherapeutic D'Arsonval, cage by Richard Heller of Paris (ca. 1890–1910)

471. Below left. Electric Solenoid bath as illustrated in *A System of Instruction in X- Ray Methods and Medical Uses of Light, Hot-Air, Vibration and High-Frequency Currents* (1902) by S.H. Monell, MD

472. Below right. Electrohydric bath from *Rational Hydrotherapy* (1902) by J.H. Kellogg, MD

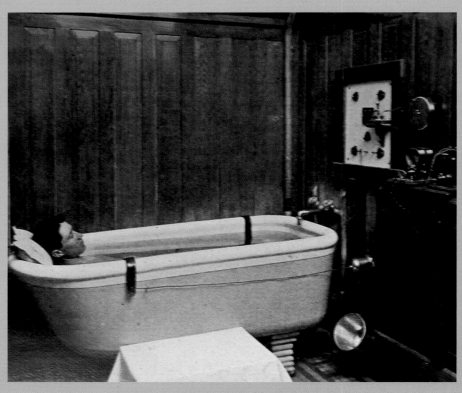

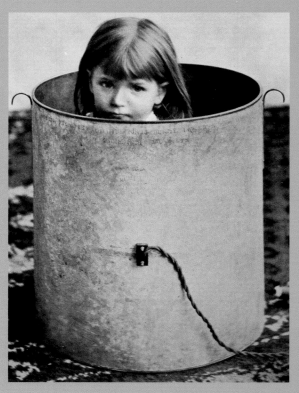

of her followers. Her technique is to find so much trouble in so many organs that usually she can say 'I told you so' when she registers an occasional lucky positive guess. In these particular tests, even her luck deserted her." Concerning her "radio-vision" device, "We find that the film images which have intrigued Mrs. Drown and her disciples are simple fog patterns produced by exposure of the film to white light before it has been fixed adequately. These images are significantly identical regardless of whether or not the film is placed in Mrs. Drown's machine before being submitted to the highly unorthodox processing which has been devised by her. In the numerous old films shown to us by Mrs. Drown we can seen no resemblance to other anatomic structures, appliances, bacteria, etc., that Mrs. Drown professes to see. In short, it is our opinion that the so-called Drown radio photographs are mere artifacts and totally without clinical value."

Two years later, Drown was fined $1,000 for interstate commerce of a misbranded device. In 1963, Mrs. Jackie Metcalf visited Drown and Chatfield in their Los Angeles clinic, though unbeknownst to the doctors, Metcalf was an undercover agent for the California State Department of Public Health, and she brought with her blood samples that she represented had been taken from her three children. The doctors told Metcalf that her children were suffering from chicken pox and mumps, though, in reality, the samples were from a turkey, a sheep, and a pig. The doctors were arrested, and two years later Drown died while still awaiting trial. Testimony in court included a diabetic who was told by Drown to reduce his insulin against the advice of his private physician and an epileptic who was told to stop his dilantin, even after having had a seizure in her office. Cases of misdiagnosed cancer that resulted in tragic consequences were also presented. Dr. Moses A. Greenfield, professor of radiology at the UCLA School of Medicine and consultant the Atomic Energy Commission, likened Drown's device to a simple flashlight battery and stated that there was no difference between any of the positions of the nine dials it contained. Drown's daughter, Cynthia Chatfield, was convicted of grand theft.

RADIOACTIVITY

The production of radium from pitchblende by Pierre and Marie Curie in 1898 was a dramatic medical advance. This was the early twentieth century, and the newly discovered wonder of radioactivity awaited commercial applications to be eagerly supplied by innovative entrepreneurs (figure 473, 474). According to the Radium Treatment Co. of Utah, "radium is truly 'THE METAL OF MYSTERY.' Its vast and almost perpetual energy offers possibilities heretofore undreamed of. It has rightly been termed 'Nature's Own Remedy.' There is scarcely a chronic disease

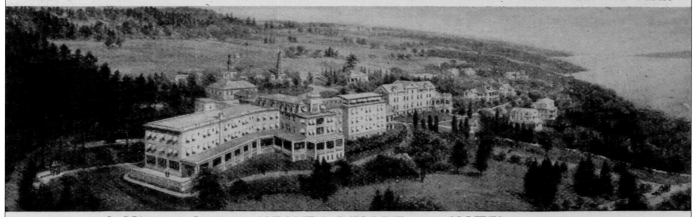

The GLEN SPRINGS

Watkins, New York on Seneca Lake.
Wm. E. Leffingwell, Pres.

OPEN ALL THE YEAR

A Mineral Springs HEALTH RESORT and HOTEL known as

THE AMERICAN NAUHEIM

Highly Radioactive Mineral Springs

Private Park. Miles of accurately graded walks for Oertel hill climbing. Five minutes walk from Watkins Glen. Sporty Golf Course. Tobogganing, Skating, Music, Dancing.

THE BATHS are DIRECTLY CONNECTED WITH THE HOTEL and are complete in all appointments for

Hydrotherapy, Electrotherapy and Mechanotherapy.

A Natural Brine—THE MOST HIGHLY RADIOACTIVE IN AMERICA—for the Nauheim Baths. Hot Brine Baths for Elimination.

WINTER CONDITIONS FOR TAKING THE "CURE" OR FOR REST AND RECUPERATION ARE ESPECIALLY DESIRABLE.

Our Illustrated Booklets and Latest Reports on our Mineral Springs will be Mailed on Request

473. Advertisement for radioactive water at the Glen Springs resort, Watkins, New York (ca. 1920)

or ailment known to mankind that does not yield to the powerful emanations from it."

From a brochure by the Radium Treatment Co.:

It has been recently discovered, however, that one of the chief effects of the radium rays is to produce an ionization of the atoms of whatever substance the rays penetrate, that is, to make these atoms electrical conductors . . . that we now possess in radio-active substances the means of carrying electrical energy into the depths of the body and there subjecting the juices, protoplasm and nuclei of the cells to an immediate bombardment by EXPLOSION OF ELECTRICAL ATOMS. . . .

The penetrative power of the gamma rays is so great that, although they resemble the X-ray in many ways, they are not available for photographing the interior portions of the body as will the X-ray, since they penetrate all substances so thoroughly . . going through solid bone without interruption and even penetrating iron to the depth of approximately six inches.

Although there is a difference of opinion regarding the exact manner in which the radium acts upon the human organism, many careful tests have shown that it exerts a marked influence, and that it has a peculiar selective, destructive action, added to its extraordinary powers of penetration, enables it to seek out and destroy elements to which it is inimical (such as dead or waste matter or diseased tissues) while passing by and leaving unharmed the normal tissues. Investigations have demonstrated that the emanations of radio active bodies promote the process of oxidation in the tissues and eliminate waste products from the body.

Few had safety concerns regarding the use of radioactive substances after reading the above advertising. An early twentieth-century advertisement for the Vita Radium Suppository illustrates that fact: "After insertion, the suppository quickly dissolves and the Radium is absorbed by the walls of the colon; then, within a few minutes, it enters the blood stream and traverses the entire body. Every tissue, every organ of the body is bombarded by its health-giving electric atoms. Thus the use of these suppositories has an effect on the human body like recharging has on an electric battery."

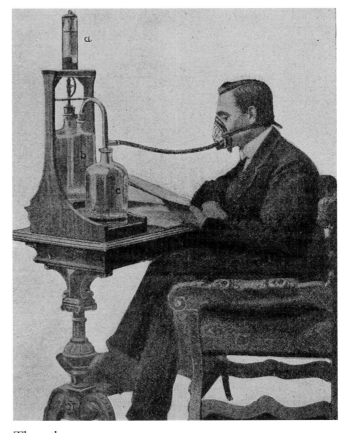

474. A therapeutic radium inhaler, *Scientific American* (June 3, 1911)

Some of the conditions supposedly treated with radium included "Blood Pressure, Rheumatism, Asthma, Appendicitis, Bright's Disease, Constipation, Diabetes, Paralysis, Prostate Gland, Female troubles, etc." Most products were accompanied by testimonials:

Ogden, Utah
October 27, 1924
 I have suffered with *Leakage of the Heart* for the past fifteen years and could get nothing to relieve me. The Doctor gave up my case and twice I was thought to be dying. I heard from your Radium Active Pad and Ore and immediately purchased them. In three weeks I gained 10 pounds and have not been in any pain since the first day I began using your appliances. I cannot praise the Ore and Pad enough for what it has done for me. My mother and sister have also purchased one and I will recommend it to all my friends.
 Yours truly,
 Mrs. Ameada Taylor

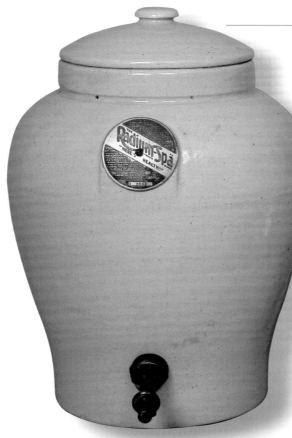

To Whom it may concern:

 Some time ago I was badly afflicted with dropsy. My lower limbs were terribly swollen and I was past going. Doctoring did me no good. Finally, I was persuaded by a friend to get a piece of uranium ore, put it in water and drink the radioactive water there from. This I did and the results were marvelous. Right away the swelling began to disappear and in a remarkably short time it had gone entirely and I have not been bothered in the slightest since that time. This has been more than a year ago.

 My daughter was similarly affected. She used the ore the same way that I did and she, too, was completely cured. . . .

Respectfully submitted,

Mrs. F.M. Shafer,

Moab, Utah, December 17, 1923

It did not take businessmen long to discover that the best way to take commercial advantage of the discovery of radiation was to market a product that could be sold in small doses. An early example was the revigator, which was a jar of weakly radioactive clay that was advertised to "cure all" if six to eight glasses of water were consumed the morning after it had been left over night in the jug (figure 475). According to an article in the 1915 *Saturday Evening Post,* "American research work has indicated that when radium water is taken as a medicine it works its way through the entire body, and proceeds to accomplish effects quite different from of the application of a little tube of radium embedded in a cancerous growth. The particular value of the radium scattered throughout the body is yet subject to a great amount of study; but it now seems to rouse all the cells of the body to greater activity—a sort of tonic for them all." Other single-dose products were clearly fraudulent on several levels, like Radol, which was an early radium treatment produced by Dr. Rupert Wells to cure all cancers. It turned out to be an acid solution of quinine sulfate and alcohol that had a blue fluorescent glow resembling a radioactive substance. According to one observer, however, it contained "exactly as much radium as dishwater."

Radithor, which was highly radioactive, was manufactured and sold by William John Aloysius Bailey, a con artist in the late 1920s who was in part responsible for the eventual regulatory controls imposed on the production and sale of radioisotopes. Bailey had entered Harvard in 1903, and, though he failed to graduate, he claimed to have a degree from that university as well as a Doctorate from the University of Vienna. Following his conviction on a mail order scam, Bailey became involved in the production of Las-I-Go for male impotence, though

475. Early twentieth-century radioactive therapy: (above) ceramic Radium Spa by the American Radium Products Company; (below) ceramic Revigator by the Radium Ore Revigator Co.

after later scrutiny, the active ingredient turned out to be strychnine. In 1915, he saw a great commercial opportunity in the new medical field of radioactive substances that were already ingredients in liniments, potions, and creams. Bailey finally hit the jackpot with his production of radithor, which was bottled radium in distilled water (figure 476). He sold almost one half million half-ounce bottles in the late 1920s. promoting it as a general curative and a form of sex therapy, as well as a treatment for the mentally ill, or the "living dead." An individual suffering from any one of one hundred and sixty diseases supposedly could be cured by the daily ingestion of a small amount of this medication. According to Bailey, "Radithor is harmless in every respect."

Eben M. Byers was a millionaire socialite who was an expert trap shooter and the 1907 US Amateur Golf Champion. He was the chairman of the A.M. Byers Iron Foundry and was a handsome and dashing figure popular in all circles of society. In 1927, while attending a Harvard-Yale game, Byers had fallen from the berth of his chartered train, injuring his arm. The pain became chronic and interfered with his golf, so he began to take an interest in radithor for relief. Byers became the poster boy for radithor and drank 1,400 bottles of it between 1927 and 1930. He subsequently developed "sinusitis," which was actually radiation poisoning of his face and skull. At the time, there were no federal regulations regarding the sale of radioactive substances, though the government was suspicious of potential toxicity because of the syndrome of bone degeneration, and the kidney and marrow failure suffered by radium chemists and dial painters (who licked their radioactive brushes to make finer lines). Eben Byers developed this syndrome, but too late for the investigation that had been initiated by the Federal Trade Commission. Robert H. Winn was an attorney in that investigation when he visited Byers in 1931 at his Long Island mansion: "A more gruesome experience in a more gorgeous setting would be hard to imagine. We went to Southhampton where Byers had a magnificent home. There we discovered him in a condition which beggars description. Young in years and mentally alert, he could hardly speak. His head was swathed in bandages. He had undergone two successive jaw operations and his whole upper jaw, excepting two front teeth, and most of his lower jaw had been removed. All the remaining bone tissue of his body was slowly disintegrating, and holes were actually forming in his skull."

Byers' condition deteriorated, and he weighed only ninety-two pounds when he died on March 31, 1932, bringing an end to the marketing of radithor. Bailey was never prosecuted for Byers' death. He went on to become the editor of the *Bloomfield Times* and came up with several inventions that were helpful to the Allies in World War II. William Bailey died of bladder cancer at the age of sixty-four in 1949, though he never

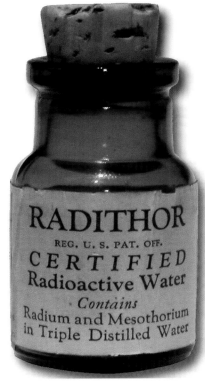

476. Radithor radioactive curative sold by William Bailey (ca. 1930)

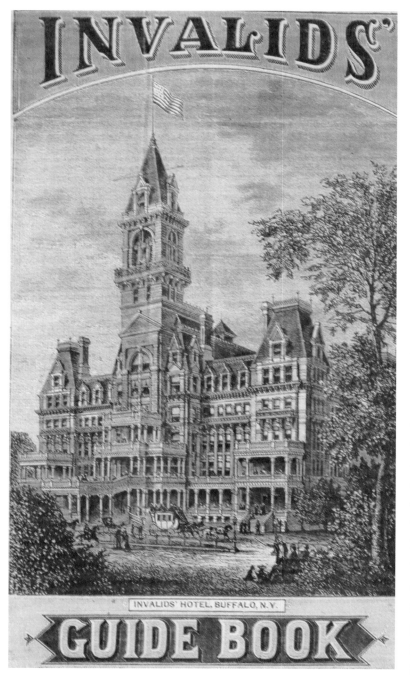

INVALIDS'

INVALIDS' HOTEL, BUFFALO, N.Y.

GUIDE BOOK

477. The Invalids' Hotel in Buffalo
(ca. 1920)

accepted the fact that his previous exposure to small doses of radioactive substances might have been harmful.

THE SANITARIUM

Retreats, or sanitariums, designed for the therapy of any number of diseases, including tuberculosis, cancer, obesity, and nervous disorders, were popular in the early part of the twentieth century (figure 477). One of the more fashionable was in Battle Creek, Michigan, where Dr. John Harvey Kellogg developed the famous Battle Creek Sanitarium. At one time or another, luminaries from all areas of American society were guests at "The San," including President William Howard Taft, Thomas Edison, George Bernard Shaw, Henry Ford, J.C. Penny, Montgomery Ward, Harvey Firestone, and Amelia Earhart, who personally flew Kellogg over the grounds of his sanitarium. Those entering The San were exposed to a full range of therapeutic options, including electricity, massage, vibration, and exercise. All had to endure rather bizarre dietary regimens, one of the more unusual involving the excess chewing of food called "Fletcherizing." The baked wheat flakes that Kellogg produced to feed his guests became so popular that they replaced the usual breakfast pork and fried potatoes of the day. John Harvey's brother, William Keith, recognized a commercial opportunity and left the sanitarium to create the Kellogg cereal empire. He was soon followed by a number of other entrepreneurs including C.W. Post (of Post Cereals) and Sylvester Graham (creator of Graham Crackers).

One of Kellogg's great obsessions was with the function of the colon. His guests spent many hours in bowel-cleansing activities, and according to Josh Clark:

From his earliest days as a doctor, Kellogg was fascinated with the bowel. . . . Ninety percent of all illness, he would calmly explain, originated in the stomach and bowel. 'The putrefactive

changes which recur in the undigested residues of flesh foods'
were to blame. . . . The bowel, poisoned by meat eating, drinking, smoking, and usually anything pleasurable was poked, prod-
ded and otherwise assaulted by attendants at the San. . . . His
favorite device was an enema machine . . . . that could run fifteen
gallons of water through an unfortunate bowel in a matter of
seconds. Every water enema was followed by a pint of yogurt—
half was eaten, the other half was administered by enema. . . . By
pumping yogurt cultures into the rectums of America's well to
do, Kellogg claimed that he had managed to cure 'cancer of the
stomach, ulcers, diabetes, schizophrenia, manic depressives . . .
migraine and premature old age. . . .' If autointoxication persisted and poisons remained, the offending stretch of intestine was
removed. Kellogg performed as many as twenty operations a day.

VICTORIAN PROHIBITIONS

Sexual activity has always been a controversial subject,
not only within the medical community, but in all aspects
of society as well. *Onanism* is another term for masturbation that came from the Bible (Genesis 38:8–10) when
Judah directed that his son Onan have intercourse with
the widow of his brother, Er, as required by law at the
time: "And Judah said unto Onan: 'Go in unto thy brother's wife, and perform the duty of a husband's brother
unto her, and raise up seed to thy brother.' And Onan
knew that the seed would not be his; and it came to pass
when he went in unto his brother's wife, he spilled it
unto the ground, lest he should give seed to his brother."
Onan was slain by the Lord for his noncompliance.

Masturbation, or spermatorrhoea (including nocturnal emissions), was a topic of great medical interest, and
had been associated with the development of weakness,
mental illness, blindness, and countless medical disorders
for generations (figure 478, 479). Moses Maimonides
(1135–1204), the great physician and philosopher of
Muslim Spain and North Africa, summarized popular
beliefs pertaining to masturbation in his *Treatise on
Asthma*:

Regarding coitus it is well known, even to the general
public, that it is harmful to most people and, when
indulged in to excess, is injurious to all of them.

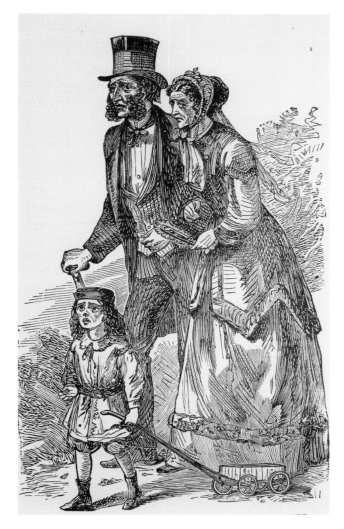

478. The effects of self-abuse on members of a family (ca. 1910)

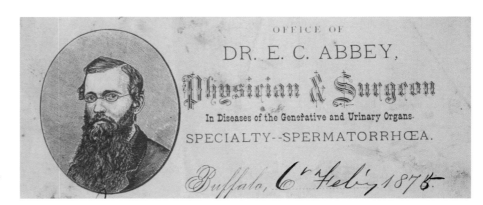

OFFICE OF
DR. E. C. ABBEY,
Physician & Surgeon
In Diseases of the Generative and Urinary Organs.
SPECIALTY--SPERMATORRHŒA.
Buffalo, 6" Feb'y 1875

479. The medical specialty of spermatorrhea

Discharge of semen as such is not counted among the salutary precepts of hygiene, except with a limited number of people with a wrong juice combination who change as time goes on. Along with the semen vital juices cannot help escaping from the body, so that its chief organs dry up and cool gradually. Only young men bear well this unavoidable nuisance, although even among them many pay for it with sickness. In any case, to old people coitus is at all times harmful since they are dependent on anything that increases their natural warmth and keeps their organs properly humid while coitus tends to extinguish and sap their strength little by little, as we pointed out above. A man of advanced age should therefore abstain from its exercise, the more strictly the better. All this is part of a healthy hygiene. Besides, this is also tied up with questions of keeping the body free of infections, purification of the spirit and of acquiring virtues through continence, modesty, and piety. If we say of coitus that it has an injurious effect on all organs it is especially true with regard to the brain because the main discharge has to do with this part of the body. All this has been discussed by Hippocrates. This is why it is so important for any one suffering from repeated headache to keep away from coitus. A man given to excessive exercise of coitus is found on inspection to suffer from lapses of memory and mental debility, with faulty digestion combined with green sickness, defective vision and bad appearance. There is a good reason for it, and, since human behavior varies greatly as well as human temperaments, there are admittedly some people, indifferent or subject to bad humor or defective digestion who actually happen to regain by it their vitality, cheerfulness, and good appetite, while others experience just the opposite. People's peculiarities vary much in this respect. Galen described one of the bad aspects of this problem, saying: There is a physical phenomenon which should be regarded as very unfortunate, namely, that some people seem to produce a lot of warm

semen which keeps them permanently excited and eager to discharge it. When they do discharge it their stomach as well as
their entire organism weaken, they dry up and grow lean, their
looks deteriorate and their eyes sink deep in their sockets. Such
people, even when they limit or suspend their coitus of their
own accord because of the discomfort that comes over them,
often suffer from a sense of heaviness in their head and pain in
their stomach, which means that even continence brings them no
relief. This results from the fact that they are harassed with nightly pollutions. Thus pollution causes them no less harm than
coitus itself.

Over five hundred years later, William Parker, MD, added the following in *The Science of Life; Self-Preservation* (1881):

In order to corroborate my own statements, I will here introduce an extract from a report on the subject of Idiocy and
Insanity, presented to the Massachusetts Senate by Dr. R.G.
Howe, in compliance with a formal resolution of that body
directing such a report to be made.

Dr. Howe makes the following forcible remarks: —

"There is another vice, a monster so hideous in mien, so disgusting in feature, altogether so beastly and loathsome, that in
very shame it hides its head by day, and vampire-like, sucks the
very life-blood from its victims by night; and it may perhaps
commit more direct ravages upon the strength and reason of
those victims than even intemperance; and that vice is SELF-
ABUSE."

Now Spermatorrhoea . . . is the secondary result of unnatural
or excessive indulgence, leading inevitably (unless stayed by the
intervention of experience and science) to the dreadful consummation so quaintly but so truthfully depictured in the following
translation from the German of Hufeland:—

"Hideous and frightful is the stamp which Nature affixes on
one of this class. He is a faded rose,—a tree withered in the
bud,—a wandering corpse. All life and fire are killed by this
secret cause, and nothing is left but weakness, inactivity, deadly
paleness, wasting of body, and depression of mind. The eye loses
its lustre and strength, the eyeball sinks, the features become
lengthened, the fair appearance of youth departs, and the face
acquires a pale, yellow, leaden tint. The whole body becomes
sickly and morbidly sensitive, the muscular power is lost, sleep
brings no refreshment, every movement becomes disagreeable,
the feet refuse to carry the body, the hands tremble, pains are felt

in all the limbs, the senses lose their power, and all gayety is destroyed. Such persons seldom speak, and only when compelled; all former activity of mind is destroyed. Boys, who before showed wit and genius, sink into mediocrity, or even become blockheads; the mind loses its taste for all good and lofty ideas, and the imagination is utterly vitiated. Every glance at a female form excites desire. Anxiety, repentance, shame, and despair of any remedy for the evil make the painful state of such a man complete. His whole life is a series of secret reproaches, distressing feelings, self-deserved weakness, indecision, and weariness of life; and it is no wonder if the inclination to suicide ultimately arises,—an inclination to which no man is more prone. The dreadful experience of a living death renders actual death a desirable consummation; for the waste of that which gives life generally produces disgust and weariness of life, and leads to that particular kind of self-destruction, *par depit*, from sheer disgust of existence, which is characteristic of our age. Moreover, the digestive power is destroyed; flatulence and pains in the stomach create constant annoyance; the blood is vitiated, the chest obstructed, eruptions and ulcers break out upon the skin, the whole body becomes dried and wasted, and in the end come epilepsy, consumption, slow fever, fainting fits, and an early death."

In *Plain Facts for Old and Young* (1886), John Kellogg, MD, suggested that one ought to suspect spermatorrhoea should the following symptoms be present: "lassitude, change in disposition, sleeplessness, bashfulness, round shoulders, acne, biting the finger nails, palpitation of the heart, wetting the bed." How embarrassed must have been individuals suffering from those rather common problems.

Many therapeutic devices to "cure" this nasty habit were available in the nineteenth century (figures 480–482), including the spermatorrhoea ring, or the "Timely Warning," patented in 1905 by Dr. Edward B. Foote and advertised in the Sears catalog. These beliefs remain popular today, and it is a common practice for athletes to refrain from sexual activity prior to competition thinking that strength would thereby be reduced.

JOHN BRINKLEY: THE GOAT GLAND DOCTOR

Affluence in America in the early twentieth century reached new heights, and without effective medical oversight, the climate was right for those who wished to take advantage of America's ambivalent sexual attitudes. Enter Dr. John Romulus Brinkley, who became the wealthiest and most powerful quack physician in the world by promoting rejuvenation

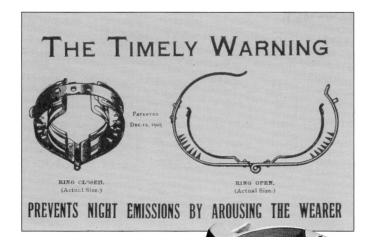

THE TIMELY WARNING

RING CLOSED.
(Actual Size.)

RING OPEN.
(Actual Size.)

PREVENTS NIGHT EMISSIONS BY AROUSING THE WEARER

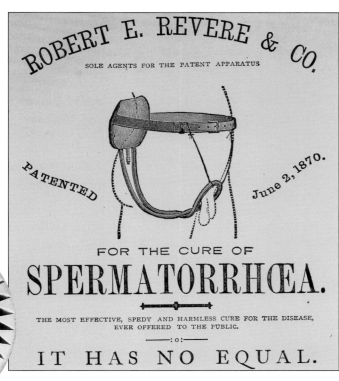

ROBERT E. REVERE & CO.

SOLE AGENTS FOR THE PATENT APPARATUS

PATENTED

June 2, 1870.

FOR THE CURE OF

SPERMATORRHŒA.

THE MOST EFFECTIVE, SPEDY AND HARMLESS CURE FOR THE DISEASE, EVER OFFERED TO THE PUBLIC.

—:o:—

IT HAS NO EQUAL.

through the transplantation of goats' gonads to his patients.

In 1885, Brinkley was born into poverty in Beta, North Carolina, where he was brought up by is aunt. He spent his early years as a telegraph operator and learned his craft as a snake oil salesman after moving to the northeastern United States. Brinkley traveled around the country, staying just ahead of the law, and eventually landed in Kansas where he obtained an MD degree from the Eclectic Medical University of Kansas City (for $500). Despite never having finished high school, Brinkley was also awarded a bogus medical diploma from the Bennett Medical College of Chicago. He became a practicing physician at the Swift & Co. meat packing company where he was exposed to the reproductive habits of goats. The theory that animal characteristics could be transmitted by transplantation had been suggested by physicians for hundreds of years, and in the early twentieth century, French physician Dr. Serge Voronoff was actually transplanting monkey glands into humans for improved potency. Brinkley's fortunes improved dramatically after one of his patients asked him to provide him with goat glands. The doctor implanted the glands from a Toggenberg goat into the farmer's testicles, and it was not long before his patient reported a dramatic improvement in his libido. He fathered a son the next year, whom he appropriately named "Billy." The popularity of Brinkley's procedure spread, and, with goats kept in a nearby pen, the Brinkley Clinic grew at an astonishing rate.

Brinkley's operation reached not only national, but international proportions following transplant surgery on *Los Angeles Times* magnate Harry Chandler. Chandler had purchased Los Angeles' first radio sta-

480. Above left. Early twentieth-century advertisement for the Spermatorrhoea Ring by Dr. Foot's Sanitary Bureau (ca. 1900)

481. Spermatorrhoea Ring (ca. 1900)

482. Above right. An iced cure for spermatorrhoea by the Robert E. Revere and Co. (ca. 1900)

tion, KHJ, and Brinkley was determined to own the first radio station in Kansas. The initial transmission was broadcast from Milford in September of 1923, and the station's 1,000 watts could be heard for over 1,000 miles. Goat testicular transplants and other medical "miracles" were advertised over KFKB 1050 ("Kansas First, Kansas Best"), along with infomercials and many shows with religious themes. Brinkley's business grew rapidly, and, by 1927, his clinic was performing about fifty operations a month, each procedure bringing in $750. He branched out into selling medications and was able to inflate prices by negotiating deals between druggists throughout the country and his National Dr. Brinkley Pharmaceutical Association. Brinkley became one of the most powerful men in the state and lived a commensurate life style that included ownership of a 115-foot yacht and a private airplane. His radio station thrived, and in 1929, KFKB won the gold cup as the most popular station in America.

The *Kansas Star* developed a rival station, and when Brinkley tried to boost his station to 5,000 watts to compete, the newspaper countered with a series of damaging articles that resulted in a state supreme court decision noting that "The licensee has performed an organized charlatanism. . . ." The Kansas Medical Society finally became involved by filing a complaint with the Kansas State Board of Medical Registration, accusing Brinkley of malpractice related to his goat testicular transplants, and other charges were filed for unprofessional conduct and alcoholism. The state board revoked his license, and at about the same time, the Federal Radio Commission shut down his radio station. Brinkley ran an unsuccessful campaign for governor and moved to the Texas boarder town of Del Rio.

Bypassing US restrictions, Brinkley crossed the boarder into Mexico and built a transmitter with towers three hundred feet high. In 1931, his new radio station, XER, initially broadcast a variety show with a powerful 75,000 watts, though after some encouragement, Mexican authorities allowed him to boost power to 500,000 watts, making it the most powerful station in the world. It was not long before XER became XERA, and he increased the power to an earth shattering one million watts, drowning out many channels over a large part of the United States. Brinkley's operations grossed twelve million dollars in Mexico, and his wealth grew to include real estate, oil wells, two more radio stations, and three yachts, one with a twenty-one–man crew. In 1937, the AMA analyzed Brinkley's formula No. 1020 and determined the composition to be one part indigo and 100,000 parts water. According to AMA representative Dr. Morris Fishbein, whom Brinkley had unsuccessfully sued twice, "The kind of genius capable of taking a body of water like Lake Erie, coloring it with a dash of bluing and then selling the stuff at $100 for six ampules represents a type which all the world up to now has never been able to equal. John R. Brinkley is the absolute apotheosis in his field. Centuries to come may never produce again such blatancy, such fertility of imagination, or such ego."

All good things must come to an end, and federal authorities played the income-tax card, billing the doctor for $200,000 in back taxes. In 1941, XERA was forced to close after negotiations between Mexico and the United States shut down all similar renegade radio stations across the boarder. The US Post Office indicted "the goat gland doctor" for mail fraud, though the case never came to trial since Brinkley suffered a severe myocardial infarction, which was followed by numerous other health problems. Dr. John Brinkley, after having risen to fabulous wealth and power for his rejuvenating goat testicular implants, died on May 26, 1942, at the age of only fifty-six.

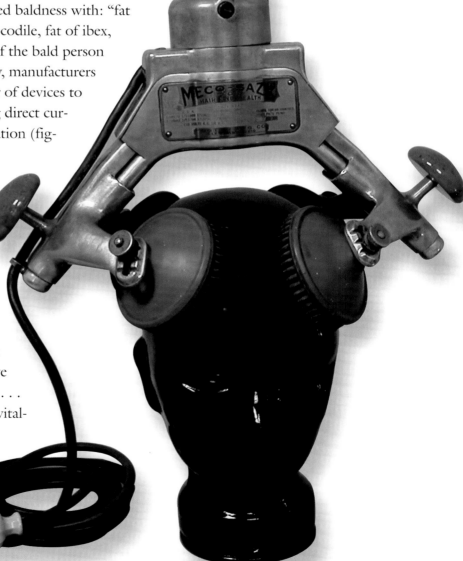

483. Meco-Sazh for Hair and Health by the Foster Manufacturing Co., Cleveland

MISCELLANEOUS THERAPIES

Personal appearance has been of interest to patients from the earliest recorded history when Egyptian physicians treated baldness with: "fat of lion, fat of hippopotamus, fat of cat, fat of crocodile, fat of ibex, fat of serpent, are mixed together and the head of the bald person is anointed with them." In the nineteenth century, manufacturers responded to the market by producing a number of devices to address the "medical problem" of hair loss, using direct current, static electricity, magnetism, heat, and vibration (figures 483–487).

"Professor" William C. Wilson recognized the difficulties people were having with their hearing and vision, so he produced the Actina Pocket Battery, which purportedly cured both blindness and deafness for a mere $10 (figure 488). The advertisement for his product read:

Physicians, Surgeons, and Oculists, from Galen down to the present time, have sought a remedy outside the Optician's skill, but have perfected none. Prof. Wilson, the Electrician . . . has discovered in 'Actina' the Odic-force and vitalizing influence, ever present in all forms of life, animal and vegetable, and after experiments upon himself and intimate friends is now in a position to meet any physician

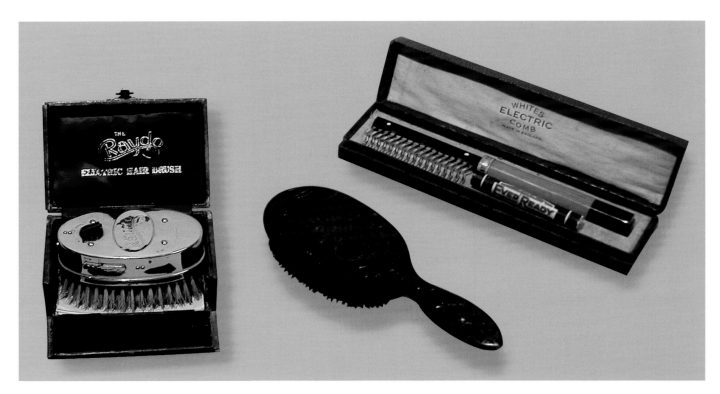

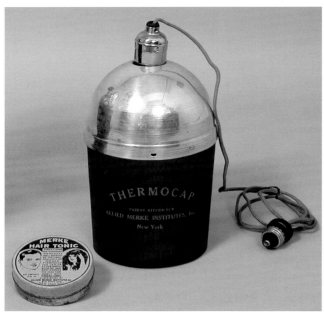

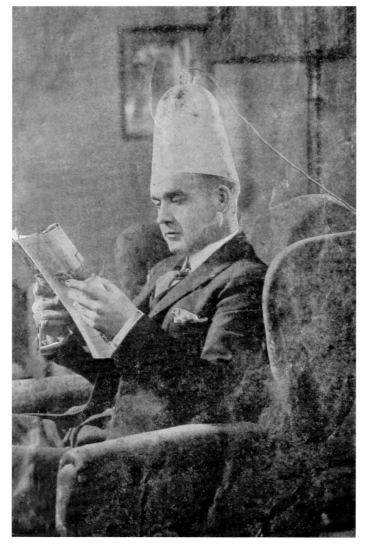

484. Top. Early twentieth-century magnetic and electric hair products: (left to right) Scott's magnetic hair brush with compass, Rayola Electric Hair Brush, White's Electric comb

485, 486. The Merke Thermocap by Allied Merke Institutes, Inc., New York, for hair growth (ca. 1920)

487. Opposite. Advertising card for products by the Dr. Scott's Electric Company (ca. 1900)

DR. SCOTT'S
ELECTRIC
CORSET.

DR. SCOTT'S
ELECTRIC
HAIR-BRUSH.

DR. SCOTT'S
ELECTRIC
HAIR-CURLER.

DR. SCOTT'S
ELECTRIC
TOOTH-BRUSH.

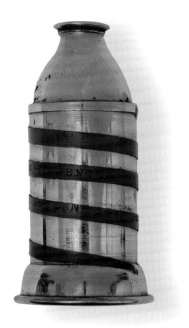

488. Actina by the New York & London Electric Association, Kansas City, Mo. (ca. 1910)

and explain the character of this great discovery. . . . The Electric Light and Telephone are mere toys in value compared with the wonderful 'Actina.' 'Oh, bosh!' say some of our thoughtless readers. But is it not a more useful and wonderful machine that will make the deaf hear and the blind see than all the steam engines and telephones? Yes, doubting reader, all is true we write and *hundreds of thousands so testify to the facts.*

Blindness, weakened vision or sore eyes:

Apply the eyecup first to one eye and then to the other, holding it to each eye until the current produces a decided burning sensation. After this, insert the small end into the nostrils and take as deep an inhalation as possible.

By this simple method Cataracts are absorbed, Abnormal growths removed, the Optic Nerve restored to healthy action, Granulated Lids and all forms of inflammation allayed, Nerves and Muscles made strong and healthy so that weakened vision cannot exist, rendering spectacles unnecessary, and all is accomplished by setting up and maintaining a perfect circulation of the blood in all parts of the eye and head. These are the certain results if the above directions are complied with at least six to twelve times daily, and as much oftener as possible.

The Actina was simply a small metal cylinder that contained a piece of muslin soaked in sassafras, mustard oil, belladonna extract, ether, and amyl nitrate. The device had to be sent back to the manufacturer three times a year to be recharged (for $1), and a "caution" was included in the package insert: "Do not allow any one under any circumstances to recharge your Actina. Our formula is a secret and we offer $1,000 to anyone who can give us the formula to Actina. Some druggists claim they can recharge our Actina—they cannot do so—and will only ruin your instrument, and perhaps put something in the Actina that will injure the eye." The pungent odor convinced the user of its effectiveness, though Samuel Hopkins Adams wrote in his expose "The Great American Fraud" in *Colliers,* "The Actina, upon being unpacked from the box in which it is mailed, comports itself like a decayed onion. It is worth the $10 to get away from the odor."

At the end of the nineteenth century, Dr. Hercules Sanche invented the Electropoise, claiming that it "forces oxygen into the blood stream," thereby treating any number of serious medical conditions (figures 489–492). Its successor was an 1896 upgrade aptly named the Oxydonor that contained a piece of carbon and sold for $35. The claim for this device was similar in that it "causes the human organism to thirst for

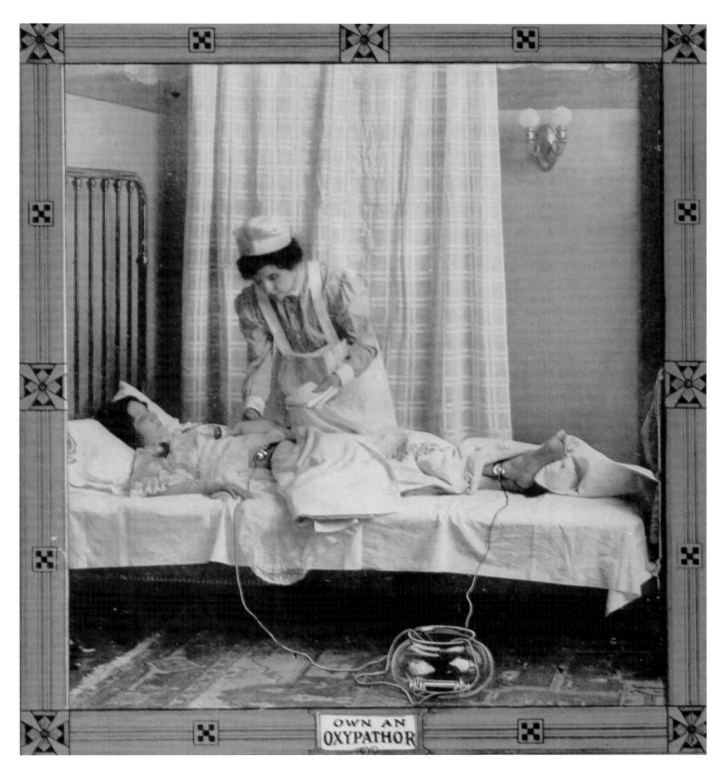

OWN AN
OXYPATHOR

and absorb oxygen, the true vitalizer of the blood, through pores in the skin." Other similar inventions, including the Oxygenator, were totally useless and provided an example of the worst in quackery since they sometimes delayed proper medical care. For example, the manufacturers of the Oxygenator offered parents false hope for the treatment of diphtheria, which is a devastating and potentially fatal disease in children.

489. Hospital use of the Oxypathor (ca. 1900)

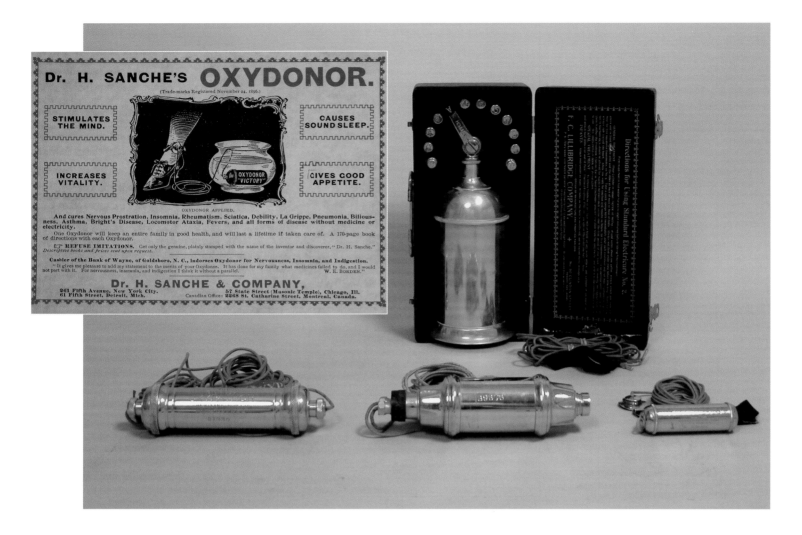

490. Above left. Advertisement of Dr. Sanche's Oxydonor (ca. 1900)

491. Above. Early twentieth-century "oxygenators": (top) Standard Electrocure No. 2 by FC Lillibridge Co., Newark; (bottom) Duplex Oxypathor by the Oxypathor Co., Buffalo, Farador by the Farador Co. of Canada, Ontario, Electropoise, Birmingham

492. Opposite. The Farador treatment at home (ca. 1910)

This was their outrageous claim: "Diphtheria. This overwhelming child's disease finds its supreme master in the Oxygenator. No earthly power except the Oxygenator can take the slowly choking child, and with speed, simplicity, and safety, bring it back to health. Don't jeopardize the health and life of your children by allowing to be injected into their veins and blood the often fearfully contaminated and death dealing serum of an animal, otherwise known as antitoxin."

A similar device sold in the early part of the twentieth century that had no therapeutic value was the Farador. It was manufactured in Canada and was touted to cure by "Thermo-magnetic Induction" such serious diseases as polio and appendicitis. According to the booklet accompanying the Farador, "Infantile Paralysis (Polio-Myelitis). In the first or acute stages of infantile paralysis the Farador operates with almost magical effect and has been the means of saving children from the paralysis and deformity that under treatment usually succeeds the acute condition." Regarding appendicitis, this disease is described as "an inflammation of the short blind duct, attached to the head of the colon or large intestine, in the lower right side of the abdomen. Abscess formation is seldom set up in a neg-

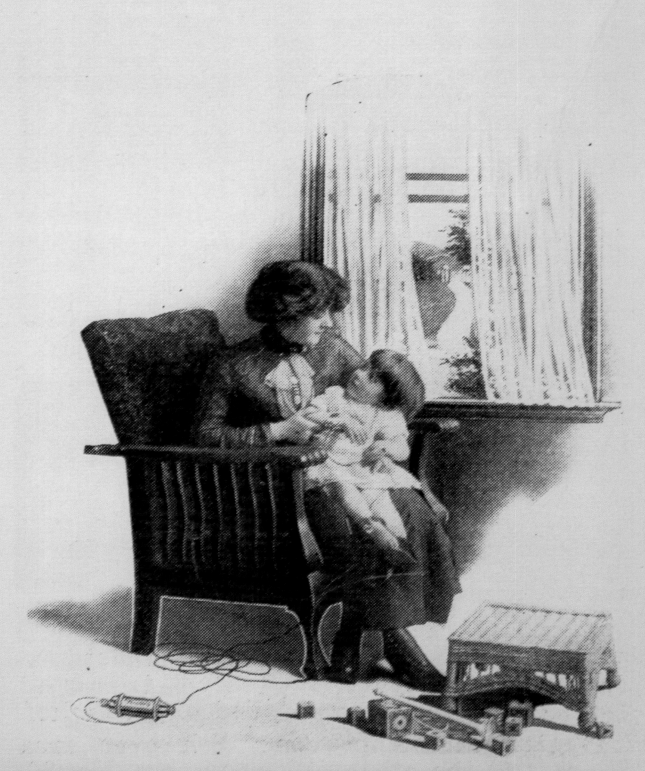

Children Especially Like the Farador Treatment. It makes Them Feel so Comfortable

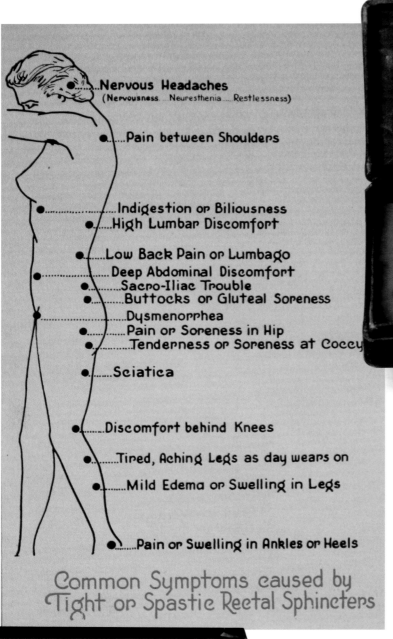

Nervous Headaches
(Nervousness Neuresthenia Restlessness)

Pain between Shoulders

Indigestion or Biliousness
High Lumbar Discomfort

Low Back Pain or Lumbago
Deep Abdominal Discomfort
Sacro-Iliac Trouble
Buttocks or Gluteal Soreness
Dysmenorrhea
Pain or Soreness in Hip
Tenderness or Soreness at Coccy

Sciatica

Discomfort behind Knees

Tired, Aching Legs as day wears on

Mild Edema or Swelling in Legs

Pain or Swelling in Ankles or Heels

Common Symptoms caused by
Tight or Spastic Rectal Sphincters

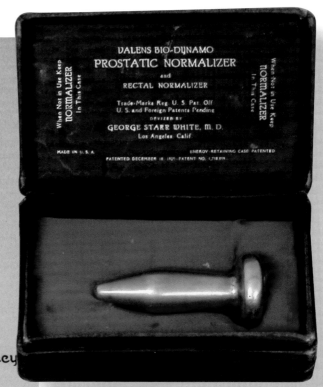

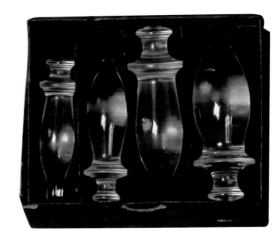

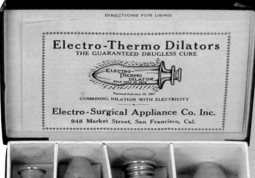

lected case within a week and with the Farador in hand when the symptoms first develop there is absolutely no danger. It is one of the easiest troubles to overcome that the Farador has to deal with."

Rectal dilators were popular in the early twentieth century, and were sold as a home device to treat any number of medical and neurological complaints, the theory being that the use of this product stimulated nerve pathways that controlled metabolic functions in various organ systems (figures 493, 494).

THE FUTURE?

All the devices previously mentioned had no scientific proof of efficacy and were marketed on the advice of a physician, manufacturer, or by the testimonial of a pleased customer. The irony of past quackery is that many abandoned practices are once again in vogue, including the use of leeches, magnets, and color therapy. Violet rays have been shown to be bacteriostatic and may be useful in treating lymphomas, electricity is used to increase circulation in diseased tissues, and leeches are beneficial in microsurgery. We await controlled studies and proof by use of the scientific method for guidance, though it is certain that until then there will always be those eager to find alternative and unproven forms of therapy. The following observation from *The Chirurgical Works of Percival Pott* (1778) remains germane: "The desire of health and ease, like that of money, seems to put all understandings, and all men upon a level; the avaricious are duped by every bubble; the lame and the unhealthy by every quack. Each party resigns his understanding; swallows greedily, and for a time believes implicitly the most groundless, ill-founded, and delusory promises. . . ."

493. Opposite. Manual for Young's Rectal Dilators (ca. 1920): Conditions related to the spastic rectal sphincter

494. Opposite. Early twentieth-century rectal dilators: (top) Young's Rectal Dilators by F.E. Young and Co., Chicago, Valens Bio-Dynamo Prostatic and Rectal Normalizer, George Starr White, MD, Los Angeles; (bottom) Curvlite glass rectal dilators and Electro-Thermo Dilators by the Electro-Surgical Appliance Co., Inc., San Francisco

"The whole problem with the world is that fools and fanatics are always so certain of themselves, but wiser people so full of doubts."

Bertrand Russell (1872-1970)

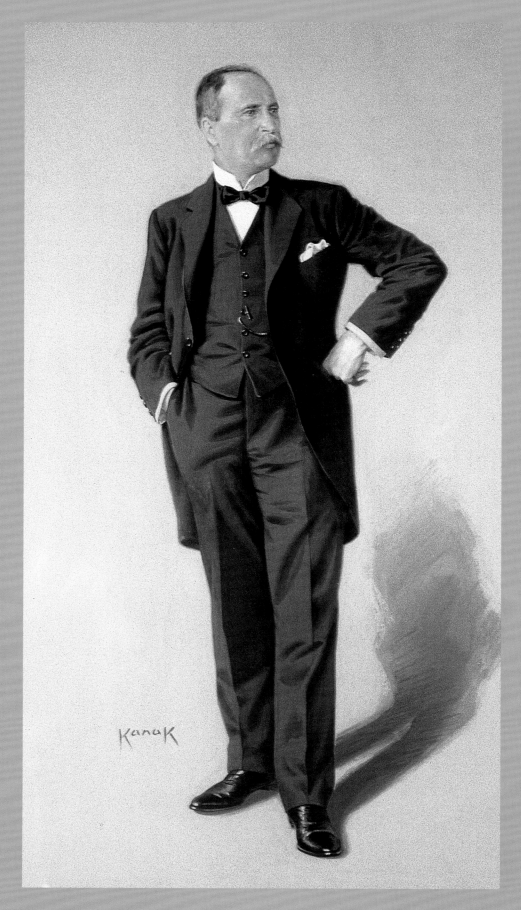

"It is easier to buy books than to read them. And easier to read them than to absorb them."
—William Osler, MD, *British Medical Journal,* 1909

GLOSSARY

Abbreviations for the glossary: G (Greek), F (French), L (Latin), and ME (Middle English)

abstract: a preparation made by mixing a powdered extract of a substance mixed with lactose

accoucheur: a male midwife

ague: intermittent chills and fever (as in malaria)

amalgam: a mixture of metals that usually includes mercury, from the Greek "malasso" meaning "to soften"

aneurism: a dilated artery

animalculist theory: the seventeenth-century belief that a totally preformed individual, called a homunculus, is produced by the male to become a fully formed individual

animism: the belief that evil spirits are the cause of disease

anodyne: a medication that soothes or relieves pain by causing sleep

antiphlogistic: anti-inflammatory

aperients: laxatives

aposteme: an abscess or a swelling filled with purulent matter

apoplexy: sudden paralysis, caused perhaps by a stroke or bleeding into the brain

astringent: an agent that arrests a discharge or contracts tissues

autointoxication: resorption of toxic substances from the bowel

axilla: the armpit

bad blood: syphilis

balm: a soothing ointment

balsam: an oily vegetable product

Black Death: bubonic plague

Bright's Disease: kidney disease that is accompanied by proteinuria and often kidney failure (described by Sir Richard Bright)

bubo: an inflamed lymph node

cadaver: a corpse

calculus: stone formed in the kidney

calomel: chloride of mercury used as a purgative

camp fever: typhus

carminative: medication that relieves gas in the alimentary tract

catamenia: menstruation

cataplexy: "shock" by fright

catarrh: upper-respiratory tract infection, mucous

cathartic: a purgative medication

caustics: substances that destroy tissue

cholera: any epidemic infectious disease characterized by diarrhea, vomiting, and cramps

chorea: jerky, involuntary movements; also called Saint Vitus Dance

cicatrize: to heal

clap, drip: gonorrhea

cinchonism: systemic effects of quinine overdose

clyster: an enema used for rectal administration of medications

collapse: failure of the vital powers

compound fracture: a broken bone protruding through the skin

consumption: tuberculosis

coryza: inflammation of the nose

couching: a cataract operation that displaces the lens into the vitreous

counterirritants: substances that irritate tissue to reduce discomfort in other areas

crisis: the turning point of a disease

debride: to remove contaminated or dead tissue

demulcent: mucilaginous substance allaying irritation

derivative bleeding: bleeding close to or over the diseased area

desiccants: substances that reduce secretions

discutient: an agent removing a swelling or effusion

diuretic: a medication that increases the flow of urine

douche: a stream of water directed against a part of the body

dropsy: fluid retention (from heart, liver, or kidney disease)

dysentery: intestinal inflammation leading to bloody evacuations

dystocia: difficult delivery

écorché: an anatomic model demonstrating musculature

elixir: a sweetened aromatic alcoholic preparation

emesis: vomiting

emollient: an agent that softens tissue

empyema: pus in the pleural cavity

emulsion: milky fluid obtained by suspending oil in water

epiglottitis: inflammation of the epiglottis (a cartilaginous plate over the larynx)

ergot: a parasitic fungus from rye used as a uterine stimulant

erysipelas: inflammation of the skin with fever, called Saint Anthony's Fire

erythema: redness of the skin

eschar: dry slough or crust of dead tissue

essence: inherent qualities of a drug

falling sickness: epilepsy

fester: (noun) a pustule or abscess; (verb) to suppurate or rot

fetid: having an offensive smell

fiacre: diseases of the rectum

first intention: healing of the lips of a wound by immediate union without suppuration

fistula-in-ano: an abnormal connection of the rectum to the skin surface resulting in a discharge of feces (also *ano-rectal fistula*)

fit: a convulsion

flux: a flow or discharge

French (or great) pox, lues: syphilis

furuncle: boil

Gallic disease: syphilis

gangrene: death of soft tissue

gangrene (dry): death of a part from insufficient blood

gangrene (hospital): contagious disease in crowded conditions where there is an absence of asepsis

gathering: an abscess

gleet: chronic gonorrhea

gravel: small kidney stones

gravid: pregnant

green sickness: anemia

grippe: influenza

hemolysis: the destruction of red cells

hemostasis: the arrest of bleeding

Hippocratic faces: pale, shrunken, and contracted features

homeopathy: a system of therapy using small doses of agents that cause symptoms similar to the diseases they treat

homunculus: a totally preformed individual produced by males

hydrops: fluid retention

hystera: the uterus or womb

hysteria: neurosis, paroxysms of abnormal behavior

humor: any secreted bodily fluid

hydrophobia: rabies (with apparent "fear of water")

ischemia: reduced blood flow

issue: caustic potash for use as a counterirritant

King's Evil: scrofula, or tuberculosis of the lymph nodes in the neck

laudable pus: purulent discharge from a wound—thought to be a good sign

laudanum: a pain medication composed of opium and alcohol

laughing gas: nitrous oxide

"mad as a hatter": mental changes from mercury poisoning (formerly used by hat makers)

liquor: a liquid solution

lockjaw: tetanus

lithotripsy: the act of crushing bladder stones

lithotomy: entering the bladder to remove a stone

lues: syphilis

lumbago: pain in the loins

mania: insanity

marasmus: wasting or emaciation

medicament: a medicine

member: any limb of the body

miasma: "diseased" air that causes illness

mortification: infection

moxa: inflammable matter used as a caustic

nostrom: a quack medication

oedema (edema): fluid retention and swelling

omentum: a fold of peritoneum that covers viscera

palsy: difficulty in muscular control

pap: bread, meal, and sugar soaked in wine, and fed to infants

percussion: diagnosis of an underlying condition by tapping the body

phlebotomy: the removal of blood

phlogistic: inflammatory

phrenology: a belief that the appearance of the skull reflects enlargements of parts of the brain, and thus reflects personality traits

physiognomy: the study of personality by body habitus

poultice: a soft emulsion for external application

puerperal fever: "childbed fever" or infection transmitted to the mother following delivery

physik: medication, or the practice of medicine

piles: hemorrhoids

plethora: abnormal fullness of the blood vessels

podagra: gout

Pott's disease: tuberculosis of the spine

proximal: toward the center of the body

puerperal fever: "childbed fever" or infection transmitted to the mother following delivery

pulsilogium: the first measuring device in medical history,

invented by Sanctrius of Padua (1561–1636) to represent the pulse rate as the length of a pendulum

purgative: an agent producing watery evacuation

putrid fever: diphtheria

quickening: the first fetal movement that occurs between the fourth and fifth month

quicksilver: mercury

quinsy: tonsillar abscess

râles: crackling sound heard in congested lungs

reins: kidneys

remitting fever: malaria

resurrectionist: a body snatcher

revulsive bleeding: bleeding far away from the diseased area

rubefacient: a counterirritant that reddens the skin

Saint Anthony's fire: contagious skin disease, erysipelas (hemolytic streptococcus)

Saint Vitas dance: involuntary jerking movements

saturnism: lead poisoning

scirrhus: indurated tissue, or tumor

scrofula: tuberculosis of the lymph nodes of the neck

second intention: healing of a wound with suppuration

seton: a strip of material threaded beneath the skin to produce a chronically draining tract for counter-irritation

shaking palsy: Parkinson's disease

ship's fever: typhus

sinapism: mustard plaster

spermatorrhea (onanism): nocturnal discharge, masturbation

strangury: painful urination in drops

styptic: an astringent or hemostatic

suppuration: the formation of pus

syncope: loss of consciousness

tertiary: the third phase of a disease (syphilis, for example)

tokology: the study of women's diseases

trepan: a large brace containing a cylindrical saw to enter the skull (also a verb)

trephine: a cylindrical saw for entering the skull cavity (also a verb)

uroscopy: observation of the characteristics of urine to determine a diagnosis

variolated: lesions resembling smallpox

venesection: bleeding

vesicant: a counterirritant that raises a blister

vitalism: the theory that an individual or animal's personality could perhaps be transferred by way of its blood

vivisection: dissection of living animals

yard: penis

MEDICAL INSTRUMENTS

basilyst: instrument used to break up the fetal head

bistoury: a long, narrow knife with a straight or curved blade for opening cavities. (F. bistouri, dagger)

bistoury cache: a spring loaded, double bladed instrument used in urology

bordeloue: a female urinal

bougie: a cylindrical instrument used for dilating tubular organs, such as the urethra or esophagus. (F. Bougie, an Algerian seaport from which candles were imported)

catlin: a long, double-edged knife, often used in amputations

cephalotribe: forcepslike instrument with a screw handle, used to crush the head in fetal abortion (G. kephale, the head + G. tribo, to bruise)

counterirritant: a substance or device that irritates one area of the body presumably to relieve pain in another part

cranioclast: a strong forceps used for crushing and extracting the fetal head after perforation (G. kranion, skull + G. klao, to break in pieces)

craniotomy forceps: forceps with a screw to crush the skull

crochet: a hooked instrument used for removing an aborted fetus (F. croche, hook)

cupping (wet and dry): the act of applying a heated cup to bring blood to the skin to act as a counterirritant (dry), or to bleed (wet)

dental key: a key-shaped instrument used to remove teeth

ecraseur: instrument used to crush tissue (F. ecraser, to crush)

elevator (dental or neurosurgical): instrument used to lift a tooth or piece of bone (L. e-levo, to lift up)

etui: a small pocket case for instruments (F.estuier, to preserve)

fleam: a sharp lancet for bloodletting (G. phleb, vein + tomon, to cut)

forceps: an instrument to grasp a structure for compression or traction (L. formus, hot + ceps, to take)

gorget: a director or guide with a wide groove used in lithitomy (ME. gorge, throat)

gutta-percha: a substance consisting of gutta hydrocarbon from Malaysian trees used in medical instruments

Hey's saw: neurosurgical instrument for removal of a section of the skull (Dr. William Hey)

ivorine: a trademark substance resembling ivory

lancet: a surgical knife with a short, wide, two-edged blade (F. lancette)

lithoclast (lithotrite): an instrument used to crush a urinary stone (G. lithos, stone + G. klastos, broken or L. tritus, to rub) ophthalmoscope: device for studying the interior of the eye through the pupil (G. ophthalmos relationship to the eye + G. skopeo, to examine)

otoscope: an instrument for examining the eardrum (G. ous, ear + G. skopea, to examine)

. . . otomy: (G. tomos, cutting)—craniotomy (G. kranion, skull), lithotomy (G. lithos, stone)

papboat: a boat-shaped dish used to hold pap (a soft food for infants) (L. pappa, food)

percussor: a small hammer used to tap part of the body in order to determine density (L. percussio, to beat)

pessary: an appliance introduced into the vagina to support the uterus (L. Pessarium, from G. pessos, an oval stone used in certain games)

perforator: obstetric instrument for making a bony opening through the cranium in abortion (L. perforare, to bore through)

pleximeter: an oblong plate placed on the body and struck with the percussor to determine density (G. plesso, to strike + metron , measure)

probang: a flexible rod with a soft tip used to advance or retrieve an esophageal foreign body (from proving, by inventor Walter Rumsey)

rachitome: instrument used for opening the spinal canal

scalpel: knife used in surgical dissection (L. scalprum, a knife)

scarificator: instrument used to make multiple superficial incisions in the skin for wet cupping (L. scarifico, to scratch)

seton needle: a straight blade used to introduce a material under the skin to act as a counterirritant (L. bristle)

shagreen: a dyed, untanned leather or sharkskin used for etuis or lancet cases

sound: an elongated, cylindrical instrument, used for exploring, dilating, or detecting a foreign body in a cavity or canal (usually urethra, or esophagus)

speculum: an instrument for opening a canal or cavity for inspection (L. a mirror, from specio to look at)

styptic: a device or instrument to stop bleeding (L. stypticus, to contract)

tenaculum: a hooked instrument used to hold a vessel that is to be tied off (L. teneo, to hold)

tortoise shell: horny (or artificial) plate from a turtle that was used in nineteenth-century instruments

trepan: a large brace with a bit for boring a hole in the cranium (also a verb) (G. trypanon, auger)

trephine: a T-shaped instrument used for removing a disk of bone, usually from the skull (also a verb) (L. tres fines, three ends)

trocar: a sharp instrument with a three cornered tip that fits into a cannula, used to remove fluid from a cavity (F. trocart, from trios, three, + carre, side of a sword blade)

vectis: a single bladed curved instrument used to aid in delivery (L. a lever or bar)

venesection: therapeutic bleeding (L. vena, vein + section, a cutting)

QUACK MEDICINE AND ELECTRICITY

arc light: light that is produced between two carbon electrodes after the application of an electric current

capacitor: device consisting of two conducting surfaces that permits the storage of electric charges

d'Arsonval current: a high-frequency, low-voltage current of comparatively high amperage

diathermy: therapeutic use of a high-frequency current, ultrasonic waves, or microwave radiation to generate heat within some part of the body

electrostatic generator (also static or influence machine): therapeutic device that creates static electricity, or a high-tension, direct current

faradic current: an intermittent, alternating current induced in the secondary winding of an induction coil

Galvanism: therapeutic use of direct current induced by a chemical reaction

high-frequency current: current having a frequency of interruption or change of direction sufficiently high so that tetanic contractions do not result when it is passed through living contractile tissues. The treatment is termed "medical diathermy" if the voltage is lower and if two electrodes are applied to the body rather than one

induction coil: transformer with open magnetic circuit, excited by an interrupted or variable current

infrared rays: radiations with wave lengths between 7,700 and 500,000 angstroms, just beyond the red end of the spectrum

leyden jar: glass jar partially coated with tinfoil that contains a salt solution that acts as a capacitor to accumulate electricity

low-frequency current: an alternating current of a frequency low enough to produce motor and sensory stimulation when passing through living tissue

ozone: a form of oxygen (O_3) that is produced by a static charge and was thought to have health benefits

radiotherapy: treatment of disease with roentgen rays, radium, ultraviolet, and other radiations

static electricity: electricity produced by friction

tension: synonym for voltage

tesla current: high-frequency current with voltage intermediate between an Oudin and d'Arsonval current

ultraviolet radiation: radiation ranging between 200 and
4,000 angstroms that is invisible and located in the electromagnetic spectrum between violet and roentgen rays

EARLY PRINTING TECHNIQUES

woodcut: The first reproducible picture was via the woodcut, a technique that allowed images to be used easily
with moveable type. Areas outside of a sketch drawn on
the side grain of wood were cut away with a sharp
knife, and the remaining flat surface was inked prior to
its use.

copperplate: The copperplate was first used in printing in
1523, and significantly improved the images that had
been produced by the woodcut. After the image was
engraved on the surface, the areas that were to remain
white were removed with a sharp implement while the
remainder was inked and printed. Pressure was required on the image, so there is a characteristic line of
indentation around the anatomic figures.

etching: The popular technique of etching was invented in
the 1630s, and the process began by covering a plate
with a coating of material that was resistant to acid.
Lines were drawn into that material, and the exposed
areas were removed by the acid, leaving a detailed
image.

mezzotint: This was a method of printing that involved
multiple layers of colors, proceeding from dark to light.
A metal plate was first abraded with a rocker, and then
areas of the plate were smoothed with a scraper. The
more the artist scraped, the lighter the tones became,
imparting effects of light and shadow, and making the
images appear similar to an oil painting.

. . . and Voltaire's (1694–1778) definition of physicians:
Doctors are men who prescribe medicines of which
they know little, to cure diseases of which they know
less, in human beings of whom they know nothing.

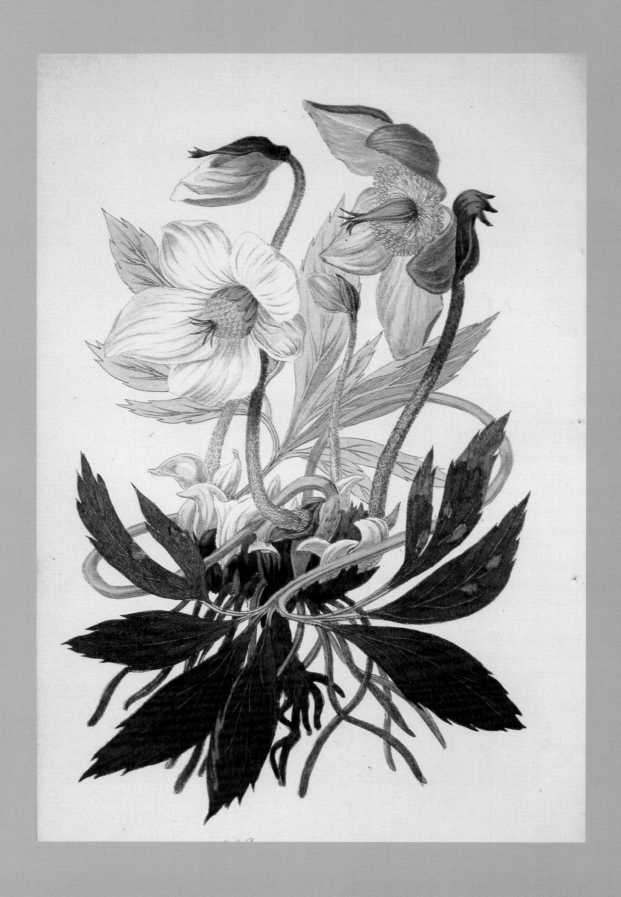

ILLUSTRATION CREDITS

Except for the figures noted below, the photographs of the instruments and art are from my personal collection.

I would like to thank the museums, art galleries, medical schools, and private collectors who have allowed their antiques and works of art to be reproduced in this book. Unless otherwise indicated, the numbers below refer to the figure numbers in the text:

Alex Peck Medical Antiques: 128

Art Resource: 1 Erich Lessing/Musée du Louvre, 21 and Anatomy introduction (detail) Scala/Mauritshuis, Haag, 41 Scala/Cigoli, Bargello, Florence 63 Scala/Museo Civico, Piacenza, Italy, 66 and Physical Diagnosis introduction (detail) Erich Lessing/Kunsthistorisches Museum, Vienna, 68 Sorbonne, Paris, Réunion dés Musees Nationaux, 74 and Book cover Erich Lessing/Kunsthistoriches Museum, Vienna, 78 Musée du Louvre, Paris, Réunion des Musées Nationaux, 105 Scala/Museo Archeologico Nazionale, Naples, 158 and Trauma introduction (detail) Erich Lessing/Museo del Prado, Madrid, 262 and back cover Musée Condé, Chantilly, France, 337 National Museum of American Art, Smithsonian Institution, Washington, Dentistry introduction

Biblioteca Apostolica Vaticana: 2

Cliché Bibliothéque national de France, Paris: 108

Biblioteca Universitá di Bologna. Riproduzione editoriale: 315

Boston Medical Library in the Francis A. Countway Library of Medicine: 147

Bridgeman Art Library: 52 Galleria Borghese, Rome, 56 Musée d'Histoire de la Medicine, Paris, 102 Musée du Louvre, Paris, 109 Koninklijk Museum voor Schine Kunsten, Antwerp, 264 and medicine introduction (detail)

© Christie's Images Limited: 8–11, 45, 46, 59

Chrysler Museum of Art, Norfolk, Va., gift of Walter P. Chrysler Jr. (71.480): 110.

Clendening History of Medicine Library, University of Kansas Medical Center: 39, 201, 253, 282

Collection of the New-York Historical Society: 89

Deutsches Museum: 240

German Museum of the History of Medicine in Ingolstadt: 365

Jefferson College, Philadephia: 140 and general surgery introduction (detail)

John Martin Rare Book Room, Hardin Library for the Health Sciences, University of Iowa: 15, 16

Massachusetts General Hospital, Archives and Special Collections, on loan to the Fogg Museum 1979-1 MGH-1: 148

Museo di Storia Naturale Universitá di Firenze, "La Specola": 42, 44, 198, 218

National Library of Medicine: 13, 14, 17, 234, 596

National Museum of Dentistry, Baltimore, Md.: 343, 365 (Bundersverband der Deutschen

Zahnarzte), 377, 385, 389 (on exhibit at the Dr. and Mrs. Edwin F. Weaver, III Historical Dental Museum at the Temple University School of Dentistry), 393

The National Museum of Health and Medicine, Armed Forces Institute of Pathology, Washington, DC (M-129 00079): 125, 127

Oak Ridge Associated Universities: 476

Reynolds Historical Library, the University of Alabama at Birmingham: 73, 112, 136, 151, 155, 159

The Rijksmuseum, Amsterdam: 370

The Royal Collection © 2000, Her Majesty Queen Elizabeth II: 5, 6, 7, 193, 194 and Obstetrics and Gynecology introduction (detail)

© The Royal College of Surgeons of England (by kind permission of the President and Council): 111, 114

Science Museum/Science and Society Picture Library: 69, 92, 214, 259,263, 274, 281, 308, 317, 318, 358, 375, 376, 399, 427, 470

Semmelweis Museum, Budapest: 43

Smithsonan Institution's Division of Science, Medicine and Society: 18, 48, 84, 197, 280, 333

Stanley B. Burns and the Burns Archive: 49, 62, 70, 88, 119, 127, 173, 174, 176, 177, 178, 239, 270, 272, 273, 364, 443, 444

Swanson, Jr., Ben Z., DDS, Baltimore, MD: 394.

© The Trustees of the British Museum: 220 and urology introduction

Universiteitsmuseum Utrech: 58

The Warren Anatomical Museum,
Francis A. Countway Library of
Medicine: 146

Wellcome Library, London: 3, 12, 19,
20, 26, 27, 28, 29, 30, 31, 32, 40, 50, 53,
54, 65, 79 and bleeding introduction
(detail), 90, 93, 100, 101, 103, 104, 141,
143, 195, 196, 199, 205, 236, 245, 254,
260, 261, 265, 268, 283, 285, 303, 307,
316, 355, 356, 366, 369, 383, 397, 423
and quack medicine introduction
(detail), 436, praying skeleton (appreciation), caricature of Sir William
Osler (across from glossary), kneeling
skeleton (bibliography)

William P. Didusch Museum of the
American Urological Association: 480

Yale University, Harvey Cushing/John
Hay Whitney Medical Library: 4, 76

Zentralbibliothek Zürich: 77

Captions

Page 572. Caricature of Sir William
Osler, watercolor gouache by Kanak
(1914)

Page 578. *Helleborus Niger* from
*Medical Botany: or, Illustrations and
Descriptions of the Medicinal Plants of
the London, Edinburgh, and Dublin
Pharmacopoeias* (1828) by John
Stephenson, MD and James
Churchill, FLS

Page 581. Kneeling skeleton from
*Nouveau recueil d'Ostéologie et de myolo-
gie* (1779) by Jacques Gamelin

Page 584. Autographed photograph of
Sir William Osler, Baltimore (ca 1900)

Page 594. Dance of death from
*Nouveau recueil d'ostéologie et de myolo-
gie* (1779) by Jacques Gamelin

BIBLIOGRAPHY

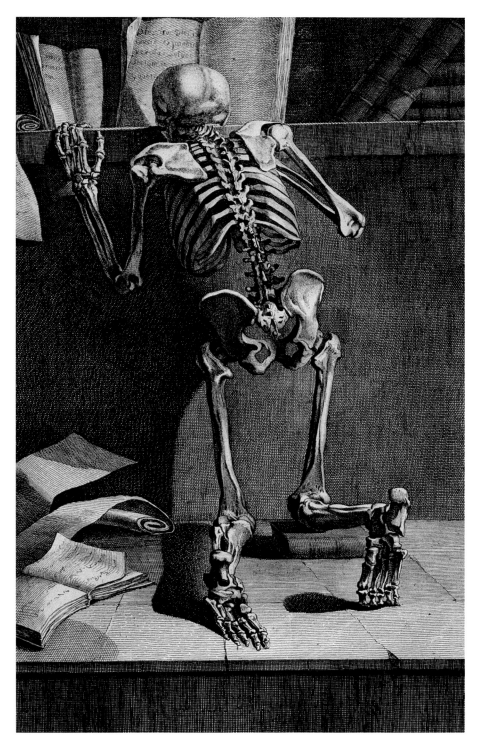

Ackerknecht, E. *A Short History of Medicine.* Baltimore and London: Johns Hopkins University Press, 1982.

Aubry, A. *Catalogue Illustre des Instruments de Chirurgie.* Paris, 1900.

Bellar, S. *Medical Practices in the Civil War.* Cincinnati: Betterway Books, 1992.

Bender, G. *Great Moments in Medicine.* Detroit: Parke-Davis, 1961.

Bennion, E. *Antique Hearing Devices.* London: Vernier Press, 1994.

Bennion, E. *Antique Medical Instruments.* London: Philip Wilson Publishers, Ltd., 1980.

Bettmann, O. *A Pictorial History of Medicine.* Illinois: Charles C. Thomas, 1956.

Burns, S. *A Morning's Work: Medical Photographs from the Burns Archive and Collection, 1843–1939.* Santa Fe, New Mexico: Twin Palms, 1998.

Carmichael, A., and Ratzan, R. *Medicine: A Treasury of Art and Literature.* New York: Hugh Lauter Levin Associates, Inc., 1991.

Castiglioni, A. *A History of Medicine.* New York: Jason Aronson, Inc., 1975.

Dammann, G. *Pictorial Encyclopedia of Civil War Medical Instruments and Equipment.* 3 Vols. Montana: Pictorial Histories Publishing Company, 1983, 1994, and 1997.

Davidson, D.C. *Spectacles, Lorgnettes, and Monocles.* Great Britain: Shire Publications, Ltd, 1989.

Davis, A., and Appel, T. *Bloodletting Instruments in the National Museum of History and Technology.* Washington, DC: Smithsonian Institution Press, 1979.

Davis, A., and Dreyfuss, M. *The Finest Instruments Ever Made*. Massachusetts: Medical History Publishing Associates I, 1986.

Davis, D. *The Principles and Practice of Obstetric Medicine*. 2 vols. London: Taylor and Watson, 1836.

Denny, R. *Civil War Medicine: Care and Comfort of the Wounded*. New York. Sterling Publishing Co., Inc., 1994.

Duffin, J. *History of Medicine: A Scandalously Short Introduction*. Toronto, Buffalo: University of Toronto Press, 2001.

Düring, M., Didi-Huberman, G., and Poggesi, M. *Encyclopaedia Anatomica*, Germany: Taschen, 1999.

Edmonson, J., and Hambrecht, F.T. *American Armementarium Chirurgicum*. San Francisco and Boston: Norman Publishing and the Printers Devil, 1989.

Edmonson, J. *American Surgical Instruments*. San Francisco: Norman Publishing, 1997.

Garrison, F. *An Introduction to the History of Medicine*. Philadelphia: W.B. Saunders, 1929.

Gordon, R. *Great Medical Disasters*. New York: Dorset Press, 1986.

Gordon, R. *The Alarming History of Medicine*. New York: St. Martin's Griffin, 1993.

Gould, G. *Gould's Pocket Pronouncing Medical Dictionary*. Philadelphia: P. Blakiston, Son and Co., 1892

Gove, P. (editor). *Webster's Third New International Dictionary*. Massachusetts: Haeger, K. *The Illustrated History of Surgery*. New York: Bell Publishing Company, 1988.

Haggard, H. *Devils, Drugs, and Doctors*. New York: Blue Ribbon Books, Inc., 1929.

Haggard, H. *The Doctor in History*. New York: Dorset Press, 1989.

Haggard, H. *The Lame, the Halt, and the Blind*. New York: Harper and Brothers, 1932.

Haggard, H. *Mystery, Magic, and Medicine*. New York: Doubleday, Doran and Company, Inc., 1933.

Hansen, J., and Porter, S. *The Physician's Art: Representations of Art and Medicine*. North Carolina: Duke University Medical Center Library and Duke University Museum of Art, 1999.

Holbrook, S. *The Golden Age of Quackery*. New York: Macmillan, 1959.

Jones, W. and Withington, E. (trans.). *Hippocrates*. 4vols. London: Heinemannn, 1923–1931.

Kail, A. *The Medical Mind of Shakespeare*. Australia: Williams and Wilkins, 1986.

Kemp, M., and Wallace, M. *Spectacular Bodies: The Art and Science of the Human Body from Leonardo to Now*. California: Haywood Gallery and the University of California Press, 2000.

Kennedy, M. *A Brief History of Disease, Science, and Medicine*. Rhode Island: Writers' Collective, 2004.

Kuz, J., and Bengtson, B. *Orthopaedic Injuries of the Civil War*. Georgia: Kennesaw Mountain Press, Inc., 1996.

Lanza, B. *Le Cere Anatomiche della Specola*. Firenze: Arnaud Edifore, 1997.

Leavitt, J.W. *Typhoid Mary: Captive to the Public's Health*. Boston: Beacon Press, 1996.

Lyons, A. and Petrucelli, R. J. *Medicine: An Illustrated History*. New York: Harry N. Abrams, Inc., 1987.

Major, R. *Classic Descriptions of Disease*. Illinois and Baltimore: Charles C Thomas, 1932.

Margotta, R. *The Story of Medicine*. New York: Golden Press, 1967.

Margotta, R. *The History of Medicine*.

New York: Smithmark Publishers, 1996.

Massengill, S. *A Sketch of Medicine and Pharmacy*. Tennessee: S.E. Massengill Company, 1943.

Mettler, C. *History of Medicine*. Philadelphia and Toronto: Blakiston Company, 1947.

Mould, R. *Mould's Medical Anecdotes*. Bristol and Philadelphia: Institute of Physics Publishing, 1996.

Nasr, S. *Science and Civilization in Islam,* 2nd ed. Cambridge: Islamix Texts Society, 1987.

Norman, J.M. (editor). *Morton's Medical Bibliography*. 5th ed. Vermont: Gower Publishing Company, 1991.

Norman, H. *One Hundred Books Famous in Medicine*. New York: Grolier Club, 1995.

Novotny, A., and Smith, C. *Images of Healing*. New York and London: Macmillan, 1980.

Nuland, S. *Medicine: The Art of Healing*. New York: Hugh Lauter Levin Associates, Inc., 1992.

O'Malley, C., and Saunders, J.B. *Leonardo da Vinci on the Human Body*. New York: Henry Schuman, 1952.

Panati, C. *Panati's Extraordinary Endings of Practically Everything and Everybody*. New York: Harper and Row, 1989.

Pettigrew, T.J. *On Superstitions connected with the history and practice of Medicine and Surgery*. London: John Churchill, 1844.

Porter, R. *Cambridge Illustrated History of Medicine*. Cambridge: Cambridge University Press, 1996.

Roddin, A., and Key, J. *Medicine, Literature, and Eponyms*. Malabar, Florida: Robert E. Krieger Publishing Company, 1989.

Root-Bernstein, R., and M. *Honey, Mud, Maggots, and Other Medical Marvels*. Boston: Houghton Mifflin, 1998.

Rousselot, J. *Medicine in Art: A Cultural History*. New York: McGraw-Hill, 1967.

Rutkow, I. *American Surgery: An Illustrated History*. Philadelphia: Lippincott-Raven, 1998.

Rurkow, I. *Surgery: An Illustrated History*. St. Louis: C.V. Mosby, 1993.

Sandbloom, P. *Creativity and Disease*. Philadelphia: G.B. Lippincott Company, 1989.

Sappol, M., and Mullen, E. *Dream Anatomy Exhibition*. Bethesda, Maryland: National Library of Medicine, 2002–2003.

Savitt, T. *Fevers, Agues, and Cures*. Virginia: Virginia Historical Society, 1990.

Stedman, T. *Stedman's Medical Dictionary*. 27th ed. Philadelphia: Lippincott Williams and Wilkins, 1999.

Thompson, C.J.S. *The History and Evolution of Surgical Instruments*. New York: Schuman, 1942.

Tonkelaar, I., Henkes, H. and van Leersum, G. *Eye and Instruments*. Amsterdam: Batavian Lion, 1996.

Weir, N. *Otolaryngology: An Illustrated History*. Cambridge: Butterworth and Company, Ltd.,1990.

Wilbur, C.K. *Antique Medical Instruments*. Philadelphia: Schiffer Publishing Ltd., 1987.

Wilbur, C.K. *Civil War Medicine, 1861–1865*. Connecticut: Globe Pequot Press, 1998.

Wilbur, C.K. *Revolutionary Medicine, 1700–1800*. Connecticut: Globe Pequot Press, 1980.

Wocher, M., and Son. *Surgical Instruments*. Cincinnati, 1904.

Youngson, A.J. *The Scientific Revolution in Victorian Medicine*. New York: Holmes and Meier Publishers, Inc., 1979.

Zimmerman, L.M., and Veith, I. *Great Ideas in the History of Surgery*. Baltimore: Williams and Wilkens Company, 1961.

PHARMACY

Bingham, A.W. *The Snake-Oil Syndrome: Patent Medicine Advertising*. Massachusetts: Christopher Publishing House, 1994.

Cowen, D., and Helfand, W. *Pharmacy: An Illustrated History*. New York: Harry N. Abrams, Inc., 1990.

Mathews, L. *Antiques of the Pharmacy*. London: G. Bell and Sons, 1971.

Richardson, L., and Richardson, C. *The Pill Rollers*. Virginia: Old Fort Press, 1992.

DENTISTRY

Bennion, E. *Antique Dental Instruments*. London: Sotheby's Philip Wilson Publishers, Ltd., 1986.

Glenner, R., Davis, A., and Burns, S. *The American Dentist*. Montana: Pictorial Histories Publishing Company, 1990.

Glenner, R. *The Dental Office: A Pictorial History*. Montana: Pictorial Histories Publishing Company, 1985.

Ring, M. *Dentistry: An Illustrated History*. New York: Harry N. Abrams, Inc., 1985.

White, S.S. *Catalogue of Dental Materials, Furniture, Instruments, etc.*, Philadelphia, 1876.

Wynbrandt, J. *The Excruciating History of Dentistry*. New York: St. Martin's Griffin, 1998.

QUACK MEDICINE

Armstrong, D., and E. *The Great American Medicine Show*. New York: Prentice Hall, 1991.

McCoy, B. *Quack! Tales of Medical Fraud from the Museum of Questionable Medical Devices*. Santa Monica: Santa Monica Press, LLC, 2000.

And finally, my use of the Internet was extensive over a four-year period, and that material supplemented information in almost every chapter of this book. My thanks (and apologies) to the many hundreds not referenced above. Quotes taken from original sources are noted in the text.

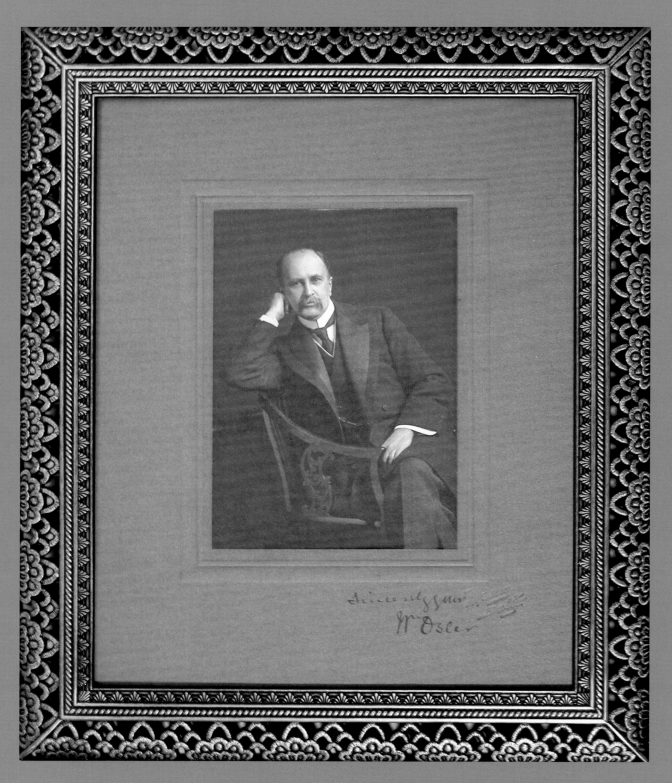

"To study the phenomena of disease without books is to sail an uncharted sea, while to study books without patients is not to go to sea at all."

—William Osler, MD, *Books and Men*, Boston Medical Surgical Journal, 1901

INDEX

Note: Illustrations are in **bold face.**

A

Abortion
    Definitions of life and death 261-263
    Medical 263
    Surgical 263-267, **264-265**
Abrams, Albert, "King of the Quacks"
    544-547, **545**
Actina 563-**566**
Acupuncture **329**
Adams, Samuel Hopkins, and "The Great
    American Fraud" 447-450
Aderlasskalender, and a calendar for blood-
    letting 337
Aegineta, Paulus, and polyp removal with
    the cautery 318
Aeneas, fresco from Pompeii **129**
Aesculapius – see Asklepios
Albarello jars **445-446**
Albinus, Bernhardus Siegfried, and
    Tabulae Sceleti e Musculorum Corporis
    Humani **32**
Albucasis in *Altasrif*
Allbutt, Thomas Clifford, and the ther-
    mometer 65
Amalgam Wars of 1840-1850 471-473
Amputation
    Circular 145-146, **147, 148**
    Civil War 221-224
    Excision 151-153, **152, 153**
    Flap 148-150, **149**
Anatomic models
    Auzoux paper-mache **42, 43**
    Bronze statuette by Cigoli **40**
    Dental **469-470**
    Flap anatomy 43-44
    Ivory model by Stephan Zwick 37, **40**
    Wax models at *La Specola* 37, **40, 41,**
    245, 272
    Wax models by Emil Kotschi and G.
    Zeiller 40-**41**
    Wax models by Gactano Zumbo and
    Clemente Susini 37
Anatomy

Dental **467-470**
Embalming 52-55
Microscopic 47-52
Models 37-43
Postmortem instruments 46-47
Renaissance art 10-23
Andry, Nicolas, and women's contribu-
    tion to the fetus 240-246
Anesthesia
    Chloroform 190-196
    Civil War 228
    Cocaine 175, 196-197
    Controversies 190-195
    Ether 180-189, **182, 184**
    Local anesthesia 196-197
    Mandragora (mandrake) 174-175
    Mastectomy **176,** 177-178
    Nitrous oxide 178-180
    Opium 173
Animism and the causes of disease 134
Apothecary trade 408-**409**
Aretaeus of Cappadocia
    Diabetes 402
    Diphtheria 318-321
    Female hysteria 516
    Liver disease 398
    Tetanus 377-**378**
    Tracheotomy 321-322
Asepsis
    Civil War 219-221, 227-228
    Lister, Joseph 170
    Surgical 164-171
Ashhurst, John, and the horrors of ampu-
    tation 150-151
Asklepios (Roman: Aesculapius)
    Bust **ii**
    Cesarean section 257
    Legend **333-334**
    Statue **333**
Astruc, John, and objection to the theory
    of infectious disease 351
Atkinson, and opposition to anesthesia
    194-195
Auenbrugger, Leopold, and auscultation
    71-72

Auscultation 66-71
Auzoux, Louis Thomas Jerôme
    Embryos **245**
    Female abdominal anatomy **41**
    History 40
    Male and female models **42-43**
Avicenna and *The Canon of Medicine*
    Bloodletting
        Indications 85-86
        Risks 91-92
    Cupping 112
    Manuscript page **407**
    Purging 393
    Surgery 132
Ayurveda, Indian medicine
    Charaka 332
    Doshas 59, 330-332
    Gem therapy 410
    Reproduction 240-242
    Susruta
        Hemostasis 164
        Rhynoplasty 211-**212**
    Tibetan (Hindu) medicine 332
    Tongue diagnosis 58-60

B

Bacon, Roger, and the use of spectacles in
    Opus Majus 311
Baltimore College of Dental Surgery 469
Barber-surgeons 132-141
Bard, Samuel, and *A Discourse upon the*
    Duties of a Physician 3
Bartisch, Georg, and *Das ist Augendienst*
    Cataract surgery **300**
    Spectacles **309**
Baunscheidism, and counterirritation 117-121
Beethoven, Ludwig van , and loss of hear-
    ing 315
Bell, Alexander Graham, and President
    Garfield's assassination 215-216
Bell, Benjamin
    Criticism of Frère Jacques in *A System*
    of Surgery 285
    Head trauma 204
Bell, Charles, and neuroanatomy 29, 31

Bell, John
  Artists' role in *Engraving of the Bones, Muscles, and Joints* 20-21
  The Principles of Surgery
    Nasal packing **317**
    Sepsis and its consequences 170
Bell, Joseph, and physical examination 61
Belladonna 416-**417**
Benedetti, Alessandro, and dissecting techniques in *The History of the Human Body* 13-14
Bhaisajyaguru, the medicine Buddha Thangka **331**
Bible
  Anesthesia in Genesis (2:21and 3:16) 192-193
  Caduceus in Numbers (21:8) 334
  Circumcision in Exodus (4:25) 124-127
  Hygiene in Leviticus (25:1-13) 165
  Leprosy in Leviticus (13:1-46) 348
  Liver forecast in Ezekiel (21:21) 58
  Onanism in Genesis (38:8-10) 557
  Urine therapy in Proverbs (5:15) 412
Bibliography 581-583
Bichat, Xavier, and a defense of abortion in *Physiological Researches upon Life and Death* 260-261
Bidloo, Govert
  Anatomia humani corporis 27-29
  Abdominal anatomy **29**
  Muscles of the arm **28**
    Skeletal system **28**
Black, Greene Vardiman, "Father of Modern Operative Dentistry" 487
Blood, uses for 106-108
Bloodletting
  Derivative and revulsive 88
  Eye diseases 306-307
  George Washington 100-103
  Indications 85-91
  Instrumentation **98-100**
  Leeches, in *A General System of Surgery* by Laurence Heister 94-97, **95, 96**
  Methods, in *A Treatise on Operative Surgery* by Joseph Pancoast 87
  Risks
    Avicenna, *The Canon of Medicine* 91-92
    Heister, *General System of Surgery* 93-94
    Maimonides page 92-93

Treatment of King Charles II 93
Blundell, James, and transfusion 106-**107**
Board, Ernest, and dissection performed by Mondino de Cuzzi **6**
Boerhaave, Hermann in *Aphorisms: Concerning the Knowledge and Cure of Diseases*
  Abortion 263
  Circular amputation 145-146
  Colic 391
  Determination of fetal demise 262-263
  Empyema 383
  Head trauma 204-205
  Kidney stones and medical treatment 279
  Normal anatomy and physiology 29
  Of Belchings and Winds 391-392
  Pneumonia 382-383
Borelli, Giovanni
  De Motu Animalium **31**
  Mechanical view of anatomy 29
Botany, medical
  Dangerous substances 429-433
  Early Eastern and Asian herbs 413-415
  Medicinal herbs in *Medical Botany: or, Illustrations and Descriptions of the Medicinal Plants of the London, Edinburgh, and Dublin Pharmacopoeias* by Stephenson and Churchill **417-428**
  Strange ingredients 409-413
Bourgery, JM, and *Traité complet d'anatomie de l'homme* second edition (1866-1871) 32
  Back muscles **34**
  Bloodletting from the extremities **90**
  Bloodletting from the head and neck **89**
  Bone excision **152**
  Cataract surgery **303**
  Chest and abdomen **36**
  Circular amputation **147**
  Dental extraction **478**
  Dupuytren's double bistoury caché **276**
  Ear **294-295, 314**
  Exploded skull **34**
  Facial anatomy **296**
  Facial muscles **34**
  Flap amputation **149**
  Head hemi-section **vii**
  Lithotripsy with bow Civiale **286**

Mastectomy **176**
Muscles of the eyes **298**
Neck sectioned **312**
Renal system **273**
Rhinoplasty **212**
Seton needle **116**
Tourniquet **163**
Trepanning **203**
Venous system of the shoulder **35**
Boyd's galvanic battery 524-**526**
Brady, Matthew, photograph **54**
Bright, Richard in *Guy's Hospital Reports, Cases and Observations* and renal failure **290**, 291-293
Brinkley, John, "the Goat Gland Doctor" 560-563
Brown Gustavus, and George Washington's death 100-103
Browne, John, and *A compleat treatise of the muscles, as they appear in the humane body, and arise in dissection* 21, **23**
Brueghel the Elder, Peter, *The Triumph of Death* 326-327, 342-343
Bullein, William, and description of a surgeon in *Bullein's Bulwarke Of Defence Againste All Sicknes, Sores, And Woundes* 123
Bullock, Walter, microscopes **51-52**
Bunts, Frank Emory, and early aseptic technique 171-173, **172**
Burke, William, and anatomic specimens 44-46
Burney, Fanny, and mastectomy in "journals and letters" 177-178
Burr, Richard, embalmer **54**

C

Caduceus 334
Canon of Medicine, see Avicenna
Cartier, Jacques, and the anatomy of scurvy in *The Principall Navigations, Voyages, Traffiques and Discoveries of the English Nation Made by Sea or Over-land to the Remote and Farthest Distant Quarters of the Earth at Any Time Within the Compasse of These 1600 Yeeres* 15
Carwardine, H.H., and the discovery of Chamberlen's lost forceps 254-255
Casseri, Giulio Cesare, *Tabulae anatomicae* 21, **22**
Cataracts

Medical therapy 299, 412
Surgery 299-306, **300, 301, 303, 304**
Cathell, Daniel, on instrumentation in *The Physician Himself* 49, 52
Catlin, George, *White Buffalo, an Aged Medicine Man (Blackfoot)* **436**
Cattell, Henry
Embalming of Willie Lincoln 53
Post-mortem Pathology: a manual of post-mortem examinations… 46, **47**
Cautery in surgery 161-**162**
Dental instrumentation 477
Otolaryngology, surgical 311
Surgery **131**-132
Celsus, Aulus Cornelius, in *De Medicina*
Attributes of a good surgeon **173-175**
Circular amputation **145**
Dissection 7
Inflammation **164**
Poppy 415-416
Toothache therapy 461
Cesarean section 257-**258**
Chamberlen, Hugh, and obstetric forceps 255-256
Chamberlen, Peter, and obstetric forceps 252-255
Charles II, King, and his medical care 93
Chartran, Theobald and Rene Laennec at the Necker hospital **68**
Chaucer, Geoffrey, and astrology in medicine **336**-337
Cheselden, William
Bladder catheterization 284
Osteographia 31, **32**
Lithotomy 286
Praying skeleton **iv**
Chinese medicine **328**-330
Chloroform 190-195
Cigoli, Ludovico, and bronze statuette **40**
Cinnabar 410
Circular amputation 145-148, **147**
Circumcision 124-127, **125**
Civil War medicine 216-237
Ambulance corps 231-232
Amputation 221-224
Anesthesia 228
Death toll 218-219
Medical advances 236-237
Surgical conditions 219-221
Clarke, W. Mitchell on bleeding 121
Clowes, William

Cautery 161
Criticism of barber-surgeons 139
Clyster
Hindu medicine 395
Hippocrates 395
Louis XI and XIII 395-**397**
Coca Cola, and John Pemberton 431-433
Cocaine
Anesthesia 175, 196-197
Coca Cola 431-433
Ophthalmology 196-197, 431
Robert Louis Stevenson 430
Sigmund Freud 430-431
Cold Harbor, Virginia
Civil War Battle 228-236
Letters
Merari 234-236
Thomas FW 232-233
Political implications 231
Coleridge, Samuel Taylor, and nitrous oxide 180
Contraria contrariis 84
Cooper, Richard Tennant, and *Diphtheria Trying to Strangle a Small Child* **319**
Corvisart, Jean Nicolas, and percussion 72
Cosmas and Damian, Saints
Transplantation 132-134. **133**
Uroscopy **73**
Counterirritaton
Blisters and caustics 109-110
Cupping 110-114
Definition and methods 108-109
Lebenswecker 117-121
Function 117-119
Testimonials 120-121
Seton needle 114-**117, 116**
Cowper, William
Anatomy 27-28
Title page of *The anatomy of humane bodies* **30**
Craik, James, and George Washington's death 100-103
Crawcour brothers, and dental amalgam 471-472
Crumpe, Samuel, and *An Inquiry into the Nature and Properties of Opium* 429-430
Cruveilhier, J., and *Anatomia Pathologique du corps Humain*
Dislocated femur **209**
Dysentery **363**
Fractured femur **208**

Pneumonia **382**
Puerperal fever **370**
Typhoid enteritis **365**
Typhoid, follicular **364**
Culpeper, Nicholas, and *Culpeper's School of Physick*
Cataracts 299
Earache 313
Hemorrhoids 398-399
Kidney stone therapy 278-279
Medical therapy of venereal disease 272
Nosebleed 317
Tooth pain 462
Tuberculosis 362
Urinary obstruction 272-**277**
Urine therapy 412-413
Cupping
Description 110-112
Diseases to be cupped in *A Treatise on the Art of Cupping* by Thomas Mapleson 110-111
Hyperemic therapy 114, **115**
Methods in *A General System of Surgery* by Laurence Heister 111-112
Monson Hills and patients' concerns 156-157
Risks in *The Canon of Medicine* by Avicenna 112

D

D'Agoty, Jacques Fabien Gautier 31-32
Circle of Willis in *Exposition anatomique des organs des sens…* **297**
Female anatomy in *Anatomie des parties de la génération de l'homme et de la femme* **33**
Female muscles of the back in *Myologie complette en couleur et grandeur naturelle composée de l'essai et de la suite de l'essai d'anatomie* **33**
Female with child in *Anatomie des parties de la génération de l'homme et de la Femme* **244**
Male anatomy in *Anatomie des parties de la génération de l'homme et de la femme* **33**
Muscular anatomy of the head in *Anatomie de la tête en tableux* **33**
Da Cortona, Pierto, and *Tabulae anatomicae* 21, **23**

Darwin, Charles, and anesthesia 178

Davey, Humphrey, and nitrous oxide 178-179

Da Vinci, Leonardo
 Anatomic advice 10-13
 Sketches
  Gravid uterus **238-239, 243**
  Muscles of the arm **11**
  Principal organs **11**
  Procreation 240, **242**
  Skeleton **12**

Davis, D., and *The Principles and Practice of Obstetric Medicine*
 Abortion with crochet forceps **265**
 Abortion with Ramsbothan cranioclast **264**

Deafness
 Hearing aids **315-316**
 Medical treatment 412

De Beaulieu, Jacques (Frère Jacques) 284-286

De Cervantes, Miguel, and the Helmet of Membrino 98

De Goya y Lucientes, Francisco José
 A caza de dientes **461**
 Loss of hearing 315

De humani corporis fabrica libri septem, by Andreas Vesalius
 Muscular system **18**
 Portrait **16**
 Skeletal system **18**
 Title page **17**

De Ketham, Johannes, and *Fasciculus Medicinae*
 Dissection **9**, 10
 Uroscopy wheel **76**

Dekkers, Frederik, and cupping in *Exercitationes practicae* **113**

Delatour H. Beeckman, and caution against sterilization in the *Brooklyn Medical Journal* 157

De Marchetti, Pietro, and prosthetics in *Observuatiomum Medico-Chirurgicarum Raiorum Sylloge* 211-212

De Medicina, see Celcus

De Montaigne, Michel, on physicians and kidney stones 281-284

Denis, Jean-Baptiste, and interspecies transfusion 104

Dental treatment
 Extraction by Benjamin Rush 465-466

Medical 461-462
 Personal hygiene **485-487**

Dental anatomy **467-470**

Dental education
 Horace Hayden and Chapin Harris 469-470
 University of Maryland 469-470

Dental furniture 482-**484**

Dental hygiene **485-487**

Dental prosthetics
 George Washington's dentures 474-**475**
 Giuseppangelo Fonzi's porcelain prosthetics 475-**476**
 Vulconite 476

Derivative bleeding 88

Diabetes mellitus, description by Aretaeus of Cappadocia 402

Dialysis 293

Dick, Elisha Cullen and George Washington's death 100-103

Dieffenbach, Johann Friedrich
 On anesthesia 195
 On vesicovaginal fistula 258-259

Dioscorides, Pedacius, and the formulary *De Materia Medica Libri Quinque* 415

Doctors' lady **59**

Donato, Marcello, supporting dissection in *De medicina historia mirabile, libri sex* 14-15

Doshas 59, 330-332

Dou, Gerrit
 The Dentist 454-455
 The Physician **74**

Doyle, Arthur Conan, and Sherlock Holmes 61

Drown, Ruth, the "Queen of Quacks" 547-551

Drug jars **444-448**

E

Eakins, Thomas, and *The Gross Clinic* **122-123, 169**

Ear, medical therapy 313-314

Ebers, Georg, papyrus
 Anatomy 4
 Gastroenterology 387-390
 Opium 173
 Surgery 127-128

Écorchés
 Auzoux, Louis, male and female **42, 43**
 Cigoli, Ludovico, bronze statuette **40**

Genga, Bernardino, copperplate muscleman **38**

La Specola, muscleman and female torso **40, 41**

Rubens, Peter Paul, chalk muscleman **39**

Rudinger, Nicolaus, in *Topographisch-chirurgische anatomie des menchen*, nude figures **43**

Zeiller, G., wax superficial muscles **41**

Zwick, Stephan, ivory manikin **40**

Edmonds, Emma, and a description of the Battle of Bull Run 218

Egyptian medicine
 Anatomy 4
 Anesthesia 173
 Bloodletting 85
 Embalming 52-55
 Eye of Horus and Rx **406**-408
 Head trauma 200-202
 Papyri
  Ebers, Georg 4, 127-128, 387-390, 406
  Kahun 240
  Smith, Edwin 128-130, **126**, 200-202
 Percussion 71
 Pharmacy 406-408
 Surgery 125-130
 Tracheotomy 321
 Women's diseases 240

Electricity
 Belts 525-527, **529-530**
 Boyd's battery 524-**526**
 Davis & Kidder magneto-electric machine 525-**527**
 Diathermy 540-**544**
 Electreat 530, **536**
 Electrostatic generators 527, **531-533**
 I-ON-A-CO body coil 525-527, **530**
 Penny arcade machines 532-533, **536**
 Violet ray generators 535-**539**

Electropoise 566-**568**

Ellsworth, Elmer, first Civil War casualty 52

Embalming
 Egyptian 52
 Holmes, Thomas, "Father of Modern Embalming" 52-53
 Lincoln, Abraham 53-55

Empedocles of Acragas, and the four humors in *On the Nature of Man* 82

Epilepsy, diagnosis and treatment 202-204

Estienne, Charles, and *La dissection des parties du corps humain* 21, **22**

Ether anesthesia 180-189, **182-185**

Eustachi, Bartolomeo
Dental anatomy 467
Opuscula anatomica 19
Tabulae anatomicae Bartolomaie Eustachi quas a tenebris tandem vindicates 19-**20**

Excision procedure 151-153, **152-153**

Exercitatio Anatomica de Motu Cordis et Sanguinis in Animalibus by William Harvey 22-**26**

Eye of Horus 406-408

F

Fabiola, and the first hospital 338

Fahrenheit, Gabriel 65

Fasciculus Medicinae **9**-10

Fauchard, Pierre, "Father of Dentistry"
Dental cavities 471
Dental chair 482
Le Chirurgien Dentiste, ou Traite des Dents 467
Urine cleanser **486**-487

Federal Pure Food and Drug Act, 1906 450

Fèlix, Charles-François and fistula-in-ano 135

Fistula-in-ano 135, 397

Flagg, Josiah
Amalgam 472
Dental chair **483**

Flap amputation 148-150, **149**

Flap anatomies 43-**44**

Flint, Austin, on Laënnec 69

Fonzi, Giuseppangelo, and porcelain teeth 475-**476**

Food, Drug, and Cosmetic Act of 1938 451-452

Forceps, obstetric 252-257, **253**

Four humors 82-85, **83**

Francken, Ambrosius, and transplantation by Saints Cosmas and Damian **133**

Frankincense 406, 413

Franklin, Benjamin
Electricity 524
On physicians 492

Frère Jacques, and kidney stones 284-286

Freud, Sigmund
Cocaine 430-431
Local anesthesia 196-197

G

Gaddesden, John of
Bladder catheterization 274
Stone removal 280

Galen, Claudius
Anatomy and circulation 7-8
Four humors 82-85
Hemostasis 159
Surgery 130
Tooth worm **456**-458

Galileo
Circulation 25
Thermometer 65

Gall, Franz, and phrenology 499

Gamelin, J., from *Nouveau recueil d'Ostéologie et de myologie*
Dance of death **594**
Kneeling skeleton **581**

Garcia, Manuel, and the discovery of the laryngoscope 323-324

Garfield, President James, and his assassination 213-216

Gastroenterology
Cathartics 392-395, **394**
Clyster 395-398, **396**, **397**
Hemorrhoids 398-399
Liver disease 398
Medical therapy 387-398
Surgery
Colectomy 400-401
Hemorrhoidectomy 399-400

Gay, John, and *The Sick Man and the Angel* 153

Ge Hong, Master, Chinese alchemist 410

Gem therapy 410

Genga, Bernardino, and a muscle écorché in *Anatomia per uso et intelligenza del disegno ricercata non solo su gl'ossi* **38**

Ghadiali, Dinshah, and the Spectro-Chrome machine 505-510, **508**

Gillray, James, etchings
Gout **174**
Vaccination **379**

Glossary 573-577

Grant, F.J., supporting anesthesia in the *Lancet* 195

Grant, Ulysses S., and the Battle of Cold Harbor 228-230, **229**

Granville, A.B.
Counterirritation 110
Definition and results of cupping in *Counter-Irritation, Its Principles and Practice* 108-109

Gray, Henry, and *Anatomy, Descriptive and Surgical* 32, **37**

Greenfield, John, and *A Compleat Treatise of the Stone and Gravel*
Kidney stones, etiology and diagnosis 277
Kidney stones, surgical treatment **282**

Greenwood, John, colonial dentist
Dental engine 482
Dental prosthetics 474
Dental teacher 469

Gross, Samuel
Asepsis 167-169
Cathartics 395
Inflammation in *System of Surgery* 168
The Gross Clinic 168-**169**

Guiteau, Charles, and the Garfield assassination 213-216

Gunshot wounds, and treatment with boiling oil 166-167

H

Hahnemann, Samuel, and homeopathy 433-**435**

Halsted, William
Cocaine addiction 431
Progress in surgery 197
Surgical gloves 173

Hamlet, and the Eustachian tube 20

Hammond, William Alexander, surgeon general 224

Hammurabi, Code of **124**, 299

Hare, William, and anatomic specimens 44-46

Harris, Chapin A.
Amalgam 472
University of Maryland Dental School 469-470

Harvey, William
Bloodletting 87
Exercitatio Anatomica de Motu Cordis et Sanguinis in Animalibus
Description of circulation 25

Landmark text 22-26
    Title page **26**
    Venous circulation **26**
Hayden, Horace H., and dental education
    469-470
Heine's osteotome **152**
Heister, Laurence in *A General System of
    Surgery*
    Amputation **142**
    Anesthesia 175
    Bleeding and its risks 93-94
    Head trauma 205
    Cataract surgery 299-306
    Cautery in surgery 162-163
    Cupping III-II2
    Infectious diseases, etiology and thera-
    py 340-341
    Leeches 95-97
    Phlebotomy in ophthalmology 306-307
    Seton needle 114-117
    Tobacco clyster 395
    Urinary catheters 274
Hemostasis 159-164
Heron of Alexandria, and temperature
    notation 65
Hesi-Re, the first dentist 461
Hills, Monson, in defense of small surgi-
    cal sets in the *Boston Medical and
    Surgical Journal* 156-157
Hinckley, Robert, and *First Operation
    under Ether* **182-183**
Hindu medicine 332
Hippocrates
    Anatomy **4**
    Art of medicine v
    Cautery 161
    Clyster 395
    Facies Hippocratica 77-78
    Female hysteria 516
    Four humors 8, 82- 85, 83
    Marble bust **4**
    Nasal polyp surgery 317-318
    Oath of Hippocrates **5**, 7
    Physical diagnosis 60
    Physician's appearance 62
    Puerperal fever 367-368
    Pulse diagnosis 63
    Tuberculosis 359
Hogarth, William, and *The Reward of
    Cruelty* 22, **24**
Holbein the Younger, Hans, and the *Act of

Union **138**
Holmes, Oliver Wendell
    Anatomic instruction 46
    Anesthesia 187
    Materia medica 453
    Pharmacopoeia 405
    Puerperal Fever 369-370
    Quackery 490
    Quote on the importance of medicine
    x
    Thoracic aneurism 357
Holmes, Sherlock, and Dr. Bell 61
Holmes, Thomas, and embalming 52-53
Homeopathy
    Samuel Hahnemann 433-**435**
    Similia similibus curantur 434
Homunculus theory 240
Horus, Eye of 406-408
Hospitals 338-339
Hunter, John, and surgery 140-141
Hunter, William
    Gravid uterus in *Anatomia Uteri
    Humani Gravidi* **241**
    Obstetric forceps 257
Hydrocele 286-288
Hygiae 334
Hyperemic treatment 114, **115**
Hysteria, female 516

I

Illustration credits 579-580
Imhotep **126**-127
Immunizaton
    Anti-vaccinationists 378-380
    Rabies **379**-380
    Smallpox
        Description by Rhazes **372**-374
        Edward Jenner 375-**376**
        Variolation 374-375
    Tetanus 377-**378**
Infectious disease
    Etiology 338-341
    Leprosy **348**-350
    Malaria 347-348
    Plague 341-347, **342-343**
    Puerperal fever 367-372, **370**
    Rabies 377
    Smallpox 373-377, **376**
    Syphilis 350-359
    Tetanus 377-**378**
    Tuberculosis 359-363

Typhoid fever 363-367
Inflammation
    Hermann Boerhaave in *Aphorisms:
    Concerning the Knowledge and Cure of
    Diseases* 340
    Samuel Gross in *System of Surgery* **169**
    Laurence Heister in *A General System of
    Surgery* 340-341
Inspection, and physical examination 58-61
Instrumentation
    Bleeding 98-100, **99**
    Dental 477-482, **477-481**
    Dissection 46-47, **48**, **50**
    Gynecologic **268-269**
    Laryngoscope 323-324
    Manufacturers 156
    Microscopes 47-52, **50**, **51**
    Neurosurgical **203-204**
    Obstetric forceps 252-257
    Ophthalmoscope **306**, 307
    Orthopedic **213**
    Stethoscope 66-71, **69**, **70**, **71**
    Surgical **147-158**
    Urologic **287**

J

Jackson, Charles, and anesthesia 181, 189
Jansen, Johannes and Zacharias, and the
    microscope 47
Janus, and the pharmacy 439- **442**
Jenner, Edward, and vaccination 375-**376**
Junod, Victor-Théodore, and dry cupping
    114

K

Kahun papyrus, and contraceptives 240
Kellogg, John H.
    Bowel preparation 556-557
    Colectomy 400-401
    Light therapy 504
    Spermatorrhea 560
    Water therapy 512-**513**
Kidney stones
    Causes 277-278
    Frère Jacques 284-286
    Medical treatment 278-279
    Surgical treatment 279-281
Kings
    Charles II and his death 93
    Henry VIII and the *Act of Union* **138**-
    139

Louis XIV and his fistula-in-ano 135, 397

Kircher, Athanasius, and microscopic organisms 49

Koch, Robert, and his postulates 380-381

Koller, Carl, and the discovery of local anesthesia 196-197

Kotschi, Emil, and a wax model of the cranial nerves **41**

Kullmaurer, H. and Meher, A., and catheterization in *Short-robed Surgeon Catheterizes a Patient* **270, 275**

L

Laënnec, Rene, and the stethoscope 66-69, **68**

Landseer, Charles, and *Chalk drawing of a flayed corpse* **48**

Larrey, Dominique-Jean, and a mastectomy 177-178

Laryngoscope, discovery 323-324

La Specola
    Anatomic collection 37-40
    Female internal anatomy **41**
    Kidneys, ureter, and bladder **272**
    Muscleman **40**
    Twins in utero **245**

Laughing gas (nitrous oxide) 178-180, **179**

Lebenswecker by Bauncheidt 117-121, **119**

LeClerc, C., and hemostasis in *The Compleat Surgeon* 159-161

Lee, Jr., Samuel, and patent medicine 437

Lee, Robert E., and the Battle of Cold Harbor 228

Leeches
    Application by physicians in *A General System of Surgery* 95-97
    Application by nurses in *The Theory & Practice of Nursing* 97-98
    Artificial, by Andrew Smith 98

Leprosy
    Anglicus, Gilbertus, and appearance 349
    Leviticus (13:1-46) 348
    Rules for behavior 349-350

Lewis, Percy, and *The Theory & Practice of Nursing* 97-98

Life awakener 117-118, **119**

Ligature, and its use 164

Light therapy 504-510, **506-508**

Lincoln, Abraham, and The Lincoln

Special 53, 55

Linden, John, and the lebenswecker in *Baunscheidtism, or a New Exanthematic Method of Cure* 117-119

Lister, Joseph
    Aseptic surgery 170
    Fracture repair 210

Liston, Robert, and limb amputation 148-150

Local anesthesia 196-197

Locke, John, and the function of anatomy 21

London Guild of Surgeons 135-139

Long, Crawford, and anesthesia 181, 187

M

Macaura Pulsocon 514-516

Mackenzie, Morell, and tonsillectomy 322

Magnetism 516-524

Maimonides
    Bleeding 92-93
    Enemas 393
    Masturbation 557-559
    Philosophy of medicine 93
    Urine examination 75

Malaria 347-348

Malpighi, Marcello, and capillary anatomy 49

Mandrake (*Mandragora officiarum*) 174-175

Mapleson, Thomas
    Cupper's complaints 112-114
    Indications for cupping 110-112

Maryland, University of
    Dental School 469-470
    Hammond, William Alexander, and *The Medical and Surgical History of the War of the Rebellion* 224
    Wood, Thomas Fanning, and a letter from Cold Harbor 232-233

Masturbation 557-561

Matthijs, Naiveu, and a patient being bled **80-81, 86**

Maygrier, J.P., in *Nouvelles Démonstrations D'Accouchemens*
    Cesarean section **258**
    Female examination **240**
    Forceps delivery **253**
    Smellie's perforator **264**

The Medical and Surgical History of the War of the Rebellion 224-227

Medicine chests 446-**448**

Meigs, J.F., on anesthesia 192-193

Melcher, S.H., and Civil War post-op care **219**

Mercury
    Amalgam 471-473
    Description and use 410, 416
    Syphilis treatment 358-359

Mesmer, Franz Anton
    Magnetic therapy and animal magnetism 516-523
    Mesmerized patients **488-489, 522**

Meyer, Edouard, and cataract surgery in *Cataract Surgery: Teaching a Student How to Make a Superior Incision* **304**

Michelangelo Buonarroti 10, **45**

Microscopes
    Bullock **51**
    Powell and Lealand **51**
    Van Leeuwenhoek **50**

Midwives
    Controversy 251-252
    Preparation for delivery 246-248
    Prerequisites 250-251
    Role in delivery 246-252

Miller, James, and the discovery of anesthesia in *The Principles of Surgery* 190

Mirfield, John of
    Bad prognoses 77
    Medications 408

Molière
    On physicians 403
    On uroscopy 75-77

Mondino de Cuzzi, and early dissection **6**, 10

Monfalcon on hemostasis in the *Boston Medical and Surgical Journal* 159

Moreau, F.J., and turning of the foot in *A Practical Treatise on Midwifery: Exhibiting the Present Advanced State of the Science* **246**

Morgagni, Giovanni Battista, and tracheal foreign body 322-323

Mortar and pestle 442-**444**

Morton, William, and anesthesia 181-187, **182-183**, 188-189

Mott, Valentine, supporting anesthesia in the *Boston Med and Surgical Journal* 195

Moveable kidney 289-291

Moynihan Berkeley, and early aseptic technique 171

Mummy powder **413**

Myrrh 406, 413-414

N

Napoléon Bonaparte

    Auscultation 72

    Autopsy instruments **50**

Nasal surgery (polyps) 317-318

Nei Ching

    Pharmacy 414

    Tao 328

Neurosurgery 200-207

Nightingale, Florence 227-228

Nose bleed and treatment 317

O

Oath of Hippocrates 4-7, **5**

Obstetric forceps 252-257

Obstetrics 240-267

Ophthalmology 296-311

Ophthalmoscope **306**, 307

Opium

    Anesthesia 173

    Experimentation 429-430

    Illustration **426**

    Manufacture and use in *De Medicina* 415-416

    Theriac **410**

Orthopedic surgery

    Compound fractures 209-210

    Palliative procedures

        Hand and leg prosthesis 211-**212, 223**

        Nose re-implantation 211-**212**

    Techniques for fracture repair 207-209, **208-209**

    Prostheses **211-212, 223**

Oscilloclast 545-**547**

Osler, William

    Harvey, William 25

    Imhotep 127

    Medicine 327

    Moveable kidney 289-291

    Physical diagnosis 57

    Quack medicine 489

    Quotes on books **572, 584**

    Rx 408

Otolaryngology 311-324, **320, 321, 323**

P

Pancoast, Joseph, and bloodletting in *A*

Treatise in Operative Surgery 87

Paper-mache models **42, 43**

Paracelsus

    Gem therapy 410

    Ideal surgeon 428-429

    Magnetism 516-517

    Pharmaceutical philosophy 428

    Signatures 434

Paré, Ambrose

    Asepsis in *Apologie* 166-167

    Delivery 248-250

    Dental caries 471

    Gangrene 143-144

    Gunshot wounds 166

    Incurable cases 139-140

    Kidney stone surgical treatment 280-**281**

    Ligature 164

    Phantom pain in *Apologie Et Voyages* 143-144

    Surgical technique 140

Passarotti, Bartolomeo, and *An Anatomy Lesson given by Michelangelo to other artists* **45**

Pasteur, Louis 380

Patent medications

    Definition and early examples 436-439, **437-438**

    Federal Pure Food and Drug Act, 1906 450-451

    Food, Drug, and Cosmetic Act, 1938 451-452

    Lydia Pinkham **437-438**

    Mark Twain's criticism 452

    Sherley amendment 450-451

Patin, Guy, and the barber-surgeon controversy 135

Paul of Aegina, and uses for blood in *Pauli Aeginetae de re medica libri septem, graece* 106-108

Pelican in dentistry 477-480

Percussion 71-**72**

Perkins Tractors **496**-499

Phrenology

    Comparative physiognomy 502-**503**

    Definition 499

    Fowler, Lorenzo and Orson 502

    Gall, Franz 499

    Twain, Mark, and a personal experience 502-504

Physical diagnosis

Auscultation 66-71

Inspection 58-61

Percussion 71-72

Psychograph 499-**502**

Pulse diagnosis 61-**63**

Temperature evaluation 63-66

Uroscopy 72-77

Pinkham, Lydia, and patent medicines **437-438**

Piorry, Pierre-Adolphe, and the pleximeter **72**

Placebo effect 408, 490-492

Plague ("The Black Death")

    Boccaccio, Giovanni, and *Decameron* 344-345

    Description 341-345

    Petrarch, Francesco, and a warning to Pope Clement VI 346-347

    Ring around the rosie 345-346

    The Triumph of Death **326-327, 342-343**

Pliny the Elder

    Dental disease 461

    Enemas 392-393

    Urine therapy *Naturalis Historia* 412

Pneumonia

    Description **382**-383

    Treatment 383-384

Pott, Percival

    Epididymitis 288-289

    Fracture repair 207-**209, 208**

    Head trauma and trepanning 204-207

    Hydrocele 288

    Pott's disease **360**

    Quack medicine 571

Powell and Lealand microscope **51**

Prohibition, and prescription whiskey **452**

Prosthetics, dental **473-476**

Puerperal Fever

    Description

        Alexander Gordon in *Essays on the Puerperal Fever and Other Diseases Peculiar to Women* 368-369

        Hippocrates' description 367-368

        Holmes, Oliver Wendell, and the physician's role in contagion 369-370

        Ignas Semmelweis 370-373

Pulmonary medicine

    Empyema 383

    Pneumonia, diagnosis and treatment **382-384**

    Tobacco 386-387, **388-389**

Pulse diagnosis
    Chinese 62-**63**
    Hippocrates 62
Purmann, Matthäus
    Technique of interspecies blood trans-
    fusion in *Chirurgia Curiosa* 105-106
    Transfusion from lamb to man in
    *Grosser und gantz neugewundener
    Lorbeer-Krantz, oder Wund Artzney* **105**

Q

Qi and Chinese medicine **328-330**
Quack medicine
    Definitions 490-492
    Electricity 524-544
    Hair loss **563-565**
    Light therapy 504-510, **506-508**
    Methods of quacks 492-495
    Radioactivity 551-556
    Vibration therapy 513-**517**
    Water therapy 510-**513**

R

Rabies 377
Radam's Microbe Killer 451
Radioactivity
    Physiology 551-552
    Radithor 554-556, **555**
    Revigator **554**
Radionics
    Oscilloclast **545-547**
    Physiology 544-546
Rectal dilators **570**
Rembrandt van Rijn, and *The Anatomy
    Lesson of Nicholaes Tulp* **2-3, 27**
Resurrectionists Hare and Burke 44-46
Revulsive bleeding 88
Rhazes, and smallpox 373
Rhinoplasty 211-**212**
Roger, Henri, on Laënnec's discovery 69
Rösslin, Eucharius, and midwives in *A
    Rose Garden for Expectant Women and
    Midwives* 246-**247**
Royal College of Surgery 139
Royal touch, and tuberculosis 360-362
Rubens, Peter Paul, and muscle écorché **39**
Rudiger, Nicolaus, and photograph of
    nude figures 40, **43**
Rueff, Jacob, and sixteenth-century deliv-
    ery 246-248
Rush, Benjamin

Bleeding 100
    Dental extraction 465-467
    Water therapy 511
Russell, Bertrand, and medical quackery
    571
Rx symbol **406-408**

S

Saint Anthony's Fire 141
Saint Apollonia, patron saint of dentistry
    457-460
Saints Cosmas and Damian
    Transplantation 132-134, **133**
    Uroscopy **73**
Saints of medicine and dentistry
    Roman Catholic saints 335
    St. Anthony's Fire 141
    St. Apollonia, patron saint of dentistry
    457-460
Salerno, School of 8
Sanitariums **456-457**
Santorio, Santorio, and use of the ther-
    mometer 65
Savage, Henry, and the repair of a vesico-
    vaginal fistula in *The surgery, surgical
    pathology, and surgical anatomy of the
    female pelvis organs* **260**
Scales, apothecary 442-**444**
Schurz, Carl, and surgery at Gettysburg
    219
Scrofula
    King's touch **360-362**
    Macbeth 360-361
Scultetus, Joannis, in *Armamentarium
    Chiruigicum*
    Bullet forceps **214**
    Mastectomy **177**
    Repair of fracture and dislocation **209**
    Trauma **209**
Self-experimentation
    Crumpe, Samuel, and *An Inquiry into
    the Nature and Properties of Opium*
    429-430
    Freud, Sigmund, and *On Cocaine* 430-
    431
    Shen Nung, and *Shen-nung pen ts'ao
    ching* 414
Semmelweis, Ignas, and puerperal fever
    370-373
Sertürner, Friedrich Wilhelm, and the dis-
    covery of morphine 175

Servetus, Michael, and the pulmonary cir-
    culation in *On the Restitution of
    Christianity* 16
Seton needle in counterirritation 114-**117**
Sexual prohibitions **557-561**
Shakespeare, William
    A Midsummer Night's Dream, and spi-
    der webs in hemostasis 159
    As You Like It, and ageing 324-325
    As You Like It, and post mortem
    changes 55
    Cariolanus, and communicable disease
    339
    Hamlet, and middle ear anatomy 20
    Macbeth, and the King's touch 360-362
    Much Ado About Nothing, and
    toothache 455
    Richard III, and rabies 377
    Romeo and Juliet, and mandrake 175
    The Life of Timon of Athens, and distrust
    of physicians 452
Shaw, George Bernard, and medical criti-
    cism 152
Shen Nung
    Acupuncture **328-329**
    Shen-nung pen ts'ao ching, and herbal
    medications 414
Sherley Amendment of 1912 450-451
Show globes 442-**443**
Sickles, Major General Daniel, amputa-
    tion **220**
Signatures, and homeopathy 434-435
Simpson, James
    Chloroform anesthesia 190-191, 193-194
    Letter from a friend on amputation
    150-151
Sims, James Marion, on the repair of vesi-
    covaginal fistula 259-261
Smallpox
    Famous patients 374
    Jenner, Edward, and vaccination 375-
    376
    Rhazes, and description 373
    Variolation 374-375
Smellie, William
    Abortion by a midwife 263-267
    Conflict with physicians 251-252
    Prerequisites for a midwife 250-251
    Proper use of forceps 256
Smith, Andrew, and the artificial leech 98,
    99

Smith papyrus
    Head trauma 200-202
    Surgery **126**, 127-130
Snake oil 439-**441**
Soranus of Ephesus, and podalic version 246
Spanish Fly 93, 109
Spectacles **308-310**, 311
Spectro-Chrome machine 505-510, **508**
Spermatorrhea and its consequences **557**-560
Spigelius, Adrianus, and pregnant woman in *De formato foetu liber singularis geneis figures exornatus in Opera quae extant omna* **244**
SS White Dental Manufacturing Company 480
Stephenson, J., and Churchill, J., and *Medical Botany: or, Illustrations and Descriptions of the Medicinal Plants of the London, Edinburgh, and Dublin Pharmacopoeias* **404-405, 417-428**
Stethoscope, and its evolution 66-**71**
Stevenson, Robert Louis, and cocaine 430
Stone of insanity **198-199, 206**-207
Stones, kidney
    Causes 277-278
    Frère Jacques 284-286
    Medical treatment 278-279
    Surgical treatment 279-281
Sulfanilamide, and the Food, Drug, and Cosmetic Act of 1938 451-452
Surgery 122-197
Surgical sets and manufacturers 153-157
Susini, Clemente, and wax models 37
Susruta
    Hemostasis 164
    Rhynoplasty 211-**212**
Susruta-samhita 332-333, 395
Swift, Jonathan, and loss of hearing 315
Sydenham, Thomas
    History taking 60-61
    Pharmacy 408-409
    Physical diagnosis 58
Syphilis
    Congenital **354**-355
    Etiology 350-351
    Famous patients 359
    Frascastro, and description in *De conta-gione Et contagiosis morbis* 351-354
    Therapy 357-359
    Thoracic aortic aneurism 355-357

T

Tait, Lawson, and operating room conditions 169-170
Taylor, John, quack oculist 299
Temperature evaluation 63-66
Teniers the Younger, David, and *The Surgeon* **136-137**
Tesla, Nikola, and alternating current 535
Tetanus 377-**378**
Theriac 409-**410**
Tibetan medicine
    Charka Samhita 332
    Yutok Yonten K Gongpo 332
Tiemann, George, instrument maker 156
Tobacco
    Advertising **388-389**
    Asbestos filters 387
    Enemas 395
    Uses 386, **422**
Tongue diagnosis 58-60
Tonsillectomy 322
Tooth worm
    Galen **456**-458
    Treatment 458
Tourniquet 163-164
Toynbee, Joseph and inner ear infection in *The Diseases of the Ear: Their Nature, Diagnosis, and Treatment* 313
Tracheotomy **320**, 321-322
Transfusion
    Method for interspecies transfusion 104-106, **105**
    Person to person *Harper's Weekly* **107**
    Vitalism 103
Trepanning, purpose and technique 200
Trotula of Salerno, and medical abortion in *A Medieval Woman's Guide to Health* 263
Tuberculosis
    Description by Thomas Sydenham 359-360
    Famous patients 362-363
    Pott's Disease
        Macbeth 360-361
        The King's Touch 360-362
    Treatment 362

Tumi knife **202**
Twain, Mark, and his observations
    Dentists 462
    Medical diagnoses 78-79
    Pharmaceutical advertising 452
    Phrenology 502-504
    Placebo effect 492
Typhoid fever, and Typhoid Mary 363-367

U

Urine therapy
    Dental treatment **486**-487
    Medical uses 412-413
Urology 270-293
Uroscopy 72-77

V

Vaccination
    Antivaccinationists 378-380
    Edward Jenner 375-377
    Etching by James Gillray **379**
    Variolation 374-375
Vaginal speculum, and objection to its use 267-268
Van Beethoven, Ludwig, and his loss of hearing 315
Van Hemessen, Jan Sanders, and *Extraction of the Fool's Stone* **198-199, 206**
Van Kalcar, Jan Stefan, and anatomic illustration 16
Van Leeuwenhoek, Antoni, and the microscope 47, 49-**50**
Van Mieris the Elder, Frans, and *The Visit of the Physician* **56-57, 64**
Van Rijn, Rembrandt, and *The Anatomy Lesson of Dr. Tulp* **2-3, 26-27**
Venereal disease, medical and surgical treatment 272-276
Vesalius, Andreas in *De humani corporis fabrica libri septem*
    Instruments used for dissection **48**
    Muscular system **18**
    Self-portrait **16**
    Skeletal system **18**
    Title page **17**
Vesicovaginal fistula
    Description 258-259
    Treatment 259-261
Vibration therapy 513-**517**
Victoria, Queen, and anesthesia 194

Violet ray therapy 535-**539**

Vitalism, and transfusion 103

Voltaire on physicians 577

Von Gersdorff, Hans, and *Feldtbüch der Wundartzney*

    Amputation and advice to physicians 141-**142**

        Fracture repair **208**

        Hemostasis **160**-161

        Trauma **201**

        Trepanning **203**

        Uroscopy **73**

Von Helmholtz, Herman, and the discovery of the ophthalmoscope **306**, 307

Von Hutten, Ulrich, and the etiology of syphilis in *De morbo Gallico* 351

Von Pfolspeundt, Heinrich, and surgical asepsis in *Buch der Bündth-Ertznei* 165-166

Vulcanite, and dentures **476**

W

Wang Shu-ho, on the pulse **63**

Warren, John Collins, and anesthesia 181-186, **182-185**

Washington, George

    Dentures 474-**475**

    Final moments 100-103

    George Washington in his last illness **102**

Water therapy

    Graefenberg cure 511-512

    Medical applications 510-511

    Physiologic bases by John Kellogg, MD 512-**513**

Wells, Horace, and anesthesia 180-181, **187-188**

Woodman, Phillip, in *The Modern Physician*

    Fever, causes and cure 63-65

    Kidney stone therapy 278

    Seizure treatment 202-204

Wunderlich, C.A., and temperature evaluation 65-66

X

X-ray diagnosis 530

Y

Yin and Yang

    Chinese medical care **328-330**

    Herbs 414

Yonge, James, and the flap amputation 148

Yutok Yonten K. Gongpo, and Tibetan medicine 332

Z

Zeiller, G., and a wax model of superficial muscles 41

Zentmayer, Joseph, and the microscope 52

Zodiac, in medical diagnosis and treatment **336**-337

Zumbo, Gaetano Guilo, and wax anatomic models 37

Zwick, Stephan, and a female anatomic manikin **40**

. . .And again for the mind, and for the heart

*"One's first step in wisdom is to question everything
— and one's last is to come to terms with everything."*
GEORG CHRISTOPH LICHTENBERG (1742-1799)

*"I wrote when I did not know life; now that I do
know the meaning of life, I have no more to write.
Life cannot be written; life can only be lived."*
OSCAR WILDE (1854-1900)

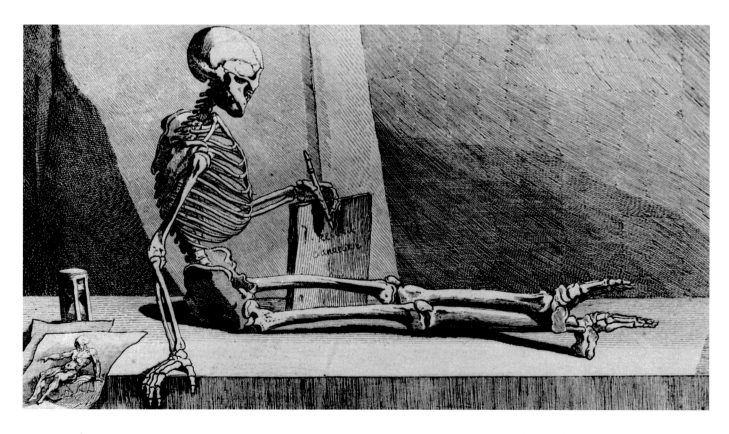

So that's that.
OLGIERD LINDAN, MD, PhD